Nutrition Manag
Metabolic Diseases

Laurie E. Bernstein • Fran Rohr
Sandy van Calcar
Editors

Nutrition Management of Inherited Metabolic Diseases

Lessons from Metabolic University

Second Edition

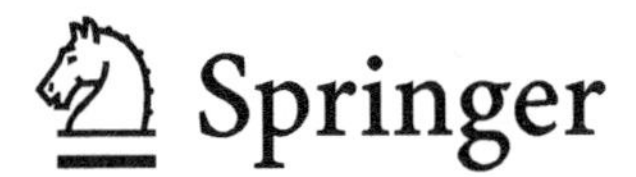

Editors
Laurie E. Bernstein
Children's Hospital Colorado
University of Colorado Hospital
Aurora, CO, USA

Fran Rohr
Met Ed Co
Boulder, CO, USA

Sandy van Calcar
Molecular and Medical Genetics
Oregon Health & Science University
Portland, OR, USA

ISBN 978-3-030-94509-1 ISBN 978-3-030-94510-7 (eBook)
https://doi.org/10.1007/978-3-030-94510-7

This Springer imprint is published by the registered company Springer Nature Switzerland AG
The registered company address is: Gewerbestrasse 11, 6330 Cham, Switzerland

Preface

Nutrition Management of Inherited Metabolic Diseases: Lessons from Metabolic University is dedicated to the nutrition management of patients with inherited metabolic diseases (IMD). It presents a compilation of topics that have been taught at Metabolic University (MU), an interactive, didactic educational program that has trained over 1000 metabolic dietitians/nutritionists, physicians, genetic counselors, and nurses since 2006. The purpose of MU, and thus the subject matter included within, is intended to assist the entry-level clinician with a broad understanding of the nutrition management of inherited metabolic diseases.

Each chapter in the book reflects both the author's literature review and insights from their clinical experience. For many disorders there is no consensus in the literature regarding the nutritional management, likely because the incidence of IMD is low and randomized clinical trials on intervention strategies are rare. In addition, each disorder has a wide spectrum of disease severity. Recognizing that there are variations in practice, the precept of MU is that nutrition management of IMD is not a "cookbook." Rather, the key to management lies in understanding how the inactivity of an enzyme in a metabolic pathway determines which components of the diet must be restricted and which must be supplemented, as well as the monitoring of appropriate biomarkers to make diet adjustments and ensure the goals of therapy are met. The goals of nutrition therapy are to correct the metabolic imbalance to lower the risk of morbidity and mortality associated with the disorder and to promote normal growth and development by providing adequate nutrition. Readers are encouraged to confer with their clinical teams regarding management protocols specific to their institutions and to recognize that management of metabolic disease is complex and guidance provided in the book may not apply to every clinical situation.

This book contains mostly subject matter covered at MU and in general the chapters are authored by the experts who presented the material. Therefore, it is not a comprehensive treatise on IMD, but rather a textbook on the most frequently encountered challenges in IMD nutrition. The book contains introductory chapters on nutrition and metabolism principles common to many metabolic disorders and disease-specific chapters on disorders of amino acid, fat, and carbohydrate metabolism.

Feedback from MU participants regarding the efficacy and effectiveness of MU confirmed that they attended MU primarily to obtain practical guidance on nutrition management for their IMD patients. Therefore, each nutrition chapter in the book highlights principles of nutrition management, how to initiate a diet, and biomarkers to monitor the diet. Diet calculations are another element of MU that appears at the end of each nutrition chapter.

The book is designed for day-to-day clinical use. We hope it proves helpful in the nutrition management of your patients with inborn errors of metabolism.

Disclaimer

The authors, editors, and publishers have made every effort to provide accurate information. However, they are not responsible for errors, omissions, or for any outcomes related to the use of the contents of this book and take no responsibility for the use of the products and procedures described. The information presented within this book is based on training, knowledge of medicine, biochemistry, nutrition, genetics, and the clinical experience of the authors. Medical and nutrition management of patients with inborn errors of metabolism varies between individuals and between management teams. The information presented within this book represents one way, among many, to manage a patient. If questions arise pertaining to the individual management of a patient with whom you are involved, it is best to discuss issues and alternative ideas with your medical team.

Aurora, CO, USA — Laurie E. Bernstein
Boulder, CO, USA — Fran Rohr
Portland, OR, USA — Sandy van Calcar

Acknowledgments

We would like to thank BioMarin Pharmaceutical, Inc. and Nutricia North America for support of Metabolic University.

We acknowledge Amanda Hamm, Morgan Drumm, DTR; and Sommer Gaughan, RD, for their contributions in bringing this book to fruition.

And to those who inspire and teach us:

- Phyllis Acosta, DrPH, RD, for her lifelong contributions to this field and to her mentorship
- Stephen Goodman, MD, PhD, for his lifelong contributions to this field and his mentorship
- Our colleagues in metabolism at Boston Children's Hospital, the University of Colorado/Children's Hospital Colorado, the University of Wisconsin-Madison/Waisman Center, and Oregon Health & Science University
- Our patients

Contents

Contributors

Ashley Andrews, MSN, CPNP Division of Medical Genetics, University of Utah School of Medicine, University of Utah Hospital, Salt Lake City, UT, USA

Peter R. Baker II, MD, FAAP Clinical Genetics and Metabolism, Children's Hospital Colorado, University of Colorado Denver – Anschutz Medical Campus, Aurora, CO, USA

Laurie E. Bernstein, MS, RD, FADA, FAND University of Colorado Hospital, Children's Hospital Colorado, Aurora, CO, USA

Curtis R. Coughlin II, MS, MBe, CGC Clinical Genetics and Metabolism, Children's Hospital Colorado, University of Colorado Denver – Anschutz Medical Campus, Aurora, CO, USA

Rebecca Gibson, MD Division of Medical Genetics, Pediatrics, Duke University School of Medicine, Durham, NC, USA

Maria Giżewska, MD, PhD Department of Pediatrics, Endocrinology, Diabetology, Metabolic Diseases and Cardiology, Pomeranian Medical University, Szczecin, Poland

Janell Kierstein, MS, CGC Clinical Genetics and Metabolism, Children's Hospital Colorado, University of Colorado Denver – Anschutz Medical Campus, Aurora, CO, USA

Priya S. Kishnani, MD Division of Medical Genetics, Pediatrics, Duke University School of Medicine, Durham, NC, USA

Aditi Korlimarla, MD Division of Medical Genetics, Pediatrics, Duke University School of Medicine, Durham, NC, USA

Kimberly A. Kripps, MD Department of Molecular and Medical Genetics, School of Medicine, Oregon Health and Science University, Portland, OR, USA

Kent Lai, PhD Division of Pediatric Genetics, University of Utah School of Medicine, Salt Lake City, UT, USA

Austin Larson, MD, PhD Clinical Genetics and Metabolism, Children's Hospital Colorado, University of Colorado Denver – Anschutz Medical Campus, Aurora, CO, USA

Nicola Longo, MD, PhD Division of Medical Genetics, University of Utah School of Medicine, University of Utah Hospital, Salt Lake City, UT, USA

Erin MacLeod, PhD, RD Rare Disease Institute – Genetics and Metabolism, Children's National Hospital, Washington, DC, USA

Ann-Marie Roberts, MS, RD Medical Genetics and Metabolism Department, Valley Children's Hospital, Madera, CA, USA

Fran Rohr, MS, RD Met Ed Co, Boulder, CO, USA

Mary Sowa, MS, RD Division of Medical Genetics, CHOC Children's, Orange, CA, USA

Janet A. Thomas, MD Department of Pediatrics, Section of Clinical Genetics and Metabolism, University of Colorado School of Medicine, Aurora, CO, USA

Sandy van Calcar, PhD, RD Oregon Health & Science University, Molecular and Medical Genetics, Portland, OR, USA

Johan L. K. Van Hove, MD, PhD, MBA Clinical Genetics and Metabolism, Children's Hospital Colorado, University of Colorado Denver – Anschutz Medical Campus, Aurora, CO, USA

Erica Wright, MS, CGC Clinical Genetics and Metabolism, Children's Hospital Colorado, University of Colorado Denver – Anschutz Medical Campus, Aurora, CO, USA

Steven Yannicelli, PhD, RD Medical and Scientific Affairs, Nutricia North America, Rockville, MD, USA

Part I

Background

Introduction to Genetics

1

Janell Kierstein

Contents

J. Kierstein (✉)
Clinical Genetics and Metabolism, Children's Hospital Colorado, University of Colorado Denver – Anschutz Medical Campus, Aurora, CO, USA
e-mail: Janell.Kierstein@childrenscolorado.org

L. E. Bernstein et al. (eds.), *Nutrition Management of Inherited Metabolic Diseases*,
https://doi.org/10.1007/978-3-030-94510-7_1

Core Messages

- Genes are short segments of DNA that carry information to make cellular proteins necessary for life.
- Mutations are heritable changes in the DNA nucleotide sequence of a gene.
- There are three broad categories of mutations: substitutions, insertions, and deletions.
- The most frequent consequence of a mutation is loss of protein function.
- Most inherited metabolic diseases are transmitted as an autosomal-recessive trait.

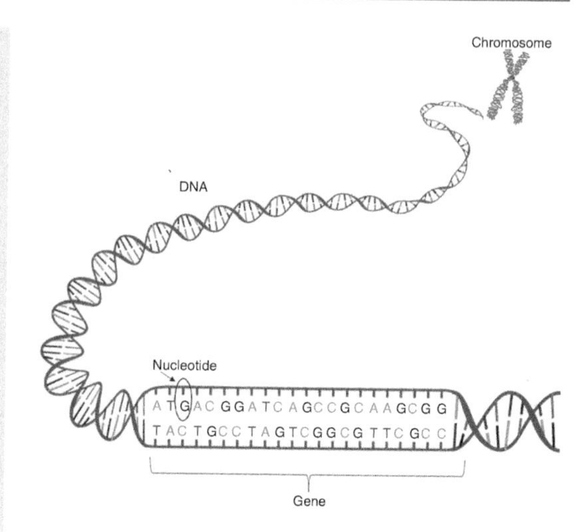

Fig. 1.1 Chromosomes are structures made of tightly coiled DNA

1.1 Background

The total number of cells in a human body is estimated to be 37.2 trillion [1]. In the nucleus of each of these cells are 46 chromosomes. One set of 23 chromosomes is inherited from an individual's mother and a second set of 23 chromosomes is inherited from their father. In every typical cell, there are 22 pairs of autosomes, which are the same in males and females. There is also one pair of sex chromosomes. Typically, females have two X chromosomes and males have one X chromosome (inherited from their mother) and one Y chromosome (inherited from their father). Each gamete (egg or sperm cell) contains only one member of each autosomal pair and one sex chromosome. When an egg cell is fertilized by a sperm cell, the result is a complete set of 46 chromosomes and unique individual.

Each chromosome is made up of tightly coiled strands of deoxyribonucleic acid (DNA). DNA is composed of long strings of nucleotides (Fig. 1.1). Each nucleotide includes a phosphate and sugar (deoxyribose) backbone attached to one of four nitrogenous bases: adenine (A), cytosine (C), guanine (G), and thymine (T) (Fig. 1.2). These bases form the chemical alphabet of DNA. The bases are complementary such that A always bonds with T on the opposing strand of DNA and C always bonds with G. Together, these matched nucleotides are referred to as base pairs. The bonds effectively create a ladder with rungs of bonded nucleotides and sides of sugar + phosphate backbones. The ladder is twisted into a double helical shape.

The vast majority of human DNA (approximately 98–99%) is considered "noncoding" DNA; its purpose is still enigmatic [2]. The remaining 1–2% of the human genome contains approximately 20,000 unique genes. Each gene represents a sequence of DNA that serves as a blueprint or code for production of a specific protein. Within each gene are segments of DNA called exons that actively encode protein production. Interspersed with exons are introns, which are composed of noncoding DNA. Genes also contain a variety of regulatory elements, which mark where a specific gene starts and ends and control in what tissues, at what point(s) in development, and how much of the final protein is produced (Fig. 1.3).

1.2 From Genes to Proteins

The process by which genes lead to production of proteins involves two key steps: transcription and translation. Transcription occurs when one DNA strand of a gene is used as the template to make a complementary strand of ribonucleic acid (RNA).

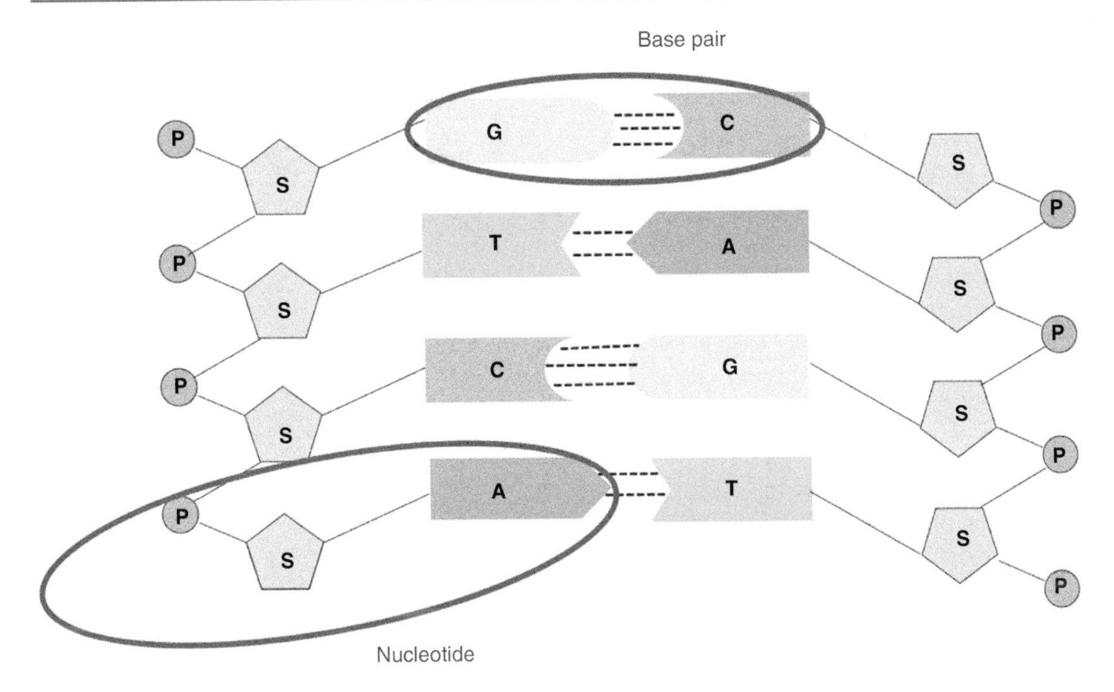

Fig. 1.2 DNA is composed of nucleotides, each of which includes a phosphate and sugar backbone and a nitrogenous base (A, C, G, or T). The bases form bonds with complementary bases on the opposite strand of DNA. The structure is twisted into a double helix

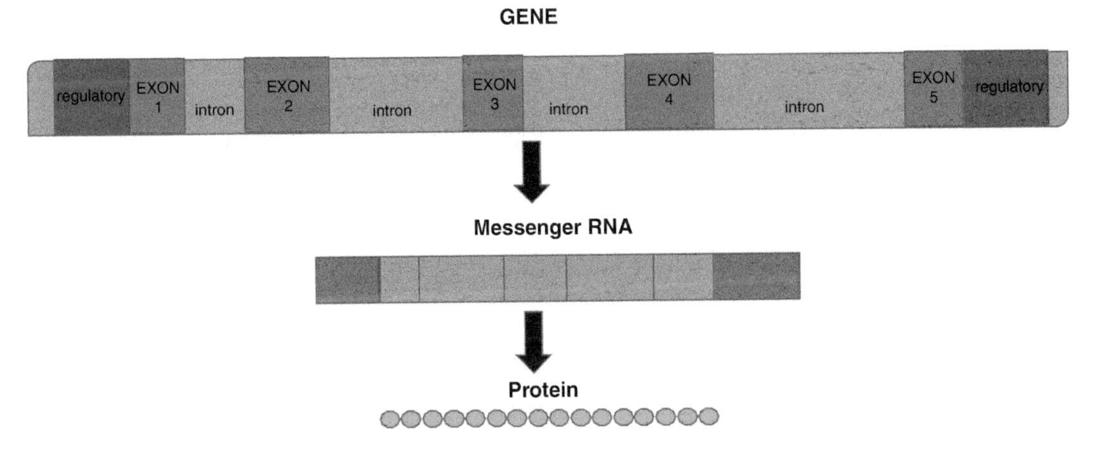

Fig. 1.3 Genes are composed of exons (protein coding regions), introns, and regulatory elements (nonprotein coding regions)

Similar to the structure of DNA, RNA is made of nucleotides composed of a phosphate and sugar (ribose) backbone, each attached to a nitrogenous base: adenine (A), cytosine (C), guanine (G), and uracil (U). The messenger RNA strand is able to leave the nucleus and attach to a ribosome where it is used as the template to assemble a protein. RNA reads three bases at a time, in a unit called a codon. Each codon corresponds to a specific amino acid. Most amino acids, however, can be encoded by more than one codon. This is described as a redundant or degenerate code. Note that there are also three termination or "stop" codons, which do not correspond to an amino acid but rather signal the end of a coding region (Table 1.1). The process by which RNA is used to assemble a specific string of amino acids into a protein is called translation (Fig. 1.4).

The order and chemical properties of amino acids within a protein (as dictated by the nucleotide sequence of the gene) determines the final shape and function of the protein. Envision a three-dimensional structure in which hydrophobic amino acids pull their part of the chain toward the center of the structure to avoid contact with water. Hydrophilic amino acids move outward in search of water. In doing so, a hydrophobic central core is created (Fig. 1.5). Positively charged amino acids then seek negatively charged amino acids, covalent bonds are formed, and accommodations are made for variances in the amino acid shapes and sizes. Subject to these intermolecular forces, the linear amino acid chain folds into a compact structure.

Table 1.1 Amino acid abbreviations and associated DNA codons

GENETIC CODE			
Amino acid (AA)	AA ABBREVIATIONS 3-letter	1-letter	DNA CODONS
Alanine	Ala	A	GCT, GCC, GCA, GCG
Arginine	Arg	R	CGT, CGC, CGA, CGG, AGA, AGG
Asparagine	Asn	N	AAT, AAC
Aspartic acid	Asp	D	GAT, GAC
Cysteine	Cys	C	TGT, TGC
Glutamine	Gln	Q	CAA, CAG
Glutamate	Glu	E	GAA, GAG
Glycine	Gly	G	GGT, GGC, GGA, GGG
Histidine	His	H	CAT, CAC
Isoleucine	Ile	I	ATT, ATC, ATA
Leucine	Leu	L	CTT, CTC, CTA, CTG, TTA, TTG
Lysine	Lys	K	AAA, AAG
Methionine	Met	M	ATG
Phenylalanine	Phe	F	TTT, TTC
Proline	Pro	P	CCT, CCC, CCA, CCG
Serine	Ser	S	TCT, TCC, TCA, TCG, AGT, AGC
Threonine	Thr	T	ACT, ACC, ACA, ACG
Tryptophan	Trp	W	TGG
Tyrosine	Tyr	Y	TAT, TAC
Valine	Val	V	GTT, GTC, GTA, GTG
Termination (stop) codons			TAA, TAG, TGA

The folding process is complex in the crowded cellular environment; hence, molecular chaperones assist. Chaperones are specialized molecules with cell housekeeping duties. They interact with a newly synthesized unfolded or partially folded amino acid chain and promote folding and stabilization of the protein structure. The resultant, folded structure is genetically designed to serve a specific function in the cell. The final protein may work autonomously in the cell, or it may join with other proteins to form a functional unit.

1.3 Genetic Variants

A variant (or mutation) is a permanent, heritable change in the nucleotide sequence of a gene. Variants can be classified based on the effect they have on the structure of the gene, the sequence of the amino acids, or the ultimate protein.

1.3.1 Variant Effects on Gene Structure

Some variants affect only one nucleotide in the DNA sequence of a gene. Whether that nucleotide is deleted or substituted for a different nucleotide, or if there is an insertion of an additional nucleotide, this single nucleotide change can be referred to as a point mutation. Other variants may involve several nucleotides or perhaps even an entire gene. In some cases, there can be deletion or translocation of multiple neighboring genes. Such variants are referred to as large-scale variants.

A substitution occurs when one or more nucleotides in the gene are mistakenly replaced with others (Table 1.2). Depending on the loca-

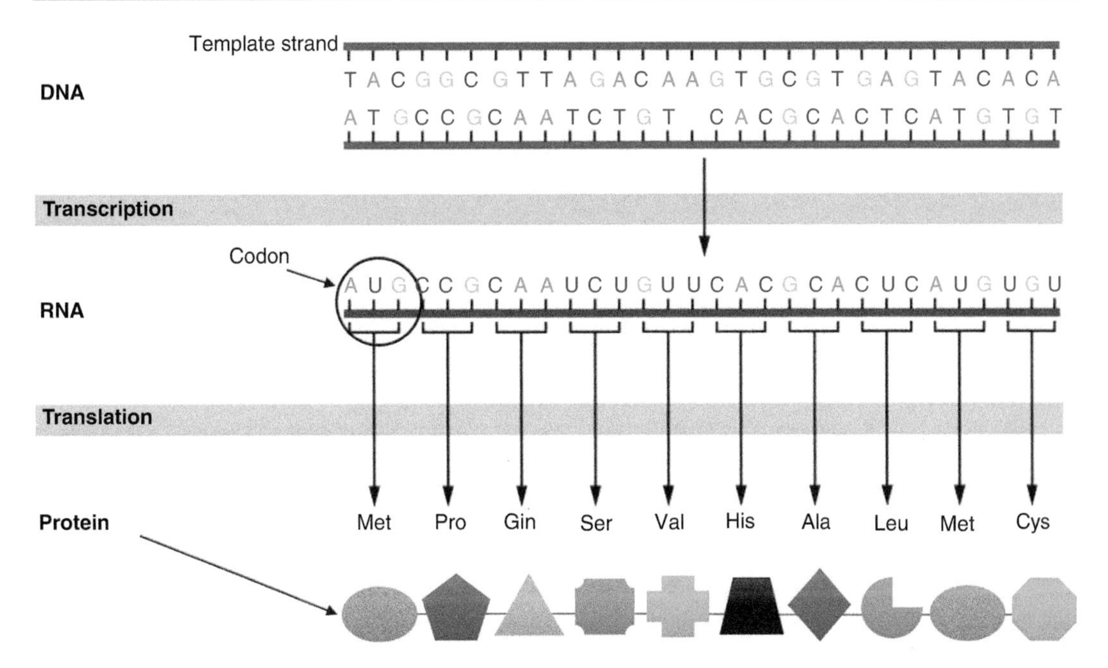

Fig. 1.4 Genes are transcribed into messenger RNA and translated into amino acids, which combine to form proteins

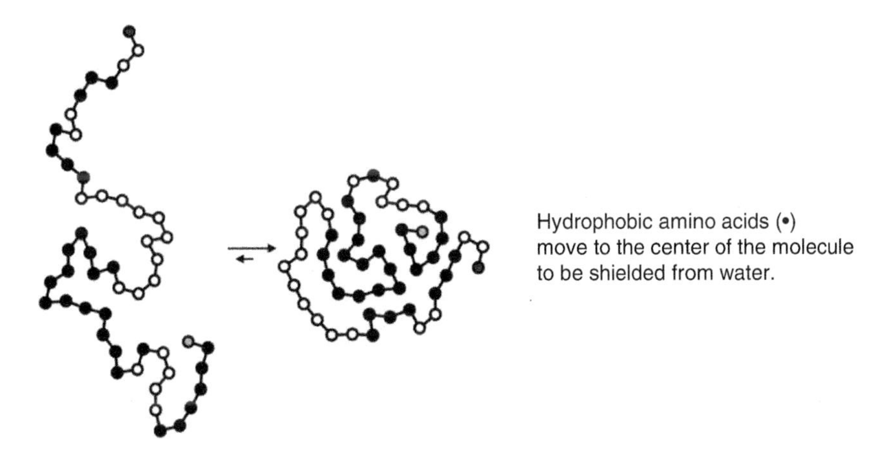

Fig. 1.5 The linear chain of amino acids (left side) assumes a compact, folded shape (right side) as hydrophobic amino acids (dark dots) gravitate toward the center core, promoting protein folding

tion of the substitution and how many nucleotides are involved, this may affect one or more codons and thus one or more amino acids in the protein sequence.

An insertion involves the addition of one or more extra nucleotides that do not belong in the typical DNA sequence of the gene. Recall that DNA is translated to RNA and then transcribed one codon (3 nucleotides) at a time. An insertion, unless it happens to occur between established codons and involve a number of nucleotides divisible by three, is likely to disrupt the codon reading frame. This variant leads to an unintended sequence of amino acids from that point on in the newly synthesized protein. The result is referred to as a frameshift variant. When the codon reading frame is shifted, it is also likely that one of the newly created codons will be a stop codon, creating a premature truncation of the protein.

Table 1.2 Variant effects on the structure of a gene

Normal DNA reference sequence	TAC GGC GTT AAA CAA GTG CGT ACG TAC ACA
Substitution	TAC **A**GC GTT AAA CAA GTG CGT ACG TAC ACA
Insertion Leading to frameshift	TAC GGC GTT AAA CAT AGT GCG TAC GTA CAC A
Deletion Of 3 nucleotides-no change in reading frame	TAC GGC GTT AAA CAA GTG ~~CGT~~ ACG TAC ACA

Table 1.3 Variant effects on the sequence of amino acids in a protein

Normal DNA reference sequence Messenger RNA Protein	TAC GGC GTT AAA CAA GTG CGT ACG TAC ACA AUG CCG CAA UUU GUU CAC GCA UCG AUG UGU Met Pro Gln Lys Val His Ala Ser Met Cys
substitution leading to **silent variant** The amino acid is not changed	TAC GGT GTA AAA CAA GTG CGT ACG TAC ACA AUG CC**A** CAA UUU GUU CAC GCA UCG AUG UGU Met Pro Gln Lys Val His Ala Ser Met Cys
substitution leading to **neutral variant** Lysine is replaced with arginine which is chemically similar	TAC GGC GTT AGA CCA AGT GCG ACG GTA CAC A AUG CCG CAA U**C**U GUU CAC GCA UCG AUG UGU Met Pro Gln **Arg** Val His Ala Ser Met Cys
substitution leading to **missense variant** Alanine is replaced with threonine which has very different chemical properties	TAC GGC GTT AAA CAA GTG TGT ACG TAC ACA AUG CCG CAA UUU GUU CAC **A**CA UCG AUG UGU Met Pro Gln Lys Val His **Thr** Ser Met Cys
substitution leading to **nonsense variant**	TAC GGC GTT AAA CAA GTG CGT ATC TAC ACA AUG CCG CAA UUU GUU CAC GCA U**A**G Met Pro Gln Lys Val His Ala **STOP**
deletion leading to **frameshift and premature protein truncation**	TAC G~~GC~~ GT TAA ACA AGT GCG TGA GTA CAC A AUG CCA AUU UGU UCA CGC ACU CAU GUG U Met Gly **STOP**

Deletions occur when one or more nucleotides are removed from the gene. As with insertions, deletions can disrupt the codon reading sequence of the gene, resulting in frameshift and/or protein truncation.

1.3.2 Variant Effects on Amino Acid Sequence

As discussed above, changing one or more nucleotides can lead to a change in the corresponding sequence of amino acids. Genetic variants can also be classified based on the functional effect of these changes (Table 1.3).

The most benign change is referred to as a silent variant. Silent variants occur when there is a change in the DNA, which does not lead to a change in the resulting codon or amino acid. For instance, a substitution that changes the sequence "GCT" to "GCC" results in a different codon, with the same reading frame, which also codes for alanine, the same amino acid encoded by the original sequence. Silent variants have no effect on the final protein.

Neutral variants involve a change in the DNA sequence that leads to a different but chemically similar amino acid at the designated place in the protein. For instance, changing an arginine to a lysine in the amino acid sequence will have little effect on the protein since both of these amino acids share similar chemical properties.

A missense variant changes the DNA in a way that leads to one or more amino acids with very different chemical properties from the intended sequence. For instance, a substitution that changes the sequence "CGT" to TGT" changes the corresponding amino acid from alanine to threonine. In this case, the intended amino acid, which is hydrophobic, is changed to a hydrophilic molecule, which could lead to changes in the conformation and thus the function of the ultimate protein. Of note, missense variants are typically most amenable to chemical chaperone therapy, which can help to restore a more normal protein conformation.

Variants that change the DNA, leading to a premature stop codon and, therefore, a truncated protein, are called nonsense variants. If a nonsense variant occurs toward the beginning of a gene, there may not be any protein made at all. If it occurs toward the end of the gene, there may or may not be a significant effect on the function of the truncated protein produced.

1.3.3 Variant Effects on the Protein

A variant's effect on health and well-being is dependent upon the gene involved and the effect of the variant on the protein it encodes. Possible effects include loss of protein function, gain of protein function, or no effect.

Variants that result in loss of function of the intended protein are the most common cause of inherited metabolic diseases. Loss of function may be due to an alteration of DNA sequences critical to the protein's activity or function, such as the catalytic properties of an enzyme. Loss of function may also be due to variants that drastically decrease the abundance of the protein in the cell. This includes variants that alter DNA sequences, which are critical to protein folding. Improper or misfolded proteins are unstable and may be flagged for destruction in the cell. Variants that result in the loss of protein expression, RNA degradation, or changes in the localization and targeting of the protein in the cell are other causes of decreased protein abundance.

Some variants alter the gene in such a way that the ultimate protein created takes on unintended functions. It may also cause the protein to be expressed in unintended cell types. This type of variant is referred to as a gain of function. Gain-of-function variants are typically associated with dominantly inherited diseases.

Variants that fully abolish the function of a protein are referred to as null variants. Null variants generally result in severe clinical disease, whereas variants that reduce, but do not abolish, protein function result in relatively less severe disease.

1.4 Variant Nomenclature

Variant nomenclature has evolved as we have learned more about the human genome and standard methods of reporting mutations have been developed [3, 4]. Describing a specific variant begins with identifying the reference sequence being used. A variant beginning with "c." refers to a change in coding DNA. Likewise, a variant beginning with "p." describes a change in the protein sequence. Other reference sequences include "g." for genomic DNA, "n." for noncoding DNA, "m." for mitochondrial DNA, and "r." for RNA.

For variants in coding DNA, "c." is followed by notation of which nucleotide(s) in the coding sequence are involved and what specific change occurred as compared to the typical or "wild type" reference sequence. The following are examples of basic variants in the *PAH* gene known to be associated with phenylketonuria (PKU) (Box 1.1):

Box 1.1: Variants in Coding DNA

Type of variant	Examples	Description
Substitution	c.1222C > T	At nucleotide number 1222, a cytosine has been replaced with a thymine.
Deletion	c.184delC	At nucleotide number 184, a cytosine has been deleted.
	c.163_165delTTT	Including nucleotides number 163, 164, and 165, there are three thymines deleted.
Duplication	c.111dupG	At nucleotide number 111, there are two guanine nucleotides (instead of one).
	c.185_188dupTGAC	Including nucleotides number 185 through 188, there is a duplication of 4 nucleotides: thymine, guanine, adenine, and cytosine.
Insertion	c.266_267insG	Between nucleotides 266 and 267, a guanine nucleotide was inserted.
	c.43_44insAG	Between nucleotides 43 and 44, an adenine and a guanine were inserted.

Source: PAHvdb http://www.biopku.org [5]

Box 1.2: Variants in the Amino Acid Sequence of a Protein

Change in gene	Resulting change in protein	Description
c.1222C > T	p. Arg408Trp p.R408W	At amino acid number 408 in the protein, an arginine is changed to a tryptophan.
c.184delC	p.Leu62Ter p.L62* or p.L62X	At amino acid number 62 in the protein, a leucine has been replaced with a termination (stop) codon.
c.163_165delTTT	p.Phe55del	At amino acid number 55 in the protein, a phenylalanine is deleted from the sequence.
c.111dupG	p.Ile38AspfsTer19	At amino acid number 38, an isoleucine was changed to an aspartate, the length of the frameshift is 19 amino acids including the termination (stop) codon.

Variants in the amino acid sequence of a protein are denoted as "p." followed by a description of the amino acid change. It is typically expressed using three letter abbreviations for the amino acids; however, former nomenclature used single letter abbreviations (Table 1.1). These examples correlate with some of the changes in coding DNA listed above (Box 1.2).

1.5 Genetic Testing

1.5.1 Genetic Testing Technologies

The origin of genetic testing dates back to the 1950s, when it was established that humans typically have 46 chromosomes in every body cell and it became possible to stain and count chromosomes in leukocyte cultures [6, 7]. By stopping cell division when the long strands of DNA are becoming most compacted into chromosomes and then applying special stains, it is possible to count the number and type of chromosomes in a cell. Areas of the DNA that are rich in adenine and thymine nucleotides stain differently than those with more cytosine and guanine nucleotides, creating "banding patterns" or darker stripes of stain along the chromosomes. For analysis, cytogeneticists line up the chromosomes based on size and match up the chromosome pairs based on banding patterns; the result is called a karyotype (Fig. 1.6). Initially, karyotypes were limited to testing for an abnormal number of chromosomes. As the resolution of chromosome analysis improved, it also became possible to detect deletions, additions, or rearrangements of relatively large segments of DNA within a chromosome or exchanged between two or more chromosomes.

In the 1980s, molecular cytogenetic technologies were developed. By using the same culture techniques as karyotyping but employing a specific nucleotide sequence designed to attach to a targeted region of a specific chromosome, fluorescent in situ hybridization (FISH) is able to identify the presence or absence and the location of that specific sequence of DNA [8]. This enables testing for specific regions of a chromosome too small to be visible by karyotype.

In 1992, comparative genomic hybridization (CGH) was first reported [9]. CGH involves combining DNA from one cell line (blood, tumor, etc.) with DNA from a normal or "wild type" reference sequence and attaching molecular labels or tags. The two sources of DNA are chemically induced to hybridize to each other where their DNA sequences match up. The molecular labels are fluorescent and can be measured at specific positions in the genome. By comparing fluorescence to a standard, CGH provides information on the relative copy number of sequences in the test cell line. By analyzing copy number variations (CNVs), it is possible to deduce whether there are small sequences of DNA that are missing or duplicated. Different versions of this technology have advanced to the chromosome microarray analysis (CMA) widely used today to detect microdeletions and microduplications, which may involve one or multiple genes.

The terms, "molecular testing" and "DNA testing," are often used interchangeably. Both

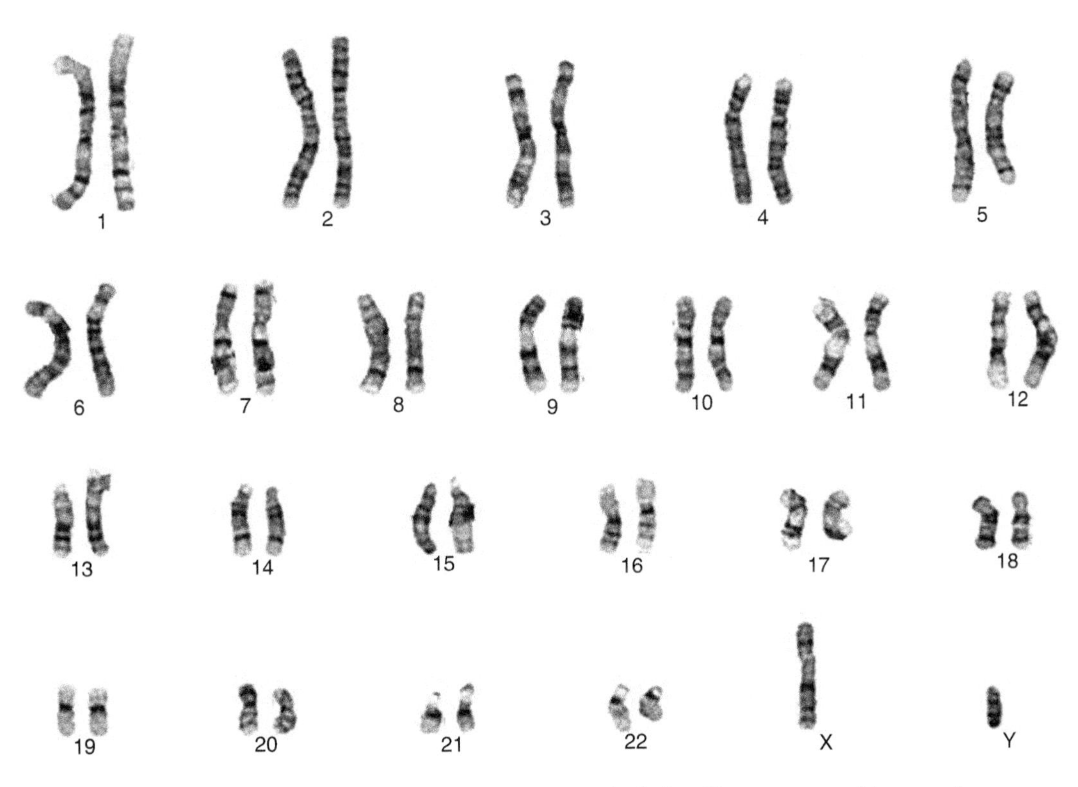

Fig. 1.6 A standard male karyotype with 46 total chromosomes including 22 autosomes and two sex chromosomes (XY)

refer to testing techniques that allow for identification of nucleotides in a gene. This allows for detection of DNA sequence variation due to substitutions, insertions, and deletions. A variety of molecular testing approaches and methods exist. For the purposes of this chapter, we will focus on two: Sanger sequencing and next-generation sequencing (NGS).

Sanger sequencing (developed by Frederic Sanger and colleagues in the 1970s) has long been a gold standard in DNA testing [10, 11]. It begins with isolating a specific gene and then using the DNA strand as a template to generate multiple copies through the use of polymerase chain reaction (PCR). As the name implies, sequencing involves reading nucleotide by nucleotide through the DNA sequence of a gene in an effort to identify changes from a normal or "wild type" reference sequence. Sanger sequencing is accurate and well suited for targeted molecular studies. Targeted variant analysis is used when looking for the presence of a specific variant in a gene. For instance, if there is a specific variant that was previously identified in another family member.

Next-generation sequencing (NGS) is a general term that involves several different technologies. NGS begins with fragmenting and amplifying millions of different DNA sequences at the same time. In this way, it can create multiple copies of hundreds to thousands of genes simultaneously. The millions of DNA fragments are then compared to a normal or "wild-type" reference sequence. Using an NGS platform allows for more automation and higher throughput. Accuracy of variant detection is also significantly improved owing to repeated sampling of the same DNA sequences.

NGS serves as the base for gene panel testing. Gene panels are a select group of genes that may be involved in a common differential diagnosis. Panel tests may be based on a specific disorder; for instance, a maple syrup urine disease (MSUD) panel that includes the different genes involved in encoding each subunit of the enzyme deficient in MSUD. Panel tests can also be built around a set of biochemical and/or clinical symptoms; for example, a panel of genes associated with ketotic hypoglycemia or developmental delay. A single panel can test for hundreds of genes, thereby eliminating the need to use Sanger sequencing to test one gene at a time.

NGS platforms also allow for broader scale testing including exome and genome sequencing. Whole exome sequencing (WES) allows for the analysis of the exons of most every gene. Collectively referred to as the exome, this is inclusive of the coding regions of most known genes. Although the exome represents <2% of the human genome, it contains an estimated 85% of known disease-causing variants [12]. Whole genome sequencing (WGS), by contrast, includes not only the exons, but also the introns and regulatory elements included in noncoding DNA. Since some disease-causing variants can occur in noncoding regions of a gene, WGS is the most comprehensive but is also the most complex to interpret. To aid in interpretation of possible variants, most WES and WGS analyses refer to DNA samples from both biological parents of an affected individual; thus, testing is often ordered as a "trio."

Importantly, both Sanger sequencing and NGS have a limited ability to detect relatively large deletions or duplications within a gene. They also cannot distinguish between two copies of the same variant (one on the maternal gene copy, one on the paternal gene copy) versus one copy of a variant paired with a deletion in that same area of the other gene copy. If a disease-causing variant is suspected in a specific gene but is not identified by sequencing, additional testing may be indicated. Microarray-based testing, multiplex ligation–dependent probe amplification (MLPA) analysis, and quantitative PCR (qPCR) analysis are all potential options to identify these variants (Fig. 1.7).

1.5.2 Interpretation of Genetic Testing

Dependent upon the testing method(s) used, there are four main categories of possible results:

Positive results are those that identify at least one specific genetic variant that accounts for all

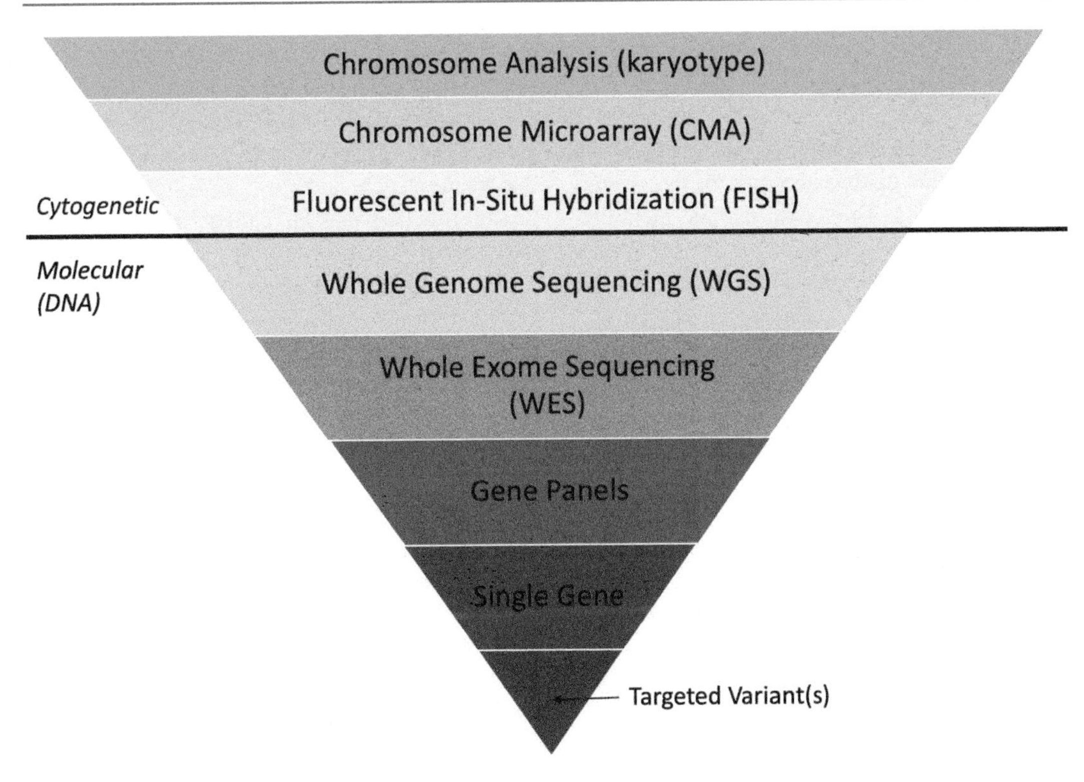

Fig. 1.7 Genetic testing methods organized from least (top) to most (bottom) specific

or part of the clinical and biochemical symptoms of the individual. Positive results involve at least one variant determined to be capable of causing disease, also referred to as a pathogenic variant. The specific variant may already be known in the scientific community and reported in association with clinical disease or, based on the type and location of the variant within the gene, it may be predicted to be disease-causing or likely disease-causing.

Negative results refer to testing that does not identify a disease-causing variant. Negative results do not necessarily rule out the possibility of the disease in question. It is possible that additional testing technologies may be required to identify the variant. It is also possible to have a gene that, in sequence, appears to be normal but is affected by a secondary genetic or epigenetic mechanism that leads to malfunction.

Genetic testing may also identify one or more variants of uncertain significance (VUS). A VUS is a variant about which we have no, limited, or conflicting information. Many DNA variants, whether inherited or unique to a given individual, may just be part of normal, benign variation and not associated with disease. Other variants may have disease-causing potential; however, the specific variant has never been reported before or has not been subject to functional studies to help clarify the potential significance. Some variants have been reported in both healthy individuals and in individuals with clinical symptoms and are therefore more difficult to interpret. In the case of a VUS, it is important to consider the clinical context of the individual. As our knowledge of genes and human disease continues to expand, VUSs are often reclassified as benign, likely benign, pathogenic, or likely pathogenic.

A fourth category of results is important to consider, especially when using more broad testing methods that can uncover unexpected results. In some cases, genetic testing can reveal that biological relationships are not as reported. For instance, it can identify misattributed paternity or consanguinity (a common ancestor as in siblings or cousins). Chromosome analysis and CMA may identify a difference between the biological sex and phenotypic or apparent sex of an individual. Since panel testing, WES, and WGS analyze more than one gene, it is possible to uncover positive results in a gene that was not part of the primary reason for testing. This could include identification of carrier status for, susceptibility to, or presence of another disorder. For instance, exome analysis completed for the purpose of identifying a cause of developmental delay may also identify that the individual is a carrier for phenylketonuria (PKU) or at increased risk to develop hereditary cancer or cardiovascular disease. These results are also referred to as secondary findings. The identification of a secondary finding in the individual being tested can also inform the risk for other family members to have the same condition or predisposition. Complex results and unsought information can raise moral and ethical challenges [13–16]. Clear expectations regarding the benefits and limitations of testing, what information could be identified, and what information will or will not be shared should be established prior to testing [17]. Therefore, an informed consent process is generally required, and genetic counseling is strongly recommended.

1.5.3 Purposes of Genetic Testing

Genetic testing may be helpful in a number of different circumstances. It can establish a genetic diagnosis in an individual, an in vitro embryo, or a pregnancy. A known diagnosis, in turn, can allow for more comprehensive management, monitoring for other anticipated findings, and potentially targeted treatments. Genetic testing can determine an inheritance pattern and allow for identification of other family members who may be at risk of developing the condition. It can determine carrier status for a specific variant or disorder, or for a broad panel of disorders. It can identify individuals who are clinically asymptomatic or presymptomatic who are at increased risk to develop a later-onset condition. Even if an affected individual already has a clinical and/or biochemical diagnosis, knowledge of the specific genetic variant(s) may lead to additional information about the expected clinical course (genotype/phenotype correlation described in Sect. 1.6) or may open doors to therapies based on a specific variant or type of variant. For example, some variants are responsive to chemical chaperone therapy such as the use of sapropterin dihydrochloride (Kuvan®) in patients with PKU who have certain missense variants [18–20]. Stop codon read-through therapy is another example currently in development, which allows cells to ignore premature termination codons induced by nonsense variants in order to restore more normal protein production. Other investigational treatments and gene therapies hold promise for the future.

1.6 Genotype and Phenotype

DNA testing determines the genotype, or genetic constitution, of an individual. The genotype is typically expressed with molecular nomenclature noting the specific variant(s). Since most genes occur in pairs (with one copy inherited from the mother and the other from the father), there are typically two versions of each gene in an individual. Each unique version of a gene is referred to as an allele. If the alleles are identical, the person is described as being homozygous at that genetic location. If the two alleles are different, they are described as being heterozygous at that location. One can be heterozygous with one variant allele and one "normal" allele. Alternatively, one can be compound heterozygous with a variant on one allele and a *different* variant on the other allele (Box 1.3).

Box 1.3: Examples of Homozygous and Heterozygous States

State	*Galactose-1-phosphate uridyltransferase (GALT) gene*
Homozygous	
Not affected	Normal/Normal
Affected	p.Q188R/p.Q188R
Heterozygous	
Carrier, not affected	Normal /p.Q188R
Compound heterozygous, affected	p.Q188R/ p.H319Q

In contrast to an individual's genotype, their phenotype refers to their observable physical and biochemical characteristics. If an individual's genotype, as noted by specific variant(s) of a certain gene, predicts a specific phenotypic outcome, there is said to be a genotype/phenotype correlation. For example, an individual with a genotype of p.Q188R/p.Q188R in the *GALT* gene is expected to have classic galactosemia. Some genotypes can predict responsiveness to various cofactors or therapies or may predict more mild or more severe clinical courses. This information, if established, can help to suggest outcome and drive management of the disease.

The term phenocopy refers to an environmentally induced variation that closely resembles a genetically determined variation. For example, dietary vitamin B_{12} deficiency is a phenocopy of the inherited disease, methylmalonic acidemia and homocystinuria, due to cobalamin C disease. Both dietary vitamin B_{12} deficiency and cobalamin C disease have the same biochemical findings of elevated plasma methylmalonic acid and homocysteine. Awareness of phenocopies is important as they can provide an alternative explanation for clinical findings. For example, in the case of elevated methylmalonic acid and elevated homocystinuria, one may want to exclude maternal vitamin B_{12} deficiency as a possible cause of these abnormal labs prior to testing for cobalamin C disease or other possible metabolic etiologies.

1.7 Single Gene Inheritance Patterns and Pedigrees

There are three main patterns of single gene inheritance (also called Mendelian inheritance, discovered by Gregor Mendel in the late 1800s): autosomal recessive, autosomal dominant, and X-linked. In autosomal-dominant and autosomal-recessive inheritance, the gene responsible for the disorder is located on one of the 22 autosomal chromosomes. For X-linked conditions, the gene involved is located on the X chromosome. Y-linked, polygenic, and mitochondrial inheritance patterns exist as well but will not be addressed in this chapter.

1.7.1 Single Gene Inheritance Patterns

In order for an individual to be affected with an autosomal-recessive disorder, he or she must have inherited a disease-causing variant from both parents. Although the variants are recessive, an affected individual has no normal copy of the gene. Parents of an affected individual are considered to be obligate carriers of the disorder, having one variant gene copy and one presumably normal gene copy. Since the variant is recessive, carriers are able to use their normal gene copy as a template to make sufficient amounts of the encoded protein so that they are not affected with the disorder. For two carriers of an autosomal-recessive disorder, there is a 1 in 4 (25%) chance that *each* pregnancy they conceive will be affected with the disorder (Fig. 1.8). Children of two carriers, who are not affected themselves, have a 2 in 3 (66%) chance to also be carriers. In the general population (individuals without a family history of the disorder in question), the carrier frequency or chance that an individual would happen to be a carrier for a given disorder varies depending on the specific disorder, gene, and sometimes ethnic population. Autosomal-recessive inheritance is the most common inheritance pattern seen in inborn errors of metabolism.

For an individual to be affected with an autosomal-dominant disorder, he or she must inherit one disease-causing variant. Since the variant is dominant, it will cause disease despite having another, normal copy of the gene. Especially with dominant variants, some variants can occur spontaneously, just by chance, and are not inherited from an affected parent. Such variants are referred to as de novo variants. Whether a dominant variant is inherited or de novo, an affected parent has a 50% chance to pass it to each of his/her children (Fig. 1.9). A child who inherits the variant will be affected with the disorder.

Sometimes, two individuals with the same variant may express different clinical features, severity, or age of onset, even within the same family. This is referred to as variable expressiv-

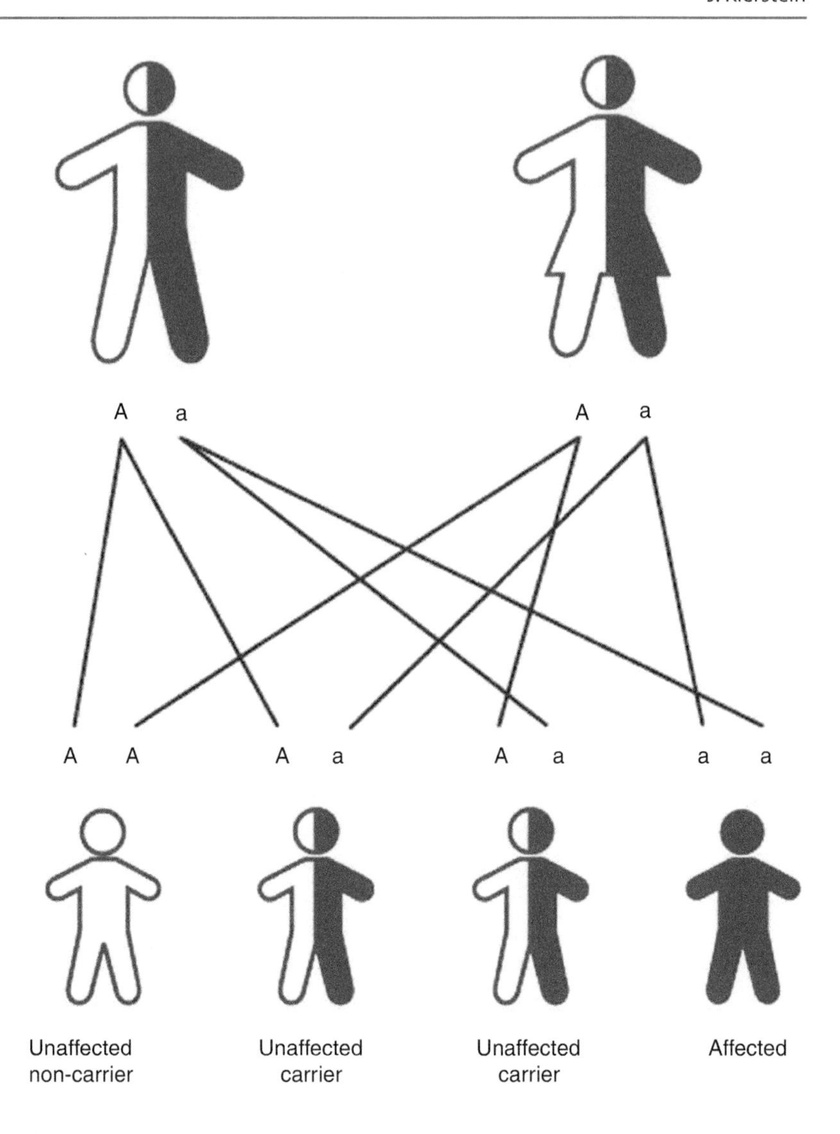

Fig. 1.8 Autosomal-recessive inheritance

ity. For some conditions, an individual with a confirmed disease-causing variant may not express any clinical symptoms at all through a phenomenon called incomplete penetrance. In that situation, the phenotype may appear to "skip a generation" but the genotype does not.

X-linked inheritance results from a variant that occurs in a gene located on the X chromosome. Recall that females have two X chromosomes (one inherited from their mother and the other from their father) and males have only one X chromosome (inherited from their mother) and one Y chromosome (inherited from their father). If a male inherits an X-linked variant, he will be affected with the disorder. Likewise, if he has a de novo, disease causing variant in an X-linked gene, he will also be affected. In either case, he will pass his variant to each daughter he has, but none of his sons (Fig. 1.10).

X-linked disorders in females are more complicated and typically variable in expression.

Since females have two X chromosomes, they also have two copies of all X-linked genes. As proven by males who only have one X chromosome, humans only need one copy of most of these genes. In order to account for this double dosage, one X chromosome in every female's cell is inactivated through a process called lyonization or X-inactivation. This process is typically random and occurs early in the embry-

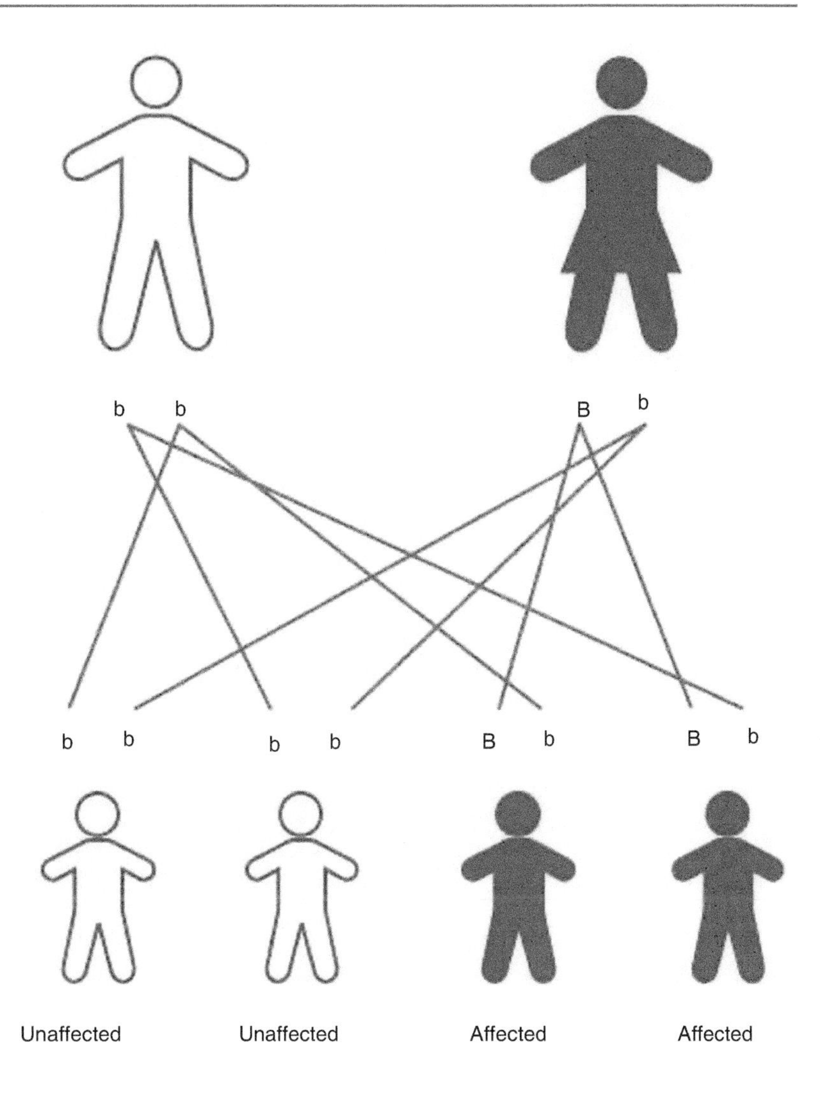

Fig. 1.9 Autosomal-dominant inheritance

onic development of a female, long before she is born. Once an X chromosome is inactivated, all new cells created from that cell line will have the same X chromosome inactivated. Inactivation does not change over time. Since this process happens early in embryonic development as different tissue types are beginning to differentiate, it is common that all cells in a given tissue will share the same X inactivation pattern. That pattern, however, can differ between tissue types. For instance, a female may have her maternally inherited X chromosome inactivated in her liver but her paternally inherited X chromosome inactivated in her brain. Occasionally, inactivation patterns may be skewed such that the vast majority of a female's cells have inactivated the same X chromosome. Skewed X-inactivation can be favorable or unfavorable if there happens to be a genetic variant on one of the X chromosomes.

If a female is affected with or is a carrier of an X-linked gene variant, she has a 50% chance to pass the variant to each child she has (Fig. 1.11). If the child who inherits the variant is a male, he will be affected with the disorder. If the child who inherits the variant is a female, her inactivation pattern will be determined after conception. Regardless of whether her mother is clinically symptomatic of the condition, a daughter who inherits the variant may be more mildly or more severely affected or, in some cases, may have no clinical symptoms at all.

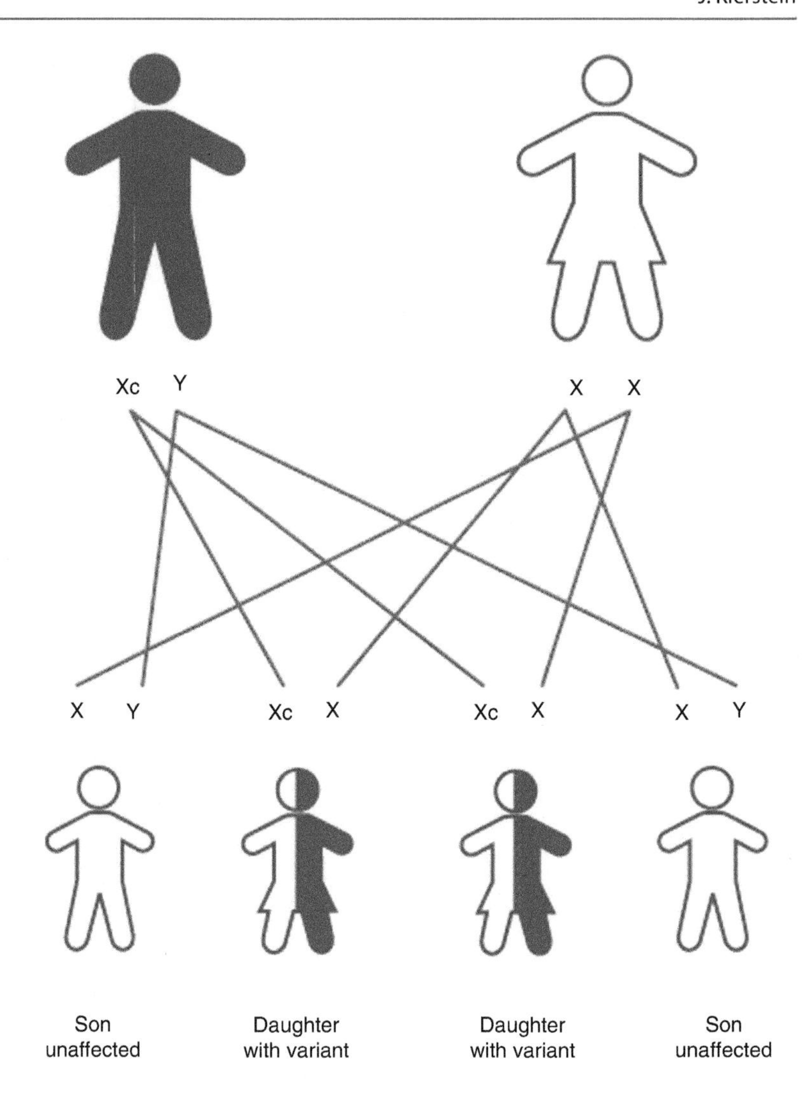

Fig. 1.10 X-linked inheritance, affected male. Note that carrier females may or may not show symptoms of the disorder depending on the disorder and their X inactivation pattern

1.7.2 Pedigrees

A genetic family history or pedigree, detailing genetic relationships and medical history of family members, can help determine the inheritance pattern of a disorder. Pedigrees can also identify individuals in the family who are at risk for developing disease or for passing on disease-causing variants in a gene. Standard symbols and terminology are used to identify individuals, relationships, and carrier or disease state (Fig. 1.12) [21]. The use of symbols allows for a concise, graphic representation of a family's genetic health history.

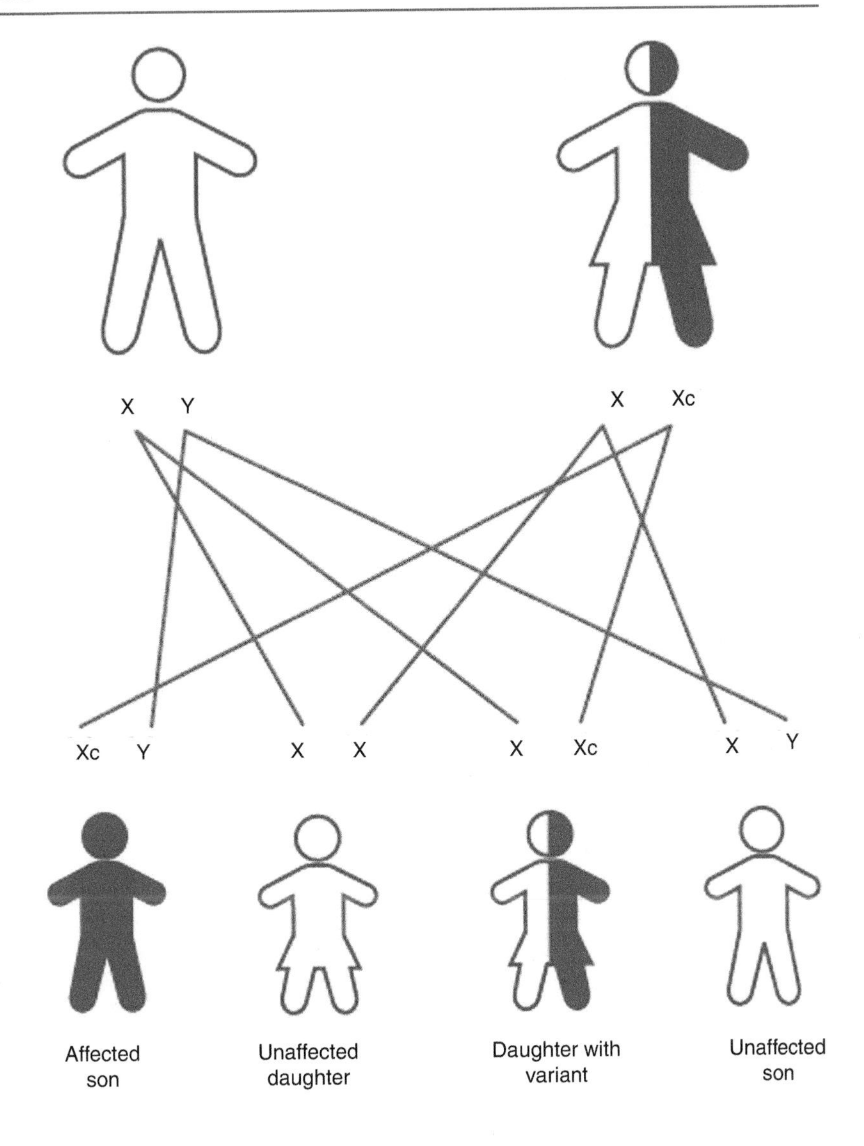

Fig. 1.11 X-linked inheritance, affected female. Due to the variability of X-linked disorders in females, a female who has the variant may or may not show symptoms of the disorder. True X-linked recessive disorders exist where carrier females are completely unaffected. X-linked dominant disorders also exist but are influenced by X inactivation patterns

The pedigree below is typical for an autosomal-recessive disorder (Fig. 1.13). Notice the carriers, all designated by the dot in the center of the square (males) or circle (females). In most cases, autosomal-recessive carrier status is not revealed until an affected individual is born into the family. Every child of an individual affected with an autosomal-recessive disorder will be an obligate carrier for the condition. They would only be at risk to be affected themselves if their other parent also happened to be a carrier of or affected with the disorder.

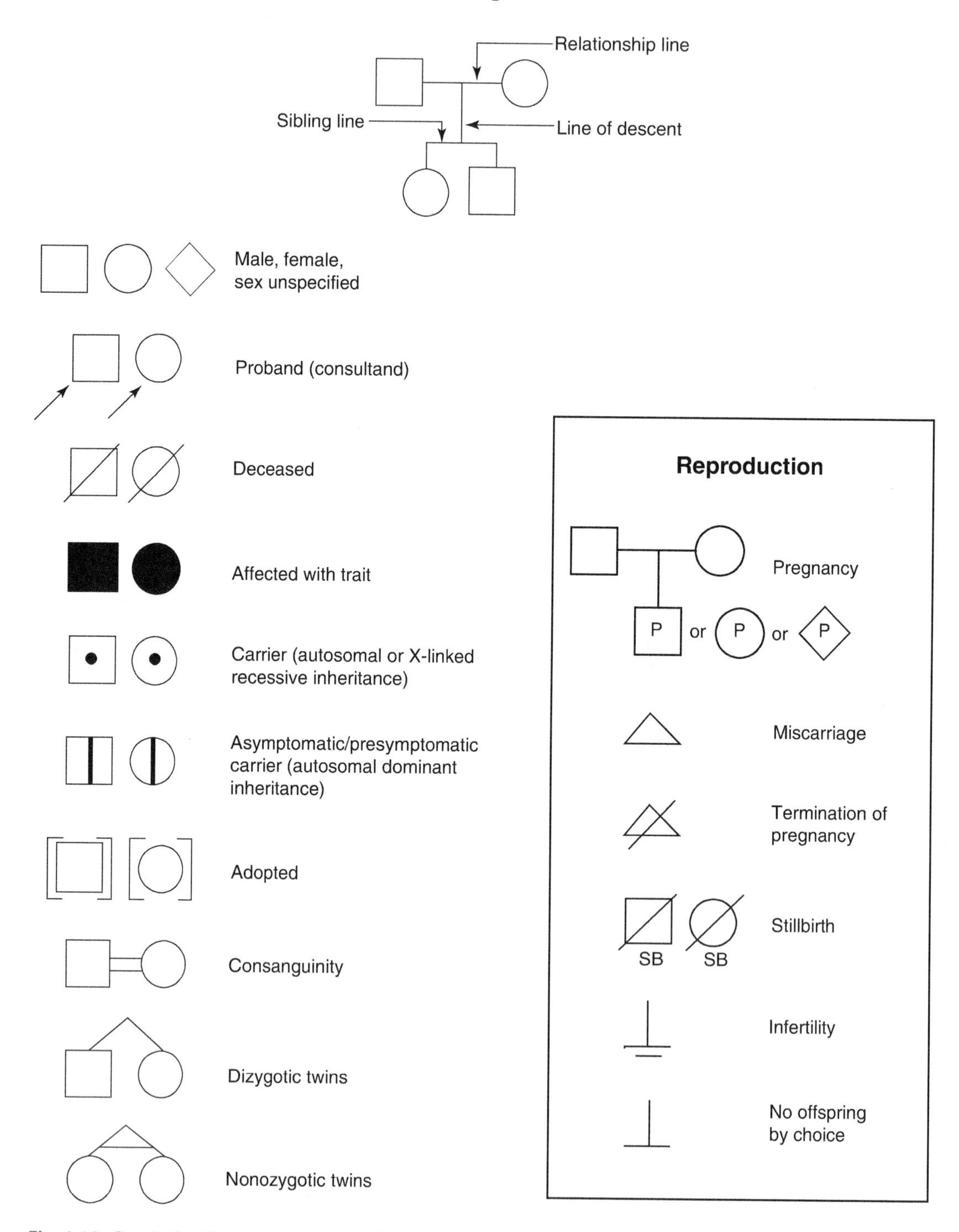

Fig. 1.12 Standard pedigree nomenclature. Common symbols are used to draw a pedigree (family tree). A pedigree shows relationships between family members and patterns of inheritance for certain traits and diseases

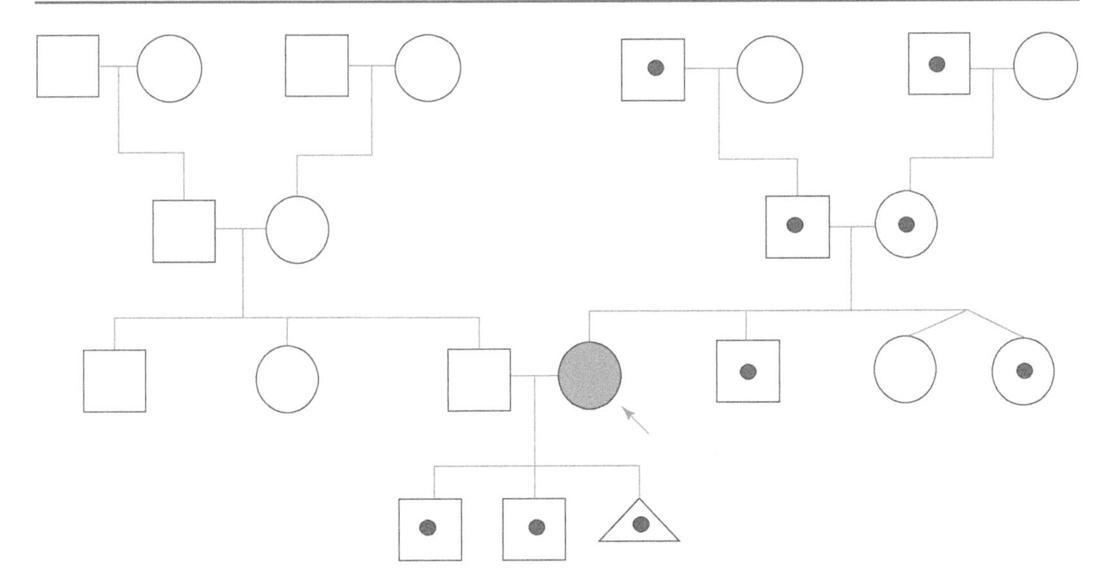

Fig. 1.13 An example of a pedigree for an autosomal-recessive disorder. The affected individual is shown as a shaded figure. Carriers are designated by a dot in the center of the figures

1.8 Summary

Our lives and well-being depend upon the function of thousands of unique proteins in each of our trillions of cells. Variants in the genes that encode these proteins disrupt cellular function and can lead to disease. The symptoms of the disease and severity are dependent upon the specific protein and the degree to which it is impacted. Genetic testing allows for the identification of the underlying genetic changes. Identifying specific variants can predict disease severity, provide risk assessment to other family members, suggest and inform on likely pathophysiology, and potentially provide strategies for intervention.

Acknowledgments Thank you to Cindy Freehauf of Children's Hospital of Colorado for her contributions to this chapter's content in the 1st Edition of Nutrition Management of Inherited Metabolic Diseases.

References

1. Bianconi E, Piovesan A, Facchin F, Beraudi A, Casadei R, Frabetti F, et al. An estimation of the number of cells in the human body. Ann Hum Biol. 2013;40(6):463–71.
2. Encode Project Consortium. An integrated encyclopedia of DNA elements in the human genome. Nature. 2012;489(7414):57–74.
3. Ogino S, Gulley ML, den Dunnen JT, Wilson RB, Association for Molecular Patholpogy T, Education C. Standard mutation nomenclature in molecular diagnostics: practical and educational challenges. J Mol Diagn. 2007;9(1):1–6.
4. den Dunnen JT, Dalgleish R, Maglott DR, Hart RK, Greenblatt MS, McGowan-Jordan J, et al. HGVS recommendations for the description of sequence variants: 2016 update. Hum Mutat. 2016;37(6):564–9.
5. PAHvdb: Phenylalanine Hydroxylase Gene Locus-Specific Database 2020. Available from: http://www.biopku.org/home/home.asp.
6. Tijo J, Levan A. The chromosome number of man. Hereditas. 2010;42(1–2):1–6.
7. Moorhead PS, Nowell PC, Mellman WJ, Battips DM, Hungerford DA. Chromosome preparations of leukocytes cultured from human peripheral blood. Exp Cell Res. 1960;20:613–6.
8. Langer-Safer PR, Levine M, Ward DC. Immunological method for mapping genes on Drosophila polytene chromosomes. Proc Natl Acad Sci U S A. 1982;79(14):4381–5.
9. Kallioniemi A, Kallioniemi OP, Sudar D, Rutovitz D, Gray JW, Waldman F, et al. Comparative genomic hybridization for molecular cytogenetic analysis of solid tumors. Science. 1992;258(5083):818–21.
10. Sanger F, Coulson AR. A rapid method for determining sequences in DNA by primed synthesis with DNA polymerase. J Mol Biol. 1975;94(3):441–8.
11. Sanger F, Nicklen S, Coulson AR. DNA sequencing with chain-terminating inhibitors. Proc Natl Acad Sci U S A. 1977;74(12):5463–7.

12. Choi M, Scholl UI, Ji W, Liu T, Tikhonova IR, Zumbo P, et al. Genetic diagnosis by whole exome capture and massively parallel DNA sequencing. Proc Natl Acad Sci U S A. 2009;106(45):19096–101.
13. Burke W, Trinidad SB, Clayton EW. Seeking genomic knowledge: the case for clinical restraint. Hastings Law J. 2013;64(6):1650–64.
14. Evans JP, Rothschild BB. Return of results: not that complicated? Genet Med. 2012;14(4):358–60.
15. Grove ME, Wolpert MN, Cho MK, Lee SS, Ormond KE. Views of genetics health professionals on the return of genomic results. J Genet Couns. 2014;23(4):531–8.
16. Yu JH, Harrell TM, Jamal SM, Tabor HK, Bamshad MJ. Attitudes of genetics professionals toward the return of incidental results from exome and whole-genome sequencing. Am J Hum Genet. 2014;95(1):77–84.
17. National Society of Genetic Counselors: NSGC Headquarters. 2013. Available from: nsgc@nsgc.org.
18. Erlandsen H, Pey AL, Gamez A, Perez B, Desviat LR, Aguado C, et al. Correction of kinetic and stability defects by tetrahydrobiopterin in phenylketonuria patients with certain phenylalanine hydroxylase mutations. Proc Natl Acad Sci U S A. 2004;101(48):16903–8.
19. Zurfluh MR, Zschocke J, Lindner M, Feillet F, Chery C, Burlina A, et al. Molecular genetics of tetrahydrobiopterin-responsive phenylalanine hydroxylase deficiency. Hum Mutat. 2008;29(1):167–75.
20. Farrugia R, Scerri CA, Montalto SA, Parascandolo R, Neville BG, Felice AE. Molecular genetics of tetrahydrobiopterin (BH4) deficiency in the Maltese population. Mol Genet Metab. 2007;90(3):277–83.
21. Bennett RL, French KS, Resta RG, Doyle DL. Standardized human pedigree nomenclature: update and assessment of the recommendations of the National Society of Genetic Counselors. J Genet Couns. 2008;17(5):424–33.

Newborn Screening for Inherited Metabolic Diseases

2

Erica Wright

Contents

E. Wright (✉)
Clinical Genetics and Metabolism, Children's Hospital Colorado, University of Colorado Denver – Anschutz Medical Campus, Aurora, CO, USA
e-mail: erica.wright@childrenscolorado.org

L. E. Bernstein et al. (eds.), *Nutrition Management of Inherited Metabolic Diseases*,
https://doi.org/10.1007/978-3-030-94510-7_2

Core Messages

- The success of newborn screening for phenylketonuria (PKU) led to the expansion of newborn screening for other disorders, including many inborn errors of metabolism, thus preventing significant morbidity and mortality.
- Newborn screening is an integrated system requiring all aspects (birthing facilities, newborn screening programs including laboratories and follow-up, confirmatory testing laboratories, primary care and specialty providers, and families) to work in conjunction with each other to ensure the best outcome of the patients and continued quality improvement of the newborn screening system.
- Limitations of newborn screening include timeliness of screening and diagnosis, false negatives, and disorders not included on the newborn screening panel.
- Expansion of newborn screening is often propelled by new testing methodologies, emerging treatments, and parent advocacy groups.

2.1 Background

For over 50 years, newborn screening has evolved to become one of the most successful public health initiatives and is considered the gold standard as a population-based screening system. Prior to newborn screening, patients were diagnosed only after symptoms manifested resulting in significant health and developmental sequelae, and even death. Other patients never received a diagnosis and therefore were never treated. Early attempts of population-based screening for inborn errors of metabolism began in the 1950s with phenylketonuria (PKU) after Dr. Horst Bickel showed that diet intervention resulted in improved outcome [1].

In 1957, Willard Centerwall developed the "diaper test" in which elevation of phenylalanine was detected in the urine of affected individuals with PKU by applying a ferric chloride solution to a wet diaper. This method was most often utilized in pediatric offices in older infants, thus still delaying the diagnosis and treatment of PKU and hindering the outcomes of the identified patients [2, 3].

In 1959, Dr. Robert Guthrie developed a bacterial inhibition assay to detect elevation of phenylalanine in dried blood spots collected on filter paper [4, 5]. The presence of elevated phenylalanine in the blood spot resulted in bacterial growth. This method was sensitive enough to detect elevations of phenylalanine greater than 180–240 μmol/L (3–4 mg/dL). With the availability of an appropriate screening test for early detection of PKU, Massachusetts became the first state in the United States to begin statewide newborn screening in 1963 (Fig. 2.1). By the late 1960s, newborn screening for PKU was mandated in a majority of the states.

The success of newborn screening for PKU led to the addition of other inborn errors of metabolism and endocrine disorders to the newborn screening panel. The bacterial inhibition technique was later implemented for newborn screening for

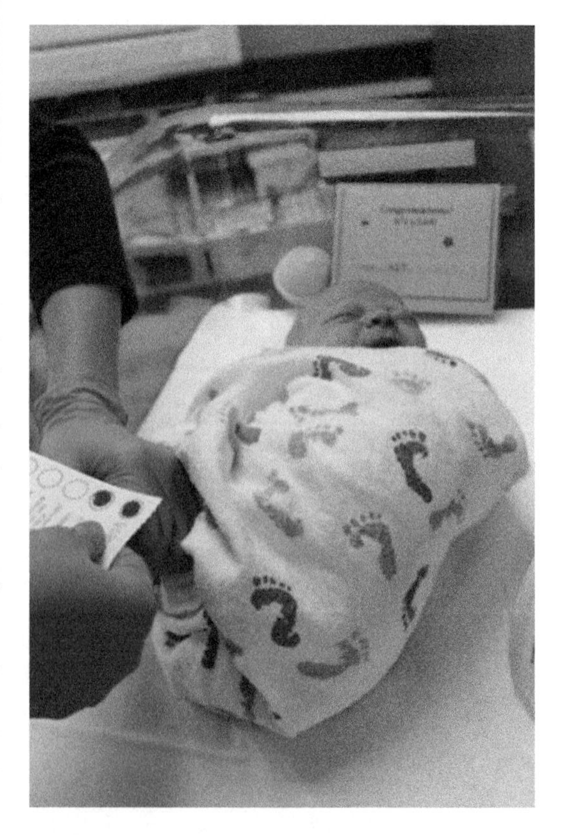

Fig. 2.1 Newborn heel-prick and spotting of blood onto filter paper for newborn screening. (Photo courtesy of Adelyn Wright)

maple syrup urine disease (elevated leucine) and homocystinuria (elevated methionine). Other laboratory techniques utilized in newborn screening in the following decades included: enzymatic assays for other inborn errors of metabolism such as galactosemia and biotinidase deficiency; immunoassays for endocrine disorders such as congenital hypothyroidism; and electrophoresis for sickle cell anemia and hemoglobinopathies [5]. Historically, each disorder required a separate screening test and was added to a panel after proving to meet the screening criteria set forth by the World Health Organization in 1968 [6]. This report "Principles and Practice of Screening for Disease" authored by James Maxwell Glover Wilson and Gunner Jungner has been the standard of screening in the public health realm. In the United States, each individual state was at liberty to add disorders to their newborn screening panel and generally followed these criteria to determine if a disorder was suitable for inclusion on the newborn screening panel (Box 2.1).

Box 2.1: Criteria for Newborn Screening

Goal:

To provide early detection of children at increased risk for disorders in which promptly initiating treatment prevents a metabolic crisis and/or irreversible sequelae, thus improving outcome.

Principles of screening based on Wilson and Jungner's criteria

- The condition is an important health problem.
- There is an acceptable treatment.
- Facilities for diagnosis and treatment are available.
- There is a recognizable latent or early symptomatic stage.
- There is a suitable screening test.
- The test is acceptable to the population.
- The natural history of the condition is adequately understood.
- There is an understanding of whom to treat as patients.
- It is cost effective.
- Identification of affected patients is a continuing process [6].

2.2 Newborn Screening by Tandem Mass Spectrometry

In 1990, the application of tandem mass spectrometry (MS/MS) to the analysis of dried blood spots was first described by David Millington [7]. During the 1990s, MS/MS proved to be a successful method for newborn screening with some states and private laboratories instituting the technology and better defining the sensitivity and specificity. MS/MS quantifies both amino acids and carnitine esters by using electrical and magnetic fields to separate and measure the mass of the charged particles. This allows for multiple biochemical parameters to be tested in a single dried blood spot, resulting in identification of over 30 inborn errors of metabolism including amino acidemias, urea cycle disorders, organic acidemias, and disorders of fatty acid oxidation [8–11] (Table 2.1). The ability to "multiplex" drastically altered the landscape of newborn screening.

The case to add MS/MS to newborn screening was driven primarily by one disorder: medium-chain acyl-CoA dehydrogenase deficiency (MCADD). MCADD meets all of the traditional criteria for newborn screening. The prevalence of MCADD is similar to PKU, with approximately 1 in 15,000 live births affected in the United States. MCADD typically presents clinically in late infancy, and/or during intercurrent illnesses with emesis or long periods of fasting. If not identified presymptomatically, mortality occurs in approximately 20% of affected individuals. With appropriate management during illness, including glucose-containing fluids, and the avoidance of fasting, mortality is reduced essentially to 0% [12, 13]. Screening for MCADD with MS/MS technology allows for the detection of multiple other inborn errors of metabolism simultaneously, without additional sampling or cost. Some disorders currently screened for by newborn screening do not meet the traditional criteria, either due to their rarity, limited understanding of natural history, or lack of an evidence-based effective treatment. Benefits argued in support of continued screening of these disorders include the ability to initiate early treatment and possibly improve out-

Table 2.1 Disorders identified by newborn screening using tandem mass spectrometry (MS/MS)

Amino acid disorders[a]	**Elevated analytes (amino acids)**[b]
Phenylketonuria (PKU) *or* Hyperphenylalaninemia	Phenylalanine, Phenylalanine/Tyrosine ratio
Maple syrup urine disease (MSUD)	Leucine
Homocystinuria (cystathionine synthase deficiency) *or* Hypermethioninemia	Methionine
Tyrosinemia, type I	Succinylacetone
Urea cycle disorders[a]	
Citrullinemia	Citrulline
Argininosuccinic aciduria (ASA)	Citrulline
Argininemia[a]	Arginine
Fatty acid oxidation disorders[a]	**Elevated analytes (acylcarnitines)**[b]
Short chain acyl-CoA dehydrogenase deficiency (SCAD)	**C4**
Isobutyryl-CoA dehydrogenase deficiency (IBCD)	**C4**
Glutaric aciduria, type 2 (GAII) *or* Multiple acyl-CoA dehydrogenase deficiency (MADD)	**C4, C5, +/– other acylcarnitines**
Medium/Short chain L-3-hydroxyacyl-CoA dehydrogenase deficiency (M/SCHAD)[a]	**C4-OH**
Medium chain acyl-CoA dehydrogenase deficiency (MCAD)	C6, **C8**, C10, C10:1
Long chain 3 hydroxyacyl-CoA dehydrogenase def. (LCHAD)	**C16-OH, C18:1-OH**
Trifunctional protein deficiency (TFPD)[a]	**C16-OH, C18:1-OH**
Very long chain acyl-CoA dehydrogenase deficiency (VLCAD)	**C14:1**, C14, C14:2
Carnitine palmitoyl transferase deficiency, type 2 (CPTII)[a]	**C16, C18:1, C18**
Carnitine palmitoyl transferase deficiency, type 1A (CPT1A)[a]	**Elevated C0,** decreased C16, C18
Carnitine/acylcarnitine translocase deficiency (CACT)[a]	**C16, C18:1, C18**
Carnitine uptake defect (CUD)[a]	**Decreased C0**
Organic acid disorders[a]	**Elevated analytes (acylcarnitines)**[b]
Propionic acidemia (PA)[a]	**C3**
Methylmalonic acidemia (MMA)[a]	**C3**
Malonic aciduria (MA)[a]	**C3-DC**
Multiple carboxylase deficiency (MCD)	**C5-OH**
3-hydroxy 3-methylglutaric-CoA lyase deficiency (3HMG)	**C5-OH**
3-methylcrotonyl-CoA carboxylase deficiency (3MCC)	**C5-OH**
3-methylglutaconic aciduria (3MGA)	**C5-OH**
Isovaleric acidemia (IVA)	**C5**
Glutaric acidemia, type 1 (GAI)	**C5-DC**
Beta-ketothiolase deficiency (BKT)[a]	**C5:1**, C5-OH
Other disorders	**Elevated analytes**
X-linked adrenoleukodystrophy (XALD)	**C26:0**

MS/MS analytes are measured in micromoles/Liter (μmol/L)
Hydroxylation is designated (-OH); dicarboxylic acids are designated (-DC); unsaturation of fatty acid is designated (:)
[a]Some genotypes of these disorders may not be detected by newborn screening or are extremely rare (1:>250,000 live births)
[b]Primary MS/MS analyte(s) in **bold** type

come, collection of long-term data on the course of the natural history of the disease, development of potential treatments, improved overall health of the affected individual, and genetic counseling for recurrence risks in future children [14, 15].

2.3 Standardization of Newborn Screening

By the start of the twenty-first century, with the advent of MS/MS newborn screening, the disorders included on the NBS panels varied from state to state. Some states were quick to implement MS/MS and began screening for more than 40 disorders, while other states lagged behind and screened for only 3 disorders [16]. National organizations, such as the March of Dimes, as well as parent advocacy groups, called for standardization of newborn screening panels across all states. At the federal level, the Health Resources and Services Administration commissioned the American College of Medical Genetics (ACMG) to conduct an analysis of the scientific literature as well as gather expert opinion to develop a recommended uniform screening panel. In 2005, the recommended uniform screening panel was released with 29 disorders initially selected as part of the core panel [17]. Many of these core disorders were inborn errors of metabolism screened for by utilizing tandem mass spectrometry. Within 5 years of the recommendation of the core screening panel, all states were utilizing the MS/MS technology. The process of adding disorders to the recommended uniform screening panel is now an undertaking of the federal Advisory Committee on Heritable Disorders in Newborns and Children (ACHDNC) as originally written in the "Newborn Screening Saves Lives Act" legislation [18]. New disorders are now nominated to the committee and undergo a lengthy evidence-based review process for inclusion on the Recommended Uniform Screening Panel (RUSP). Once recommended by the committee, the Secretary of Health and Human Services can either recommend or decline that a disorder be added to a states' newborn panel [19, 20]. States currently retain the ability to add disorders at their own discretion as the RUSP merely serves as guidance and not a federal mandate.

2.4 The Newborn Screening Process

Newborn screening is an integrated system involving multiple entities including the birthing facility, public health department (newborn screening program), confirmatory testing laboratories, subspecialists, primary care providers, and families [21]. The process begins with the collection of blood via a heel prick, typically obtained at 24–48 hours of age at the birthing facility. The blood spots are collected on filter paper called the newborn screening card. The newborn screening card is then sent to either a state public health laboratory or a commercial laboratory via courier or overnight shipment [22]. States with smaller birth frequencies might utilize another state's newborn screening lab or a commercial lab. Newborns also receive point-of-care screening at the birth hospital including a hearing screen and pulse oximetry for critical congenital heart disease (CCHD). Once the lab has received the newborn screening card, the specimen is run in a timely manner with results optimally available within 24–48 hours of receipt of the specimen. If a specimen has an abnormal (out of range) result, the public health department or subspecialists familiar with the flagged disorder conduct appropriate follow-up of the infant. In inborn errors of metabolism, timely follow-up is needed to ensure appropriate diagnosis and initiation of treatment prior to onset of symptoms. Many inborn errors of metabolism are considered time-critical results, needing prompt diagnosis and treatment [23, 24]. In cases of severe disease or concerning newborn screening results, the infant will require immediate evaluation by a metabolic specialist to determine if the infant is symptomatic and if immediate treatment is necessary. Biochemical studies may prove to be diagnostic, or additional studies such as gene sequencing or enzymatic studies may be indicated.

Terminology used in newborn screening includes true positive, false positive, and false negative. An infant determined to have a disorder based on a positive newborn screening result and follow-up confirmatory studies is called a "true positive." An infant that has an abnormal newborn screening result but deemed not to have the disorder based on confirmatory studies is called a "false positive." An infant that has a normal newborn screen but later is determined to have a disorder is called a "false negative." Newborn screening programs attempt to identify all true positives while limiting false positives and false negatives by selecting appropriate cut-offs of the metabolites measured. Programs will track their "positive predictive values" as a quality indicator: a measurement of the true positives (the numerator) divided by the number of abnormal screens reported (the denominator) [5]. Newborn screening programs track these quality indicators as essential components for continuing quality improvement efforts [25].

2.5 Limitations of Newborn Screening

2.5.1 Disorders That Present Early in Life

Some inborn errors of metabolism on the current newborn screening panel, such as organic acidemias and disorders of fatty acid oxidation, have severe forms that may present as metabolic emergencies within the first days of life before newborn screening results are available. Timeliness of newborn screening is essential in order to limit morbidity and mortality. Turn-around time for newborn screening results will vary from state to state because most states utilize their own newborn screening labs with their own rules and regulations and hours of operation. Use of couriers and overnight shipping for timely transit of specimens to the newborn screening laboratory will improve turn-around time of time-critical results [26]. A worst-case scenario is presented in the highlighted box below (Box 2.2).

Box 2.2: Case Example of Delayed Newborn Screening

Mary, a female newborn, is born at a rural hospital. Her newborn screen is collected at 24 hours of age on a Friday, and the specimen is dried overnight. The specimen is then put in an envelope and remains at the hospital lab for the next 5 days. Eventually, there are two other babies born at that small hospital resulting in the hospital bundling all three specimens in one package, a practice known as "batching." The hospital calls the courier for the specimens to be brought to the newborn screening lab the following Thursday for analysis.

The sample is run overnight and reported out to the local metabolic clinic on Friday with elevated propionylcarnitine (C3). The differential diagnosis includes propionic acidemia, methylmalonic acidemias, maternal B_{12} deficiency, hyperbilirubinemia, and false-positive results.

The metabolic clinic immediately calls out the results to the provider of the infant, now 8 days old. The baby is in a neonatal intensive care unit due to prematurity but is reportedly doing well. However, the day the results are reported, the infant is no longer feeding well. The metabolic clinic requests that confirmatory testing of plasma acylcarnitine profile and urine organic acid screen be obtained.

Due to concern of the recent changes to the status of the infant, additional labs including a metabolic panel and plasma ammonia are recommended immediately. These labs show the baby is extremely acidotic as well as hyperammonemic. The infant is airlifted to a children's hospital for tertiary care by the metabolic team. However, due to the extent of the acidosis and hyperammonemia as well as the prematurity, care is terminated.

Postmortem studies indicate that the infant had methylmalonic acidemia, cobalamin A. Treatment with cobalamin injections and diet typically yields a good outcome.

2.5.2 Disorders That Have Risk of False Negatives

Newborn screening is not diagnostic. The cut-offs for a disorder to be "flagged" are established in order to ascertain all true positives while limiting the number of false positives. Metabolite levels (analytes) for affected infants may overlap significantly with levels from unaffected infants. Case in point is the low-excretor phenotype of glutaric acidemia, type I (GA-1) in whom affected individuals often do not excrete glutaric acid and 3-hydroxyglutaric acid metabolites and thus are not detected with abnormal elevations of glutarylcarnitine (C5DC) by MS/MS. [14] Newborn screening can miss other organic acidemias, aminoacidopathies, and fatty acid oxidation disorders. Also, the timing of the newborn screening will affect certain metabolites, resulting in false positives and false negatives. If a newborn screen specimen is obtained earlier than the recommended 24–48 hours in aminoacidopathies, an affected infant may be missed, as the concentration of the metabolites has not yet become elevated in the blood to screen above the threshold [27, 28]. The opposite also holds true. If a newborn screen specimen is obtained later, such as at a week or later of life, an affected individual with a long-chain fatty acid oxidation disorder can be missed as long-chain carnitine esters decrease with age and long-chain carnitine esters are less likely to flag in the well-fed state.

Many labs utilize second tier (2TT) testing to limit false positives, while avoiding false negatives. Second tier analysis is based on more conservative cut-offs, in order for more newborn screens to initially flag as abnormal. Abnormal newborn screens in tier one will undergo more specialized studies immediately from the same newborn screening card. Only those specimens that have abnormal second tier studies will be reported as abnormal. This limits the number of infants requiring additional confirmatory studies and thus parental anxiety [29]. Second tier testing also allows for refined cut-offs, particularly important for some inherited metabolic diseases that prove difficult to screen for with current limitations of tandem mass spectrometry [30] (Box 2.3).

Box 2.3: Case Example of a Missed Diagnosis During Newborn Screening

James is an 8-year-old boy being evaluated by an ophthalmologist due to recent changes in his vision noted by his teacher. He is otherwise generally healthy. James was born at full term following an uncomplicated pregnancy and delivery. He has mild developmental delay for which he receives additional assistance in school for both math and reading. He is tall for his age for which his parents believe is from his mother's side of the family as maternal grandfather is over 6 feet tall.

The ophthalmologist notes that in addition to myopia, James also has a dislocated lens (ectopia lentis). Given his young age of this eye finding, she suggests that James be evaluated by the Children's Hospital Genetics team. The geneticist evaluates James in the following weeks and notes his marfanoid habitus. She determines that the constellation of symptoms is most suggestive of homocystinuria. She sends James to the lab for a plasma total homocysteine and plasma amino acids. Later that day, the geneticist calls the parents to discuss that the biochemical studies confirm homocystinuria with a significantly elevated total plasma homocysteine and elevated methionine on the amino acid panel. James returns to the Children's Hospital later in the week to begin the treatment for homocystinuria: a methionine-restricted diet, and vitamin B_6 (pyridoxine), and folate supplementation.

James' pediatrician was surprised to learn the diagnosis of homocystinuria given that James had a normal newborn screen. He calls the newborn screening lab to inquire of this "mistake" or false-negative result. The pediatrician learns that only some patients with homocystinuria are detected via newborn screening as the tandem mass spectrometry measures methionine, not homocysteine. Methionine is only elevated in some patients, typically those patients with pyridoxine nonresponsive homocystinuria. In individuals with pyridoxine-responsive homocystinuria, the type James is diagnosed with have normal methionine during the initial days of life. Some newborn screening labs have instituted second tier testing of homocysteine in order to decrease the number of infants with homocystinuria missed by current limitations of screening [30, 31].

The cut-offs for newborn screening are re-evaluated by the newborn screening lab based on data collected and clinical experience. In recent years, worldwide collaboration has resulted in improved cut-off values based on cumulative data of true-positive cases, thus improving sensitivity and specificity [32].

2.5.3 Metabolic Disorders Not Included on Newborn Screening

With the expansion of newborn screening in the last two decades, many providers who are not familiar with inborn errors of metabolism are under the assumption that a "normal" newborn screen excludes all inborn errors of metabolism in their differential diagnosis. While newborn screening is a very helpful tool, it is only one piece of the puzzle of a diagnostic work-up. If clinical concerns arise for an inherited metabolic disease, one should not rely on newborn screen results, but rather pursue further diagnostic work-up to investigate the possibility of a metabolic disorder (Box 2.4).

Box 2.4: Case Example of a Metabolic Disorder Not Included on the Newborn Screening Panel

Camilla, a newborn female, was delivered in a forcep-assisted vaginal after a normal pregnancy. The infant did well for the first 3 days of life but began showing seizure-like activity. A CT scan showed a small trauma from the forcep-assisted birth including a small bleed and skull fracture. Laboratory studies obtained showed mild metabolic acidosis and mild hyperammonemia. The infant was transferred to children's hospital for further tertiary care. Repeat plasma ammonia showed increasing hyperammonemia.

The metabolic team was consulted and obtained STAT biochemical labs including plasma acylcarnitine profile, plasma amino acids, urine organic acids, and urine orotic acid. Labs showed elevated orotic acid as well as a plasma amino acid pattern consistent with ornithine transcarbamylase (OTC) deficiency. The newborn screen was normal. The infant was placed on a protein-restricted diet, supplemented with arginine, and started on nitrogen-scavenging medications.

OTC deficiency is the most common urea cycle disorder and is not routinely screened for on most states' newborn screening panel as it is difficult to establish cut-off for low concentrations of citrulline and arginine.

2.6 Future of Newborn Screening

The trend of expansion of newborn screening continues at a rapid pace. Many factors and contributors including technology, industry, researchers, parents and advocacy groups, and politics drive this expansion. Multiple inherited metabolic diseases are currently under investigation for the potential of utilizing newborn screening for early diagnosis and initiation of treatment. With the continued development of enzyme replacement therapies for lysosomal disorders as well as options for screening methodologies, Pompe Disease and Mucopolysaccharidosis type 1 (MPS1) are now on the RUSP with multiple states implementing screening within the last 5 years [33]. Other lysosomal disorders are being considered in some states as these disorders can be multiplexed to current screening methodologies. With multiple gene therapies for inherited metabolic diseases and other pediatric disorders on the horizon, newborn screening will continue to be an essential tool for early diagnosis and treatment, thus allowing for full utility of these new treatment options. With the ability to perform whole exome sequencing (WES) and whole genome sequencing (WGS) on dried blood spots, development of screening methodologies for other disorders becomes possible [34]. However, despite the feasibility of WES/WGS for newborn screening, there are still multiple issues that need to be addressed including clinical utility, cost-effectiveness, variant interpretation, and the ethical and policy issues that utilizing this technology on newborns brings [35].

Parent advocacy groups are strong lobbyists for the addition of new disorders to states' newborn screening panels. Legislators sometimes bypass the public health departments and pass laws mandating the addition of new disorders without, in some cases, an available screening methodology or proven treatment. The development of new screening methodologies including WES/WGS, emerging treatments such as gene therapies, and strong support from parent advocates, researchers, and industry opens up opportunities for new disorders to be added to newborn screening panels at an unprecedented rate. While newborn screening continues to progress forward, those in the field continue to advocate for strengthening the current system with continuous quality improvement.

References

1. Bickel H, Gerrard J, Hickmans EM. The influence of phenylalanine intake on the chemistry and behaviour of a phenyl-ketonuric child. Acta Paediatr. 1954;43(1):64–77.
2. Centerwall WR. Phenylketonuria. J Am Med Assoc. 1957;165(4):392.
3. Koch J. Robert Guthrie--the Pku story: crusade against mental retardation: hope publishing house; 1997. 190 p.
4. Guthrie R, Susi A. A simple phenylalanine method for detecting phenylketonuria in large populations of newborn infants. Pediatrics. 1963;32: 338–43.
5. Sahai I, Marsden D. Newborn screening. Crit Rev Clin Lab Sci. 2009;46(2):55–82.
6. Wilson JM, Jungner YG. Principles and practice of mass screening for disease. Bol Oficina Sanit Panam. 1968;65(4):281–393.
7. Millington DS, Kodo N, Norwood DL, Roe CR. Tandem mass spectrometry: a new method for acylcarnitine profiling with potential for neonatal screening for inborn errors of metabolism. J Inherit Metab Dis. 1990;13(3):321–4.
8. Fearing MK, Marsden D. Expanded newborn screening. Pediatr Ann. 2003;32(8):509–15.
9. Frazier DM, Millington DS, McCandless SE, Koeberl DD, Weavil SD, Chaing SH, et al. The tandem mass spectrometry newborn screening experience in North Carolina: 1997-2005. J Inherit Metab Dis. 2006;29(1):76–85.
10. Jones PM, Bennett MJ. The changing face of newborn screening: diagnosis of inborn errors of metabolism by tandem mass spectrometry. Clin Chim Acta. 2002;324(1–2):121–8.
11. Wilcken B, Wiley V, Hammond J, Carpenter K. Screening newborns for inborn errors of metabolism by tandem mass spectrometry. N Engl J Med. 2003;348(23):2304–12.
12. Iafolla AK, Thompson RJ Jr, Roe CR. Medium-chain acyl-coenzyme A dehydrogenase deficiency: clinical course in 120 affected children. J Pediatr. 1994;124(3):409–15.
13. Wilson CJ, Champion MP, Collins JE, Clayton PT, Leonard JV. Outcome of medium chain acyl-CoA dehydrogenase deficiency after diagnosis. Arch Dis Child. 1999;80(5):459–62.
14. Kolker S, Garbade SF, Greenberg CR, Leonard JV, Saudubray JM, Ribes A, et al. Natural history, outcome, and treatment efficacy in children and adults with glutaryl-CoA dehydrogenase deficiency. Pediatr Res. 2006;59(6):840–7.
15. Schulze A, Lindner M, Kohlmuller D, Olgemoller K, Mayatepek E, Hoffmann GF. Expanded newborn screening for inborn errors of metabolism by electrospray ionization-tandem mass spectrometry: results, outcome, and implications. Pediatrics. 2003;111(6 Pt 1):1399–406.
16. National Newborn Screening & Genetics Resource Center (NNSGRC). Screening Programs 2013. Available from: http://genes-r-us.uthscsa.edu/screening.
17. American College of Medical Genetics Newborn Screening Expert G. Newborn screening: toward a uniform screening panel and system--executive summary. Pediatrics. 2006;117(5 Pt 2):S296–307.
18. Newborn Screening Saves Lives Act. 2007.
19. Calonge N, Green NS, Rinaldo P, Lloyd-Puryear M, Dougherty D, Boyle C, et al. Committee report: method for evaluating conditions nominated for population-based screening of newborns and children. Genet Med. 2010;12(3):153–9.
20. Kemper AR, Green NS, Calonge N, Lam WK, Comeau AM, Goldenberg AJ, et al. Decision-making process for conditions nominated to the recommended uniform screening panel: statement of the US Department of Health and Human Services Secretary's Advisory Committee on Heritable Disorders in Newborns and Children. Genet Med. 2014;16(2):183–7.
21. Therrell BL Jr, Schwartz M, Southard C, Williams D, Hannon WH, Mann MY, et al. Newborn screening system performance evaluation assessment scheme (PEAS). Semin Perinatol. 2010;34(2):105–20.
22. Clinical and Laboratory Standards Institute. Blood Collection on Filter Paper for Newborn Screening Programs; Approved Standard—Fifth Edition. CLSI document NBS01-A5. 5th ed. CLSI, editor. Wayne; 2007.

23. Disorders SfIM. SIMD Position statement: identifying abnormal newborn screens requiring immediate notification of the health care provider; 2014.
24. Tanksley S. Timeslines of newborn screening: recommendations from advisory committee on heritable disorders in newborns and children. 2015. Available from: https://www.aphl.org/conferences/proceedings/Documents/2015/Annual-Meeting/26Tanksley.pdf.
25. Yusuf C, Sontag MK, Miller J, Kellar-Guenther Y, McKasson S, Shone S, et al. Development of national newborn screening quality indicators in the United States. Int J Neonatal Screen. 2019;5(3):34.
26. Sontag MK, Miller JI, McKasson S, Sheller R, Edelman S, Yusuf C, et al. Newborn screening timeliness quality improvement initiative: impact of national recommendations and data repository. PLoS One. 2020;15(4):e0231050.
27. Hanley WB, Demshar H, Preston MA, Borczyk A, Schoonheyt WE, Clarke JT, et al. Newborn phenylketonuria (PKU) Guthrie (BIA) screening and early hospital discharge. Early Hum Dev. 1997;47(1):87–96.
28. Tang H, Feuchtbaum L, Neogi P, Ho T, Gaffney L, Currier RJ. Damaged goods?: an empirical cohort study of blood specimens collected 12 to 23 hours after birth in newborn screening in California. Genet Med. 2016;18(3):259–64.
29. Matern D, Tortorelli S, Oglesbee D, Gavrilov D, Rinaldo P. Reduction of the false-positive rate in newborn screening by implementation of MS/MS-based second-tier tests: the Mayo Clinic experience (2004-2007). J Inherit Metab Dis. 2007;30(4):585–92.
30. Keller R, Chrastina P, Pavlikova M, Gouveia S, Ribes A, Kolker S, et al. Newborn screening for homocystinurias: recent recommendations versus current practice. J Inherit Metab Dis. 2019;42(1):128–39.
31. Sacharow SJ, Picker JD, Levy HL. Homocystinuria caused by cystathionine beta-synthase deficiency. In: Adam MP, Ardinger HH, Pagon RA, Wallace SE, LJH B, Mirzaa G, et al., editors. GeneReviews((R)). Seattle; 1993.
32. McHugh D, Cameron CA, Abdenur JE, Abdulrahman M, Adair O, Al Nuaimi SA, et al. Clinical validation of cutoff target ranges in newborn screening of metabolic disorders by tandem mass spectrometry: a worldwide collaborative project. Genet Med. 2011;13(3):230–54.
33. Advisory committee on heritable disorders in newborns and children: previously nominated conditions 2020. Available from: https://www.hrsa.gov/advisory-committees/heritable-disorders/rusp/previous-nominations.html.
34. Roman TS, Crowley SB, Roche MI, Foreman AKM, O'Daniel JM, Seifert BA, et al. Genomic sequencing for newborn screening: results of the NC NEXUS project. Am J Hum Genet. 2020;107(4):596–611.
35. Friedman JM, Cornel MC, Goldenberg AJ, Lister KJ, Senecal K, Vears DF, et al. Genomic newborn screening: public health policy considerations and recommendations. BMC Med Genet. 2017;10(1):9.

3 Pathophysiology of Inherited Metabolic Diseases

Peter R. Baker II

Contents

P. R. Baker II (✉)
Clinical Genetics and Metabolism, Children's
Hospital Colorado, University of Colorado
Denver – Anschutz Medical Campus, Aurora, CO, USA
e-mail: peter.baker@childrenscolorado.org

L. E. Bernstein et al. (eds.), *Nutrition Management of Inherited Metabolic Diseases*,
https://doi.org/10.1007/978-3-030-94510-7_3

Core Messages

- The liver, brain, heart, muscle, and kidney are the organs most often affected by inherited metabolic diseases.
- As the primary site of amino acid, lipid, and glucose metabolism, the liver has a disproportionally high involvement in inherited metabolic diseases.
- The brain, heart, and muscle have high-energy demands and are therefore susceptible to disorders of fatty acid, ketone, or glucose metabolism.
- Several metabolic diseases affect kidney function leading to chronic complications including osteoporosis, hypertension, anemia, and electrolyte abnormalities.

3.1 Background

Inborn errors of metabolism are a large, diverse set of disorders in which genetic abnormalities at the cellular level result in pathophysiology at the tissue and organ level. For every disorder and corresponding enzyme affected, there may be one or (more often) more than one tissue and organ system involved. While the enzyme itself may be tissue specific, factors including systemic metabolite circulation and tissue energy requirements result in damage to the primary tissue as well as tissues far removed from the enzymatic defect. Therefore, inborn errors of metabolism typically have a multisystemic clinical presentation.

This chapter will explore the pathophysiology of key organs affected in various inherited metabolic disorders, specifically the normal structure and function of the liver, skeletal and cardiac muscle, kidney, and central nervous system.

The effects of physiologic damage to these organs at the biochemical level and key clinical and laboratory abnormalities associated with damage in the setting of metabolic disease will be examined. Finally, a multisystemic perspective highlighting the role of each organ in particular inborn errors of metabolism is provided.

3.2 Pathophysiology of Organs

3.2.1 The Liver

The liver is arguably the most biochemically unique and multifunctional organ in the body. It is located in the right upper quadrant of the abdomen, with afferent blood flow from the intestine and systemic circulation and efferent flow to systemic circulation. As blood passes through the liver, it traverses sinusoids, exposing the blood to hepatocytes. These cells, the basic functional cells of the liver, serve to detoxify exogenous metabolites through biochemical modifications carried out by various cytochrome p450 enzymes. These enzymes facilitate excretion through conjugation with hydrophilic molecules like taurine, glycine, glucuronide, and sulfate. Additionally, ammonia, a by-product of protein catabolism and a potential neurotoxin, is turned into urea for excretion in the urine. Hepatocytes have primary synthetic function including the synthesis of bile, bile conjugates, cholesterol, proteins (including clotting factors and albumin), and glycoproteins, as well as processing of metals (including iron and copper) and heme (Fig. 3.1).

Biochemically, the liver serves a primary role in glucose metabolism. Alanine is used to create glucose by gluconeogenesis, and glycogen (a branching glucose polymer) is stored for release of glucose in times of fasting. It also is involved in turning alternative carbohydrates including fructose and galactose into useable forms. The liver also plays a key role in lipid metabolism, ketogenesis, and energy metabolism in the fasting state. Further, in amino acid metabolism, it serves as an important organ of catabolism to allow utilization of amino acids as an alternative fuel source, via transamination and formation of ketoacids. This again highlights the role of the liver in both energy metabolism as well as ammonia elimination. Finally, other amino acids, including glycine, are exclusively metabolized here.

In many inborn errors of metabolism, the liver's ability to accomplish some or most of these tasks may be diminished. Synthetic dysfunction can manifest by coagulopathy (including low clotting factors V, VII, VIII) and results in prolonged coagulation times (INR and partial pro-

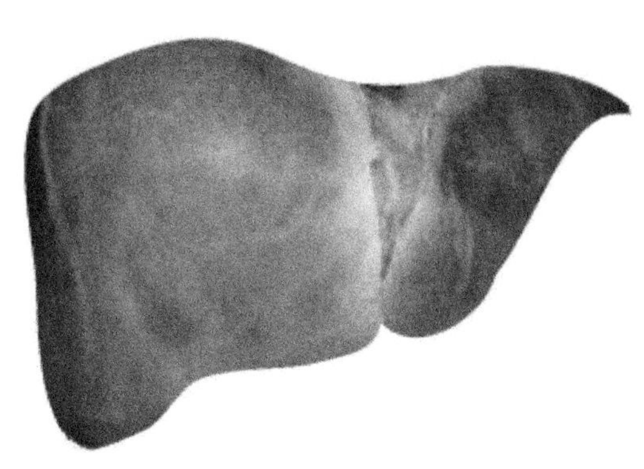

Fig. 3.1 Functions of the Liver

thrombin time). Conversely, problems with glycosylation (including Proteins C and S) can result in a hypercoagulable state. Clinically, coagulopathy manifests as excess bleeding and bruising, which can be complicated by ectopic clot formation if there is a hypercoagulable component. Deficient production of albumin results in lower oncotic pressure in the blood, which in turn results in water seeping from the blood into surrounding tissues and cavities. This seepage creates edema, and in severe cases ascites and/or anasarca. The inability to make bile and conjugate bilirubin (the main heme breakdown product) results in high serum concentrations of bilirubin and jaundice, or a yellowing of the skin and eyes (which may be accompanied by itching). Failure to transport the bile to the intestine (via the gall bladder) results in cholestasis, which in turn may result in fat-soluble vitamin (A, D, E, K) malabsorption and steatorrhea (fatty stool). In specific disorders of metal metabolism, copper or iron may also be stored here (as well as other tissues), creating localized damage. This can also be found in disorders of heme catabolism (certain porphyrias). Cellular damage may be followed with elevated blood transaminase concentrations, including aspartate/alanine aminotransferase (AST, ALT) and gamma-glutamyl transferase (GGT), as well as synthetic markers of function including serum albumin, bilirubin, and coagulation times (Box 3.1).

Box 3.1: Manifestations and Laboratory Markers of Liver Failure

- Hepatocyte insufficiency/dysfunction
  - Hypoglycemia
  - Lactic acidosis
  - Hyperammonemia
  - Low albumin, edema
  - Abnormal or low coagulation factors (factor V, long INR/PT/PTT)
  - Failed bilirubin conjugation (jaundice)
- Hepatocyte lysis / damage
  - Release of intracellular hepatocyte content
  - Elevated liver enzymes (AST, ALT, and GGT)
- Biliary dysfunction
  - Cholestasis (increased bilirubin, abnormal bile acids)
  - Intestinal malabsorption (water- and fat-soluble vitamins)

In energy metabolism, loss of liver function results in low blood sugar as a result of dysfunctional gluconeogenesis and/or abnormal glycogen storage or release. This in turn may lead to elevations in the gluconeogenic precursors alanine and lactate. Lipids and triglycerides, which cannot be converted to ketones, may be stored in the form of fatty vesicles or result in increased levels of circulating lipids (either as free fatty acids, triglycerides, or lipoproteins). Amino acid catabolism, especially in the setting of liver disease, may result in elevated amino acids in the serum. This includes branched chain amino acids (leucine, isoleucine, and valine), tyrosine, homocysteine, and methionine. More critically, dysfunction of the urea cycle may lead to elevations in ammonia, glutamine, alanine, and/or glycine. Glycine may also be elevated due to defects in the glycine cleavage complex, housed only in the liver and brain.

Chronic liver damage, by inflammation, toxic metabolite exposure, and/or intracellular storage, may result in a predictable path toward liver failure. This usually begins with hepatomegaly, contributed to by ectopic lipid storage or storage of compounds like mucopolysaccharides, oligosaccharides, or cholesterol. After years of exposure, this gives way to fibrosis and eventually cirrhosis (Box 3.2). Most of the liver's volume becomes occupied by scar tissue, while patches of hepatocytes have limited functionality and a potential for oncogenic transformation (including hepatoblastoma or hepatocellular carcinoma). This results in vascular problems and many of the aforementioned functional abnormalities. Ultimately, and without transplant, longstanding and severe liver dysfunction can lead to death.

With the liver as a hub of metabolism, inborn errors of metabolism have a disproportionately high involvement of the liver itself. While other organ systems may be affected, one or more functions of the liver may be compromised, resulting in a spectrum of organ damage (Box 3.3) (Fig. 3.2). For example, in storage disorders like Wolman Syndrome (or Cholesterol Ester Storage Disease), several mucopolysaccharidoses, and Niemann-Pick (A, B, and C), storage material is trapped in macrophages, which are, in turn, trapped within the parenchyma of the liver. This leads to mechanical enlargement but can also lead to functional disturbances manifesting as cellular damage, synthetic dysfunction, and cholestatic jaundice. In glycogen storage diseases (especially type I), patients have an enlarged liver, profound hypoglycemia, severe and chronic lactic acidosis, and increased long-term risk for liver cancer.

Carbohydrate metabolism disorders such as hereditary fructose intolerance and galactosemia result in acute, leading to chronic, liver damage through depletion of available ATP (by depleting the total phosphate pool) as well as aberrant glycosylation [1, 2]. Gluconeogenic defects like pyruvate carboxylase or 1,6-fructose-bis-

Box 3.2: Manifestations of Chronic Liver Injury

- *Hepatomegaly* – lipid, glycogen, or saccharide storage can lead to enlargement and slowly diminish liver function.
- *Steatosis* – reversible fat storage.
- *Fibrosis/Cirrhosis* – scar tissue formation with portal hypertension, varicosities, bleeding, and splenomegaly.

Box 3.3: Inborn Errors of Metabolism Associated with Liver Damage

Examples include

- Tyrosinemia type 1
  - Hepatocellular dysfunction
  - Cirrhosis
- Galactosemia
  - Hepatomegaly
  - Hepatocellular dysfunction/cholestasis
- Glycogen storage diseases
  - Hepatomegaly
  - Cirrhosis (esp. GSD type IV)
- Fatty acid oxidation disorders
  - Hepatocellular damage (MCAD, VLCAD, LCHAD)
  - Cholestasis
- Urea cycle disorders
  - Hepatocellular damage (ornithine transcarbamylase deficiency)
  - Steatosis/cholestasis
  - Fibrosis/cirrhosis (argininosuccinic aciduria)

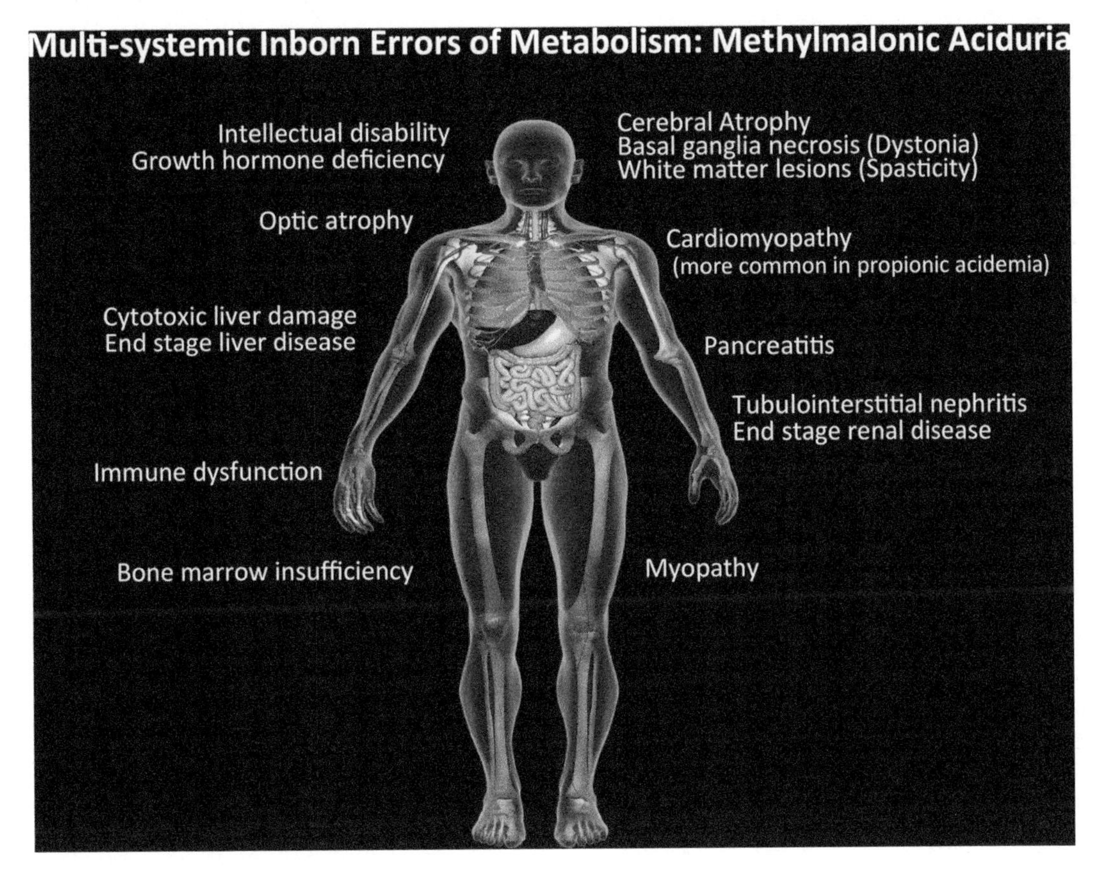

Fig. 3.2 Multisystemic complications due to methylmalonic acidemia

phosphatase deficiency manifest with hypoglycemia and profound lactic acidosis. In urea cycle disorders, dysfunction of ammonia clearance may lead to direct hepatotoxic damage (as in ornithine transcarbamylase (OTC) deficiency) or long-term cirrhosis (as in arginosuccinic aciduria). Primary disorders of bile acid synthesis as well as disorders of bilirubin conjugation like Crigler-Najjar, Gilbert, Rotor, and Dubin-Johnson Syndromes lead to hyperbilrubinemia and jaundice. Citrin deficiency (Citrullinemia Type 2) causes cholestatic jaundice, as does the fatty acid oxidation disorder long-chain hydroxyacyl-CoA dehydrogenase (LCHAD) deficiency. This disorder, along with other fatty acid oxidation and ketolytic defects, can also lead to direct cytotoxic damage in the liver manifesting as acute liver failure. Maple syrup urine disease (MSUD), in which branched-chain amino acids cannot be catabolized, causes cellular damage in the liver as well as a build-up of the toxic amino acid leucine that affects the brain. Toxic organic acid disorders, such as methylmalonic acidemia and propionic acidemia, lead to acute and chronic hepatocellular damage. Other amino acidopathies, such as tyrosinemia type 1, result in hepatocellular damage and abnormal synthetic function through toxic intermediates (e.g., succinylacetone), leading to cirrhosis and liver cancer risk early in life. Finally, the broad category of mitochondrial disorders, most specifically depletion disorders (e.g., *DGUOK* and *POLG1* defects), can lead to early and severe liver damage.

As a primary player in metabolism, many inborn errors affect liver function and health. Many harm the liver acutely, and some predispose to chronic liver disease. Unfortunately, many of these disorders are not amenable to dietary or medical therapies, making the only means of treatment liver (or sometimes bone marrow) transplantation. Transplantation can alternatively serve as a means of effective treatment. In disorders including ornithine transcarbamylase deficiency, liver transplantation is thought to be curative. Bone marrow transplantation helps with visceral symptoms in many storage disorders as well, providing an adjunct to enzyme or substrate replacement therapies. Gene therapies targeting the liver specifically are also being developed for a variety of inborn errors of metabolism (Chap. 8).

3.2.2 The Muscle

Skeletal and cardiac muscles have unique properties, making them susceptible to pathology in inborn errors of metabolism. As organs of high-energy utilization, they may be damaged in biochemical disorders of fatty acid, ketone, or glucose metabolism. By necessity, skeletal and cardiac muscles carry their own glucose stores in the form of glycogen, so in glycogen storage disorders, these organs may be affected. While muscle is a hardy tissue, it is susceptible to toxic damage as well.

Manifestations of metabolic disorders in skeletal muscle include easy fatigue, exercise intolerance, myopathy (muscle weakness), pain, atrophy, and cellular breakdown (rhabdomyolysis). Biochemically, this is manifested in the serum with elevated creatine kinase (CK). Transaminase enzymes (ALT and AST) are elevated (as in the liver), with the exception of gamma-glutamyl transferase (GGT) that is found in the liver alone. Aldolase A, an enzyme in carbohydrate metabolism in muscle, may also be elevated. This should not be confused with Aldolase B, the liver isoform that is deficient in hereditary fructose intolerance. In the urine, specifically in rhabdomyolysis, myoglobin can be detected. Finally, in some disorders of muscle metabolism, abnormal muscle pathology may be seen on biopsy. This may include storage material (e.g., glycogen), abnormal fiber distribution, or abnormal mitochondrial morphology or number indicative of a respiratory chain or mitochondrial depletion defect. Activity of the respiratory chain components may also provide clues to disorders of mitochondrial energy metabolism (Box 3.4).

Box 3.4: Manifestations and Laboratory Markers of Muscle Dysfunction

- Early and easy fatigue with exercise intolerance
- Myopathy (muscle weakness)
- Muscle pain/muscle atrophy
- Rhabdomyolysis (muscle cell breakdown)
- Elevated creatine kinase (CK)
- Myoglobinuria
- Elevated AST/ALT (not GGT)
- Aldolase A (not Aldolase B)
- Abnormal pathology of the muscle (requires a muscle biopsy)

Rhabdomyolysis may be seen in disorders of fatty acid oxidation, specifically in disorders of long-chain metabolism, as well as more subtly in some muscle glycogenoses. Myopathy or muscle wasting may also manifest in these disorders, as well as in primary mitochondrial defects. Muscle fatigue and exercise intolerance is found in energy metabolism disorders including fatty acid oxidation disorders, carnitine metabolism defects, and primary mitochondrial defects. In glycogen storage disorders in which exercise intolerance may be the primary manifesting symptom, useful diagnostic tools include biopsy with evidence of glycogen storage or diastase resistance, as well as the ischemic forearm test [3]. In the ischemic forearm test, useful in diagnosing muscular glycogen storage disorders, ammonia production rises above lactate production in an exercised anaerobic muscle of affected patients. A rise in lactate without ammonia indicates myoadenylate deaminase deficiency, and a rise in both together is normal [4].

Cardiac muscle may have much of the same pathophysiology; however, laboratory values and clinical manifestations may differ. Depending on the inborn error of metabolism, effects on the heart may involve a weakened heart muscle seen as decreased ejection fraction on echocardiogram. The heart, in this case, may be large and floppy (dilated cardiomyopathy) or thick and rigid (hypertrophic cardiomyopathy). In either case, the muscle is not strong enough to pump blood adequately. Damage to the heart muscle in both instances may manifest as elevated CK, lactate, and/or troponin levels in the blood. Basic natriuretic peptide (BNP) is also a sign of cardiac muscle strain indicative of cardiomyopathy. Finally, an electrocardiogram (ECG) may indicate hypertrophy as well as arrhythmogenic potential in individuals at risk.

Dilated cardiomyopathy can be found in many metabolic disorders including fatty acid oxidation defects, carnitine metabolism defects (e.g., CPT1 and primary carnitine deficiency), congenital disorders of glycosylation, and primary mitochondrial disorders [5]. Organic acidemias, including propionic acidemia, 2-methyl-3-hydroxybutyric aciduria, and Barth syndrome (X-linked 3-methylglutaconic aciduria and neutropenia), all manifest with dilated cardiomyopathy. Nutritional deficiencies including carnitine and thiamin deficiency as well as storage disorders including some of the mucopolysaccharidoses can also present in this manner (Box 3.5).

Hypertrophic cardiomyopathy, a thick, rigid cardiac muscle, is also seen in inborn errors of metabolism, with some overlap with the disorders associated with a dilated phenotype. This includes carnitine deficiency, primary respiratory chain defects, Barth syndrome, several glycogenoses (e.g., GSD III, IV, and IX), and lysosomal storage disorders. In lysosomal storage disease, cardiac valves are typically more affected than the muscle itself. In the neonate, there should be high suspicion for GSD type II or Pompe Disease. Tyrosinemia type 1, which mainly affects the liver and kidney, also manifests with hypertrophic cardiomyopathy. Conduction defects predisposing to arrhythmia are typically found in disorders of fatty acid oxidation (especially long chain disorders, CPTII, and carnitine-acylcarnitine translocase deficiency), Kearn-Sayre, and other primary mitochondrial defects.

Box 3.5: Dilated Cardiomyopathy Associated with Inborn Errors of Metabolism

- Energy defect
  - Primary carnitine deficiency (transporter)
  - Mitochondrial defects
  - Some fatty oxidation defects (VLCAD, LCHAD)
- Storage/transport
  - Congenital disorders of glycosylation
- Toxicity
  - Organic acid disorders
  - Nutritional
  - Dietary carnitine deficiency
  - Thiamin deficiency

3.2.3 The Kidney

The kidneys act to filter toxins out of blood for excretion in the urine. There are complex mechanisms to recover electrolytes, carbohydrates, and amino acids. The kidney is also an endocrine organ, regulating vitamin D metabolism and signaling red blood cell proliferation through erythropoietin. While each of these unique roles is not specifically tied to an inborn error of metabolism, the kidneys are affected by several disorders and may be the source of chronic complications of disease. Symptoms of chronic kidney disease include osteoporosis, hypertension, anemia, and electrolyte abnormalities with the primary therapies of hemodialysis or transplant (Box 3.6).

Renal filtration involves blood flow to the kidney through renal arteries, filtering of small molecules through the glomerulus (a fine network of capillaries abutting renal tubules), and the passing of that filtrate past active and passive transporters to concentrate the urine and salvage small molecules for continued use in the body. Dysfunction in the proximal renal tubules, as may be found in mitochondrial diseases, may lead to renal Fanconi Syndrome. This is an inability to resorb electrolytes, carbohydrates, and amino acids, resulting in low serum levels of sodium, potassium, bicarbonate, phosphorous, and glucose, as well as generalized aminoacid-

Box 3.6: Manifestations and Laboratory Markers of Kidney Dysfunction

- Decreased glomerular filtration
  - Renal insufficiency (electrolyte and pH imbalance, hypertension, uremia)
  - Proteinuria/hematuria
- Decreased tubular reabsorption
  - Generalized loss of amino acids, glucose, phosphate, bicarbonate (Fanconi syndrome)
  - Excessive urinary cysteine, ornithine, lysine, and arginine (Cystinuria)
  - Excessive urinary ornithine, lysine, and arginine (lysinuric protein intolerance)
- Anemia and loss of bone density
  - Calcium and phosphorus imbalance
- Elevated serum creatinine, blood urea nitrogen
- Metabolic acidosis (decreased serum phosphate, serum bicarbonate)
- Glucosuria

Box 3.7: Inborn Errors of Metabolism Associated with Kidney Damage

Examples include

- Tyrosinemia type 1
  - Glomerular/Renal tubular dysfunction
- Methylmalonic acidemia
  - Interstitial nephropathy
- Galactosemia and Hereditary Fructose Intolerance
  - Renal tubular dysfunction
- Glycogen storage disease type 1
  - Glomerular/renal tubular dysfunction
- Fabry's disease
  - Storage disorder
- Amino acid transporter defects
  - Cystinosis
  - Lysinuric protein intolerance

uria. Renal Fanconi Syndrome is a major cause of renal tubular acidosis, and may also be present in disorders of glycosylation, cystinosis (a lysosomal transport defect causing systemic crystal accumulation), galactosemia, hereditary fructose intolerance, and tyrosinemia type 1 [6].

Other, more specific, transporter dysfunctions lead to distinct inborn errors of metabolism. Oxaluria and cystinuria, defects in oxalate and cysteine transport respectively, manifest with renal stones. Cystinuria specifically presents with cysteine, ornithine, lysine, and arginine in the urine. The latter should not be confused with cystinosis. Lysinuric protein intolerance (LPI) is a defect in the dibasic amino acid transporter. This results in a specific amino aciduria pattern (ornithine, lysine, and arginine), which in turn results in secondary inhibition of the urea cycle. Individuals affected by LPI are at risk for hyperammonemia, and also have a unique susceptibility to macrophage activation syndrome, an exaggerated systemic inflammatory response, and alveolar proteinosis. Renal damage secondary to other inborn errors of metabolism, and their circulating metabolites, can result in parenchymal damage and loss of renal function over time (Box 3.7).

Methylmalonic acidemia is well known to cause renal damage that eventually necessitates transplantation. The mechanism is not well understood, but it may be oxidative damage from mitochondrial electron transport chain dysfunction, and not necessarily methylmalonic acid concentration itself, that ultimately leads to renal failure [7, 8]. In tyrosinemia type 1 (the hepatorenal form), renal parenchyma is damaged by high levels of succinylacetone. This may be mitigated with Nitisinone (NTBC) therapy, even after liver transplantation [9]. Glycogen storage disease (specifically type 1a) may lead to long-term impairment of renal function and result in hyperfiltration. If the disorder is treated by liver transplant, this risk is diminished, but not eliminated, and early medical intervention may prevent or slow renal damage [10]. Chronic complications in treated GSD1a patients include risk for primary renal tumors. Finally, Fabry disease is one of the few lysosomal storage disorders to affect the kidney; proteinuria is one of the earliest signs of renal involvement, but over years can progress to renal failure due to deposition of globotriaosylceramide (Gb3) glycolipids.

3.2.4 The Brain

The brain is a high-energy-requiring organ, and so, it is particularly susceptible to disorders of energy metabolism, as in mitochondrial disorders and disorders of fatty acid oxidation. It is also one of the major organs damaged in disorders of intoxication both acutely (in urea cycle disorders, organic acidemias, maple syrup urine disease, and glutaric acidemia type 1), subacutely (in X-linked adrenoleukodystrophy and severe lysosomal disorders), and chronically (in phenylketonuria as well as most intoxication disorders). Functionally, damage to the brain can lead to loss of vision, hearing, motor coordination, and movement inhibition (leading to movement disorders and abnormal posturing), as well as seizures and intellectual disability. Clinical signs and symptoms of inborn errors affecting the brain depend largely on the nature and location of injury (Box 3.8).

Box 3.8: Inborn Errors of Metabolism Affecting the Brain
Examples include

- Phenylketonuria
  - Abnormal myelination
  - Neurotransmitter deficiency
- Fatty acid oxidation disorders
  - Hypoglycemia without ketones leading to seizures and brain injury
- Maple syrup urine disease
  - Cerebral edema
  - Abnormal myelination
- Urea cycle defects
  - Cerebral edema
- Organic acid disorders
  - Metabolic stroke (particularly in the basal ganglia)

Mitochondrial diseases are a broad group of disorders affecting the function of the electron transport chain, proliferation of mitochondria, or transport of molecules into mitochondria to enable function. There are over 200 specific disorders involving over 1000 genes, both in the nuclear DNA as well as the circular mitochondrial DNA (mtDNA) found in multiple copies within the mitochondrial matrix. A common final pathophysiology in many of these disorders is Leigh disease. This phenotype, marked by characteristic MRI findings including T2 hyperintensity of the basal ganglia, deep white matter, and brain stem, is found in a large number of specific mitochondrial disorders. The most common genetic causes include SURF1-associated complex IV deficiency and ATP6-associated NARP mutation T8993C; however, there are at least 26 known genetic causes of Leigh disease including mtDNA deletions and duplications, point mutations, and mitochondrial DNA depletion (one of the most common of which is POLG1 deficiency) [11, 12]. The clinical course typically involves severe hypotonia and muscle weakness, leading to respiratory failure. Damage to the basal ganglia can lead to severe dystonia as well.

Brain atrophy and nonspecific demyelination may be phenotypes in mitochondrial disease, thought to result from a combination of energy depletion and oxidative stress. Symptoms include cognitive decline, motor disabilities, and/or seizures. A less common presentation of mitochondrial disease in the brain is metabolic stroke, as typified by the condition Mitochondrial Encephalopathy, Lactic Acidosis, and Stroke (MELAS). The most common cause of MELAS is the well-known A3243G mtDNA mutation affecting the mitochondrial leucine tRNA. The mechanism is thought to be a combination of mitochondrial energy depletion, oxidative stress, lactate production, and angiopathy with poor nitrous oxide responsiveness [13]. The eye is often considered an extension of the brain, and therefore is also susceptible to mitochondrial dysfunction. POLG1, the only mitochondrial DNA polymerase, as well as several other mitochondrial-depletion-associated genes, can cause specific paralysis of the extraocular muscles. Mitochondrial disorders also result in pigmented retinopathy.

Other energy depletion disorders include disorders of fatty acid oxidation, ketone disorders (both synthesis and ketolysis), and disorders of glucose metabolism. These often present with a global neurologic phenotype, resulting in altered mental status and/or seizures. Often these present in the setting of fasting, vomiting, or generalized illness. Damage is not chronic or progressive, unless there are multiple and/or severe metabolic crises.

Acute disorders of intoxication that affect the brain include urea cycle disorders, some amino acidopathies, and organic acidemias. Urea cycle disorders and organic acidemias result in hyperammonemia, which directly causes cerebral edema and damage to neurons. Too much or too little glutamine in these conditions also contributes to neurotoxicity. Multiple repeated events can lead to more global, chronic damage. Maple syrup urine disease, resulting from a defect in branched chain ketoacid dehydrogenase, results in the buildup of branched-chain amino acids and their associated alpha-ketoacids. The most damaging of these molecules is leucine, which causes acute cerebral edema and neuronal damage [14]. Oxidative damage may also play a role [15]. In the absence of hyperammonemia, organic acidemias including propionic acidemia and methylmalonic acidemia can also result in chronic damage to the white matter and basal ganglia. This is thought to occur even in the setting of well-controlled disease. [16] The underlying mechanism is not known.

The organic acidemia, glutaric acidemia type 1 (GA-1), is confined to the brain alone. It is set apart from other organic acidemias by its natural history. The primary lesion in GA-1 is acute and permanent necrosis of the basal ganglia associated with catabolism and fevers. Children are at highest risk between 6 months and 2 years of age. After the age of 6-years, acute cerebral events are extremely rare [17]. Some adults may present with headaches and white matter changes [18], and some (including those in families with known, severe, symptomatic disease) are completely unaffected. Classic MRI findings include lesions in the basal ganglia, macrocephaly, subdural bleeding, and frontotemporal atrophy.

Another condition, in which pathophysiology is primarily manifested in the brain, is nonketotic hyperglycinemia (NKH), a disorder of glycine metabolism. As mentioned above, the glycine cleavage complex resides in cells of the liver and brain only. While the liver is unaffected in this condition, increased amounts of glycine in the brain are associated with severe neonatal seizure activity thought to be caused by glycine's excitatory effects on the NMDA receptor [19].

Subacute to chronic damage in the white matter (demyelination) or poor development of the white matter (hypomyelination) are associated with storage diseases. Hypomyelinating disorders include Tay Sachs, Salla, and some forms of Neimann-Pick and Gaucher disease. Peroxisomal disorders (specifically those involved in peroxisomal biogenesis) result in Zellweger-like phenotypes, in which children are affected with severe hypotonia, vision and hearing loss, and difficult to control seizures. Phenotypically similar, but biochemically unrelated, the neuronal ceroid lipofuscinoses (NCL) tend to be more rapidly progressive with a marked deterioration of neuronal function over the course of several years. Lysosomal diseases including Krabbe and metachromatic leukodystrophy present with both hypo- and demyelination [20]. Demyelination, or leukodystrophy, is likely a result of innate immune activation [21]. One of the more severe and rapidly progressive demyelinating disorders is X-linked adrenoleukodystrophy. Here, very-long-chain fatty acids (VLCFAs) cannot enter the peroxisome. Through mechanisms not yet defined, this build-up of VLCFA [22] results in a rapidly progressive loss of myelination, typically in the midline occipital region moving distally and anteriorly. This is characterized by a "leading edge" of enhancement, indicating inflammation on gadolinium-contrast MRI. Treatment for this is bone marrow transplantation before symptoms progress.

In most of these disorders, white matter damage is patchy, and the basal ganglia are not affected. Treatments to protect the brain are few.

In some disorders, enzyme replacement or substrate reduction is possible, but the efficacy in the brain, an organ "protected" by the blood-brain barrier, is often poor.

Finally, chronic damage may occur in intoxication disorders. In addition to the organic acidemias mentioned above, the most classic example of this is phenylketonuria (PKU). Untreated, PKU results in severe cognitive impairment, anxiety, motor impairment, spasticity, and seizures. Damage is thought to result from phenylalanine toxicity directly, oxidative damage to neuronal tissue, and decreased dopamine, norepinephrine, and serotonin production (Chap. 9).

Understanding the underlying pathophysiology has made it possible to effectively manage inborn errors of metabolism with the goal of preserving quality of life and preventing mortality. The organ(s) affected by each disorder determine(s) the target of therapy and the impact a disorder has on the body as a whole.

References

1. Liu Y, Xia B, Gleason TJ, Castaneda U, He M, Berry GT, et al. N- and O-linked glycosylation of total plasma glycoproteins in galactosemia. Mol Genet Metab. 2012;106(4):442–54.
2. Latta M, Kunstle G, Leist M, Wendel A. Metabolic depletion of ATP by fructose inversely controls CD95- and tumor necrosis factor receptor 1-mediated hepatic apoptosis. J Exp Med. 2000;191(11):1975–85.
3. Sinkeler SP, Wevers RA, Joosten EM, Binkhorst RA, Oei LT, Van't Hof MA, et al. Improvement of screening in exertional myalgia with a standardized ischemic forearm test. Muscle Nerve. 1986;9(8):731–7.
4. Kost GJ, Verity MA. A new variant of late-onset myophosphorylase deficiency. Muscle Nerve. 1980;3(3):195–201.
5. Gilbert-Barness E. Review: metabolic cardiomyopathy and conduction system defects in children. Ann Clin Lab Sci. 2004;34(1):15–34.
6. Saudubray JM, Van den Berghe G, Walter J. Inborn metabolic diseases : diagnosis and treatment, vol. xxv., 656 p. 5th ed. Berlin: Springer; 2012.
7. Manoli I, Sysol JR, Li L, Houillier P, Garone C, Wang C, et al. Targeting proximal tubule mitochondrial dysfunction attenuates the renal disease of methylmalonic acidemia. Proc Natl Acad Sci U S A. 2013;110(33):13552–7.
8. Zsengeller ZK, Aljinovic N, Teot LA, Korson M, Rodig N, Sloan JL, et al. Methylmalonic acidemia: a megamitochondrial disorder affecting the kidney. Pediatr Nephrol. 2014;29(11):2139–46.
9. Larochelle J, Alvarez F, Bussieres JF, Chevalier I, Dallaire L, Dubois J, et al. Effect of nitisinone (NTBC) treatment on the clinical course of hepatorenal tyrosinemia in Quebec. Mol Genet Metab. 2012;107(1–2):49–54.
10. Araoka T, Takeoka H, Abe H, Kishi S, Araki M, Nishioka K, et al. Early diagnosis and treatment may prevent the development of complications in an adult patient with glycogen storage disease type Ia. Intern Med. 2010;49(16):1787–92.
11. Finsterer J. Leigh and Leigh-like syndrome in children and adults. Pediatr Neurol. 2008;39(4): 223–35.
12. The United Mitochondrial Disease Foundation. 2014 [cited 2014. Available from: http://www.umdf.org.
13. Koga Y, Povalko N, Nishioka J, Katayama K, Yatsuga S, Matsuishi T. Molecular pathology of MELAS and L-arginine effects. Biochim Biophys Acta. 2012;1820(5):608–14.
14. Kasinski A, Doering CB, Danner DJ. Leucine toxicity in a neuronal cell model with inhibited branched chain amino acid catabolism. Brain Res Mol Brain Res. 2004;122(2):180–7.
15. Barschak AG, Sitta A, Deon M, de Oliveira MH, Haeser A, Dutra-Filho CS, et al. Evidence that oxidative stress is increased in plasma from patients with maple syrup urine disease. Metab Brain Dis. 2006;21(4):279–86.
16. Harting I, Seitz A, Geb S, Zwickler T, Porto L, Lindner M, et al. Looking beyond the basal ganglia: the spectrum of MRI changes in methylmalonic acidaemia. J Inherit Metab Dis. 2008;31(3):368–78.
17. Strauss KA, Puffenberger EG, Robinson DL, Morton DH. Type I glutaric aciduria, part 1: natural history of 77 patients. Am J Med Genet C Semin Med Genet. 2003;121C(1):38–52.
18. Sonmez G, Mutlu H, Ozturk E, Sildiroglu HO, Keskin AT, Basekim CC, et al. Magnetic resonance imaging findings of adult-onset glutaric aciduria type I. Acta Radiol. 2007;48(5):557–9.
19. McDonald JW, Johnston MV. Nonketotic hyperglycinemia: pathophysiological role of NMDA-type excitatory amino acid receptors. Ann Neurol. 1990;27(4):449–50.
20. Di Rocco M, Rossi A, Parenti G, Allegri AE, Filocamo M, Pessagno A, et al. Different molecular mechanisms leading to white matter hypomyelination in infantile onset lysosomal disorders. Neuropediatrics. 2005;36(4):265–9.
21. Snook ER, Fisher-Perkins JM, Sansing HA, Lee KM, Alvarez X, MacLean AG, et al. Innate immune activation in the pathogenesis of a murine model of globoid cell leukodystrophy. Am J Pathol. 2014;184(2):382–96.
22. Berger J, Forss-Petter S, Eichler FS. Pathophysiology of X-linked adrenoleukodystrophy. Biochimie. 2014;98:135–42.

4 Metabolic Intoxication Syndrome in a Newborn

Maria Giżewska

Contents

M. Giżewska (✉)
Department of Pediatrics, Endocrinology,
Diabetology, Metabolic Diseases and Cardiology,
Pomeranian Medical University, Szczecin, Poland

L. E. Bernstein et al. (eds.), *Nutrition Management of Inherited Metabolic Diseases*,
https://doi.org/10.1007/978-3-030-94510-7_4

Core Messages

- Inborn errors of metabolism should be considered alongside other diagnoses in all neonates with unclear, severe, or progressive illness.
- The course of inborn errors of metabolism presenting with intoxication syndrome is often very sudden and severe.
- Without timely and proper diagnosis and treatment, metabolic intoxication syndrome can often lead to irreversible organ damage or death.
- Prevention of accumulation of metabolic toxins and promotion of anabolism are the most important steps in treatment in metabolic intoxication.

4.1 Background

The term inborn errors of metabolism (IEMs) was introduced over a hundred years ago and, still today, these diseases are responsible for many diagnostic and therapeutic dilemmas [1]. Metabolic disorders are often undiagnosed due to the erroneous belief that they are very rare. While particular metabolic disorders occur infrequently, when combined, inborn errors of metabolism become a large group of diagnoses, with a worldwide incidence of approximately 1:1000 live births [2–6]. Inborn errors of metabolism can result from all types of genetic inheritance patterns, including mitochondrial, with most diseases having an autosomal-recessive type of inheritance [4, 6–8].

4.2 Classification

There are many ways to categorize inborn errors of metabolism [5, 6, 9, 10]. When considering the effectiveness of therapeutic procedures in acute illness, they can be classified into 5 groups: (1) disorders presenting with intoxication syndrome, (2) disorders of reduced tolerance to fasting, (3) disorders of mitochondrial energy metabolism, (4) disorders of neurotransmission, and (5) disorders with limited therapeutic options in illness [9].

4.2.1 Disorders Presenting with Intoxication Syndrome

Intoxication disorders include urea cycle disorders, organic acidurias, aminoacidopathies, fatty acid oxidation disorders, and carbohydrate disorders such as galactosemia or hereditary fructose intolerance. In these disorders, a partial or complete lack of enzymatic activity causes the accumulation of substances proximal to the metabolic block in tissues and body fluids, where they act as toxins (Fig. 4.1). Treatment is based on limiting the substances that are the source of the toxic metabolites and introducing alternatives (e.g., drugs, procedures) that speed the elimination of those toxic metabolites [5].

4.2.2 Disorders of Reduced Tolerance to Fasting

Some inborn errors of metabolism present with hypoglycemia, occurring after periods of extended fasting. Disorders of reduced tolerance to fasting include glucose homeostasis disorders such as glycogen storage disorders, gluconeogenesis disturbances, and inborn hyperinsulinism. Mitochondrial fatty acid oxidation disorders are also considered part of these diseases; however, due to the accumulation of toxic acylcarnitines, the traits that typically present with intoxication syndromes may also manifest. The main treatment is to supply glucose and stop fat oxidation.

4.2.3 Disorders of Mitochondrial Energy Metabolism

Pyruvate dehydrogenase complex (PDHC) deficiency and electron transport chain disorders are examples of mitochondrial energy disorders. The primary goal with treatment is to minimize acidosis by supplementing with a steady infusion of

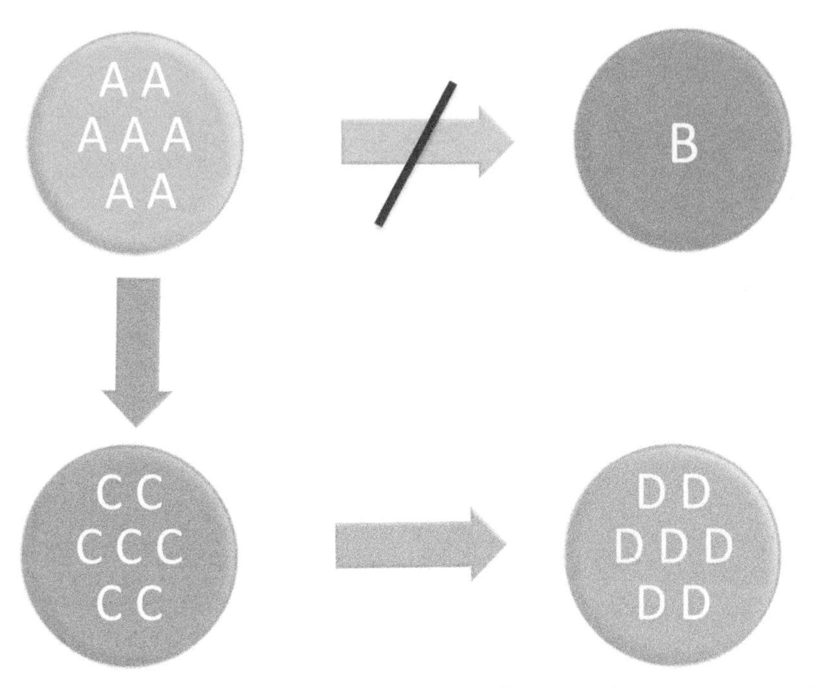

Fig. 4.1 The acute and progressive intoxication from a metabolic block, leading to accumulation of compound A, C, and D while providing insufficient quantities of B

glucose to avoid negative consequences, such as lactic acidosis in PDHC.

4.2.4 Disorders of Neurotransmission

These disorders, such as pyridoxine dependent epilepsy, present with seizures that can be treated with vitamin B_6 and lysine restriction.

4.2.5 Disorders with Limited Therapeutic Options in Acute Illness

For some diseases (nonketotic hyperglycemia, sulfite oxidase deficiency), progressive encephalopathy is the presenting symptom. In others (peroxisomal diseases, some glycosylation disorders), aggravation of the chronic disease is caused by illness (e.g., infections).

4.3 Suspicion of an Inborn Error of Metabolism in a Neonate

During pregnancy, the placenta provides a protective environment for fetal development. Both mother and child are generally unaffected by most inborn errors of metabolism that present after birth [5]. There are, however, certain disorders that disturb the energy metabolism of the affected fetus, including intracerebral metabolism, with secondary penetration of inappropriate metabolites from brain tissue into body fluids (e.g., nonketotic hyperglycemia). An inborn error of metabolism should also be suspected in the case of nonimmunological fetal edema or if there are any signs that fetal metabolism is negatively influencing the mother [6]. Noteworthy examples include HELLP syndrome (hemolysis, elevated liver enzymes, and low platelets) and acute fatty liver of pregnancy (AFLP) in the mother. Both are suggestive of an infant affected with a fatty acid oxidation disorder and the neonate born

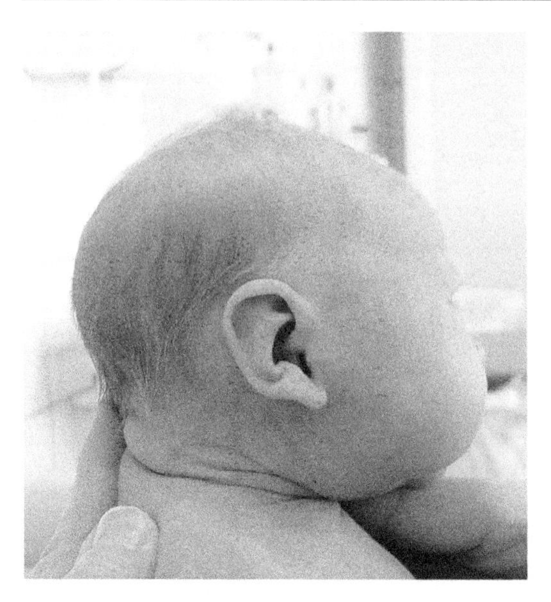

Fig. 4.2 Microcephaly in a newborn with maternal PKU syndrome (MPKU) born from a mother with classical phenylketonuria treated since 33 weeks' gestation. (Photo courtesy of Dr. Maria Giżewska)

from such a pregnancy should be treated as potentially affected, until inherited mitochondrial fatty acid metabolism disorders can be excluded [11, 12].

Immediately after birth and during the first days of life, infants with an inborn error of metabolism usually appear asymptomatic. However, the presence of dysmorphic features often indicates a metabolic disorder (e.g. coarse facial features in some lysosomal storage disorders) [6]. Characteristic facial features of children born with glutaric aciduria type II, hyperinsulinism, or offspring of mothers with phenylketonuria, such as microcephaly, are prime examples [2, 3, 13, 14] (Fig. 4.2).

Seizures are another frequent clinical manifestation of inborn errors of metabolism in the neonate. This may be a leading or progressive symptom (especially in disorders with intoxication syndrome) appearing after the child is comatose or together with other progressive neurological changes [5].

Muscle hypotonia is a trait demonstrated by many children born with an inborn error of metabolism. "Floppy baby syndrome," typical for such disorders as Prader-Willi syndrome and severe motor neuron diseases, may also be present in inborn lactic acidosis, some respiratory chain disorders, nonketotic hyperglycemia, molybdenum cofactor deficiency, sulfite oxidase deficiency, peroxisomal disorders, glycosylation disorders, Pompe disease, and many others [2, 5, 7].

Inborn errors of metabolism should be considered in children with cardiovascular pathology as well. Cardiac insufficiency in a child with cardiomyopathy and/or arrhythmia, acute life-threatening episodes (ALTEs), or sudden infant death (SIDS) can be indicative of a fatty acid oxidation defect, respiratory chain disorder, glycosylation disorder (frequently with pericardial exudation), or Pompe disease [2, 3, 6, 7, 13].

It is important to remember that a small child will respond to illness in similar ways regardless of whether the cause is acquired or genetic. Therefore, inherited metabolic disorders should be suspected in all sick children, especially neonates. Placing metabolic disorders at the very end of the list of differential diagnostic possibilities can be a mistake. They should be considered along with other, more frequent causes of sudden health deterioration of the neonatal or pediatric patient, especially if the child presents with one or a combination of signs such as encephalopathy, liver damage, or cardiomyopathy [2, 4, 5, 7, 13, 15]. Only intensive, multidirectional diagnostic and therapeutic processes will ensure that we *"... do not miss a treatable disorder,"* Professor JM Saudubray [2, 15] (Box 4.1).

4.4 Presentation of a Newborn with Intoxication Syndrome

A disorder presenting with intoxication syndrome is often very sudden and severe in its course. Without timely and proper diagnosis and treatment, it can lead to irreversible organ damage or death. On the other hand, if diagnosed and treated properly and urgently, the short- and long-term consequences of the intoxication syndrome may be prevented or ameliorated [2, 15, 16].

Box 4.1: Consideration of an IEM in a Neonate

- The neonate has a limited repertoire of responses to a severe illness, regardless of whether the disease has an infectious, genetic, or traumatic background as the cause. [13]
- In the first few days of life, an infant with an undiagnosed inborn error of metabolism may not show any symptoms of the metabolic disorder.
- A metabolic disorder should be considered in all neonates with an unexplained, overwhelming, or progressive disease, particularly after a normal pregnancy and delivery [5].
- The time between the first symptoms of metabolic intoxication and the initiation of effective treatment is often associated with the infant's prognosis and/or survival.
- Suspect that any neonatal death, particularly those who have been attributed to sepsis, may have been due to an inborn error of metabolism [2, 5, 13].

Box 4.2: Examples of Metabolic Toxins

- Ammonia in urea cycle disorders
- Leucine and its branched chain ketoacids, such as 2-oxoisocaproic acid, in maple syrup urine disease
- Isovaleryl-CoA and its metabolites in isovaleric aciduria
- Galactose-1-phosphate in galactosemia
- Acylcarnitines in fatty acid oxidation diseases

There are many metabolic toxins that accumulate due to enzymatic dysfunction (Box 4.2).

While inborn errors of metabolism with intoxication syndrome can occur in a preterm neonate, they are most frequently diagnosed in term delivery neonates born from uneventful pregnancies and uncomplicated births. Patients typically have normal birth weight, a high Apgar Scale score, and no dysmorphic features. During the first days, or even weeks of life, they are considered healthy. However, if the patient is of a specific ethnic group or has a history of parental consanguinity, a family history may reveal unexplained deaths in young children or similar illness in a sibling or other blood relatives.

After an asymptomatic period, typical signs of intoxication or "poisoning" as a result of the accumulation of harmful metabolites begin. The length of time of the apparent health can vary across the spectrum of disorders and is shorter if the accumulating metabolite is particularly toxic. For example, ammonia can accumulate to toxic concentrations within hours in cases of severe urea cycle disorders or can manifest over a few days in organic acidemias. At times, the relationship between feeding (breast milk or infant formula) and onset of the first symptoms can be noted. Catabolism occurs as part of the normal adaptation to living outside the womb and causes the child's condition to deteriorate even prior to the introduction of oral feeding [3, 5].

The symptoms of acute intoxication may be very similar to that of other diseases (Box 4.3) and may often lead to a misdiagnosis and at times, death. On the other hand, some metabolic disorders can predispose a neonate to frequent neonatal period complications such as infections such as *E. coli* sepsis in children with galactosemia, or hematological complications such as central nervous system hemorrhage in hyperammonemia or thrombocytopenia in aminoacidurias due to the suppression of bone marrow production [2, 5].

Box 4.3: Disorders in Neonates That Present with Symptoms Similar to IEM

- Generalized infection
- Birth trauma
- Respiratory distress syndrome
- Congenital cardiac disorders
- Endocrine diseases (e.g., congenital adrenal hyperplasia or neonatal diabetes) [8]

Box 4.4: Clinical Presentation of Neonates with Metabolic Intoxication [2, 5, 7]

- Poor sucking reflex resulting in feeding difficulties and poor oral intake
- Vomiting leading to dehydration and weight loss
- Muscle tone abnormalities
- Involuntary movements (boxing or pedaling)
- Seizures
- Increasing somnolence, progressing to stupor and coma, ultimately leading to death

The first symptoms that typically appear in an infant with an inborn error of metabolism with intoxication syndrome are similar to other illnesses yet often change dramatically in severity within a short period of time (Box 4.4).

Neonates presenting with intoxication syndromes and who are comatose often have neurovegetative symptoms including breathing disorders with apnea, hiccups, bradycardia, and hypothermia. Some patients may emit a characteristic scent, which can be detected in the presence of the child and during an examination of a urine, blood, stool, cerumen, or cerebrospinal fluid sample [2, 5, 13] (Table 4.1).

Neonates may also present with symptoms of hepatic failure including jaundice, elevated transaminases, hypoalbuminemia with ascites, and clotting disturbances [5, 17]. This presentation, often with accompanying tubulopathy, may suggest the diagnosis of tyrosinemia type 1, or in the presence of hypoglycemia, *E. coli* infection, kidney enlargement, and glaucoma may be suggestive of the diagnosis of galactosemia.

Table 4.1 Characteristic odor detected in patients with selected inborn errors of metabolism [6, 13, 18]

Inborn errors of metabolism	Odor
Isovaleric acidemia Glutaric acidemia type II 3-Hydroxy-3-methylglutaric aciduria	Sweaty feet
Maple Syrup Urine Disease (MSUD)	Maple syrup, burnt sugar
Phenylketonuria (PKU)	Musty, mousy
Tyrosinemia type I	Cabbage-like
3-Methylcrotonylglycinuria Multiple carboxylase deficiency	Tomcat urine
Hypermethioninemia	Rancid butter, rotten cabbage
Trimethylaminuria	Fishy
Cystinuria	Sulfurous

4.4.1 Biochemical Diagnostics

When suspecting an inborn error of metabolism, especially those with metabolic intoxication, specific laboratory testing should be conducted simultaneously while excluding other causes of a sudden or progressive deterioration of a neonate. This should include four basic biochemical blood tests: electrolytes, blood glucose, liver function tests, ketones, lactic acid, and ammonia [2, 10, 16, 17]. An anion gap should also be considered when accessing biochemical test results (Chap. 7). In a healthy, full-term baby, the anion gap should not exceed 15 mmol/L. A value higher than 16 mmol/L suggests a metabolic disorder, most frequently an organic aciduria [16].

A careful analysis of the medical history including family background, pregnancy, first days of life, history of present illness, and clinical condition of the patient, backed up with the interpretation of basic biochemical test results, often allows for establishing the reasonable initial suspicion of an inborn error of metabolism and directs further diagnostic and therapeutic actions [18–20] (Table 4.2).

It is crucial to provide proper conditions for collecting samples of blood and other biological materials to obtain reliable tests results. It is especially important when measuring ammonia and lactic acid, both of which require free flowing blood (no tourniquet), and transportation on ice to the lab for immediate analysis. Other conditions causing elevated lactic acid (hypoxia, infection, trauma, or stress when obtaining a sample from the child) should be excluded [2, 3, 13, 16]. When possible, blood samples should be secured prior to beginning a specific treatment or before ceasing oral feeding to preclude false-negative results.

Table 4.2 Basic biochemical tests performed in sick neonates and examples of possible interpretation in the direction of inborn errors of metabolism [2, 18, 19]

Tests	Example of possible clinical interpretation
Blood cell count with blood smear	Pancytopenia-thrombocytopenia-leukopenia in organic acidurias; hemolytic anemia in galactosemia, congenital erythropoietic porphyria, glycolytic and pentose-phosphate enzymes deficiencies; macrocytic anemia in inborn errors of cobalamin and folate metabolism
Blood gases pH, pCO_2, HCO_3, pO_2	Metabolic acidosis in organic acidurias (anion gap); respiratory alkalosis in hyperammonemias
Glucose	↓ in organic acidurias (*possible transient hyperglycemia with ketones in the urine can lead to an incorrect diagnosis of diabetes mellitus type 1*), fatty acid oxidation disorders, galactosemia, tyrosinemia type 1, hereditary fructose intolerance, glycogen storage disease type 1, hyperinsulinism
Electrolytes	Hypocalcemia in organic acidurias
Urea	↓ in urea cycle disorders, lysinuric protein intolerance ↑ in malonyl-CoA decarboxylase deficiency, cystinosis, hyperoxaluria type 1
Creatinine	↓ in creatinine biosynthesis defects
Ammonia	↑ in urea cycle disorders, organic acidurias, fatty acid oxidation disorders, maple syrup urine disease, biotinidase deficiency, hyperinsulinism + hyperammonemia syndrome
Lactate	↑ in respiratory-chain disorders, pyruvate dehydrogenase and carboxylase deficiency, fatty acid oxidation disorders, glycogen storage disorder type 1, sometimes in organic acidurias and urea cycle defects, biotinidase deficiency
Uric acid	↓ in molybdenum cofactor deficiency ↑ in glycogen storage disease type 1
Transaminases (and other liver tests)	↑ in urea cycles disorders, fatty acid oxidation disorders, galactosemia, tyrosinemia type 1, hereditary fructose intolerance, alpha-1-antitripsin deficit, peroxisomal disorders, congenital disorders of glycosylation
Creatine kinase	↑ in fatty acid oxidation disorders
Cholesterol	↓ in Smith-Lemli-Opitz syndrome, 3-methylglutaconic aciduria, methylmalonic aciduria
Ketones in urine	*Absent* together with hypoglycemia in fatty acid oxidation disorders *Present* with metabolic acidosis (ketoacidosis) in organic acidurias

Elevated ammonia, resulting from the increased production and/or disturbed detoxification of waste nitrogen, warrants particularly urgent identification and action. Ammonia is highly toxic to the brain, and hyperammonemia is considered to be a medical emergency with a high risk of irreversible neurological damage or death. Primary hyperammonemia is caused by the defect of one of six urea cycle enzymes, an ornithine transporter, or due to an asparaginate/glutamate transporter defect. Secondary elevation of ammonia can be observed in other metabolic disorders such as organic acidurias, fatty acid oxidation disorders, disturbances of some respiratory chain disorders, inborn hyperinsulinism, and conditions causing liver damage and/or infections. Temporary hyperammonemia can occur in preterm newborns as transient hyperammonemia (*THAN*), as a result of maintained blood flow through ductus venosus where the hepatic portal vein (and detoxification in liver) is being bypassed [2, 10, 19].

The symptoms of hyperammonemia are nonspecific, in most cases, and the leading manifestation is a neurological presentation with fast progressing encephalopathy. Ammonia should be assessed in every neonate suspected of septicemia, especially with neurological symptoms and respiratory alkalosis present and in children with a loss of appetite and vomiting that suffer from a loss of consciousness [19]. In healthy neonates, the ammonia concentration should not exceed 110 μmol/L; however, a sick neonate can have values as high as 180 μmol/L. Higher values, especially ones greater than 200 μmol/L, as well as ammonia values that rise rapidly, have a high likelihood of a diagnosis of an inborn error of metabolism. About 50% of children who have ammonia concentrations higher than 200 μmol/L suffer from a metabolic disorder [13, 20] (Fig. 4.3) [3].

Newborn screening results with analysis of amino acid and carnitine esters using tandem mass spectrometry (MS/MS) are helpful in determining if a sick neonate has an inborn error of metabolism and should be performed in any infant who has not been tested. Children with intoxication syndromes may already be ill by the time the newborn screening results are available. The urine organic acid analysis with gas chroma-

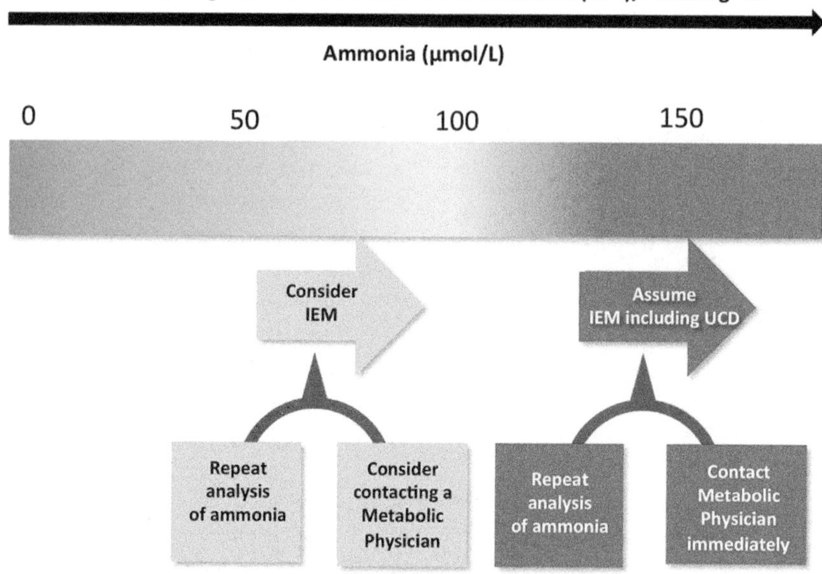

Fig. 4.3 Increasing consideration of an inborn error of metabolism as ammonia concentrations increase [3]

tography mass spectrometry (GC-MS), as well as analysis of the amino acid profile in plasma and cerebrospinal fluid should also be considered for additional testing. Therefore, while obtaining a sample of cerebrospinal fluid in a child diagnosed with a probable central nervous infection, but with suspicion of a metabolic disorder, an additional 1–2 mL of fluid should be taken and frozen for later diagnostic testing should it be needed. Enzymatic activity in various tissues or molecular examinations may also be necessary in advanced stages of diagnostic testing.

Sometimes, despite the best efforts, it is impossible to save an ill neonate and they pass before a final diagnosis is made. To ensure proper genetic counseling, detailed information for the parents regarding the causes of their child's death, and for further family planning, it is helpful to collect biological samples *peri mortem* [21].

4.5 Treating a Neonate with Intoxication Syndrome

Every severely ill neonate should be treated immediately, even before a final diagnosis is made. The first stages of treatment are nonspecific and are aimed at ensuring the patient's survival and preventing irreversible damage [5, 8, 9, 16, 22] (Box 4.5).

The successful treatment of a neonate with severe metabolic intoxication is not possible without securing a vascular catheter (often central venous catheter) that is essential for (1) administering glucose in high concentrations, (2) providing intensive hydration and managing bio-

Box 4.5: Goals of Emergency Treatment in a Neonate Suspected to Have an Inborn Error of Metabolism

- Ensure basic life functions (ventilator and circulatory support)
- Provide sufficient energy supply
- Prevent accumulation of toxic metabolites
- Correct acid-base balance
- Introduce supporting therapies, such as
  - Treating infections
  - Managing seizures
  - Supply (even empirically) cofactors

chemical disturbances, (3) total or partial parenteral feeding, and (4) toxin elimination.

The section below describes steps that are often introduced in infants where the presentation, course of the disease, and biochemical testing results suggest an inborn error of metabolism, especially with intoxication syndrome, keeping in mind that clinical scenarios differ, treatment decisions are based on the clinical judgment of the metabolic team, and should be always considered on an individual basis. Many therapeutic procedures are conducted simultaneously.

4.5.1 Stage 1 – Provision of Glucose, Cessation of Feedings

When taking care of a neonate suspected of having an inborn error of metabolism, especially if the patient suffers from encephalopathy or severe liver dysfunction, administration of any substance that may act as a toxin must be ceased. The first step is the immediate discontinuation of oral feeding as well as protein and fat supplementation. However, an energy-deprived neonate will become catabolic, leading to degradation of tissues, resulting in intoxication from the metabolites coming from endogenous proteins and fat. This makes it critical to provide adequate energy in the form of glucose. This should be done as quickly as possible, but not before obtaining samples for laboratory testing.

At first, a 10% glucose solution in an amount of 150 mL/kg/24 hours can be administered, using peripheral vascular catheters. This solution in a volume of 10 mg/kg/min delivers about 60 kcal/kg every 24 hours. This may be sufficient temporarily in some diseases where the patient has a lower tolerance to fasting (e.g., fatty acid oxidation disorders), but may be too low in children suffering from intoxication syndrome. Patients with intoxication syndrome require higher doses of glucose (12–15 mg/kg/min) not only to prevent hypoglycemia but also to stop catabolism and promote anabolism. Excessive fluid administration is avoided when providing a high glucose concentration solution by administering the glucose via a central venous catheter. If hyperglycemia occurs, with blood glucose concentrations above 150–160 mg/dL, then it should be corrected with insulin provided intravenously in doses of 0.05–0.1 units/kg/hour. The dose should be modified according to the blood glucose results [2, 9].

Due to the risk of increased lactic acidosis, the administration of glucose can be potentially dangerous in some energy metabolism disorders, particularly in pyruvate dehydrogenase complex deficiency. However, pyruvate dehydrogenase complex deficiency is very rare with a very poor prognosis except in those patients who respond to thiamin supplementation. Considering the number of metabolic disorders in which glucose supplementation can improve a patient's clinical condition, such a course of action is justified. However, the aforementioned procedure should be accompanied by regular monitoring of arterial blood gas. In the case of severe lactic acidosis, the glucose infusion should be limited to 3–5 mg/kg/minute. After the exclusion of fatty acid oxidation disorders, intravenous lipid solution should be introduced [9] (Appendix A).

4.5.2 Stage 2 – Medical Management

Correct the Acid-Based Balance If blood pH is <7.0–7.2, provide a slow administration of IV 8.4% $NaHCO_3$ in a dose of 0.25–0.5 mEq/kg/hour (up to 1–2 mEq/kg/h) keeping in mind the potential risk of hyponatremia, brain edema, and hemorrhage into the central nervous system. In the case of severe lactic acidosis, hypernatremia can occur when sodium concentrations are above 160 mmol/L that limits the use of sodium bicarbonate ($NaHC0_3$). Trometamol (THAM) and/or dialysis should be considered as a solution.

Ensure Proper Hydration Hydration is important not only to correct dehydration that often accompanies metabolic intoxication, but also to provide a way to eliminate toxins. Recommended amounts of fluids are 150/ml/kg/day, and higher doses may require forced diuresis to avoid cerebral edema. Proper hydration status should not be corrected suddenly and, depending on the level of dehydration, should be planned out over 24–48 hours [5, 23].

The correction of electrolytes, blood glucose, and hydration in the neonate is based on recent biochemical test results, performed as frequently as every 1–2 hours during the initial illness. It is also important to monitor diuresis and weight changes. The concentrations of potassium (K+) should range above 3.5 mmol/L and sodium (Na+) from 135 to 140 mmol/L.

4.5.3 Stage 3 – Detoxification

Hyperammonemia (especially in neonates) is a condition requiring prompt attention. After ceasing protein intake, supplying high concentrations of IV glucose, and restoring proper hydration status while being mindful of the risk of cerebral edema, the next step is to reduce ammonia concentrations. Certain drugs help to eliminate ammonia through different modes of action. Arginine and citrulline increase the elimination of ammonia by the urea cycle. Nitrogen-scavenging drugs, such as sodium benzoate and sodium or glycerol phenylacetate, bind with glycine and glutamine to create hippurate and phenylacetylglutamine that can be excreted with urine (Chap. 16). Carglumic acid is similar in its structure to N-acetylglutamate – natural activator of the cofactor for carbamoyl phosphate synthetase, the first enzyme of the urea cycle – and normalizes ammonia levels. It is especially helpful in patients with N-acetylglutamate synthase (NAGS) and carbamoyl phosphate synthase (CPS1) deficiency, but it is also used in secondary hyperammonemias associated with several organic acidemias, making the drug useful even when the final diagnosis has not yet been determined [13, 19, 20].

Sodium benzoate and sodium phenylbutyrate/phenylacetate can be toxic, especially with a concentration exceeding 2 and 4 mmol/L, respectively. There is also a possibility of increased sodium and decreased potassium, especially when sodium phenylbutyrate or sodium benzoate is administered together; therefore, electrolytes should be closely monitored.

In the case of rapidly increasing hyperammonemia, with ammonia values exceeding 400–500 µmol/l or if there is no significant decrease in ammonia concentrations (after 4 hours of treatment, or if after 12–24 hours of treatment, the ammonia concentration still exceeds 200 µmol/L), a swift decision should be made to eliminate ammonia with extracorporeal methods. The limitation of peritoneal dialysis or blood transfusion is that these procedures induce catabolism. Hemofiltration or hemodialysis should be started, and the best method to use depends upon the patient's body mass and experience of the medical staff. If it is not possible to perform hemodialysis, the patient should be immediately transferred to another center. If a transfer is not possible, peritoneal dialysis can be considered as a relatively simple method of extracorporeal filtration [9, 10, 19, 21, 23].

4.5.4 Stage 4 – Promotion of Anabolism

Proper caloric intake is crucial from the first moments of treating a neonate with an intoxication syndrome. Aside from glucose, lipids are an important energy source when promoting anabolism in a patient with hyperammonemia, organic aciduria, or aminoacidopathy. Lipids can be administered only after fatty acid oxidation disorders are ruled out. The recommended dose for lipids ranges from 1.0 to 3.0 g/kg/day or higher [9, 19].

After 24–48 hours of the initial cessation of oral feeding and stopping parenteral protein and lipids, intact protein should be reintroduced into the diet starting with 25–50% of daily requirement, and gradually increasing over the course of next few days. If protein is eliminated for longer than 24–48 hours, endogenous protein turnover begins, and the synthesis of toxic metabolites increases. The administration of amino acid substitutes using a gastrostomy tube may become necessary. In many cases, partial breast-feeding is possible.

4.5.5 Stage 5 – Other Supportive Treatment

Treating of infections will reduce one potential promoter of catabolism and prevent further episodes of decompensation. Treatment should be administered with an effective antipyretic and seizure management and, in some cases, antiemetic drugs, such as ondansetron. When treating seizures, avoid drugs that may inhibit mitochondrial function such as valproic acid [23].

L-carnitine is given in many metabolic disorders as a supplement or to correct a carnitine deficiency. The dose of carnitine can vary between 25 and 100 mg/kg/d, and in some organic acidurias, as much as 200–300 mg/kg/d may be necessary. In some of the long-chain fatty acid oxidation disorders, use of carnitine is controversial and with the concern of potential adverse effects from formation of cardiotoxic acylcarnitines, supplementation at time of metabolic decompensation should be avoided [24].

In propionic and methylmalonic aciduria, oral metronidazole is recommended by some clinicians and inhibits the production of propionic acid by gut bacteria. In isovaleric aciduria and methylcrotonyl-CoA carboxylase deficiency, glycine accompanied by carnitine supplementation increases the elimination of toxic metabolites. In many severe conditions, empiric administration of substances that act as cofactors proves to be helpful and this treatment option should not be neglected (Table 4.3) [25].

Table 4.3 Examples of cofactor responsive inborn errors of metabolism [2, 18, 19]

Cofactors use in inborn errors of metabolism with metabolic intoxication			
Disorder	Cofactor	Therapeutic dose	Frequency of responsive variants
Biotinidase deficiency	Biotin	5–10 mg/day	All cases
Folinic acid-responsive seizures	Folinic acid	5–15 mg/day	All cases
Glutaric aciduria type 1	Riboflavin	20–40 mg/day	Rare
Homocystinuria	Pyridoxine	50–500 mg/day	~50%
Hyperphenylalaninemia due to disorders of biopterin	Tetrahydrobiopterin	5–20 mg/day	All, but no improvement in CNS neurotransmitter levels
Methylmalonic aciduria	Vitamin B_{12}	1 mg im/day	Some
Maple syrup urine disease (MSUD)	Thiamin	10–15 mg/day	Rare
Multiple carboxylase deficiency	Biotin	10–40 mg/day	Most
Ornithine aminotransferase deficiency (OAT)	Pyridoxine	200–600 mg/day	~30%
Propionic aciduria	Biotin	5–10 mg/day	Possible never
Pyridoxine-responsive seizures	Pyridoxine	50–100 mg/day	All cases

Adapted from Walter and Wraith [25]

4.6 Summary

Individual inborn errors of metabolism are very rare, but as a group, they represent a quite common cause of acute deterioration in newborns. In the first days to weeks of life, neonates with metabolic intoxication may be asymptomatic or present with symptoms similar to more common manifestations of disorders of early infancy, including generalized infection, birth trauma, and respiratory distress syndrome. A careful analysis of medical history of present illness and clinical condition of the patient, backed up with the interpretation of basic biochemical test results, often allows for establishing a reasonable suspicion of an inborn error of metabolism and directs further diagnostic and therapeutic actions. Late effects of the treatment depend on the time between the first symptoms of metabolic intoxication and the initiation of the effective treatment. Prevention of the accumulation of metabolic toxins and promotion of anabolism are the most important steps in the treatment of metabolic intoxication.

References

1. Scriver CR. Garrod's Croonian Lectures (1908) and the charter 'Inborn Errors of Metabolism': albinism, alkaptonuria, cystinuria, and pentosuria at age 100 in 2008. J Inherit Metab Dis. 2008;31(5):580–98.
2. Saudubray JM, Van den Berghe G, Walter J. Inborn metabolic diseases: diagnosis and treatment. 5th ed. Berlin: Springer; 2012.
3. Leonard JV, Morris AA. Diagnosis and early management of inborn errors of metabolism presenting around the time of birth. Acta Paediatr. 2006;95(1):6–14.
4. Physician's guide to the treatment and follow-up of metabolic diseases. New York: Springer/Berlin/Heidelberg; 2014.
5. Saudubray JM, Garcia-Cazorla A. Inborn errors of metabolism overview: pathophysiology, manifestations, evaluation, and management. Pediatr Clin N Am. 2018;65(2):179–208.
6. Gilbert-Barness E, Farrell PM. Approach to diagnosis of metabolic diseases. Transl Sci Rare Dis. 2016;1(1):3–22.
7. Saudubray JM, Nassogne MC, de Lonlay P, Touati G. Clinical approach to inherited metabolic disorders in neonates: an overview. Semin Neonatol. 2002;7(1):3–15.
8. Hoffmann GF, A. S. Organic acidurias. In: Sarafoglu K, Roth KS, editors. Pediatric endocrinology and inborn errors of metabolism. New York: McGraw Hill Medical; 2009. p. 83–118.
9. Prietsch V, Lindner M, Zschocke J, Nyhan WL, Hoffmann GF. Emergency management of inherited metabolic diseases. J Inherit Metab Dis. 2002;25(7):531–46.
10. Rice GM, Steiner RD. Inborn errors of metabolism (metabolic disorders). Pediatr Rev. 2016;37(1):3–15; quiz 6–7, 47
11. Walter JH. Inborn errors of metabolism and pregnancy. J Inherit Metab Dis. 2000;23(3):229–36.
12. Gutierrez Junquera C, Balmaseda E, Gil E, Martinez A, Sorli M, Cuartero I, et al. Acute fatty liver of pregnancy and neonatal long-chain 3-hydroxyacyl-coenzyme A dehydrogenase (LCHAD) deficiency. Eur J Pediatr. 2009;168(1):103–6.
13. Zschocke J, Hoffman GF, Milupa AG. Vademecum metabolicum: manual of metabolic paediatrics. 2nd ed. Friedrichsdorf, Stuttgart, Milupa, editors: Schattauer; 2004.
14. Platt LD, Koch R, Hanley WB, Levy HL, Matalon R, Rouse B, et al. The international study of pregnancy outcome in women with maternal phenylketonuria: report of a 12-year study. Am J Obstet Gynecol. 2000;182(2):326–33.
15. Saudubray JM, Sedel F, Walter JH. Clinical approach to treatable inborn metabolic diseases: an introduction. J Inherit Metab Dis. 2006;29(2–3):261–74.
16. Schillaci LP, DeBrosse SD, McCandless SE. Inborn errors of metabolism with acidosis: organic acidemias and defects of pyruvate and ketone body metabolism. Pediatr Clin N Am. 2018;65(2):209–30.
17. Clayton PT. Inborn errors presenting with liver dysfunction. Semin Neonatol. 2002;7(1):49–63.
18. Blau N, Milan E, Blaskovics MD. Simple tests. In: Blau N, Blaskovics ME, Gibson KE, editors. Physician's guide to the laboratory diagnosis of metabolic diseases. Berlin: Springer-Verlag; 2014. p. 3–10.
19. Haberle J, Boddaert N, Burlina A, Chakrapani A, Dixon M, Huemer M, et al. Suggested guidelines for the diagnosis and management of urea cycle disorders. Orphanet J Rare Dis. 2012;7:32.
20. Chow SL, Gandhi V, Krywawych S, Clayton PT, Leonard JV, Morris AA. The significance of a high plasma ammonia value. Arch Dis Child. 2004;89(6):585–6.
21. Grunevald S, Davison J, Martinelli D, Duran M, Dionisi-Vici C. Emergency diagnostic procedures and emergency treatment. In: Blau N, Marinus Duran K, Gibson M, Dionisi-Vici C, editors. Physician's guide to the diagnosis, treatment, and follow-up of inherited metabolic diseases. Springer; 2014.
22. Alfadhel M, Al-Thihli K, Moubayed H, Eyaid W, Al-Jeraisy M. Drug treatment of inborn errors of metabolism: a systematic review. Arch Dis Child. 2013;98(6):454–61.

23. Dionisi-Vici C, OdB H. Emergency treatment. In: Saudubray JM, Walter J, editors. Inborn metabolic diseases diagnosis and treatment. Berlin: Springer; 2012. p. 104–11.
24. Spiekerkoetter U, Lindner M, Santer R, Grotzke M, Baumgartner MR, Boehles H, et al. Treatment recommendations in long-chain fatty acid oxidation defects: consensus from a workshop. J Inherit Metab Dis. 2009;32(4):498–505.
25. Walter J. Present status and new trends. In: Fernandes SJ, Van der Berghe J, editors. Inborn metabolic diseases diagnosis and treatment 2000. p. 75–84.

Anabolism: Practical Strategies

5

Kimberly A. Kripps and Johan L. K. Van Hove

Contents

K. A. Kripps (✉)
Department of Molecular and Medical Genetics, Oregon Health and Science University, Portland, OR, USA
e-mail: kripps@ohsu.edu

J. L. K. Van Hove
Clinical Genetics and Metabolism, Children's Hospital Colorado, University of Colorado Denver – Anschutz Medical Campus, Aurora, CO, USA
e-mail: johan.vanhove@childrenscolorado.org

L. E. Bernstein et al. (eds.), *Nutrition Management of Inherited Metabolic Diseases*,
https://doi.org/10.1007/978-3-030-94510-7_5

Core Messages

- Anabolism is a metabolic state of protein synthesis.
- In the immediate postprandial period, carbohydrates are the preferred source of energy. After 12–15 hours of fasting, energy is derived from the breakdown of fat and protein stores.
- In order to maintain an anabolic state, energy sources must be supplied, which includes the provision of essential amino acids.

5.1 Background

Anabolism is an energy-rich metabolic state in which the body synthesizes new components, including proteins. It is the opposite of catabolism, an energy-poor state where the body breaks down self-stores to supply the energy and constitutive components needed to drive life-sustaining reactions. Since many metabolic diseases stem from deficiencies in catabolic pathways, in particular, the breakdown of proteins, fats, and carbohydrates, avoiding catabolism is an important aspect of management for these conditions. Sustaining an anabolic state is particularly important during illness, in which adequate intake of nutrition is often compromised. To support anabolism, both energy and constituent components are needed. Provision of sufficient energy is the first consideration. Energy can be derived from carbohydrates or from fat. Obtaining energy from protein is limited by the nitrogen load. Other required components include essential amino acids as well as vitamins, minerals, and essential fatty acids. The management strategies to maintain anabolism described in this chapter reflect the authors' experiences and practices.

5.2 Importance of Anabolism in Metabolic Diseases

Many metabolic disorders stem from defects in the pathways involved in the breakdown of macronutrients: carbohydrates, proteins, and fats. In an anabolic state, in which the body does not rely on these breakdown pathways, patients are most stable. However, when catabolism is induced and these breakdown processes are triggered, the consequences may be life threatening.

Generally, in a stressed state, these disorders will lead to energy deficiency and/or a buildup of toxic metabolites. Thus, this class of diseases is often termed "disorders of energy metabolism." In the case of disorders of carbohydrate metabolism, the inability to properly store or break down glycogen will lead to hypoglycemia and energy failure when an exogenous source of glucose is not supplied. Similarly, defects in fatty acid beta-oxidation will lead to energy deficiency when the body becomes reliant on fat sources for energy. A buildup of fatty-acid substrates is also thought to be toxic to mitochondrial function [1, 2]. Disorders of amino acid metabolism often result in the accumulation of toxic intermediates upstream of the block in the pathway. These disorders of amino acid metabolism are often controlled through the dietary limitation of protein or of the particular amino acids that cannot be properly metabolized. By decreasing the substrate for the reaction, less toxin is produced. During times of catabolism, when the body starts breaking down self-proteins, the flood of amino acids into the system is uncontrolled, resulting in a significant substrate load and toxin accumulation.

Mitochondria are centers for energy production; thus, conditions leading to a primary impairment of mitochondrial function also lead to energy deficiency. Energy deficiency can be present in mitochondrial disorders even in a well-fed state. However, mitochondrial diseases may be further exacerbated in the catabolic state. Catabolic stress may lead to increased production of reactive oxygen species, toxic metabolites, and a greater energy deficit, leading to cellular injury and worsening of baseline symptoms [3]. Therefore, maintaining anabolism is equally as important for mitochondrial diseases.

5.3 Fasting and Postprandial Metabolism

An understanding of normal metabolism and metabolic processes is key to understanding how to support anabolism for each particular disorder of energy metabolism.

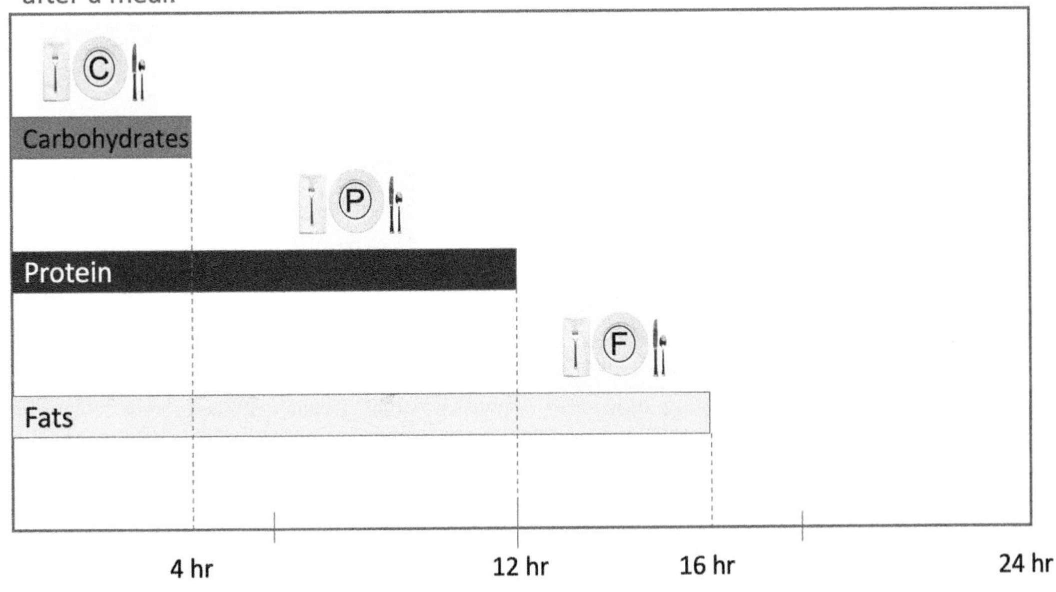

Fig. 5.1 Time for digestion of the macronutrients [14]. (Bernstein L et al. Visual Teaching Aids, Vitaflo USA)

In the immediate postprandial period, human metabolism prefers the use of carbohydrates for energy. The meal is digested and absorbed over the course of 3–4 hours, supplying the body with a source of glucose during this time (Fig. 5.1).

Thereafter, energy will be provided by glycogenolysis (breakdown of glycogen) from glycogen stores in the liver. Patients with glycogen storage or glycogen utilization defects will manifest with symptoms in this time period. As glycogen stores are depleted, usually within about 8–12 hours following a meal, the body will gradually turn to gluconeogenesis to synthesize glucose from noncarbohydrate sources, such as amino acids and fatty acids.

After 12–15 hours of fasting, lipolysis will start, and metabolism will gradually switch to the use of fat as the primary energy source. Free fatty acids increase after 12 hours, and ketones start to increase after 15 hours of fasting [4]. Disorders that affect the metabolism of fat or protein will become problematic within this timeframe of fasting. Indeed, the earliest time recorded for the onset of hypoglycemia in a fatty acid oxidation disorder such as medium chain acyl-CoA dehydrogenase (MCAD) deficiency was at 12 hours fasting time [5]. Thus, for these disorders, fasting longer than 12–15 hours should be avoided.

It should be noted that tolerated fasting times do show an age dependency [5]. Thus, for infants and younger children, especially those with low weight and decreased reserves, the time until the onset of glycogenolysis, gluconeogenesis, and lipolysis may be shortened, although the extent has not been measured. Energy needs also increase during acute illnesses, thus drawing more from body stores and decreasing the fasting times normally tolerated at baseline.

5.4 Daily Management

Guidance for the daily maintenance of anabolism in metabolic patients is derived from the above knowledge of normal energy metabolism. Patients and families should be taught to always consider the duration of fasting since the last good meal and

Table 5.1 Glucose polymer guidelines for illness

Glucose Solution	Age for use	Grams of glucose polymer per 100 mL	Amount of glucose polymer in 4 fluid ounces	Energy per 100 mL	Energy per ounce
15%	0–12 months	15	8 tsp	60	16.8
20%	1–3 years	20	11 tsp	80	22.4
25%	3–6 years	25	4.5 TBSP	100	28
30%	6+ years	30	5.5 TBSP	120	33.6

Adapted from van Hove et al. (2009) [8]

ensure that regular meals and snacks are provided so that these fasting intervals are not exceeded.

During the night when the patient sleeps, there is a natural fasting time, often of 10–12 hours for young children. For most metabolic disorders, this is an acceptable period of fasting; however, if either the evening or morning meal is missed, the fasting allowance is easily surpassed. For disorders of glycogen metabolism, in which the fasting allowance is much less, an overnight snack or overnight feeds are often necessary. Uncooked cornstarch provides a slow release of glucose after ingestion, thus extending the enteral absorption phase, and can be utilized to help stabilize blood glucose levels and extend fasting times between meals, including for patients with glycogen storage defects [6, 7].

5.5 Acute Episodes and Hospitalization

5.5.1 Home Management

Practical strategies must be established for times in which meals are missed or there is a risk for exceeding fasting parameters. If the evening meal is not consumed due to poor appetite or a vomiting illness, then patients or caregivers should note the time since the last meal, often lunch. In this case, the maximum fasting duration of 15 hours will likely occur during the night. Thus, the patient should be awakened at night to attempt to feed and if unsuccessful should be brought to the hospital for care. If the problem occurs in the morning, the patient has already been fasting overnight, and the maximum fasting duration is only a few hours off.

Often, during times of feeling unwell, frequent small meals are better tolerated than a single large amount. If solid foods are not tolerated, a high concentrated carbohydrate drink can be offered to the patient to supply a source of glucose. High carbohydrate solutions can be made using table sugar (sucrose); however, concentrated solutions of alpha-dextrin maltose are often better tolerated [8]. These alpha-dextrin maltose solutions have a low osmolality and are easily digested. The concentration of alpha-dextrin maltose that can be tolerated increases with age: a 15% solution is recommended for infants less than 1 year, 20% at 1–3 years, 25% at 3–6 years, and 30% from age 6 years on. Table 5.1 provides instructions for calculating and preparing these mixtures (Appendix C).

For most patients, drinking 60 mL of a concentrated dextrose solution each hour results in adequate intake of energy. This solution is rapidly absorbed, often within 30–60 minutes. Giving a tablespoon (15 mL) every 15 minutes is usually tolerated the best. Caution should be taken during diarrheal illnesses as these solutions may exacerbate diarrhea. Osmotic diarrhea induced by high carbohydrate loads during diarrheal illness may result in hyponatremia.

Glucose or alpha-dextrin maltose solutions are incomplete sources of nutrition and should not be used for long durations (24–36 hours maximum). These solutions can also be used to shorten the duration of fasting required for medical procedures such as anesthesia. Stomach clearing in 2 hours after an alpha-dextrin maltose solution has been documented [9].

5.5.2 Hospital Management

If patients are unable to tolerate oral feeds or solutions at home, it is critical that they be brought to the hospital so that intravenous nutrition and adequate fluids can be supplied (Appendix B).

When formulating intravenous nutritional management, not only should one consider the amount of glucose needed to prevent hypoglycemia but also the total calories provided to the patient. During most acute illnesses, the energy needs are unchanged at 100% of normal. Caloric needs can be estimated from published tables [10] or the DRI [11].

It is usually safe to start the provision of calories with intravenous glucose, but this often does not provide sufficient calories. To fulfill energy needs, usually a combination of intravenous glucose and fat (for instance, Intralipid®, Baxter International Inc., Deerfield, IL) should be provided. Optimal energy is provided by a mixture of carbohydrates and lipids in infants [12]. In the case of most fatty acid oxidation disorders, the use of intralipids is contraindicated, and glucose provision may need to be increased to meet energy needs in these patients. Total fluid administration and the risks for inducing hyperglycemia should always be considered when giving intravenous dextrose and may limit the amount of dextrose that can be safely provided.

For maintenance of anabolism, essential amino acids must be provided in addition to energy sources. Despite appropriate energy sources, in the setting of essential amino acid deficiency, the body will start breaking down protein stores to supply the necessary components for protein synthesis. This has the potential to lead to toxin accumulation, particularly for those patients with defects in protein or amino acid metabolism. Many patients are already deficient in essential amino acids upon admission due to poor intake or vomiting [13]. Provision of essential amino acids should commence immediately on admission even in the setting of existing hyperammonemia or the presence of another toxin. Essential amino acid requirements vary with age and can be estimated from published sources [10]. Certain metabolic disorders may create conditionally essential amino acids, which should also be taken into account.

Careful consideration must be made for the provision of essential amino acids to patients whose disorders necessitate a restriction of specific amino acids, such as organic acidemias, or for those with a limitation of general protein intake, such as urea cycle defects. Specialized medical foods administered enterally are the preferred method for providing essential amino acids to these patients. Medical foods depleted of particular amino acids provide a safe first source of protein to patients unable to metabolize particular amino acids, to be further adjusted with intact protein sources based on plasma amino acid concentrations. For patients with urea cycle disorders, for whom there is a generalized protein restriction, medical foods composed of only essential amino acids can be used. This allows for essential amino acid requirements to be met without causing protein overload from the accompanying nonessential amino acids found in intact protein sources. For ill patients unwilling to eat by mouth or with nausea or vomiting, nasogastric feeding can be utilized and given by slow drip to help improve tolerance.

If enteral feeding is not possible, then intravenous protein should be given without delay to provide the essential amino acids. Unfortunately, specialized intravenous protein solutions are not widely available. Readily available solutions contain complete amino acid mixtures, and thus must be carefully titrated in patients so as to meet essential amino acid needs without causing overload of the offensive amino acids or total protein. Plasma amino acid concentrations should be monitored regularly to guide the titration of these intravenous protein mixtures. In some cases, specialized parenteral nutrition depleted of specific amino acids is required, and must be specially ordered, such as branched-chain amino-acid-free parenteral nutrition for patients with maple syrup urine disease.

Finally, sufficient amounts of vitamins must be provided. Patients often have poor nutrition intake or chronic vomiting before their admission. This creates risk of thiamin deficiency. Thiamin is an integral cofactor for a number of enzymes involved in energy metabolism. Its deficiency exacerbates the energy deficit, increasing the risk for neurological damage. Extra thiamin should be provided to avoid neurological problems when large quantities of carbohydrates are given during early phases of treatment, which exacerbates thiamin requirement in metabolism.

5.6 Summary

The promotion of anabolism is key in the treatment and prevention of illness in many inherited metabolic diseases. Many metabolic disorders affect catabolic processes, such as disorders of the breakdown of fatty acids, amino acids, or glycogen. As a result of these metabolic defects, patients are at risk for energy failure and/or toxicity when stressed into a catabolic state. Maintaining anabolism is thus important to prevent this risk. Anabolism further decreases the accumulation of toxins in metabolic disorders, such as those involving protein metabolism, by promoting synthesis and the use of amino acids to build new proteins, thereby decreasing the amount of toxin-producing substrate.

The risk for catabolism is significantly increased during times of acute illness. Patients, families, and providers must have a plan in place to address times of illness so that anabolism can be maintained. The most important component needed for anabolism is calories. Synthetic processes are energy-dependent, and a positive caloric state is needed to provide an environment conducive to anabolism.

When normal oral intake is compromised, such as with vomiting illnesses, filling energy needs with carbohydrates can be addressed by providing multiple small meals, frequent intake of alpha-dextrin maltose solutions, or with gastric drip-feeding to minimize metabolic decompensation. In cases where enteral nutrition is not tolerated, hospital admission for intravenous administration of energy sources is necessary.

Constitutive components for protein synthesis and energy production are additionally required to support anabolism. Careful administration of essential amino acids and vitamins should be started early for ill patients, as delay will induce catabolism, even in the setting of sufficient energy sources.

Acknowledgments Thank you to Johan L. K. Van Hove of Children's Hospital of Colorado for his contributions to this chapter's content in the 1st Edition of Nutrition Management of Inherited Metabolic Diseases.

References

1. Ribas GS, Vargas CR. Evidence that oxidative disbalance and mitochondrial dysfunction are involved in the pathophysiology of fatty acid oxidation disorders. Cell Mol Neurobiol. Springer Nature: 2020. https://link.springer.com/article/10.1007/s10571-020-00955-7#rightslink
2. Wajner M, Amaral AU. Mitochondrial dysfunction in fatty acid oxidation disorders: insights from human and animal studies. Biosci Rep. 2015;36(1):e00281.
3. Parikh S, Goldstein A, Koenig MK, Scaglia F, Enns GM, Saneto R, et al. Diagnosis and management of mitochondrial disease: a consensus statement from the Mitochondrial Medicine Society. Genet Med. 2015;17(9):689–701.
4. Bonnefont JP, Specola NB, Vassault A, Lombes A, Ogier H, de Klerk JB, et al. The fasting test in paediatrics: application to the diagnosis of pathological hypo- and hyperketotic states. Eur J Pediatr. 1990;150(2):80–5.
5. Derks TG, van Spronsen FJ, Rake JP, van der Hilst CS, Span MM, Smit GP. Safe and unsafe duration of fasting for children with MCAD deficiency. Eur J Pediatr. 2007;166(1):5–11.
6. Kishnani PS, Austin SL, Abdenur JE, Arn P, Bali DS, Boney A, et al. Diagnosis and management of glycogen storage disease type I: a practice guideline of the American College of Medical Genetics and Genomics. Genet Med. 2014;16(11):e1.
7. Saudubray JM, Baumgartner MR, Walter J. Inborn metabolic diseases: diagnosis and treatment. Springer Berlin, Heidelberg; 2016.
8. Van Hove JL, Myers S, Kerckhove KV, Freehauf C, Bernstein L. Acute nutrition management in the prevention of metabolic illness: a practical approach with glucose polymers. Mol Genet Metab. 2009;97(1):1–3.
9. Nygren J, Thorell A, Jacobsson H, Larsson S, Schnell PO, Hylen L, et al. Preoperative gastric emptying. Effects of anxiety and oral carbohydrate administration. Ann Surg. 1995;222(6):728–34.
10. American Academy of Pediatrics Committee on N. Pediatric Nutrition. 8th ed. American Academy of Pediatrics Committee on N, editor; 2019.
11. Institute of Medicine (U.S.). Panel on Macronutrients., Institute of Medicine (U.S.). Standing Committee on the Scientific Evaluation of Dietary Reference Intakes. Dietary reference intakes for energy, carbohydrate, fiber, fat, fatty acids, cholesterol, protein, and amino acids. Washington, D.C.: National Academies Press; 2005. xxv, 1331 p.
12. Bresson JL, Narcy P, Putet G, Ricour C, Sachs C, Rey J. Energy substrate utilization in infants receiving total parenteral nutrition with different glucose to fat ratios. Pediatr Res. 1989;25(6):645–8.
13. Boneh A. Dietary protein in urea cycle defects: how much? Which? How? Mol Genet Metab. 2014;113(1–2):109–12.
14. Wright E, Thomas J, Bernstein LB, Helm J. Medium chain Acyl-CoA dehydrogenase deficiency (MCADD): Children's Hospital of Colorado; 2017.

Protein Requirements in Inherited Metabolic Diseases

6

Steven Yannicelli

Contents

S. Yannicelli (✉)
Medical and Scientific Affairs, Nutricia North America, Rockville, MD, USA
e-mail: steven.yannicelli@nutricia.com

L. E. Bernstein et al. (eds.), *Nutrition Management of Inherited Metabolic Diseases*,
https://doi.org/10.1007/978-3-030-94510-7_6

Core Messages

- Protein is a critical part of the diet in individuals with inherited metabolic diseases (IMDs).
- Current Dietary Reference Intakes may underestimate protein needs for individuals with IMD.
- Distributing protein intake throughout the day facilitates anabolism.
- Additional protein and energy is required for catch-up growth in patients with growth failure.
- Proper use of protein substitutes (medical foods) is essential in assuring adequate balance of serum amino acids and promoting growth and development.

6.1 Background

Protein is found in all cells and has multiple functions in the human body including structural, hormonal, enzymatic, immunologic, and regulation of acid: base balance. There are 20 amino acids used for protein function in humans. These are divided into three categories: indispensable amino acids (also called essential amino acids) that cannot be synthesized in the body and must be supplied from the diet; dispensable (also called nonessential amino acids) that are synthesized endogenously; and conditionally indispensable amino acids (Table 6.1). An example of a conditionally indispensable amino acid is in phenylketonuria (PKU), where tyrosine is not sufficiently hydrolyzed from phenylalanine, making tyrosine an indispensable amino acid.

6.2 Biological Value and Digestibility of Protein Composition

Protein composition and quality influence the rate of digestion, absorption, and ability to provide enough nitrogen and indispensable amino acids for protein synthesis and growth. Protein quality is determined by digestibility and amino acid composition, with indispensable amino acids of high importance. An imbalance of indispensable amino acids or an insufficient amount of a single indispensable amino acid ("limiting amino acid") will negatively affect protein synthesis and protein turnover. Consequently, all indispensable amino acids must be provided in sufficient quantities to meet protein requirements and drive protein synthesis.

Table 6.1 Classification of amino acids in the human diet

Indispensable, dispensable, and conditionally indispensable amino acids in the human diet		
Indispensable (essential)	Dispensable (non-essential)	Conditionally indispensable
Histidine	Alanine	Arginine
Isoleucine	Aspartic Acid	Cysteine
Leucine	Asparagine	Glutamine
Lysine	Glutamic Acid	Glycine
Methionine	Serine	Proline
Phenylalanine		Tyrosine
Threonine		
Tryptophan		
Valine		

Protein digestibility and amino acid composition differ among the various forms of protein. Standard infant formulas and human milk contain intact protein where all amino acids form a complex bond or polypeptide. Other infant formulas contain protein hydrolysates, where protein is broken into specific chain lengths of dipeptides and tripeptides, whereas other formulas contain free amino acids (Fig. 6.1). Medical foods, also referred to as "protein substitutes," prescribed for aminoacidopathies, organic acidemias, and urea cycle disorders, are elemental and contain free amino acids. An exception is glycomacropeptide (GMP), a bioactive 64-chain polypeptide produced during cheese processing by action of chymosin on bovine-κ-casein. GMP is naturally low in phenylalanine and tyrosine, and used in certain medical foods for individuals with PKU and tyrosinemia (TYR) [1].

Protein contains 16% nitrogen. Studies have reported that the protein source affects nitrogen retention and whole-body nitrogen [2, 3]. Luiking and others reported in humans fed soy protein compared to casein that casein resulted in increased protein synthesis, whereas soy was

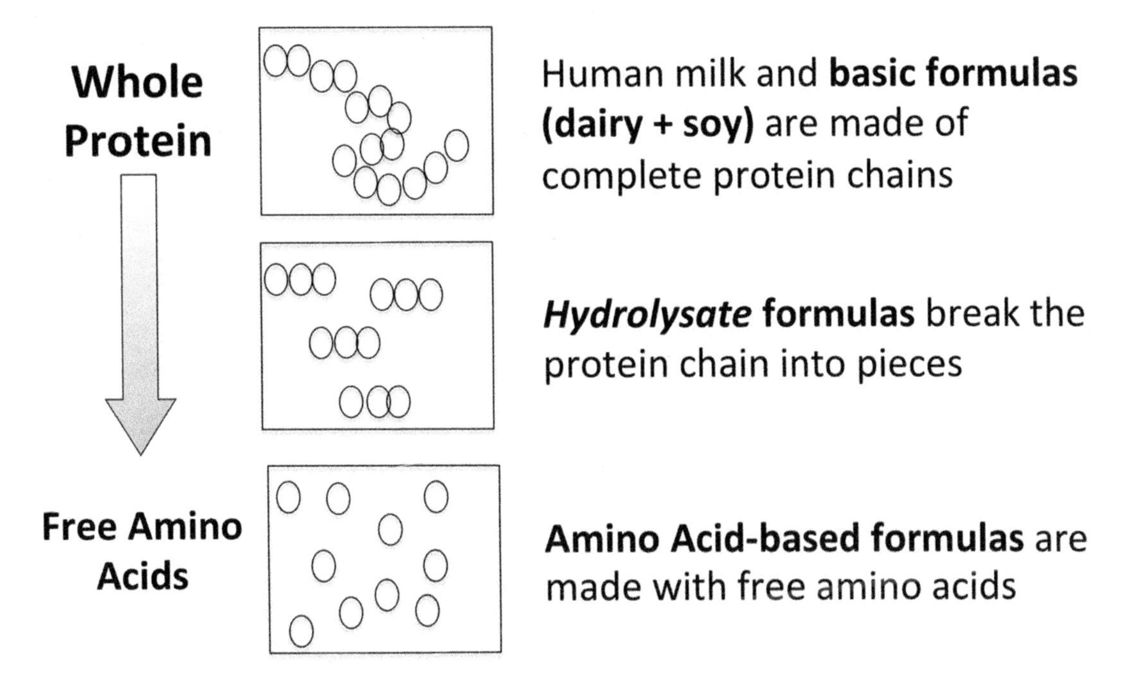

Fig. 6.1 Complexity of protein in human milk/standard formulas, hydrolysate formulas, and amino-acid-based formulas

degraded to urea in higher percentage [4]. Dangin and colleagues (2001) reported that protein digestion rates regulate protein retention in fast-acting (whey) and slow-acting (casein) proteins [5]. Whey is rapidly digested and results in a quick rise in plasma amino acids, stimulating protein synthesis [3]. One study in rats compared casein with free amino acids [6] and found increased weight gain and decreased renal nitrogen excretion in rats fed casein compared to free amino acids, indicating improved whole body nitrogen homeostasis. Monchi and associates (1993) also reported that rats fed a casein hydrolysate compared to those fed free amino acids had significantly higher body nitrogen, weight gain, and net protein utilization [7]. Children with PKU fed free amino acids compared to age-matched controls fed whole soy protein showed poorer growth and lower total body nitrogen, despite consuming the same amount of total dietary protein [8]. In another study, Jones and colleagues (1983) reported lower nitrogen retention in adults fed free amino acids compared to intact protein despite similar nitrogen consumption [9]. Total body nitrogen and height z-scores were significantly lower in PKU children who consumed free amino acids as their main protein source compared to non-PKU children consuming intact protein despite similar intakes in protein.

Compared to intact protein, free amino acids have increased rates of absorption and oxidation, partly due to rate of digestion [10–12]. Free amino acids bypass the digestive phase and can be quickly absorbed in the small intestine, which leads to rapid absorption. Researchers have reported increases in plasma amino acid concentrations up to 120 minutes postprandial in subjects fed free amino acids compared to intact protein [5]. Extensively hydrolyzed formulas compared to free amino acid–based formulas and human milk show different plasma amino acid patterns [13].

Due to the differences in nitrogen retention, along with differences in digestion and rapid absorption of free amino acids compared to intact protein, greater total protein intake above the Recommended Dietary Intakes (RDA) [14] has been suggested in patients who consume a significant percentage of their daily protein intake from medical foods. Typically, a 20–25 percent correction is recommended due to decreased nitrogen retention when using free amino acid–based medical food [15].

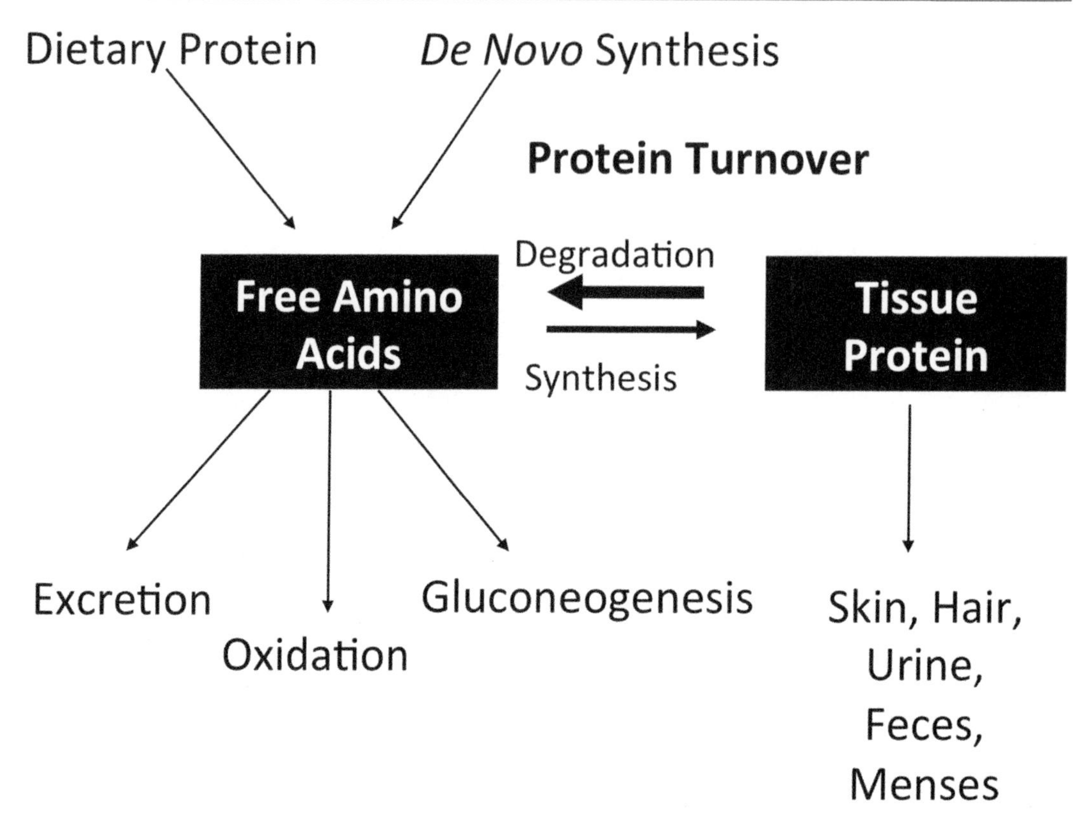

Fig. 6.2 Dietary and de novo protein synthesis. (Adapted from Dietary Reference Intakes for Energy, Carbohydrate, Fiber, Fat, Fatty Acids, Cholesterol, Protein, and Amino Acids (Macronutrients). National Academy of Sciences, 2005: pg. 598 [20])

Based on differences in digestibility and absorption of protein sources, clinicians should be cognizant as to whether a patient consumed free amino acid–based medical food alone or in combination with intact proteins prior to blood draws when assessing plasma amino acid concentrations, especially when dietary modifications are being considered.

6.3 Protein Turnover

Protein turnover is the process by which the body contributes to the free amino acid pool through a balance of synthesis and degradation. This constant turnover, or resynthesizing of endogenous protein, occurs in all cells. The majority of protein turnover is in the liver and intestines with less occurring in skeletal muscle [16, 17]. Rates of protein turnover and deposition differ through the lifespan, with infants having about four times greater daily protein turnover rate compared to adults [18, 19]. Consequently, protein requirements (based on body weight) are highest in infants. When protein synthesis is equal to degradation, the body is in "balance" (Fig. 6.2) [20].

Borsheim and colleagues (2002) reported that protein synthesis is driven by the indispensable amino acid content and not dispensable amino acid content of the diet [21]. Increasing the concentration of extracellular indispensable amino acids, particularly leucine, initiates protein synthesis. [22]

During catabolic crisis, protein degradation is more active than synthesis, resulting in negative protein balance. In patients with severe metabolic disorders, this is a concern and creates a challenge to clinicians to reduce de novo protein degradation. During acute metabolic crises, the goal is to maintain an adequate amino acid pool by ensuring that protein/amino acids are not eliminated from the diet for prolonged periods and adequate calories are provided.

6.4 Other Factors Influencing Protein Utilization

Dietary amino acid adequacy is markedly influenced by energy balance. Sufficient energy intake must be provided in diets for patients with inherited metabolic diseases to preserve protein for synthesis and adequate growth. Insufficient calories will result in amino acids being metabolized for energy instead of protein. Energy requirements for healthy patients with inherited metabolic disease should, in most cases, be similar to typical individuals. In cases of acute metabolic decompensation, additional energy is required to reduce catabolism and promote anabolism. Approaches to providing the amount and type of nonprotein energy will be discussed in disease-specific chapters of this book.

Protein, as well as nonprotein energy (i.e., carbohydrates and fats), must be provided in sufficient amounts to drive protein synthesis and prevent protein-energy deficiency [23]. Protein synthesis is dependent on supplying adequate amounts of indispensable amino acids. Insulin, in response to glucose and amino acids, especially leucine, signals anabolic pathways that drive protein synthesis in skeletal muscle. Leucine upregulates skeletal protein synthesis by enhancing activity and synthesis of proteins involved in mRNA translation [24]. A combination of intact protein, carbohydrate, and leucine has been shown to increase protein synthesis, decrease protein oxidation, and increase net whole body protein balance compared to just providing carbohydrate [25].

Excess nonprotein calories will increase weight but not lean body mass, which may be the case in certain patients with inherited metabolic disorders on low protein, high caloric intakes. The type of nonprotein energy can make a difference on protein status. Human studies have indicated that carbohydrate, and not fat, can reduce postprandial protein degradation [26, 27]. Net protein utilization improved by 5% and nitrogen retention by 14% when carbohydrate was offered. Excess carbohydrate without protein stimulates postabsorptive proteolysis and protein synthesis [28].

Early studies in infants and children on free amino acid–based diets reported 20% to 25% additional nonprotein energy was required to support nitrogen balance [29, 30]. However, in patients with metabolic disorders who have limited mobility or are nonambulatory, fewer calories may suffice in maintaining growth and weight maintenance [31].

Distributing protein throughout the day positively influences protein synthesis [32–34]. Suggested optimal protein distribution in one study is shown in Fig. 6.3 [35].

Paddon-Jones et al. (2009) reported optimal protein synthesis when dietary protein was provided in equal amounts three times per day compared with the same total amount of protein given in varying amounts [33, 35, 36]. In patients with PKU, providing amino acid–based medical food throughout the day compared to a single dose of similar protein equivalents had a positive effect on protein synthesis [37]. A positive effect on plasma phenylalanine concentrations was also reported [37]. For patients with a metabolic disorder, providing medical food along with limited intact protein foods is most beneficial to optimize protein synthesis [38] and reduce oxidation of L-amino acids [39].

6.5 Protein Requirements for the General Population

Protein requirements for both the general populace and for patients with a metabolic disease need to be used as benchmarks only. Recommended Dietary Allowances (RDA) and Dietary Reference Intakes (Appendix D) for age are determined by a number of factors, including minimum requirements for age. The RDA is the "average daily dietary intake sufficient to meet the nutrient requirements of nearly all (97–98%) healthy individuals in a group" [23]. The Estimated Average Requirement (EAR) is "the average daily nutrient intake estimated to be nec-

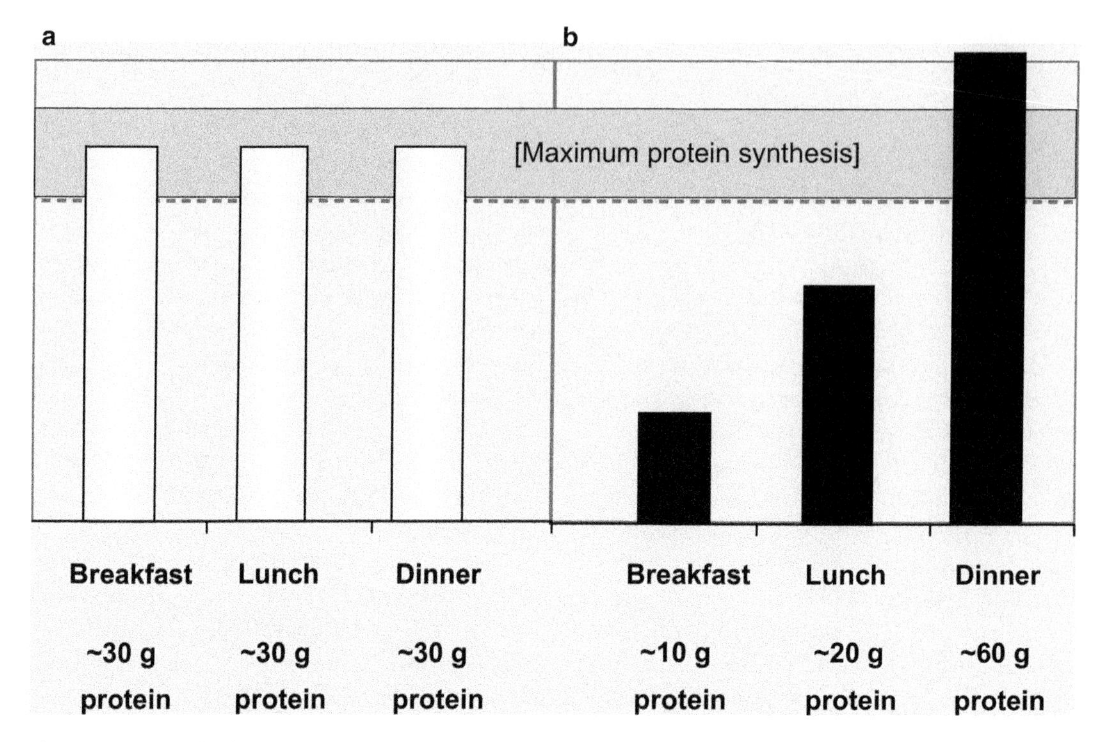

Fig. 6.3 Optimal distribution of daily protein intake. (**a**) Optimal protein distribution. (**b**) Skewed protein distribution. (Adapted from Paddon-Jones and Rasmussen [35])

essary to meet the requirements of half of the healthy individuals in a group" [23].

Protein requirements have been determined primarily by traditional nitrogen balance studies wherein calculation of intake versus excretion of nitrogen reflects either synthesis or catabolism. The EAR of protein (approx. 0.66 g/kg/day for adults) is derived from the amount of nitrogen necessary for nitrogen balance to equal zero in balance studies. The RDA for protein is based on the EAR plus a safety factor resulting in a protein recommendation of 0.8 g/kg/d for adults [20, 23]. No tolerable upper limits have been set for either protein or indispensable amino acids, due to insufficient data.

Limitations of the nitrogen balance method include difficulty in accurate measurements, chance of falsely positive nitrogen balance, and underestimation of requirements. A more precise method of determining amino acid and protein requirements is the indicator amino acid oxidation technique (IAAO) [40]. The IAAO method utilizes a carbon-labeled isotope (L-[1-^{13}C]) tracer that is ingested orally, and oxidation of this labeled carbon is measured in expired breath as $^{13}CO_2$. The IAAO method is based on the assumption that if one indispensable amino acid is deficient, all other amino acids will be oxidized until that particular indispensable amino acid is available in adequate amounts, at which point oxidation of the amino acid pool, including the tracer, will be the lowest [41]. Using the IAAO, researchers report that protein recommendations are as much as 30% higher than the Food and Agriculture Organization/World Health Organization (FAO/WHO) recommendations that are based on nitrogen balance studies [42]. Current protein recommendations (DRI 2005) of 0.76 g/kg/day (EAR) and 0.95 g/kg/day (RDA) for children may be underestimated as much as 70% compared to 1.3 g/kg/day (mean) and population safe 1.55 g/kg/day (upper 95% confidence interval) determined by the IAAO method [43]. The IAAO method may help researchers re-evaluate current protein requirements [40, 44]. In addition to assessing protein requirements, the IAAO method has been used to quantify amino acid requirements in maple syrup urine disease (MSUD) [45] and PKU [46].

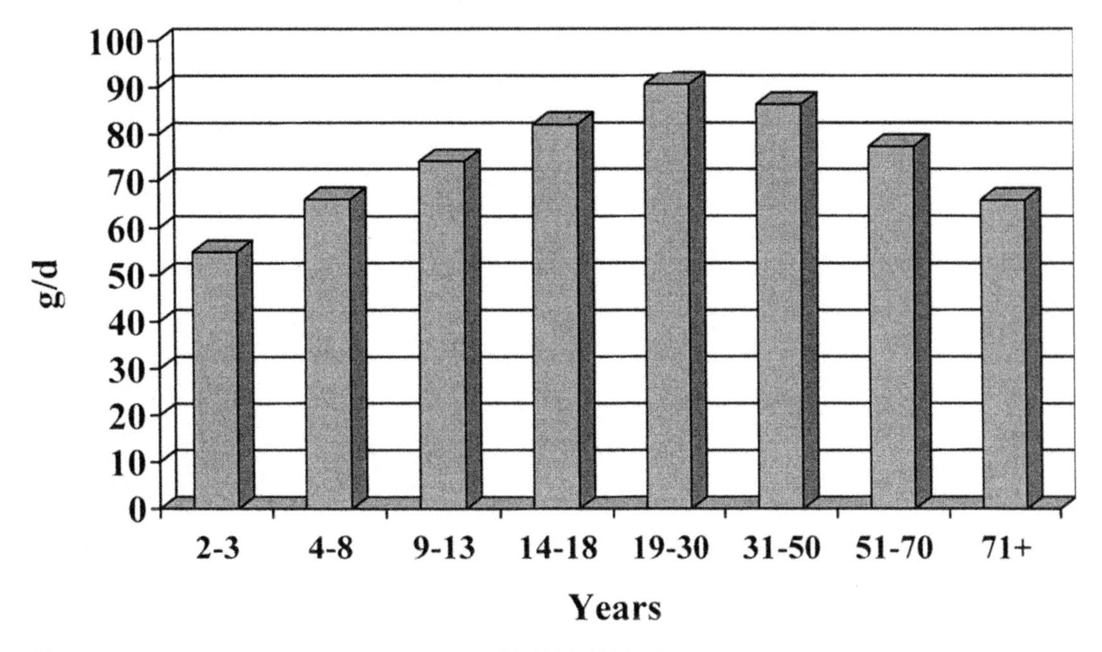

Fig. 6.4 Daily protein intake (g/d) by age – NHANES, 2003–2004 [47]

Variability in protein recommendations among different countries and within countries indicates that recommendations continue to evolve based on research and understanding of needs [47–49]. Figure 6.4 shows that actual protein intake in the United States is greater than current recommended intakes.

6.6 Protein Requirements in Inherited Metabolic Diseases

For patients with metabolic disorders requiring amino-acid-based medical foods, the RDA may not be the best indicator for protein adequacy because the nitrogen balance studies used to establish these requirements are based on healthy individuals with free access to foods. The optimal amount of protein to provide patients with metabolic disorders is not well established. Comparing the FAO/WHO protein recommendations to a standard protocol often used by metabolic dietitians [50], a significant variance can be observed in patients with phenylketonuria (PKU) [51]. For example, currently, the FAO/WHO recommendation for infants is 0.9 g protein/kg versus the updated guidelines for PKU that recommend an intake of 2.5–3.5 g protein/kg [52, 53]. FAO/WHO recommendations, like the US RDA, reflect the consumption of high biological value protein sources and not amino-acid-based formulas. In one example, infants with PKU were fed two amino-acid-based formulas, one with slightly lower protein equivalents (2.74 g/100 kcal) than the other formula (3.12 g/100 kcal). Protein content of both formulas was significantly higher than the Infant Formula Act guidelines of 1.7 g/100 kcal. After 6 months, the infants receiving the higher protein formula showed significantly greater weight, length, and head circumference and improved tolerance (38%) to restricted dietary phenylalanine [54].

Using the IAAO method, protein recommendation in children with mild PKU may be higher than current recommendations [55]. Turki and associates reported that for 6- to 18-year-old children, protein requirement may be as high as 1.85 g total protein/kg/day, or approximately 19% of total energy from protein [55], which is higher than current recommendations for patients with PKU [53]. Protein requirements will be influenced by the heterogeneity of possible variants in the PKU gene causing severe versus mild forms of the disease.

Normal growth acceleration and protein status indices were reported in infants and toddlers with organic acidemias treated for 56 months with an amino-acid-based medical food [56]. Subjects with normal linear growth consumed nearly 120% of the FAO/WHO protein requirements and slightly less than 100% of recommended energy. However, despite normal linear growth and protein status indices, plasma isoleucine and valine remained significantly below normal reference values. When comparing protein and energy intake in patients with propionic acidemia who were growing adequately versus those who suffered from poor growth, it was shown that higher protein intakes from both intact protein and amino-acid-based formulas were beneficial [56, 57].

In patients with metabolic disorders, adequate protein and indispensable amino acid intakes are needed to promote anabolism, prevent protein and amino acid insufficiency, and promote normal growth and development. Risk of protein overrestriction is a serious concern and can lead to protein-energy malnutrition and poor growth [57–62]. In patients with urea cycle disorders, overrestriction of protein can result in higher serum ammonia concentrations compared to patients consuming too much dietary protein. In contrast, too much intact protein may be contraindicated and result in metabolic decomposition.

Historically, in the United States, the recommended protein intakes for infants with PKU and other inborn errors of metabolism ranged from 3.0 to 3.5 g/kg body weight or higher [51, 52], which is significantly greater than the DRI for age [20]. These higher recommended intakes may not be fully supported by some practicing metabolic clinicians. Van Rijn et al. measured whole body protein metabolism in healthy adults with PKU compared to healthy adult controls. Using primed-continuous infusion methods with [1-^{13}C] valine, whole body protein metabolism in PKU adults was not significantly different from healthy controls when given the RDA for protein [44]. The nutrition guidelines for PKU developed by Genetic Metabolic Dietitians International (GMDI) (www.gmdi.org) and the Southeast Regional Screening and Genetics Network (SERN) (www.southeastgenetics.org) recommend protein intakes closer to the RDA with an added safety factor of 120–140% [53]. The new recommended intakes for infants are more in line with Dutch guidelines (unpublished data, 2009) of 2.5 g protein/kg body weight [52, 53] (Table 6.2).

Table 6.2 GMDI/SERN recommended intakes of phenylalanine, tyrosine, and protein for individuals with PKU [52, 53]

Age	Phenylalanine (mg/day)	Tyrosine (mg/day)	Protein[a] (g/kg)
Infants to < 4 years[b]			
0 to < 3 months[b,c]	130–430	1100–1300	3-3.5
3 to < 6 months[b]	135–400	1400–2100	3–3.5
6 to < 9 months[b]	145–370	2500–3000	2.5–3
9 to < 12 months[b]	135–330	2500–3000	2.5–3
1 to < 4 years[b,d]	200–320	2800–3500	≥30
>4 years to adults[e]	200–1100	4000–6000	120–140% RDA for age[f]

[a]Protein recommendations for individuals consuming phenylalanine-free amino-acid-based medical foods as part of their protein source

[b]Recommended intakes for infants and children <4 years of age are adapted from Acosta [51] and are for individuals with the classical form of phenylketonuria treated with a phenylalanine-restricted diet alone

[c]Phenylalanine requirements for premature infants with phenylketonuria may be higher

[d]Tolerance is usually stable by 2–5 years of age as phenylalanine requirements are based on a combination of size (increasing with age) and rate of growth (decreasing with age). For any individual, phenylalanine intake is adjusted based on frequent blood phenylalanine monitoring

[e]Adapted from van Spronsen et al. [63] Range of phenylalanine intake is for the entire spectrum of phenylketonuria (mild to classical)

[f]Recommended protein intake from hydrolyzed-protein medical food is greater than the RDA and necessary to support growth in individuals with phenylketonuria

In inherited metabolic diseases, not only is total protein a major consideration, but also the balance of individual amino acids. Excessive or imbalanced plasma amino acid concentrations negatively affect absorption, protein synthesis, and brain concentrations of indispensable amino acids. In PKU, high blood phenylalanine concen-

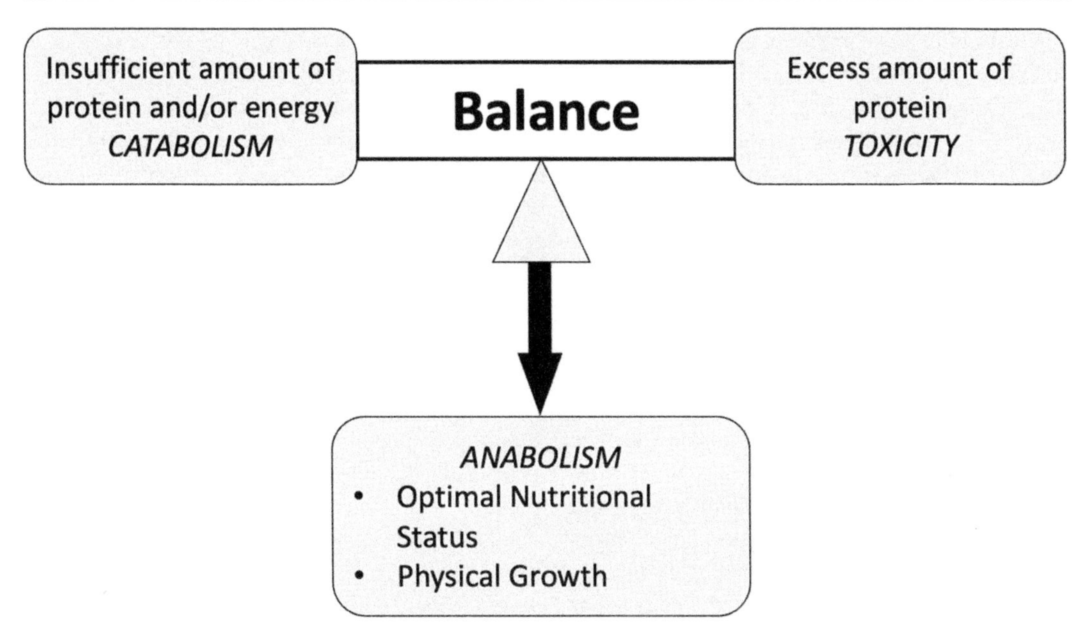

Fig. 6.5 Protein balance is obtained by providing sufficient protein and/or energy for anabolism while preventing excessive intake, which can result in toxicity

trations cause high phenylalanine concentrations in the brain [64, 65]. In organic acidemias and maple syrup urine disease (MSUD), imbalances in several or more indispensable amino acids can significantly affect protein synthesis (Fig. 6.5).

Providing sufficient protein and energy in patients with severe metabolic disorders, such as organic acidemias, can be a challenge in maintaining optimal nutrition status. Failure to thrive, anorexia, compromised immune functions, vomiting/diarrhea, and metabolic decompensation are not uncommon [58, 66]. Severe feeding difficulties are also common [66]. In patients with organic acidemias and urea cycle disorders, protein from both intact sources and amino acid–based medical foods must be carefully balanced. Both inadequate and excess dietary protein may contribute to metabolic decompensation. The exact amount of restricted indispensable amino acids and intact protein is determined by age, disease severity, blood analytes, and growth rate [58] (Table 6.3).

Quantifying an optimal protein: energy ratio (P:E) in inborn errors of metabolism has not been intensely studied. As a benchmark, the Infant Formula Act of 1980 mandated that standard

Table 6.3 Potential nutritional consequences of an imbalance or inadequacy of protein and/or energy intake

Protein and energy intakes	Possible effects
Adequate protein/ adequate energy	Normal growth
Adequate protein/ inadequate energy	Dietary protein used for energy rather than protein synthesis
	Adults: Loss of body protein
	Children: Suppressed growth
Inadequate protein/ adequate energy	Reduced body protein stores and weight loss
	Children: Suppressed growth
	Potential increased body fat
Inadequate protein/ inadequate energy	Weight loss or poor growth if too low
	"Adaptation" resulting in slow growth
Excessive protein/ adequate or inadequate energy	May impact bone health if too disproportionate
	Infants: Risk of metabolic and renal stress
	High protein/low CHO diets have benefits during weight loss
Excessive protein/ excessive energy	Overweight and obesity

Adapted from Humphrey et al. (2014) [49]

infant formula must contain a minimum of 1.8 g protein/100Kcal (7.2% of calories from protein) [67]. The goal of providing an adequate P:E ratio is to identify a safe minimum ratio for infant formula to support growth as observed in human milk–fed infants. The protein quality of the protein sources of infant formula needs to be considered. Hydrolysates and amino acid–based infant formulas contain >1.8 g protein/100 Kcal to adjust for digestibility and protein quality.

Consideration of using a P:E ratio rather than meeting recommendations for protein and energy alone may be a better approach to meet growth and nutrition goals in infants and children with compromised health status, including critically ill children. For example, infants and children with growth failure will require significantly higher protein than recommended intakes. For example, infants with growth failure require 9–12% of total energy as protein to support lean tissue gain [15]. Infant formulas for low birth-weight infants have considerably higher protein energy percentage (12%) compared to standard formulas (8%) [68].

One study in children with PKU reported that a P:E ratio of 3.0–4.5 g protein/100 kcal was associated with appropriate growth outcomes. In these same patients, a total-protein intake of 1.5–2.6 grams/kg/day (intact-protein >0.5 grams/kg/day) was associated with improved body composition [69]. In a separate study, intact protein rather than total protein (including medical food/protein substitutes) influenced head circumference but not linear growth in children with PKU [70]. As with all inborn errors of metabolism, maximizing intact protein to tolerance is a goal. Future prospective studies to identify disease-specific safe P:E ratios are warranted [49].

In patients with organic acidemias and urea cycle disorders, approximately 50% of total protein has historically been consumed as amino acid–based medical foods. The amount of total protein and percentage of amino acid–based medical foods is variable [56, 71] as are reported clinical outcomes based on dosage of amino acid–based medical foods. Touati et al. (2006) reported near-normal growth velocity in patients with propionic acidemia on diets containing total protein intakes lower than recommended [71]. The amount of whole protein consumed per age was 0.92 g/kg at age 3, 0.78 g/kg at age 6, and 0.77 g/kg at 11 years. After 3 years of age, most patients in this study received some amino acid–based medical foods. Most patients suffered from feeding disorders, and many were given nocturnal feedings.

6.6.1 Special Considerations in Protein Requirements

Medications as part of medical management may affect tolerance to both intact protein and amino acids. Administration of N-carbamylglutamate in patients with either propionic or methylmalonic acidemia resulted in increased intake of intact protein between 20% and 50% with gain in body weight [72]. In patients with PKU, it is a well-established that sapropterin can increase phenylalanine tolerance while maintaining plasma phenylalanine concentrations in recommended range [73].

Medications may also have an impact on plasma amino acid concentrations. In patients with a urea cycle disorder, administration of sodium phenylbutyrate can lead to depletion of the branched-chain amino acids [74]. Intervention with either increasing intact protein – if tolerated – or supplementation with L-amino acids or medical foods as a source of branched-chain amino acids will be required to prevent long-term effects of deficiency and promote protein synthesis.

The need for additional protein in athletes with an inborn error of metabolism has not been extensively studied. The need for additional protein in athletes in general is still controversial [75]. Currently, researchers involved in establishing dietary guidelines have not identified that athletes or individuals engaging in regular physical activity require significantly more protein than those who are sedentary. In strength-trained athletes, there is no concrete evidence to suggest a benefit of additional protein, and an intake consistent with the general protein guidelines ranging from 12% to15% of total energy is recommended [76]. Suggested protein intake in endurance athletes is between 1.2 and 1.4 g/kg/day, and slightly higher, between 1.2 and 1.7 g/

kg/d, in strength athletes. More recently, researchers used the IAAO method to assess protein requirements in male endurance athletes: they reported a higher estimated adequate requirement of 2.1 g/kg/day [77].

A series of case studies in individuals with PKU with an active exercise regimen showed no effect of exercise on blood phenylalanine concentrations [78]. Mazzola and colleagues also reported a lack of correlation of acute exercise and blood phenylalanine concentrations in nine adults with PKU [79].

Dietary suggestions to support active patients with PKU indicate the importance of maintaining a high carbohydrate intake, need for adequate hydration, and providing medical food (protein substitute) immediately postexercise [78].

Anecdotally, increased intake in protein from either intact protein and/or medical foods has been suggested. The author of this chapter noted a significant increase in both protein and energy requirement in a competitive female swimmer with PKU, along with improved tolerance to phenylalanine. When medical food was reduced, plasma phenylalanine concentrations increased, but decreased again when additional medical food was reintroduced. Appropriate energy intake is a major factor in athletes because it supports optimal function. Factors influencing the need for increased energy are dependent on several factors including level of intensity, duration, frequency, and degree of training.

The benefits of physical activity in individuals with inherited metabolic diseases are the same as the general population, including bone health, cardiovascular benefits, building lean body mass, and maintaining mobility. In a study of 59 children and 27 adults, Jani and peers reported that physical activity and protein intake can influence body mass in individuals with PKU [80] . In adult patients, higher intact protein intake was associated with higher fat-free mass, and in children, medical food intake was directly proportional to fat-free mass. The level of activity was associated with fat-free mass in adults. In children, light activity was associated with higher fat mass compared to intense activity. These results demonstrate the importance of maximizing total and intact protein intake, as tolerated, to support lean body mass in individuals with PKU [80].

6.7 Medical Foods/Protein Supplements in Management of Aminoacidopathies, Organic Acidemias, and Urea Cycle Disorders

Medical Foods, also known as "food for special medical purposes" outside the United States, are an integral part of a number of inherited metabolic diseases. Medical foods are defined by Section 5(b) of the Orphan Drug Act (1983) as "*A food formulated to be consumed or administered enterally under the supervision of a physician, and which is intended for the specific dietary management of a disease or condition for which distinctive nutritional requirements, based on recognized scientific principles, are established by medical evaluation.*" Medical foods for infants are defined as "exempt infant formula". By definition, exempt infant formula "*…is an infant formula intended for commercial or charitable distribution that is represented and labeled for use by infants who have inborn errors of metabolism or low birth weight, or who otherwise have unusual medical or dietary problems* "(21 CFR 107.3). Medical foods are NOT dietary supplements which are defined as "products taken by mouth that contain a dietary ingredient that is intended to supplement the diet."

In 1958, "Lofenalac®" (Mead Johnson Nutritionals, Evansville, IN), a powdered infant formula with iron, low phenylalanine, casein enzymatic hydrolysate for individuals with PKU, was introduced. Lofenalac was the predecessor to current medical foods and exempt infant formulas. There are currently over 200 medical foods sold in the United States. Medical foods come in many forms and flavors, including powders, liquids, and capsules with varying nutrient profiles. Some medical foods are more nutritionally adequate than others, containing a full profile of macro- and micronutrients to meet a person's needs based on age and prescribed usage. Medical foods may be more modular with little to no micronutrients.

Medical foods for inherited metabolic diseases where an essential nutrient is removed (e.g., phenylalanine for PKU) are not nutritionally complete and should not be used as the sole source of nutrition. Providing medical foods as a sole source of nutrition for disorders where a specific essential nutrient(s) is either removed, or in such small amounts as to not meet recommended intakes for age, can result in severe nutrient deficiency and significant growth failure. By definition, medical foods are to be used only under close medical supervision. Monitoring nutritional adequacy, including selected micronutrients, is indispensable. Use of medical foods must always be under strict medical supervision.

Prescribing the adequate amount of medical food as part of nutrition management in disorders requiring modification in either total protein (e.g., urea cycle disorders), or restriction of specific amino acids (e.g., PKU, MSUD, propionic acidemia), is dependent on age, disease severity, total protein requirements, and tolerance to restricted amounts of intact protein. Medical foods for these disorders function as a source of elemental amino acids providing "protein equivalents," containing either none, or little of the restricted amino acid(s), in addition to energy and micronutrients. For patients with low tolerance to intact protein, the range of medical foods prescribed as part of total protein can range widely from as little as 21% in propionic acidemia [81] to approximately 80% for those with severe PKU (nonsapropterin responders). A survey of European clinics managing patients with urea cycle disorders reported the percentage of medical foods as part of total protein ranged from 45% in infants <6 months of age to 16% (range 10–20%) in patients over 16 years of age [82].

Use of medical foods in management of organic acidemias and urea cycle disorders is not unanimously applied in clinical practice [71, 83, 84]. Evidence shows that proper use of medical food in nutrition management can result in positive clinical outcomes in patients with propionic acidemia and urea cycle disorders [56, 85, 86]. In some patients with organic acidemias, positive clinical outcomes have been reported with little-to-no medical foods, depending on disease severity. Luder and colleagues (1989) reported normal growth and development in an infant with severe propionic acidemia on an unrestricted diet [87].

A case study of a 13- to 17-month-old patient with tyrosinemia type 1 (treated with NTBC), managed only on a low intact protein diet (0.9–1.0 g/kg/day), revealed elevated plasma tyrosine+phenylalanine, with poor appetite and growth. Introduction of medical food at 17 months of age (total protein 1.8–2.3 grams/kg/day with 0.8 grams/kg/day from medical food) resulted in normalized weight with subsequent reduction in plasma tyrosine+phenylalanine concentrations [88].

Historically, and especially in organic acidemias and urea cycle disorders, clinicians would initiate a diet plan using approximately 50% medical food and 50% intact protein, depending on age, genotype, disease severity, and absence or presence of comorbidities. With careful and constant monitoring, these ratios would necessitate modification to assure appropriate growth, development, and nutrient status, including review of protein status indices. Guidelines for calculating the optimal amount of intact protein include titrating to 100–120% of either FAO/WHO/UNU or RDA recommendations for age [89–92]. If tolerance to intact protein is below the recommended range for age, then medical food should be added to provide additional protein equivalents to support nitrogen balance and protein synthesis.

Balancing medical foods and titrating intact protein to optimal levels in patients with organic acidemias is a challenge. Quantifying the right balance between intact protein required for growth and development while averting toxicity is complicated and can lead to imbalanced use of medical foods [93]. Several reasons for possible overprescription of medical foods and challenges to optimizing intact protein include episodic acute illnesses during early childhood, imprecise causal relationship of bioanalytes with diet composition, diet adherence, and feeding difficulties. In severe metabolic disorders, intermittent illnesses often require reduction or removal of intact protein to reduce risk of toxicity. In response, medical foods are often continued as sources of nitrogen (without offending amino acids), energy, macronutrients, and micronutrients. Since the transition back to the patient's usual diet after an illness may be slow, reliance on medical food as the main source of protein equivalents continues. Families who have children with chronic intermittent illness and who are managed at home may improperly dilute the formula mixture for extended periods of time, further exacerbating the imbalance of intact protein and medical food. Frequent communication with families and reassessment of the diet regimen, assuring that adequate intact protein is consumed, is paramount.

Overprescription of medical foods can alter serum amino acid concentrations in patients with organic acidemias [93–95]. In 2016, Manoli and peers reported that reduction in disease-specific medical foods and increase in intact protein significantly and positively improved the ratio of serum branched-chain amino acids in patients with methylmalonic acidemia and cobalamin C disease. Bernstein and others (2020) reported similar findings along with normalization of serum isoleucine and valine concentrations allowing for reduction in the need for additional isoleucine and valine supplements [95]. Optimizing intact protein by improving the protein: energy ratio has been shown to positively impact height z-score in patients with either methylmalonic or propionic acidemia, or urea cycle disorder [96].

Patients with severe phenotypes of either PKU (sapropterin nonresponsive) or MSUD will require a significant percentage of total protein from medical food. For patients with inborn errors of metabolism who are prescribed only low/moderate intact protein diets without medical food require vigilance to assure that adequate nonprotein energy is given to support protein synthesis, growth, and development. The quality of the diet must also be assessed as patients will often avoid high biological value sources of protein. Consequently, patients may not consume sufficient quantities of vitamin B_{12} given the primary source of this vitamin is animal protein. Supplementation of other vitamins and minerals, especially calcium and vitamin D, may be required to maintain normal nutrient status (Box 6.1).

Box 6.1: Tips for Using Medical foods/Protein Substitutes

- Provide sufficient medical food to meet total protein intake requirements for age based on tolerance to intact protein.
- Do not overprescribe medical foods.
- Individualize medical food requirements for each patient based on disease severity, age, protein, and energy requirements.
- Provide intact protein along with medical food to supply all essential amino acids needed to promote protein synthesis throughout the day.
- Provide sufficient energy from medical food and foods to support optimal use of amino acids for protein accretion rather than as an energy source.
- Closely monitor patient sustainability (adherence) to medical foods. Patients should consume entire volume of medical food each day.

6.8 Assessing Protein Sufficiency and Plasma Amino Acids

Protein status can be assessed by several biomarkers, including plasma amino acid profiles, and transthyretin (prealbumin) [53]. No marker alone is sufficient to determine protein status (Box 6.2).

For patients with inborn errors of metabolism, plasma amino acid profiles are important biomarkers necessary to prevent toxicity or deficiency of any indispensable amino acid. Routine assessment is recommended, with more frequent measurement recommended during times of metabolic crisis or rapid periods of growth. However, plasma amino acid profiles measure immediate dietary protein intake and protein status may be difficult to assess without using additional bio-

Box 6.2: Assessing Protein Sufficiency

- Biochemical
  - Plasma amino acids
  - Prealbumin (48 h half-life)
- Blood urea nitrogen
- Anthropometrics (length, height, weight, head circumference)
- Nutrition-focused physical findings
  - Hair (loss of pigment, alopecia, dull, dry, brittle)
  - Muscle wasting (interosseous muscle, clavicle, biceps/triceps)
  - Poor healing (e.g., severe diaper rash in infants)

markers [97]. Transthyretin (prealbumin) is a protein marker reflecting short-term changes in protein status; however, the inflammation that is associated with illness causes the concentration of prealbumin to be lower than would be seen in a healthy state [98]. In PKU, prealbumin can be an important biomarker for evaluating protein status [99]. Low concentrations of prealbumin have been reported in treated patients with PKU [99] and may be inversely related to linear growth in protein-insufficient patients with PKU [100].

Protein insufficiency may result in poor growth, hair loss, muscle wasting, and bone demineralization. Many of these signs and symptoms have been reported in treated patients with various metabolic disorders, especially in those with severe genotypes [57, 101]. In certain patients with inherited metabolic diseases, the increased risk of infections, anorexia, and frequent acute metabolic crises make it difficult to provide sufficient nutrients to promote growth and support good nutritional status. The impact of clinical comorbidities that may affect plasma amino acid concentrations should be assessed. Plasma amino acids may be affected by, but not limited to, chronic liver failure [102, 103], renal failure [104], and preprandial meal composition. In adults with liver-induced encephalopathy and/or cirrhosis, elevations in plasma aromatic amino acids and decreases in branched-chain amino acids have been reported [102]. In children with end-stage liver disease awaiting organ liver transplantation, supplementation with branched-chain amino acids showed improved nutrition status [105]. Mager and others reported higher requirements for branched-chain amino acids in children with chronic cholestatic liver disease compared to healthy children [106].

Patients with inborn errors of metabolism and end-stage renal disease may be at risk for malnutrition. In adults undergoing hemodialysis, a significant negative effect on plasma amino acid concentrations was reported [107]. Hendriks and others reported a loss of nearly 12.0 grams of amino acids into dialysate, of which 3.69 grams were indispensable amino acids and 1.64 grams were branched -chain amino acids, resulting in significant reduction in plasma concentrations of these amino acids. For patients with inherited metabolic diseases, it is vital to carefully monitor plasma amino acid status in patients undergoing acute or chronic hemodialysis and provide sufficient intact protein sources to prevent deficiency.

Using fasting versus 2- to 4-hour postprandial blood draws when assessing plasma amino acid concentrations has been an ongoing discussion for many years. A report from the European Prospective Investigation into Cancer and Nutrition (EPIC study) did not find statistical difference in fasting versus nonfasting amino acids when measured reliability over a 2 year period [108]. The difference in fasting versus nonfasting for some of the plasma amino acids might be significant to those with an inborn error of metabolism. However, in clinical management of patients, it is important to use only one method for each patient to assure reliability over time.

In patients with restriction in intact protein, it is important to assess actual intake before making any dietary adjustments. Clinicians must not assume that recommendations for total intact protein are adhered to, especially in conditions like urea cycle disorders where patients may have an aversion to protein intake. Boneh and peers reported a significant decrease in intake of both protein and energy (24-hour recall) compared to prescription [109]. A similar, but less significant, decrease in actual intake compared to prescribed protein and energy was shown in adult females with UCD [110].

6.9 Summary

In summary, to achieve optimal growth and development in inherited metabolic diseases, total protein recommendations are higher than DRI requirements when the majority of protein is provided by amino acid–based medical foods. To maintain balanced amino acid profiles and nitrogen retention for growth, patients who are dependent on amino acid–based medical foods should consume greater amounts of protein and calories than standard recommendations and protein synthesis is optimized if medical food is distributed evenly throughout the day. Numerous studies have found reduced nitrogen retention, reduced protein synthesis, and increased digestion rate and oxidation of free amino acids compared to intact protein sources provide evidence that those with metabolic disorders require a greater total protein intake than established recommendations for the normal populace. Attention to assessing protein status and supplying adequate protein is paramount to support adequate growth and reduce comorbidities.

References

1. Neelima SR, Rajput YS, Mann B. Chemical and functional properties of glycomacropeptide (GMP) and its role in the detection of cheese whey adulteration in milk: a review. Dairy Sci Technol. 2013;93(1):21–43.
2. Fouillet H, Mariotti F, Gaudichon C, Bos C, Tome D. Peripheral and splanchnic metabolism of dietary nitrogen are differently affected by the protein source in humans as assessed by compartmental modeling. J Nutr. 2001;132(1):125–33.
3. Boirie Y, Dangin M, Gachon P, Vasson MP, Maubois JL, Beaufrere B. Slow and fast dietary proteins differently modulate postprandial protein accretion. Proc Natl Acad Sci U S A. 1997;94(26):14930–5.
4. Luiking YC, Deutz NE, Jakel M, Soeters PB. Casein and soy protein meals differentially affect whole-body and splanchnic protein metabolism in healthy humans. J Nutr. 2005;135(5):1080–7.
5. Dangin M, Boirie Y, Garcia-Rodenas C, Gachon P, Fauquant J, Callier P, et al. The digestion rate of protein is an independent regulating factor of postprandial protein retention. Am J Physiol Endocrinol Metab. 2001;280(2):E340–8.
6. Daenzer M, Petzke KJ, Bequette BJ, Metges CC. Whole-body nitrogen and splanchnic amino acid metabolism differ in rats fed mixed diets containing casein or its corresponding amino acid mixture. J Nutr. 2001;131(7):1965–72.
7. Monchi M, Rerat AA. Comparison of net protein utilization of milk protein mild enzymatic hydrolysates and free amino acid mixtures with a close pattern in the rat. JPEN J Parenter Enteral Nutr. 1993;17(4):355–63.
8. Allen JR, Baur LA, Waters DL, Humphries IR, Allen BJ, Roberts DC, et al. Body protein in prepubertal children with phenylketonuria. Eur J Clin Nutr. 1996;50(3):178–86.
9. Jones BJ, Lees R, Andrews J, Frost P, Silk DB. Comparison of an elemental and polymeric enteral diet in patients with normal gastrointestinal function. Gut. 1983;24(1):78–84.
10. Gropper SS, Acosta PB. Effect of simultaneous ingestion of L-amino acids and whole protein on plasma amino acid and urea nitrogen concentrations in humans. JPEN J Parenter Enteral Nutr. 1991;15(1):48–53.
11. Herrmann ME, Brosicke HG, Keller M, Monch E, Helge H. Dependence of the utilization of a phenylalanine-free amino acid mixture on different amounts of single dose ingested. A case report. Eur J Pediatr. 1994;153(7):501–3.
12. Pennings B, Boirie Y, Senden JM, Gijsen AP, Kuipers H, van Loon LJ. Whey protein stimulates postprandial muscle protein accretion more effectively than do casein and casein hydrolysate in older men. Am J Clin Nutr. 2011;93(5):997–1005.
13. Burks W, Jones SM, Berseth CL, Harris C, Sampson HA, Scalabrin DM. Hypoallergenicity and effects on growth and tolerance of a new amino acid-based formula with docosahexaenoic acid and arachidonic acid. J Pediatr. 2008;153(2):266–71.
14. Aggett PJ, Bresson J, Haschke F, Hernell O, Koletzko B, Lafeber HN, et al. Recommended dietary allowances (RDAs), recommended dietary intakes (RDIs), recommended nutrient intakes (RNIs), and population reference intakes (PRIs) are not "recommended intakes". J Pediatr Gastroenterol Nutr. 1997;25(2):236–41.
15. Joint WHO, FAO UNU. Expert consultation. Protein and amino acid requirements in human nutrition. World Health Organ Tech Rep Ser. 2007;935:1–265.
16. Ten Have GA, Engelen MP, Luiking YC, Deutz NE. Absorption kinetics of amino acids, peptides, and intact proteins. Int J Sport Nutr Exerc Metab. 2007;17(Suppl):S23–36.
17. Waterlow JC. Protein turnover with special reference to man. Q J Exp Physiol. 1984;69(3):409–38.
18. Young VR, Steffee WP, Pencharz PB, Winterer JC, Scrimshaw NS. Total human body protein synthesis in relation to protein requirements at various ages. Nature. 1975;253(5488):192–4.
19. Butte NF, Hopkinson JM, Wong WW, Smith EO, Ellis KJ. Body composition during the first 2 years of life: an updated reference. Pediatr Res. 2000;47(5):578–85.

20. Trumbo P, Schlicker S, Yates AA, Poos M. Food, Nutrition Board of the Institute of Medicine TNA. Dietary reference intakes for energy, carbohydrate, fiber, fat, fatty acids, cholesterol, protein and amino acids. J Am Diet Assoc. 2002;102(11):1621–30.
21. Borsheim E, Tipton KD, Wolf SE, Wolfe RR. Essential amino acids and muscle protein recovery from resistance exercise. Am J Physiol Endocrinol Metab. 2002;283(4):E648–57.
22. Wilson J, Wilson GJ. Contemporary issues in protein requirements and consumption for resistance trained athletes. J Int Soc Sports Nutr. 2006;3:7–27.
23. Institute of Medicine Food and Nutrition Board. Dietary reference intakes for energy, carbohydrate, fiber, fat, fatty acids, cholesterol, protein and amino acids. Washington, DC: N.A. Press; 2002.
24. Anthony JC, Anthony TG, Kimball SR, Jefferson LS. Signaling pathways involved in translational control of protein synthesis in skeletal muscle by leucine. J Nutr. 2001;131(3):856S–60S.
25. Koopman R, Wagenmakers AJ, Manders RJ, Zorenc AH, Senden JM, Gorselink M, et al. Combined ingestion of protein and free leucine with carbohydrate increases postexercise muscle protein synthesis in vivo in male subjects. Am J Physiol Endocrinol Metab. 2005;288(4):E645–53.
26. Mariotti F, Mahe S, Luengo C, Benamouzig R, Tome D. Postprandial modulation of dietary and whole-body nitrogen utilization by carbohydrates in humans. Am J Clin Nutr. 2000;72(4):954–62.
27. Gaudichon C, Mahe S, Benamouzig R, Luengo C, Fouillet H, Dare S, et al. Net postprandial utilization of [15N]-labeled milk protein nitrogen is influenced by diet composition in humans. J Nutr. 1999;129(4):890–5.
28. Welle S, Matthews DE, Campbell RG, Nair KS. Stimulation of protein turnover by carbohydrate overfeeding in men. Am J Phys. 1989;257(3 Pt 1): E413–7.
29. Pratt EL, Snyderman SE, Cheung MW, Norton P, Holt LE Jr, Hansen AE, et al. The threonine requirement of the normal infant. J Nutr. 1955;56(2):231–51.
30. Rose WC, Wixom RL. The amino acid requirements of man. XIV. The sparing effect of tyrosine on the phenylalanine requirement. J Biol Chem. 1955;217(1):95–101.
31. Thomas JA, Bernstein LE, Greene CL, Koeller DM. Apparent decreased energy requirements in children with organic acidemias: preliminary observations. J Am Diet Assoc. 2000;100(9):1074–6.
32. Layman DK. Dietary guidelines should reflect new understandings about adult protein needs. Nutr Metab (Lond). 2009;6:12.
33. Mamerow MM, Mettler JA, English KL, Casperson SL, Arentson-Lantz E, Sheffield-Moore M, et al. Dietary protein distribution positively influences 24-h muscle protein synthesis in healthy adults. J Nutr. 2014;144(6):876–80.
34. MacDonald A, Rylance G, Davies P, Asplin D, Hall SK, Booth IW. Administration of protein substitute and quality of control in phenylketonuria: a randomized study. J Inherit Metab Dis. 2003;26(4):319–26.
35. Paddon-Jones D, Rasmussen BB. Dietary protein recommendations and the prevention of sarcopenia. Curr Opin Clin Nutr Metab Care. 2009;12(1):86–90.
36. Paddon-Jones D, Leidy H. Dietary protein and muscle in older persons. Curr Opin Clin Nutr Metab Care. 2014;17(1):5–11.
37. MacDonald A, Rylance G, Hall SK, Asplin D, Booth IW. Factors affecting the variation in plasma phenylalanine in patients with phenylketonuria on diet. Arch Dis Child. 1996;74(5):412–7.
38. Acosta PB. Recommendations for protein and energy intakes by patients with phenylketonuria. Eur J Pediatr. 1996;155(Suppl 1):S121–4.
39. Metges CC, El-Khoury AE, Selvaraj AB, Tsay RH, Atkinson A, Regan MM, et al. Kinetics of L-[1-(13) C]leucine when ingested with free amino acids, unlabeled or intrinsically labeled casein. Am J Physiol Endocrinol Metab. 2000;278(6):E1000–9.
40. Elango R, Ball RO, Pencharz PB. Indicator amino acid oxidation: concept and application. J Nutr. 2008;138(2):243–6.
41. Elango R, Ball RO, Pencharz PB. Recent advances in determining protein and amino acid requirements in humans. Br J Nutr. 2012;108(Suppl 2):S22–30.
42. Humayun MA, Elango R, Ball RO, Pencharz PB. Reevaluation of the protein requirement in young men with the indicator amino acid oxidation technique. Am J Clin Nutr. 2007;86(4):995–1002.
43. Elango R, Humayun MA, Ball RO, Pencharz PB. Protein requirement of healthy school-age children determined by the indicator amino acid oxidation method. Am J Clin Nutr. 2011;94(6):1545–52.
44. van Rijn M, Hoeksma M, Sauer P, Szczerbak B, Gross M, Reijngoud DJ, et al. Protein metabolism in adult patients with phenylketonuria. Nutrition. 2007;23(6):445–53.
45. Riazi R, Rafii M, Clarke JT, Wykes LJ, Ball RO, Pencharz PB. Total branched-chain amino acids requirement in patients with maple syrup urine disease by use of indicator amino acid oxidation with L-[1-13C]phenylalanine. Am J Physiol Endocrinol Metab. 2004;287(1):E142–9.
46. Courtney-Martin G, Bross R, Raffi M, Clarke JT, Ball RO, Pencharz PB. Phenylalanine requirement in children with classical PKU determined by indicator amino acid oxidation. Am J Physiol Endocrinol Metab. 2002;283(6):E1249–56.
47. Fulgoni VL 3rd. Current protein intake in America: analysis of the National Health and Nutrition Examination Survey, 2003-2004. Am J Clin Nutr. 2008;87(5):1554S–7S.
48. Panel on Dietetic Products NaA. Scientific opinion on dietary reference values for protein. Eur Food Saf Authority. 2012;10(2):66.
49. Humphrey M, Truby H, Boneh A. New ways of defining protein and energy relationships in

inborn errors of metabolism. Mol Genet Metab. 2014;112(4):247–58.
50. Acosta PB. Nutrition management of patients with inherited metabolic disorders. Sudbury: Jones and Bartlett Publishers, LLC; 2010. 476 p.
51. Acosta PB, Yannicelli S. Nutrition protocols updated for the US. 4th ed. A. Laboratories: Columbus; 2001.
52. Vockley J, Andersson HC, Antshel KM, Braverman NE, Burton BK, Frazier DM, et al. Phenylalanine hydroxylase deficiency: diagnosis and management guideline. Genet Med. 2014;16(2):188–200.
53. Singh RH, Rohr F, Frazier D, Cunningham A, Mofidi S, Ogata B, et al. Recommendations for the nutrition management of phenylalanine hydroxylase deficiency. Genet Med. 2014;16(2):121–31.
54. Acosta PB, Yannicelli S. Protein intake affects phenylalanine requirements and growth of infants with phenylketonuria. Acta Paediatr Suppl. 1994;83:66–7.
55. Turki A, Ueda K, Cheng B, Giezen A, Salvarinova R, Stockler-Ipsiroglu S, et al. The indicator amino acid oxidation method with the use of l-[1-13C]leucine suggests a higher than currently recommended protein requirement in children with phenylketonuria. J Nutr. 2017;147(2):211–7.
56. Yannicelli S, Acosta PB, Velazquez A, Bock HG, Marriage B, Kurczynski TW, et al. Improved growth and nutrition status in children with methylmalonic or propionic acidemia fed an elemental medical food. Mol Genet Metab. 2003;80(1–2):181–8.
57. van der Meer SB, Poggi F, Spada M, Bonnefont JP, Ogier H, Hubert P, et al. Clinical outcome of long-term management of patients with vitamin B12-unresponsive methylmalonic acidemia. J Pediatr. 1994;125(6 Pt 1):903–8.
58. Yannicelli S. Nutrition therapy of organic acidaemias with amino acid-based formulas: emphasis on methylmalonic and propionic acidaemia. J Inherit Metab Dis. 2006;29(2–3):281–7.
59. Hanley WB, Linsao L, Davidson W, Moes CA. Malnutrition with early treatment of phenylketonuria. Pediatr Res. 1970;4(4):318–27.
60. Dhondt JL, Largilliere C, Moreno L, Farriaux JP. Physical growth in patients with phenylketonuria. J Inherit Metab Dis. 1995;18(2):135–7.
61. Verkerk PH, van Spronsen FJ, Smit GP, Sengers RC. Impaired prenatal and postnatal growth in Dutch patients with phenylketonuria. The National PKU Steering Committee. Arch Dis Child. 1994;71(2):114–8.
62. de Baulny HO, Benoist JF, Rigal O, Touati G, Rabier D, Saudubray JM. Methylmalonic and propionic acidaemias: management and outcome. J Inherit Metab Dis. 2005;28(3):415–23.
63. van Spronsen FJ, van Rijn M, Dorgelo B, Hoeksma M, Bosch AM, Mulder MF, et al. Phenylalanine tolerance can already reliably be assessed at the age of 2 years in patients with PKU. J Inherit Metab Dis. 2009;32(1):27–31.
64. Moller HE, Ullrich K, Weglage J. In vivo proton magnetic resonance spectroscopy in phenylketonuria. Eur J Pediatr. 2000;159(Suppl 2):S121–5.
65. Weglage J, Wiedermann D, Denecke J, Feldmann R, Koch HG, Ullrich K, et al. Individual blood-brain barrier phenylalanine transport in siblings with classical phenylketonuria. J Inherit Metab Dis. 2002;25(6):431–6.
66. Evans S, Alroqaiba N, Daly A, Neville C, Davies P, Macdonald A. Feeding difficulties in children with inherited metabolic disorders: a pilot study. J Hum Nutr Diet. 2012;25(3):209–16.
67. Newberry RE. Infant formula act of 1980. J Assoc Off Anal Chem. 1982;65(6):1472–3.
68. Pencharz PB. Protein and energy requirements for 'optimal' catch-up growth. Eur J Clin Nutr. 2010;64(Suppl 1):S5–7.
69. Evans M, Truby H, Boneh A. The relationship between dietary intake, growth and body composition in phenylketonuria. Mol Genet Metab. 2007;122(1–2):36–42.
70. Hoeksma M, Van Rijn M, Verkerk PH, Bosch AM, Mulder MF, de Klerk JB, et al. The intake of total protein, natural protein and protein substitute and growth of height and head circumference in Dutch infants with phenylketonuria. J Inherit Metab Dis. 2005;28(6):845–54.
71. Touati G, Valayannopoulos V, Mention K, de Lonlay P, Jouvet P, Depondt E, et al. Methylmalonic and propionic acidurias: management without or with a few supplements of specific amino acid mixture. J Inherit Metab Dis. 2006;29(2–3):288–98.
72. Burlina A, Cazzorla C, Zanonato E, Viggiano E, Fasan I, Polo G. Clinical experience with N-carbamylglutamate in a single-centre cohort of patients with propionic and methylmalonic aciduria. Mol Genet Metab Rep. 2016;8:34–40.
73. Trefz FK, Burton BK, Longo N, Casanova MM, Gruskin DJ, Dorenbaum A, et al. Efficacy of sapropterin dihydrochloride in increasing phenylalanine tolerance in children with phenylketonuria: a phase III, randomized, double-blind, placebo-controlled study. J Pediatr. 2009;154(5):700–7.
74. Scaglia F, Carter S, O'Brien WE, Lee B. Effect of alternative pathway therapy on branched chain amino acid metabolism in urea cycle disorder patients. Mol Genet Metab. 2004;81(Suppl 1):S79–85.
75. Phillips SM, Moore DR, Tang JE. A critical examination of dietary protein requirements, benefits, and excesses in athletes. Int J Sport Nutr Exerc Metab. 2007;17(Suppl):S58–76.
76. Phillips SM. Protein requirements and supplementation in strength sports. Nutrition. 2004;20(7–8):689–95.
77. Bandegan A, Courtney-Martin G, Rafii M, Pencharz PB, Lemon PWR. Indicator amino acid oxidation protein requirement estimate in endurance-trained men 24 h postexercise exceeds both the EAR and current athlete guidelines. Am J Physiol Endocrinol Metab. 2019;316(5):E741–E8.

78. Rocha JC, van Dam E, Ahring K, Almeida MF, Belanger-Quintana A, Dokoupil K, et al. A series of three case reports in patients with phenylketonuria performing regular exercise: first steps in dietary adjustment. J Pediatr Endocrinol Metab. 2019;32(6):635–41.
79. Mazzola PN, Teixeira BC, Schirmbeck GH, Reischak-Oliveira A, Derks TGJ, van Spronsen FJ, et al. Acute exercise in treated phenylketonuria patients: physical activity and biochemical response. Mol Genet Metab Rep. 2015;5:55–9.
80. Jani R, Coakley K, Douglas T, Singh R. Protein intake and physical activity are associated with body composition in individuals with phenylalanine hydroxylase deficiency. Mol Genet Metab. 2017;121(2):104–10.
81. Daly A, Pinto A, Evans S, Almeida MF, Assoun M, Belanger-Quintana A, et al. Dietary practices in propionic acidemia: a European survey. Mol Genet Metab Rep. 2017;13:83–9.
82. Adam S, Almeida MF, Assoun M, Baruteau J, Bernabei SM, Bigot S, et al. Dietary management of urea cycle disorders: European practice. Mol Genet Metab. 2013;110(4):439–45.
83. Walter JH, MacDonald A. The use of amino acid supplements in inherited metabolic disease. J Inherit Metab Dis. 2006;29(2–3):279–80.
84. Aguiar A, Ahring K, Almeida MF, Assoun M, Belanger Quintana A, Bigot S, et al. Practices in prescribing protein substitutes for PKU in Europe: no uniformity of approach. Mol Genet Metab. 2015;115(1):17–22.
85. Acosta PB, Yannicelli S, Ryan AS, Arnold G, Marriage BJ, Plewinska M, et al. Nutritional therapy improves growth and protein status of children with a urea cycle enzyme defect. Mol Genet Metab. 2005;86(4):448–55.
86. Singh RH. Nutritional management of patients with urea cycle disorders. J Inherit Metab Dis. 2007;30(6):880–7.
87. Luder AS, Yannicelli S, Green CL. Normal growth and development with unrestricted protein intake after severe infantile propionic acidaemia. J Inherit Metab Dis. 1989;12(3):307–11.
88. Shkurko T. Metabolic university. MetEd: Denver; 2020.
89. Baumgartner MR, Horster F, Dionisi-Vici C, Haliloglu G, Karall D, Chapman KA, et al. Proposed guidelines for the diagnosis and management of methylmalonic and propionic acidemia. Orphanet J Rare Dis. 2014;9:130.
90. Haberle J, Burlina A, Chakrapani A, Dixon M, Karall D, Lindner M, et al. Suggested guidelines for the diagnosis and management of urea cycle disorders: first revision. J Inherit Metab Dis. 2019;42(6):1192–230.
91. Jurecki E, Ueda K, Frazier D, Rohr F, Thompson A, Hussa C, et al. Nutrition management guideline for propionic acidemia: an evidence- and consensus-based approach. Mol Genet Metab. 2019;126(4):341–54.
92. Mobarak A, Dawoud H, Nofal H, Zoair A. Clinical course and nutritional management of propionic and methylmalonic acidemias. J Nutr Metab. 2020;2020:8489707.
93. Manoli I, Myles JG, Sloan JL, Carrillo-Carrasco N, Morava E, Strauss KA, et al. A critical reappraisal of dietary practices in methylmalonic acidemia raises concerns about the safety of medical foods. Part 2: cobalamin C deficiency. Genet Med. 2016;18(4):396–404.
94. Molema F, Gleich F, Burgard P, van der Ploeg AT, Summar ML, Chapman KA, et al. Evaluation of dietary treatment and amino acid supplementation in organic acidurias and urea-cycle disorders: on the basis of information from a European multicenter registry. J Inherit Metab Dis. 2019;42(6):1162–75.
95. Bernstein LE, Burns C, Drumm M, Gaughan S, Sailer M, Baker PR, 2nd. Impact on isoleucine and valine supplementation when decreasing use of medical food in the nutritional management of methylmalonic acidemia. Nutrients. 2020;12(2).
96. Molema F, Gleich F, Burgard P, van der Ploeg AT, Summar ML, Chapman KA, et al. Decreased plasma l-arginine levels in organic acidurias (MMA and PA) and decreased plasma branched-chain amino acid levels in urea cycle disorders as a potential cause of growth retardation: options for treatment. Mol Genet Metab. 2019;126(4):397–405.
97. Pencharz PB. Assessment of protein nutritional status in children. Pediatr Blood Cancer. 2008;50(2 Suppl):445–6. discussion 51
98. Evans DC, Corkins MR, Malone A, Miller S, Mogensen KM, Guenter P, et al. The use of visceral proteins as nutrition markers: an ASPEN position paper. Nutr Clin Pract. 2021;36(1):22–8.
99. Rocha JC, Almeida MF, Carmona C, Cardoso ML, Borges N, Soares I, et al. The use of prealbumin concentration as a biomarker of nutritional status in treated phenylketonuric patients. Ann Nutr Metab. 2010;56(3):207–11.
100. Arnold GL, Vladutiu CJ, Kirby RS, Blakely EM, Deluca JM. Protein insufficiency and linear growth restriction in phenylketonuria. J Pediatr. 2002;141(2):243–6.
101. Aldamiz-Echevarria L, Bueno MA, Couce ML, Lage S, Dalmau J, Vitoria I, et al. Anthropometric characteristics and nutrition in a cohort of PAH-deficient patients. Clin Nutr. 2014;33(4):702–17.
102. Dejong CH, van de Poll MC, Soeters PB, Jalan R, Olde Damink SW. Aromatic amino acid metabolism during liver failure. J Nutr. 2007;137(6 Suppl 1):1579S–85S; discussion 97S–98S
103. Rossi-Fanelli F, Angelico M, Cangiano C, Cascino A, Capocaccia R, DeConciliis D, et al. Effect of glucose and/or branched chain amino acid infusion on plasma amino acid imbalance in chronic liver failure. JPEN J Parenter Enteral Nutr. 1981;5(5):414–9.

104. Ceballos I, Chauveau P, Guerin V, Bardet J, Parvy P, Kamoun P, et al. Early alterations of plasma free amino acids in chronic renal failure. Clin Chim Acta. 1990;188(2):101–8.
105. Chin SE, Shepherd RW, Thomas BJ, Cleghorn GJ, Patrick MK, Wilcox JA, et al. Nutritional support in children with end-stage liver disease: a randomized crossover trial of a branched-chain amino acid supplement. Am J Clin Nutr. 1992;56(1):158–63.
106. Mager DR, Wykes LJ, Roberts EA, Ball RO, Pencharz PB. Mild-to-moderate chronic cholestatic liver disease increases leucine oxidation in children. J Nutr. 2006;136(4):965–70.
107. Hendriks FK, Smeets JSJ, Broers NJH, van Kranenburg JMX, van der Sande FM, Kooman JP, et al. End-stage renal disease patients lose a substantial amount of amino acids during hemodialysis. J Nutr. 2020;150(5):1160–6.
108. Carayol M, Licaj I, Achaintre D, Sacerdote C, Vineis P, Key TJ, et al. Reliability of serum metabolites over a two-year period: a targeted metabolomic approach in fasting and non-fasting Samples from EPIC. PLoS One. 2015;10(8):e0135437.
109. Boneh A. Dietary protein in urea cycle defects: how much? Which? How? Mol Genet Metab. 2014;113(1–2):109–12.
110. Hook D, Diaz GA, Lee B, Bartley J, Longo N, Berquist W, et al. Protein and calorie intakes in adult and pediatric subjects with urea cycle disorders participating in clinical trials of glycerol phenylbutyrate. Mol Genet Metab Rep. 2016;6:34–40.

7 Laboratory Evaluations in Inherited Metabolic Diseases

Curtis R. Coughlin II

Contents

C. R. Coughlin II (✉)
Clinical Genetics and Metabolism, Children's Hospital Colorado, University of Colorado Denver - Anschutz Medical Campus, Aurora, CO, USA
e-mail: curtis.coughlin@childrenscolorado.org

L. E. Bernstein et al. (eds.), *Nutrition Management of Inherited Metabolic Diseases*, https://doi.org/10.1007/978-3-030-94510-7_7

Core Messages

- Routine laboratory tests are commonly available and include electrolytes, ammonia, lactate, ketones, and carnitine; these are helpful in evaluating whether a patient may have a metabolic disorder.
- Metabolic laboratory tests are specialized tests that are reviewed by a biochemical geneticist and include amino acids, acylcarnitines, and organic acids that are helpful for pinpointing a metabolic diagnosis and/or monitoring treatment.
- Evaluation of laboratory findings should always include consideration of the patient's clinical status, such as presence of illness and length of fasting.

7.1 Background

Although individually rare, collectively, the incidence of inherited metabolic diseases is estimated at 1:2500 live births [1, 2]. The clinical presentation is often nonspecific and may be indistinguishable from more common findings such as sepsis [3]. Furthermore, the phenotype within a given disease can be heterogenous, making it difficult to establish a diagnosis for even the most experienced clinician. As a result, the ability to obtain various laboratory tests is crucial to establishing the diagnosis of an inherited metabolic disease.

In this chapter, the laboratory evaluations are separated into "routine laboratories," which refer to those tests available in most clinical laboratories, and "metabolic laboratories," which refer to those tests typically performed under the purview of a biochemical geneticist. This is an artificial separation for the benefit of the reader as often multiple laboratories are utilized for both the diagnosis and management of inherited metabolic diseases. The reader should use the information in this chapter, and the reference material within, to gain an understanding of the laboratories integral to working within the field of metabolism. The chapter will focus on laboratory tests used in the diagnosis of inherited metabolic disorders; many of these are also used for monitoring nutrition management and will be discussed in disease-specific nutrition management chapters.

7.2 Routine Laboratory Tests

The routine laboratories covered in this section are not unique to inherited metabolic diseases and are performed in most major medical centers. These laboratory studies provide valuable information to the clinician and can suggest a diagnosis of an inherited metabolic disease (Table 7.1). Also, the results of these laboratory tests may be available at the bedside or within a few hours and may guide the clinician in treating an acute episode before a specific diagnosis can be confirmed.

7.2.1 Acidosis

An acidosis refers to a disturbance of the patient's acid-base balance and infers that the pH is below that of blood's physiologic pH (7.4), with a pH <7.35 indicating acidemia and a pH >7.45 indicating alkalemia. When a metabolic acidosis is identified, an anion gap should be calculated to determine if an unmeasured anion (or acid) is present. The calculated anion gap is based upon an assumption that the values of the major cation (sodium) are relatively equal to that of the major anions (bicarbonate and chloride) [4]. Although other cations (potassium, calcium, magnesium) exist in blood, it is convenient to group these together and assume the variation among this unmeasured group is minimal. Therefore, the anion gap can be calculated by subtracting the major anions ($Cl^- + HCO_3^-$) from the major cation (Na^+). A normal anion gap should equal 12 ± 4 mEq/L.

A *non-anion gap acidosis* (hyperchloremic acidosis; anion gap <16 mEq/L) is characterized by an acidosis where the anion gap is unchanged from the patient's baseline. This occurs as the decrease in serum bicarbonate is equaled by the rise in serum chloride [5]. Bicarbonate is typically

Table 7.1 Routine laboratory studies and inherited metabolic diseases

Disorder	pH	Ammonia	Glucose	Ketonuria	Lactate	Other
Urea Cycle Disorder	↑	↑↑↑	Normal	Normal	Normal	Increased glutamine, orotic acid in some UCD
Organic Acidemias	↓↓↓	↑↑	↓ Normal	↑↑↑	↑↑	Anion gap, neutropenia, thrombocytopenia
MSUD	Normal	Normal	Normal	↓ Normal	Normal	
FOD	↓	↑	↓↓↓	↓↓↓	↑	Elevated CK, Transaminases
GSD	↓	Normal	↓↓↓	Normal	↑↑	Elevated triglyceride, uric acid and ALT
Mito Disorders	↓↓	Normal	Normal	Normal	↑↑↑	Increased lactate, pyruvate, alanine
Tyrosinemia	↓ Normal	Normal	↓ Normal	Normal	Normal	Liver failure, increased AFP, renal fanconi syndrome

lost from the gastrointestinal tract (i.e., diarrhea) or through the kidneys (i.e., renal tubular acidosis) [6]. Although a few metabolic disorders result in a non-anion gap acidosis (i.e., Fanconi-Bickel syndrome, OMIM# 227810), a non-anion gap acidosis is typically not the result of an inborn error of metabolism.

An *anion gap acidosis* (anion gap > 16 mEq/L) suggests an increase in unmeasured anions and a significantly elevated anion gap (>20 mEq/L) should always be evaluated further as there are no physiologic processes to generate unmeasured anions. An anion gap acidosis is highly suggestive of an inherited metabolic disease, although an anion gap acidosis may also be iatrogenic or the result of an ingestion, that is, overdose of salicylic acid (aspirin). Whenever an acidosis is identified, it is important to determine the presence or absence of an anion gap. After establishing the anion gap, relatively few tests are indicated in order to identify the cause of the acidosis (Fig. 7.1).

7.2.2 Ammonia

An elevated ammonia concentration can be the result of a primary or secondary defect of the urea cycle. Ammonia is mainly a by-product of amino acid metabolism, although it is also produced by intestinal urease-positive bacteria. The urea cycle converts ammonia (or ammonium, NH_4^+) to urea, which is excreted by the renal system to keep the serum concentration of ammonia low. An impairment of the urea cycle results in decreased excretion of urea and increased retention of ammonia. Hyperammonemia appears to be toxic to the central nervous system (CNS), and hyperammonemia may result in cognitive disabilities, seizures, cerebral palsy, and irreversible brain damage [7, 8]. The pathophysiology of hyperammonemia resulting in CNS damage is unclear. Glutamine accumulation, resulting in impaired cerebral osmoregulation or excitotoxic injury, or energy failure, may play a major role in the resultant cognitive impairments, although ammonia remains an important biomarker for diagnosis and a surrogate for both disease control and prognosis [9].

Primary urea cycle defects are caused by a deficiency of any of the six urea cycle enzymes (Chap. 16) and result in insufficient disposal of waste nitrogen. As a result, nitrogen accumulates in the form of ammonia and, as its precursors, glutamine and glycine. Primary defects in an enzyme of the urea cycle typically result in higher ammonia levels than secondary impairments of the urea cycle, although exceptions occur.

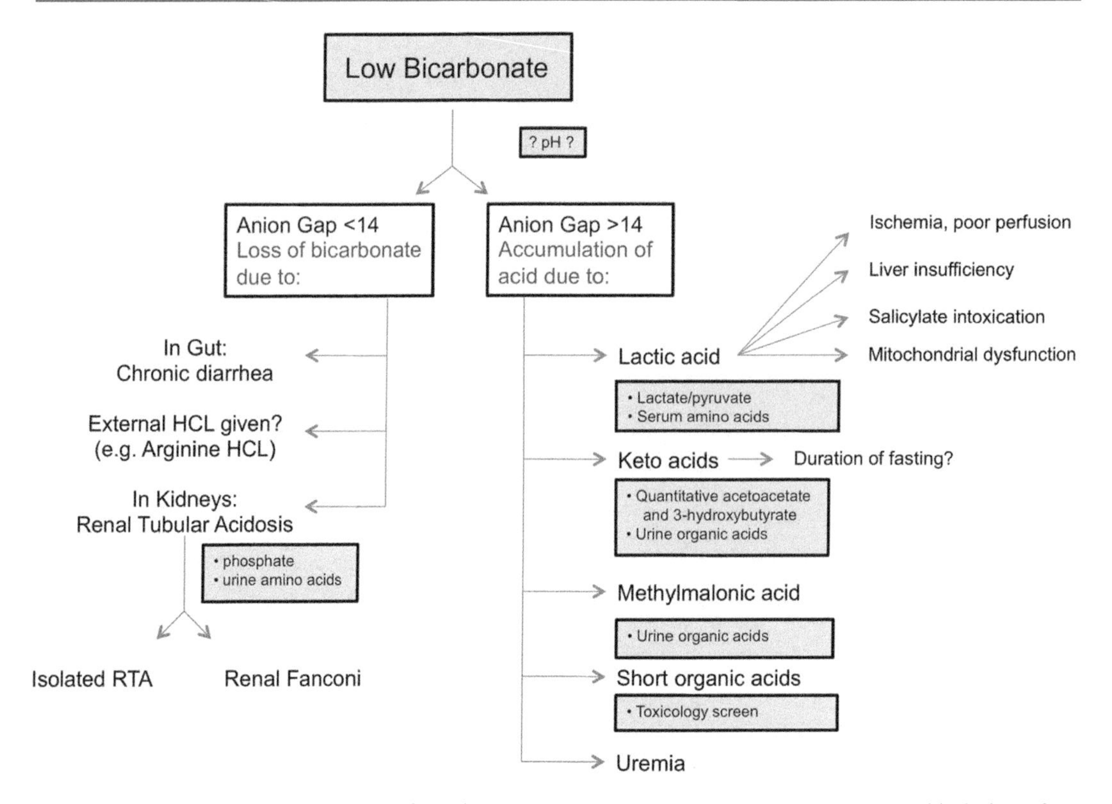

Fig. 7.1 Flow diagram for the evaluation of a patient with an acidosis due to low pH or an apparent acidosis due to low bicarbonate depending on the absence or presence of an anion gap

In secondary defects of the urea cycle, such as in disorders of organic acid and fatty acid metabolism, the buildup of toxic metabolites impairs the function of the urea cycle [10]. For example, propionyl-CoA, which accumulates in patients with propionic acidemia and methylmalonic acidemia, is hypothesized to competitively inhibit N-acetylglutamate synthetase, resulting in decreased activity of the urea cycle [11]. Hyperammonemia due to secondary defects is usually less severe than in primary defects and is often resolved by treating the underlying disorder. Ammonia scavengers, which are a standard therapy in primary urea cycle defects, may not be needed or be even dangerous in these disorders [12]. Hyperammonemia may be an underappreciated finding in fatty acid oxidation disorders and is the predominant biochemical finding in patients during an episode of metabolic decompensation [13].

It is important for the clinician to discern whether hyperammonemia is a result of a primary or secondary urea cycle defect in order to provide appropriate treatment. For example, the use of standard treatments for urea cycle disorders, such as Intralipid®, could be fatal if a patient had a fatty acid oxidation disorder. The clinical presentation and other laboratory studies may aid the clinician in discerning between various possible inherited metabolic diseases when elevated ammonia is identified (Appendix F).

Hyperammonemia may also result from congenital or acquired causes that are not related to inherited metabolic diseases. Examples of congenital causes include malformations such as portosystemic shunts, extrahepatic portal vein obstructions, and cirrhosis with portal hypertension [14, 15]. Transient hyperammonemia of the newborn (THAN) is typically identified in premature infants and does not appear to have a neurologic effect on those asymptomatic preterm infants [16]. Liver failure may also result in fulminant hyperammonemia. In severe liver failure, all of the enzymes expressed in the liver are deficient, resulting in complete impairment of the urea cycle as well as a deficiency of other important liver-specific enzymes such as the glycine cleavage enzyme [17, 18].

7.2.3 Glucose and Ketones

Hypoglycemia is a hallmark of disorders of energy metabolism, such as fatty acid oxidation disorders. Hypoglycemia is typically defined by blood glucose concentration below 55 mg/dL (3 mmol/L) in children and is often associated with clinical symptoms, such as shakiness, pale skin, sweating, confusion, and, in extreme cases, seizures and coma. Normally, as glycogen stores are depleted, beta-oxidation of fatty acids produces both glucose and ketones, with ketones being utilized preferentially over glucose in some tissues, including the brain [19].

Defects of fatty acid oxidation interfere with the production of ketones because of impaired beta-oxidation. Hypoglycemia results from excessive use of glucose by peripheral tissues and the inability to synthesize ketone bodies that can be used as alternative fuels [19]. Patients with fatty acid oxidation defects often have significant hypoketotic hypoglycemia, although it is important to note that there may be minimal ketone production, and, in rare circumstances, significant ketonuria. Patients with fatty acid oxidation disorders, even those with significant residual enzyme activity, can experience severe or fatal hypoglycemia in the setting of extreme fasting or a significant illness [20].

Glycogen storage diseases also present with hypoglycemia, but in contrast to disorders of fatty acid oxidation, relatively normal ketone production is noted. In general, hypoglycemia in these disorders is due to either the defects in the synthesis of liver glycogen (glycogen synthase deficiency) or defects in the metabolism of liver glycogen (glycogen storage).

Hypoglycemia is also a hallmark of inborn errors of ketogenesis and ketone body utilization. These disorders are typically characterized by metabolic decompensation with ketoacidosis [21]. Quantification of ketone bodies, such as acetoacetic acid and beta-hydroxy-butyric acid, is critical to understanding the etiology of hypoglycemia. Idiopathic ketotic hypoglycemia is a relatively common diagnosis in children with hypoglycemia and normal ketone production. Idiopathic ketotic hypoglycemia should only be considered when known causes of hypoglycemia have been reasonably excluded. Ketone production is a normal physiologic process that occurs when blood glucose is low. Obtaining a detailed history including the length of fasting [22, 23] as well as a physical exam to determine if there is hepatomegaly or cardiac involvement can help in understanding the cause of hypoglycemia (Fig. 7.2).

7.2.4 Lactate

Lactate exists as two stereoisomers, L-lactate and D-lactate, although L-lactate is the predominant physiologic anion and mainly discussed in the information below. The majority of plasma lactate is derived from glucose metabolism (65%) and amino acid metabolism through the degradation of alanine (15–20%) [24]. Lactic acidemia refers to blood lactate levels that are above those typically seen in blood (approximately <2.0 mM).

A lactic acidosis may result from increased lactate production, which is a by-product of compensatory mechanisms in disorders of energy metabolism. In defects of pyruvate metabolism, such as pyruvate dehydrogenase deficiency, glucose cannot enter the tricarboxylic acid (TCA) cycle and is diverted to glycolysis [25]. Similarly, in disorders of the mitochondrial respiratory chain, ATP generation is impaired, and cells become dependent on glycolysis. Glycolysis rapidly generates ATP, although the by-product of this reaction is the accumulation of lactate. Lactic acidemia may also be a result of defects in lactate removal. The gluconeogenesis pathway is the major pathway for lactate clearance and defects in the enzymes involved in this pathway (pyruvate carboxylase, phosphoenolpyruvate carboxykinase (PEPCK), fructose 1,6-bisphosphatase, and glucose 6-phosphatase) will result in a lactic acidosis [26].

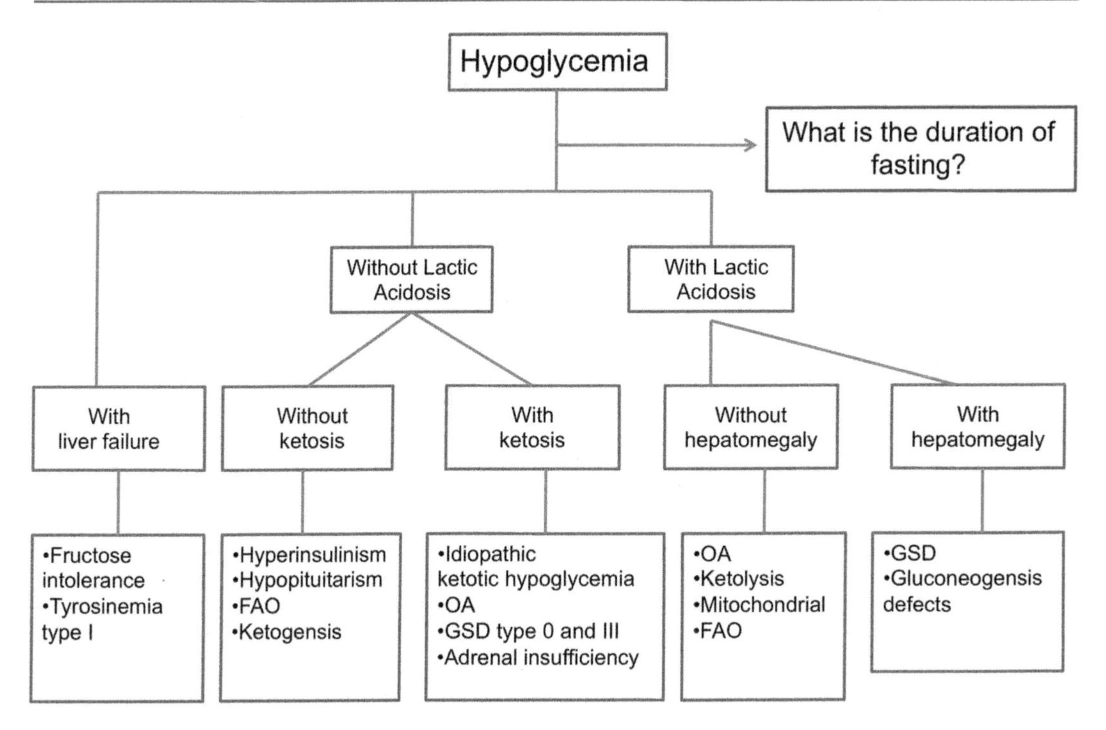

Fig. 7.2 Flow diagram for the evaluation of a patient with hypoglycemia depending on the absence or presence of lactic acid. FAO fatty acid oxidation, OA organic academia, GSD glycogen storage disease

Lactic acidemia is also reported in a variety of conditions including sepsis, chronic liver disease, and tissue hypoxia. It is also important to note that mild lactate evaluations may be due to inappropriate sample collection such as the stress (struggle) of the patient during the blood draw. Also, significant lactate elevations in healthy individuals have been documented after anaerobic exercise or prolonged exercise of fast-twitch muscle [27].

In conclusion, it should be evident that there is nothing "routine" about the above laboratories. These laboratory studies provide valuable and timely information, which is especially important in the acute setting. The astute clinician can utilize the results of these laboratory results and often prioritize the diagnosis of an inherited metabolic disease into a specific category (i.e., a fatty acid oxidation disorder). Although a suspicion of a metabolic disease can be discerned with routine laboratory studies, it is often difficult to establish a specific diagnosis, such as very long-chain acyl-CoA dehydrogenase (VLCAD) deficiency as opposed to long-chain 3-hydroxyacyl-CoA dehydrogenase (LCHAD) deficiency. The metabolic laboratories discussed below are useful in establishing a specific diagnosis.

7.3 Metabolic Laboratory Tests

The tests discussed within this section refer to those studies that typically occur within a specialized metabolic laboratory and are reviewed by a biochemical geneticist. The information stated below is general and the techniques, platforms, cut-offs, and interpretation of these tests will vary among laboratories. It is always important to interpret a laboratory test within the context of a patient's history. These laboratory studies are also impacted by diet, timing of the laboratory study with the last meal, and current medications. Unlike the routine laboratories noted above, a single metabolite does not always correlate with a specific disease, which is why interpretation of these studies by a trained biochemical geneticist is integral to the testing process.

7.3.1 Amino Acid Analysis

In many ways, the modern field of metabolism can be traced back to the identification and quantification of a single amino acid, most notably through the identification of phenylketonuria (PKU) and the development of an accurate and cost-effective analysis for phenylalanine [28–30]. Tests for single amino acid tests eventually were replaced by the ability to automatically evaluate multiple amino acids [31]. A number of amino acid analyzers are now available [32]. Regardless of the method used, amino acid analysis is typically diagnostic for all aminoacidopathies, such as PKU, maple syrup urine disease, and tyrosinemia. An abnormal amino acid profile can also aid in the diagnosis of non-aminoacidopathies such as urea cycle disorders and pyruvate carboxylase deficiency.

Blood specimens are recommended for investigation of aminoacidopathies as amino acid concentrations are fairly stable in blood. Urine amino acids analysis, on the other hand, is appropriate for disorders of amino acid renal transport such as cystinuria. Amino acid analysis in cerebral spinal fluid may be appropriate to aid in diagnosis (i.e., nonketotic hyperglycinemia) and management (i.e., cerebral amino acid disorders) of various inborn errors of metabolism. The composition of an amino acid profile is highly dependent on the nutritional intake of essential and nonessential amino acids [33]. Other clinical conditions are associated with abnormal amino acid profiles such as significant protein restriction and certain medications (Table 7.2).

Table 7.2 Clinical presentation associated with abnormal amino acids

Catabolism	↑ Leucine, isoleucine, valine
Protein restriction	↓ Leucine, isoleucine, valine
Lactic acidemia	↑ Alanine
Hyperammonemia	↑ Glutamine
Seizure medication	↑ Glycine

7.3.2 Organic Acid Profile

Disorders of organic acidemia (or aciduria) are characterized by excretion of organic acids, or acids that do not contain an amino group. As a result, organic acids historically could not be analyzed by the same techniques that were performed for amino acid analysis and are measured using a stable-isotope gas chromatography–mass spectrometry (GC-MS) [34]. Of note, organic acids bound to carnitine can be identified by other methods described below. Organic acid profiles are similar to other metabolic laboratory tests where an elevated metabolite is suggestive of an inherited metabolic disease (Fig. 7.3), although examining the pattern of organic acid excretion is paramount. Organic acids do accumulate in the serum, although they are poorly reabsorbed by the kidney, resulting in much higher concentrations of organic acids in urine than serum [34]. Similar to the other testing already discussed, causes other than a metabolic disorder, such as medications or physiologic ketosis, can result in an abnormal organic acid profile.

7.3.3 Carnitine Profile

Carnitine is a hydrophilic molecule that plays a pivotal role in both the normal physiologic process of beta-oxidation and the elimination of abnormal organic acids [35]. The majority of carnitine (approximately 75%) is derived from dietary sources such as meat and dairy products with the reminder of carnitine requirements provided through endogenous synthesis [36]. Carnitine is highly conserved through renal tubular reabsorption. Therefore, renal tubular loss of carnitine can result in significant, and pathologic, loss of carnitine.

The carnitine profile quantifies the amount of carnitine present (total carnitine) as well as the carnitine that is free or bound by an ester link to acyl-CoA (acyl or esterified carnitine) (Box 7.1) (Appendix E).

Box 7.1: Carnitine Profile

Total carnitine	All carnitine species – both free carnitine and carnitine bound to acyl-CoA
Free carnitine	Carnitine species that are *not* bound to acyl-CoA
Acyl (or esterified) Acylcarnitine	Carnitine species that *are* bound to acyl-CoA

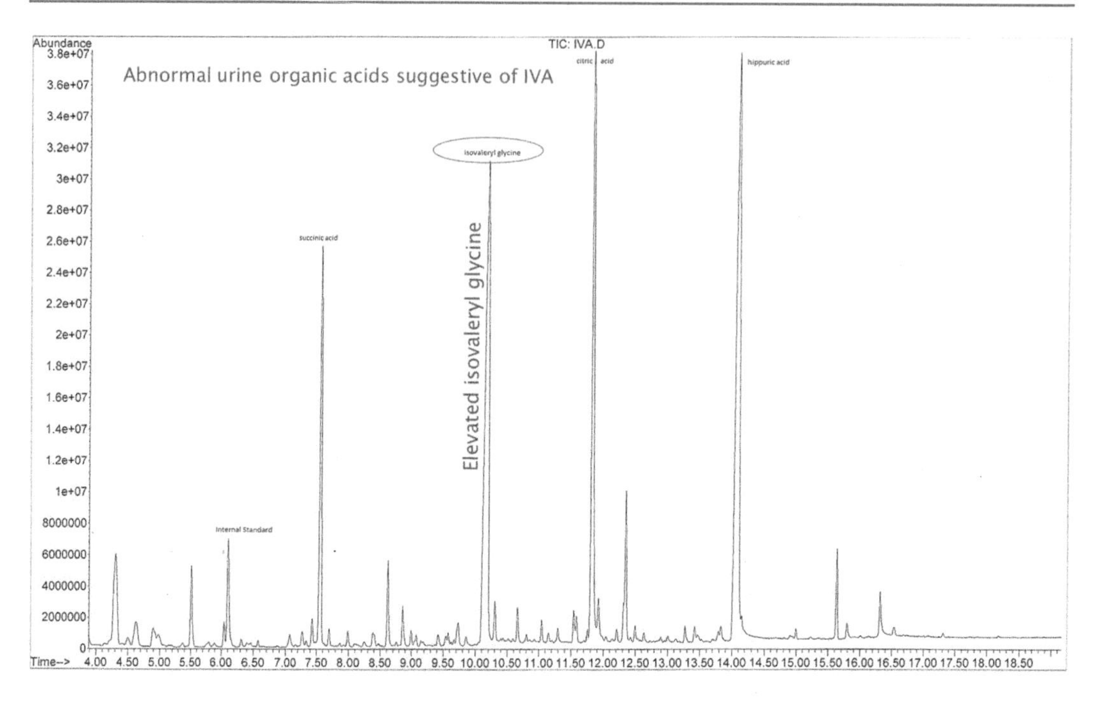

Fig. 7.3 An abnormal urine organic acid profile indicating abnormal accumulation of isovalerylglycine (indicated with a red circle). This is suggestive of isovaleric acidemia (an organic acid disorder of leucine metabolism). Organic acid profile courtesy of the Goodman Biochemical Genetics Laboratory

Primary carnitine deficiency results from a defect in the carnitine transporter within the plasma membrane resulting in the inability to reabsorb carnitine and in significant loss of urinary carnitine. As a result, extremely low serum carnitine concentrations are present and are reflected with very low free carnitine concentrations (<5 μM compared to normal value of 25–50 μM) [35]. Carnitine plays an important role in aiding the transfer of long-chain fatty acids into the mitochondria and in binding to acyl residuals to aid in the elimination of abnormal organic acids. If a significant amount of carnitine is bound to an acyl-CoA, the percentage of bound carnitine (acylcarnitine) will be high, suggesting a disorder of fatty acid or organic acid metabolism. Also, if a significant percentage of carnitine is bound to an acyl-CoA, a secondary deficiency of free carnitine may occur (i.e., low free carnitine). Except when a primary carnitine disorder is suspected, an abnormal carnitine panel should prompt the clinician to request an acylcarnitine profile and/or urine organic acids (Appendix J, Table 2).

7.3.4 Acylcarnitine Profile

Carnitine is esterified to a fatty acid molecule to form an acylcarnitine, which can then be transported across the mitochondrial membrane to provide a substrate for beta-oxidation. Carnitine can also esterify large organic molecules within the mitochondria due to a defect in fatty acid or organic acid metabolism. In defects of fatty acid oxidation, a fatty acyl-CoA molecule will be metabolized through beta-oxidation until it reaches the enzymatic defect. At the metabolic block, the acyl-CoA will continue to accumulate within the mitochondria. Organic acids are also conjugated to coenzyme A, and abnormal organic acids will also accumulate due to a metabolic block. These accumulating acyl-CoAs can esterify carnitine into acylcarnitines, which are then transported out of intracellular compartments into the blood where they can be easily detected [37].

Acylcarnitine analysis can be performed by various methods, although the introduction of liquid chromatography with tandem mass spectrometry (LC-MS/MS) revolutionized the use of

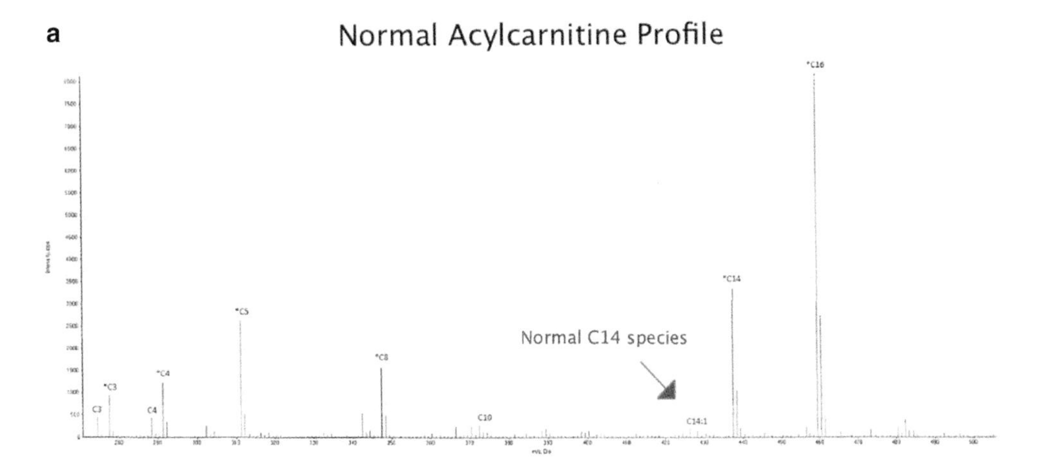

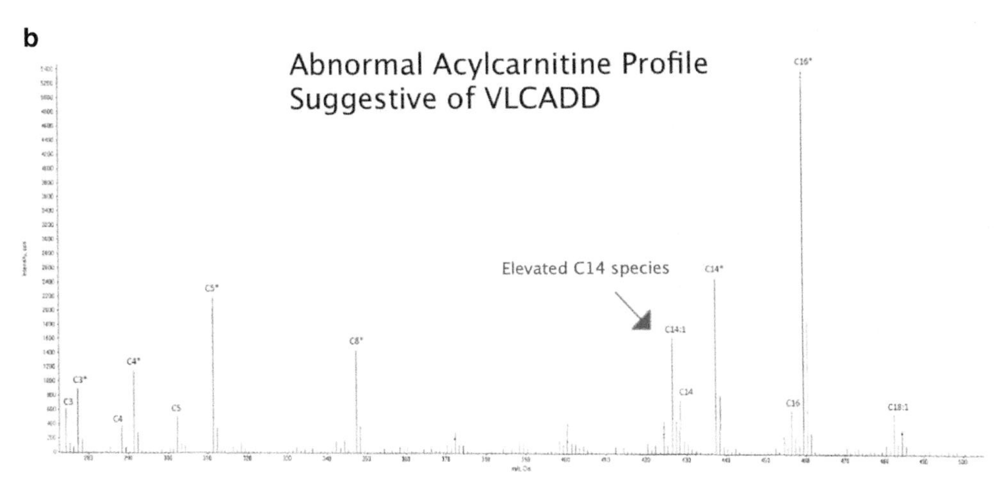

Fig. 7.4 Acylcarnitine profiles with examples of a normal acylcarnitine profile (**a**) and an acylcarnitine profile with elevated C14 esters suggestive of VLCAD deficiency (**b**). Acylcarnitine profiles are courtesy of the Goodman Biochemical Genetics Laboratory

acylcarnitine analysis for inherited metabolic diseases [38, 39]. LC-MS/MS-based acylcarnitine analysis can identify the accumulation of acyl-CoA esters with 2–18 carbons (C2-C-18) and, when compared to internal standards, the specific pattern of elevated carnitine esters can be diagnostic of an inherited metabolic disease (Fig. 7.4).

It is important to emphasize that an informative result is typically characterized by a specific pattern of acylcarnitine species as opposed to a single abnormal metabolite [40]. Although both the overall pattern of the profile and the interpretation by a biochemical geneticist are extremely important, the metabolic provider should still be familiar with the associations of specific metabolites and inherited metabolic diseases (Table 7.2).

7.3.5 Metabolomics

Unless there is a high suspicion for a specific disorder, multiple metabolic laboratory tests are often required to establish a diagnosis. Targeted testing of amino acids, organic acids, and/or acylcarnitines is often performed for disease management, although this also suggests (incorrectly) that other metabolic disturbances are relatively unimportant. Untargeted metabolomic platforms aim to identify >10,000 metabolites in a single sample using high-resolution liquid chromatography quadrupole time of flight methods (LC-QTOF) [41]. Currently, there is an imbalance between the large number of metabolites identified and the ability to quantify an important metabolite for treatment monitoring [42, 43]. Like with all testing platforms, clinicians and laboratorians should work together to determine the best testing strategy.

Interpretation of metabolic laboratories: As mentioned throughout this chapter, various factors may impact the interpretation of metabolic laboratories. For example, a patient may have normal metabolic laboratories when well, but may have significantly abnormal metabolic laboratories when catabolic [19]. Conversely, metabolism may be compromised when a patient is severely ill, such as in severe heart failure [44], which can make discerning a primary inborn error of metabolism from a secondary impairment of metabolism difficult. As a result, a patient may require metabolic laboratory studies in both the well and catabolic state. Nutritional intake and medications can significantly alter metabolic laboratory profiles. Therefore, a regimen may be initiated prior to obtaining a sample, especially when following laboratory values for treatment. This may require the laboratories to be collected following a significant fast or at a prescribed time after a meal. The timing of the sample draw may differ among metabolic clinics, although consistent timing for sample collection may allow the clinician to follow laboratory trends over time.

7.4 Confirmatory Testing

Confirmatory testing is often pursued after a probable diagnosis is made based upon the above basic and metabolic laboratories. Confirmatory testing typically consists of genetic or enzymatic analysis. Each of these testing modalities has limitations. For example, complete genetic analysis may require multiple tests (i.e., sequencing and copy number variation analysis). In certain diseases, genetic testing may only identify a subset of affected individuals. For example, in ornithine transcarbamylase deficiency (OTCD), a proximal urea cycle disorder, genetic testing is only informative in 80% of affected individuals [45, 46]. Enzyme testing is considered the gold standard of confirmatory testing. Enzyme testing also has limitations as it may require a cell line requiring a skin biopsy or may require a specific tissue where the enzyme is expressed. For example, OTCD enzyme analysis requires a liver biopsy for measurement of the hepatic enzyme activity. Enzyme activity is often a continuum and there may be an overlap between the enzyme activity in milder patients and heterozygotes (carriers) of a metabolic disease [47]. This can lead to difficulty with interpretation of the enzyme result. Many of these limitations will be discussed in disease-specific nutrition management chapters.

The clinical presentations of inherited metabolic diseases are often nonspecific, and various laboratory tests provide the information necessary to establish a diagnosis. Often multiple routine and metabolic laboratory studies are needed, and these laboratory studies are complementary. The astute clinician can use the combination of these laboratory studies to initiate emergency treatment in an acute setting, to make a probable diagnosis and to evaluate the long-term treatment of patients with an inborn error of metabolism.

References

1. Dionisi-Vici C, Rizzo C, Burlina AB, Caruso U, Sabetta G, Uziel G, et al. Inborn errors of metabolism in the Italian pediatric population: a national retrospective survey. J Pediatr. 2002;140(3):321–7.
2. Applegarth DA, Toone JR, Lowry RB. Incidence of inborn errors of metabolism in British Columbia, 1969-1996. Pediatrics. 2000;105(1):e10.
3. Saudubray JM, Sedel F, Walter JH. Clinical approach to treatable inborn metabolic diseases: an introduction. J Inherit Metab Dis. 2006;29(2–3): 261–74.
4. Carmody JB, Norwood VF. A clinical approach to paediatric acid-base disorders. Postgrad Med J. 2012;88(1037):143–51.
5. Kraut JA, Madias NE. Approach to patients with acid-base disorders. Respir Care. 2001;46(4):392–403.
6. Kraut JA, Madias NE. Differential diagnosis of nongap metabolic acidosis: value of a systematic approach. Clin J Am Soc Nephrol. 2012;7(4):671–9.
7. Enns GM. Neurologic damage and neurocognitive dysfunction in urea cycle disorders. Semin Pediatr Neurol. 2008;15(3):132–9.

8. Braissant O, McLin VA, Cudalbu C. Ammonia toxicity to the brain. J Inherit Metab Dis. 2013;36(4):595–612.
9. Gropman AL, Prust M, Breeden A, Fricke S, VanMeter J. Urea cycle defects and hyperammonemia: effects on functional imaging. Metab Brain Dis. 2013;28(2):269–75.
10. Gauthier N, Wu JW, Wang SP, Allard P, Mamer OA, Sweetman L, et al. A liver-specific defect of Acyl-CoA degradation produces hyperammonemia, hypoglycemia and a distinct hepatic Acyl-CoA pattern. PLoS One. 2013;8(7):e60581.
11. Coude FX, Sweetman L, Nyhan WL. Inhibition by propionyl-coenzyme A of N-acetylglutamate synthetase in rat liver mitochondria. A possible explanation for hyperammonemia in propionic and methylmalonic acidemia. J Clin Invest. 1979;64(6):1544–51.
12. Al-Hassnan ZN, Boyadjiev SA, Praphanphoj V, Hamosh A, Braverman NE, Thomas GH, et al. The relationship of plasma glutamine to ammonium and of glycine to acid-base balance in propionic acidaemia. J Inherit Metab Dis. 2003;26(1):89–91.
13. Baruteau J, Sachs P, Broue P, Brivet M, Abdoul H, Vianey-Saban C, et al. Clinical and biological features at diagnosis in mitochondrial fatty acid beta-oxidation defects: a French pediatric study of 187 patients. J Inherit Metab Dis. 2013;36(5):795–803.
14. Beard L, Wymore E, Fenton L, Coughlin CR, Weisfeld-Adams JD. Lethal neonatal hyperammonemia in severe ornithine transcarbamylase (OTC) deficiency compounded by large hepatic portosystemic shunt. J Inherit Metab Dis. 2017;40(1):159–60.
15. Sokollik C, Bandsma RH, Gana JC, van den Heuvel M, Ling SC. Congenital portosystemic shunt: characterization of a multisystem disease. J Pediatr Gastroenterol Nutr. 2013;56(6):675–81.
16. Batshaw ML, Wachtel RC, Cohen L, Starrett A, Boyd E, Perret YM, et al. Neurologic outcome in premature infants with transient asymptomatic hyperammonemia. J Pediatr. 1986;108(2):271–5.
17. Holecek M. Ammonia and amino acid profiles in liver cirrhosis: effects of variables leading to hepatic encephalopathy. Nutrition. 2015;31(1):14–20.
18. Jayakumar AR, Norenberg MD. Hyperammonemia in hepatic encephalopathy. J Clin Exp Hepatol. 2018;8(3):272–80.
19. Saudubray JM, de Lonlay P, Touati G, Martin D, Nassogne MC, Castelnau P, et al. Genetic hypoglycaemia in infancy and childhood: pathophysiology and diagnosis. J Inherit Metab Dis. 2000;23(3):197–214.
20. Ficicioglu C, Coughlin CR 2nd, Bennett MJ, Yudkoff M. Very long-chain acyl-CoA dehydrogenase deficiency in a patient with normal newborn screening by tandem mass spectrometry. J Pediatr. 2010;156(3):492–4.
21. Sass JO. Inborn errors of ketogenesis and ketone body utilization. J Inherit Metab Dis. 2012;35(1):23–8.
22. Lamers KJ, Doesburg WH, Gabreels FJ, Lemmens WA, Romsom AC, Wevers RA, et al. The concentration of blood components related to fuel metabolism during prolonged fasting in children. Clin Chim Acta. 1985;152(1–2):155–63.
23. Bonnefont JP, Specola NB, Vassault A, Lombes A, Ogier H, de Klerk JB, et al. The fasting test in paediatrics: application to the diagnosis of pathological hypo- and hyperketotic states. Eur J Pediatr. 1990;150(2):80–5.
24. Adeva-Andany M, Lopez-Ojen M, Funcasta-Calderon R, Ameneiros-Rodriguez E, Donapetry-Garcia C, Vila-Altesor M, et al. Comprehensive review on lactate metabolism in human health. Mitochondrion. 2014;17:76–100.
25. Adeva M, Gonzalez-Lucan M, Seco M, Donapetry C. Enzymes involved in l-lactate metabolism in humans. Mitochondrion. 2013;13(6):615–29.
26. van den Berghe G. Disorders of gluconeogenesis. J Inherit Metab Dis. 1996;19(4):470–7.
27. Robinson BH. Lactic acidemia and mitochondrial disease. Mol Genet Metab. 2006;89(1–2):3–13.
28. Centerwall WR, Centerwall SA. Phenylketonuria (FOLLING's disease). The story of its discovery. J Hist Med Allied Sci. 1961;16:292–6.
29. Guthrie R. Blood screening for phenylketonuria. JAMA. 1961;178(8):863.
30. Guthrie R, Susi A. A simple phenylalanine method for detecting phenylketonuria in large populations of newborn infants. Pediatrics. 1963;32:338–43.
31. Moore S, Stein WH. Chromatographic determination of amino acids on sulfonated polystyrene resins. J Biol Chem. 1951;192:663–81.
32. Woontner M, Goodman S. Chromatographic analysis of amino and organic acids in physiological fluids to detect inborn errors of metabolism. Curr Protoc Hum Genet. 2006. https://doi.org/10.1002/0471142905.hg1702s51
33. Nasset ES, Heald FP, Calloway DH, Margen S, Schneeman P. Amino acids in human blood plasma after single meals of meat, oil, sucrose and whiskey. J Nutr. 1979;109(4):621–30.
34. Goodman SI. An introduction to gas chromatography-mass spectrometry and the inherited organic acidemias. Am J Hum Genet. 1980;32(6):781–92.
35. Longo N, di San A, Filippo C, Pasquali M. Disorders of carnitine transport and the carnitine cycle. Am J Med Genet C Semin Med Genet. 2006;142C(2):77–85.
36. Stanley CA. Carnitine deficiency disorders in children. Ann N Y Acad Sci. 2004;1033:42–51.
37. Santra S, Hendriksz C. How to use acylcarnitine profiles to help diagnose inborn errors of metabolism. Arch Dis Child Educ Pract Ed. 2010;95(5):151–6.
38. Millington DS, Kodo N, Norwood DL, Roe CR. Tandem mass spectrometry: a new method for acylcarnitine profiling with potential for neonatal screening for inborn errors of metabolism. J Inherit Metab Dis. 1990;13(3):321–4.

39. Van Hove JL, Zhang W, Kahler SG, Roe CR, Chen YT, Terada N, et al. Medium-chain acyl-CoA dehydrogenase (MCAD) deficiency: diagnosis by acylcarnitine analysis in blood. Am J Hum Genet. 1993;52(5):958–66.
40. Rinaldo P, Cowan TM, Matern D. Acylcarnitine profile analysis. Genet Med. 2008;10(2):151–6.
41. Coene KLM, Kluijtmans LAJ, van der Heeft E, Engelke UFH, de Boer S, Hoegen B, et al. Next-generation metabolic screening: targeted and untargeted metabolomics for the diagnosis of inborn errors of metabolism in individual patients. J Inherit Metab Dis. 2018;41(3):337–53.
42. Ismail IT, Showalter MR, Fiehn O. Inborn errors of metabolism in the era of untargeted metabolomics and lipidomics. Meta. 2019;9(10):242.
43. Almontashiri NAM, Zha L, Young K, Law T, Kellogg MD, Bodamer OA, et al. Clinical validation of targeted and untargeted metabolomics testing for genetic disorders: a 3 year comparative study. Sci Rep. 2020;10(1):9382.
44. Pierpont ME, Judd D, Goldenberg IF, Ring WS, Olivari MT, Pierpont GL. Myocardial carnitine in end-stage congestive heart failure. Am J Cardiol. 1989;64(1):56–60.
45. Tuchman M, Jaleel N, Morizono H, Sheehy L, Lynch MG. Mutations and polymorphisms in the human ornithine transcarbamylase gene. Hum Mutat. 2002;19(2):93–107.
46. Caldovic L, Abdikarim I, Narain S, Tuchman M, Morizono H. Genotype-phenotype correlations in ornithine transcarbamylase deficiency: a mutation update. J Genet Genomics. 2015;42(5):181–94.
47. Hesse J, Braun C, Behringer S, Matysiak U, Spiekerkoetter U, Tucci S. The diagnostic challenge in very-long chain acyl-CoA dehydrogenase deficiency (VLCADD). J Inherit Metab Dis. 2018;41(6):1169–78.

Gene Therapy for Inherited Metabolic Diseases

8

Nicola Longo and Kent Lai

Contents

N. Longo (✉)
Division of Medical Genetics, University of Utah School of Medicine, University of Utah Hospital, Salt Lake City, UT, USA
e-mail: Nicola.Longo@hsc.utah.edu

K. Lai
Division of Pediatric Genetics, University of Utah School of Medicine, Salt Lake City, UT, USA
e-mail: kent.lai@hsc.utah.edu

L. E. Bernstein et al. (eds.), *Nutrition Management of Inherited Metabolic Diseases*,
https://doi.org/10.1007/978-3-030-94510-7_8

Core Messages

- Gene-based therapies, defined as the transfer of genetic materials to treat a disease, can potentially restore the function of the missing enzyme in individuals with inborn errors of metabolism.
- Gene-based therapies consist of gene replacement therapy, oligonucleotide-based therapy, mRNA therapy, and genome editing.
- A few gene replacement and oligonucleotide-based therapies have been approved by FDA and the European Medicines Agency, and many others are currently at clinical trial stage.

8.1 Background

Gene-based therapy is promising to revolutionize the field of medicine by providing treatment for previously untreatable conditions [1, 2]. For inborn errors of metabolism (IEMs), gene therapy could potentially offer a cure with a single treatment that replaces the function of the defective gene [2]. In contrast to enzyme replacement therapies that require repeated infusions, gene-based therapies in long-lived cells might afford sustained production of endogenous proteins, including enzymes or transporters defective in inherited metabolic disorders.

Initial attempts at gene-based therapy in humans did not provide much clinical benefit or produced severe toxicities, including patient deaths [3]. After the development of new vectors that allowed more targeted gene delivery in the early 2000s, sustained gene expression and, in some cases, clinical benefits could be observed [4, 5]. New problems became evident such as insertional genotoxicity, immune destruction of genetically modified cells, and immune reactions related to administration of certain vectors [6].

Further developments in the past 10 years have improved safety and the efficacy of gene delivery, bringing some of the gene-based therapies to approval [1]. Here we will focus on therapies for inborn errors of metabolism and their potential to improve the life of patients with rare genetic conditions.

8.2 Inborn Errors of Metabolism

Inborn errors of metabolism (IEMs) are genetically determined disorders affecting an individual's ability to convert nutrients or to use them for energy production [7]. They are caused by pathogenic variants in genes that code for specific enzymes or transporters involved in metabolic pathways. The majority of IEMs are inherited as autosomal-recessive traits and are caused by loss-of-function pathogenic variants that impair the activity of the gene product.

IEMs result in accumulation of abnormal metabolites (substrates) proximal to the metabolic block or lack of necessary products or production of abnormal by-products, all of which contribute to the clinical presentation and severity of each condition [7]. In many of the IEMs, the substrate derives from the digestion of normal food, for which therapeutic strategies using diet, cofactors, supplements, and other therapies such as enzyme replacement therapy (ERT) try to minimize the impact of the metabolic block on the body. Examples include galactose removal in galactosemia [8] and phenylalanine restriction in phenylketonuria [9]. Cofactor therapy has been employed in treating molybdenum cofactor deficiency [10], various mitochondrial disorders [11], and disorders of biopterin synthesis [12]. Pharmacological amounts of vitamins and cofactors can partially rescue defective enzymatic activity caused by some pathogenic variants, such as pyridoxine in cystathionine beta-synthase deficiency and tetrahydrobiopterin in phenylketonuria [13, 14]. Finally, enzyme replacement therapy (ERT) has been used to mitigate the nonneurological phenotypes of lysosomal diseases [15, 16]. Although these approaches prevent the acute toxicity syndromes and improve the quality of life of the patients, they do not address the genetic causes of the diseases and require lifelong administration. In theory, restoration of gene function should cure the IEM. For these reasons, IEMs are prime candidates for therapies capable of restoring the function of the defective gene.

8.3 Overview of Gene-Based Therapy

Gene-based therapy is the transfer of genetic material to treat a disease. In metabolic disorders caused by loss-of-function pathogenic variants, the long-term expression of the transduced gene at sufficient levels should restore the function of the missing enzyme/transporter. The transduced gene is usually the transcribed portion (a complementary DNA copy of the mature mRNA) of the affected gene that will replace the missing protein. The transferred gene is either integrated in the host genome of the recipient cell or, in most cases, retained without integration. Theoretically, a single gene transfer should be sufficient to cure a given genetic condition. As an alternative, exogenously delivered mRNA for the missing protein can be used in lieu of the complementary DNA, but this will need to be given repeatedly, since the mRNA will eventually be degraded and the cells will be deprived of the function of the protein once the exogenously delivered mRNA is no longer present (Fig. 8.1).

Gene-based therapy can also be designed to suppress expression of a detrimental gene by employing RNA interference (RNAi), but this is not usually the case in common metabolic disorders (with the exception of porphyrias [17]). Antisense-oligonucleotide-directed therapy can also be used to correct pre-mRNA splicing for specific genes, such as the correction of exon 7 splicing of the endogenous *SMN2* pre-mRNA in spinal muscular atrophy [18, 19].

Genome editing techniques can potentially correct a mutated gene in its precise genomic location through homologous recombination with a donor template or via base editing. This is not yet in clinical trials, due to uncertainties about possible secondary alterations of the genome caused by the technology. Here we will largely focus on gene-based therapy for IEMs that use nucleic acids to replace the functions of the missing proteins.

8.4 Routes of Administration for Gene-Based Therapy

Gene-based therapy can be performed through in vivo and ex vivo routes.

8.4.1 Ex Vivo Gene Replacement Therapy

Cells are taken from the recipient, stem cells are selected and modified in vitro with the gene of interest, in some cases the modified cells are amplified in vitro before readministration to the recipient. Since the cells in which the gene is introduced are obtained from the recipient, there is usually no immune response to their reintroduction. A conditioning regimen is necessary before reinfusion to create space for these genetically modified cells that will replace cells with the faulty gene. This type of approach requires integrating vectors that insert their DNA (usually the DNA complementary to the mRNA for the missing protein also called cDNA or minigene) into the genome of the recipient stem cells. The stem cell will retain their own endogenous genes, including the one with pathogenic variants causing the genetic disease, but will have an additional (replacement) minigene capable of producing a normal version of the defective pro-

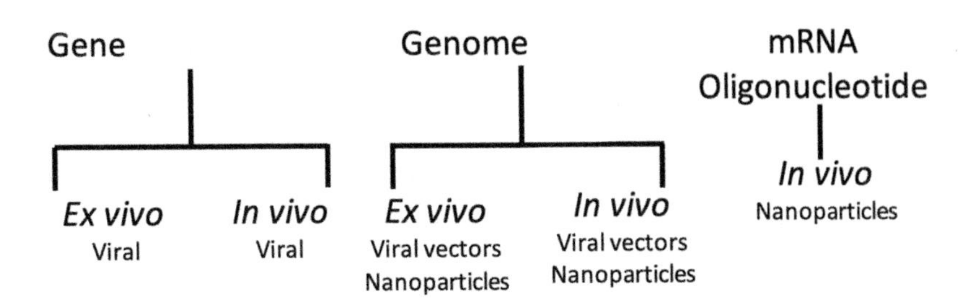

Fig. 8.1 Overview of gene-based therapies

tein integrated randomly in the DNA. This replacement gene will be replicated when the cell undergoes division and is passed to daughter cells. This explains why such therapy requires vectors capable of integrating stably in the recipient genome because nonintegrating vectors carrying the replacement gene will be lost when the cell divides. An example is ex vivo gene replacement therapy in hematopoietic stem cells (HSCs).

The success of allogeneic bone marrow transplantation for many genetic immunodeficiencies and blood disorders has driven the pursuit of gene replacement therapies targeting HSCs using ex vivo approaches. The transplantation of autologous patient stem cells in which the underlying genetic defect is corrected has an advantage over allogeneic transplants in that they do not require a histocompatible donor that, in many cases, is hard to find. Indications for this approach include, but are not limited to, adenosine deaminase deficiency causing one form of severe combined immunodeficiency (SCID) and various hemoglobinopathies and thalassemias. These approaches also eliminate the need for immune suppressants because they can avoid the immune complications of graft-versus-host disease (GVHD).

Initial clinical trials using γ-retroviral vectors showed improvement in immune function in patients with SCID caused by loss-of-function mutations in the genes encoding interleukin-2 receptor γ or adenosine deaminase. There was low HSC transduction efficiency, but the gene-modified T-lineage cells had a selective growth advantage and were able to expand and fill the empty T cell compartment, improving immune function despite minimal levels of gene-corrected cells [20, 21]. Unfortunately, a few years after the treatment, patients in the X-SCID trials, as well as those for chronic granulomatous disease and Wiskott-Aldrich syndrome, developed acute myeloid and lymphoid leukemias due to activation of proto-oncogenes adjacent to the site of proviral insertions. This was later found to be linked to strong enhancers present in γ-retroviral vectors and the propensity of these vectors to insert near promoters [22–25]. These severe toxicities led to the design of enhancer-deleted vectors that are still effective in improving Wiskott-Aldrich syndrome [26] and X-SCID [27], without causing leukemia or uncontrolled clonal expansion of transduced cells.

New lentiviral vectors in combination with pretransplant cytoreductive conditioning (to create space for the transduced cells to occupy in the human body) and better techniques for ex vivo HSC manipulation [28] are now part of the newest clinical trials for the metabolic disorder adrenoleukodystrophy and the lysosomal storage disorders metachromatic leukodystrophy and Fabry disease.

8.4.2 In Vivo Gene Replacement Therapy

In vivo gene replacement therapy targets long-lived postmitotic cells, such as those in the liver or muscle that rarely undergo cell division, at least after a certain age. The transduced gene is not integrated into genomic DNA but persists as an episome for the cell's life span. Targeting different organs in vivo is appealing because it eliminates the practical and regulatory hurdles of ex vivo cell-based gene therapies, which require the cumbersome cell collection, culture, and manipulation and transplantation steps. On the other hand, in vivo approaches require special consideration on tissue-specific targeting or local delivery and/or target cell-specific gene expression. There are also other challenges, many of which are related to the inflammatory response elicited by the virus carrying the gene of interest, with new measures now emerging to overcome some of these concerns (Sect. 8.8). Table 8.1 summarizes some of the preclinical studies, as well as clinical trials of in vivo gene replacement therapy targeting different organs for various indications.

Table 8.1 Clinical and preclinical studies targeting different organs/tissues with in vivo gene replacement therapy [29–37]

Organ/system	Stage	Indications	References
Liver	Preclinical	Hemophilia B	[29]
Liver	Clinical trials	Hemophilia B	[30]
Liver	Preclinical	Hemophilia A	[31]
Muscle	Preclinical	Hemophilia B	[32]
Eye	Clinical trials	RPE65 deficiency – induced retinal dystrophy	[32–34]
CNS	Clinical trials	AADC deficiency	[35]
CNS	Clinical trials	Spinal muscular atrophy	[36]
CNS	Clinical trials	Parkinson's disease	[37]

CNS Central nervous system

Table 8.2 Viral vectors used in the past and currently in human clinical trials

	Adenovirus	Adeno-associated virus (AAV)	Lentivirus	Retrovirus
Family	Adenoviridae	Parvoviridae	Retroviridae	Retroviridae
Genome	dsDNA	ssDNA	ssRNA	ssRNA
Pathogenic	Yes	No	Yes	Yes
Target cell types	Dividing and nondividing	Dividing and nondividing	Dividing and nondividing	Dividing
Integration into host genome	No	No	Yes	Yes
Transgene expression	Transient	Long term	Long term	Long term
Packaging capacity of the viral vector it derives	Up to 8 kb	Up to 4.5 kb	Up to 8.5 kb	Up to 8 kb
Indications targeted in preclinical studies and clinical trials	Ornithine transcarbamylase deficiency, but no longer used	Spinal muscular atrophy, RPE65-mutation-associated retinal dystrophy, many others	Fabry disease, Gaucher disease	Severe combined immunodeficiency, Wiskott-Aldrich syndrome, but no longer used

8.5 Delivery Vehicles for Gene-Based Therapy

8.5.1 Viral-Mediated Gene-Based Therapy

Historically, multiple families of viruses have been exploited as viral vectors to deliver the DNA cargo to the target cells in both in vivo and ex vivo settings. Each virus has unique characteristics, strengths, and limitations (Table 8.2). The last two decades witnessed rapid advancements in the design and delivery of the viral vectors derived from these viruses, although adeno-associated virus (AAV) and lentivirus emerged as the most popular and effective platforms that are now used in almost all clinical trials.

8.5.2 Nonviral Gene Transfer

Nonviral gene delivery has several advantages when compared to viral vectors. For instance, the nonviral vectors are often less immunogenic. Not only are they easier to produce, but they also have a larger packing capacity [38]. The major drawback for nonviral vectors is the low transfer efficacy, which is not currently sufficient to be therapeutic for most genetic diseases.

8.6 Other Gene-Based Therapies

8.6.1 Oligonucleotide Therapy and Genome Editing

Oligonucleotides (short sequence of nucleotides synthesized in the laboratory) can be used to treat metabolic disorders by affecting RNA levels of target genes. They can cause RNA degradation, reduce expression of genes causing a toxic effect, or modulate the splicing of genes with pathogenic variants or promoting formation of usable RNA by genes not normally utilized [39].

Antisense oligonucleotides bind to their cognate mRNA transcripts and favor their degradation by RNase H. Fomivirsen injected into the eye can fight cytomegalovirus retinitis [40]. Mipomersen can reduce *APOB* mRNA in the liver and ameliorate homozygous familial hypercholesterolemia [41]. Inotersen targets the *TTR* gene to reduce formation of amyloid in hereditary transthyretin amyloidosis and polyneuropathy [42].

Antisense oligonucleotides can also mask specific sequences within a target transcript blocking interactions with other RNAs or with proteins (such as the spliceosome complex), without enhancing RNA degradation. This type of approach can induce splicing of abnormal exons in Duchenne muscular dystrophy (eteplirsen, golodirsen) [43, 44] or modify the splicing of SMN2 to ameliorate spinal muscular atrophy (nusinersen) [45].

Oligonucleotides can be used to silence gene expression. siRNA binds to the target transcript to guide it to the Argonaute 2 protein, which is part of the RNA-induced silencing complex [46]. This approach is useful in acute hepatic porphyrias in which givosiran reduces expression of *ALAS1* [47]. This reduces formation of delta amino levulinic acid and abnormal porphyrins, which dramatically improves the phenotype of affected patients. In amyloidosis, patisiran targets the *TTR* gene [48].

All oligonucleotide-based therapies need to be delivered on an ongoing basis and, although attractive, do not represent a cure for genetic conditions. By contrast, genome editing in theory can be used to remove pathogenic variants and permanently correct the defective gene in a way that it will be maintained in corrected cells [49]. As with gene replacement therapy, the correction of genes can be performed in vivo or ex vivo in cells taken from the patients. The pathogenic variant of interest is corrected using site-specific endonucleases (such as zinc-finger nucleases) and the CRISPR/Cas9 system, in combination with delivery vectors engineered to target disease tissue. The major drawbacks are the low efficiency of gene correction, the need to utilize viral vectors to deliver the machinery needed for correction, and the possibility of modifying the genome in regions other than the target gene. Despite these theoretical drawbacks, gene correction therapy using CRISPR–Cas9-associated base editors, which enable nucleotide conversion independent of double-strand DNA break formation and homology-directed repair, was effective in providing sufficient phenylalanine hydroxylase activity (>20% of normal) in Pah^{enu2} mice (a model of phenylketonuria) to restore physiological blood phenylalanine concentrations without producing unwanted changes in other genes [50].

8.6.2 mRNA Therapy

In addition to the successes seen in the development of COVID-19 vaccines [51–54], exogenously delivered mRNA therapy, which essentially shares the same principle as gene replacement therapy, has the potential to treat a variety of disorders including methylmalonic acidemia [55], classic galactosemia [56], arginase and citrin deficiency [57, 58], propionic acidemia [59], acute intermittent porphyria [60], Fabry disease [61], or even cancers [62]. In contrast to viral-mediated gene therapy, mRNA therapy involves systemic administration of mRNA encapsulated in lipid nanoparticles (LNPs), which primarily target the liver [63–65], although the tropism of such nanoparticles can expand to other organs like the lungs [66]. The limited organ exposure could be advantageous in some cases when we consider undue adverse effects. Unlike gene therapy where the transgene expression is long term, mRNA has a relatively short half-life and, therefore, repeated injections will be required.

Experimental mRNA therapy for a handful of indications in humans is at different stages of development [67]. In preparation for clinical trials, extensive toxicological and immunogenicity studies have demonstrated the safety of lipid nanoparticles [55, 61, 68]. There is no increase of plasma cytokines (IL-6, IFN-γ, TNF-α, IL-1β) or antidrug antibody levels in mice following 3 and 5 weekly IV bolus injections [69]. Minimal elevations in inflammatory markers including complement and cytokines have been observed in repeat dose toxicology studies conducted in cynomolgus monkeys receiving a different mRNA encapsulated with similar lipid nanoparticles (1 mg/kg) [68, 69]. mRNA therapy can be an ideal alternative for the *significant* number of patients who cannot use AAV-based gene therapy and can be discontinued at any time if it causes undesirable side effects.

8.7 Approved Gene Therapies

Table 8.3 lists gene therapies that have received regulatory approval to treat genetic disorders (some were approved only in Europe). The first gene therapy to be approved in the European Union under the "exceptional circumstances" pathway was alipogene tiparvovec to treat lipoprotein lipase deficiency. This is a rare disorder in which triglycerides cannot be released to peripheral tissues after intestinal absorption, resulting in severe hypertriglyceridemia. The excess fat causes enlargement of liver and spleen and can cause severe pancreatitis that can be lethal. The AAV1 vector containing lipoprotein lipase was given intramuscularly and caused a transient 40% reduction in triglycerides and improvements in postprandial chylomicron triglyceride content [70]. Due to poor demand, marketing authorization was not renewed in 2017.

Table 8.3 Gene therapies approved for metabolic/genetic disorders

Name of therapeutics	Gene	Disease
Alipogene tiparvovec	Lipoprotein lipase	Lipoprotein lipase deficiency (withdrawn from market)
Betibeglogene autotemcel	Beta-globin	Beta thalassemia
Onasemnogene abeparvovec	Survival motor neuron 1	Spinal muscular atrophy (type 1)
Strimvelis	Adenosine deaminase	Adenosine deaminase deficiency
Voretigene neparvovec	Retinoid isomerohydrolase RPE65	RPE65-associated retinal dystrophy (Leber congenital amaurosis)

Voretigene neparvovec (AAV2-hRPE65v2) was approved by the FDA in 2017 for the treatment of retinal dystrophy caused by biallelic *RPE65* mutation–associated retinal dystrophy (Leber's congenital amaurosis). The *RPE65* gene encodes retinoid isomerohydrolase, an enzyme that converts light to electrical signals necessary for normal vision. Voretigene neparvovec containing a functional copy of *RPE65* injected in the subretinal space improved functional vision in affected patients [34].

Onasemnogene abeparvovec was approved in May 2019 by the FDA for children younger than 2 years with spinal muscular atrophy, a severe neuromuscular disorder usually resulting in death or the need for permanent ventilation by age 2 years. It is caused by deficiency of the gene affecting motor neuron survival (Survival Motor Neuron 1 (*SMN1*) gene). A one-time intravenous infusion of a copy of the healthy gene produced rapid and significant motor improvements in infants with severe SMA1 [71].

Adenosine deaminase deficiency is a metabolic disorder that causes the accumulation of purine nucleotides affecting lymphocyte function, resulting in severe combined immunodeficiency. Other manifestations include skeletal abnormalities, neurodevelopmental defects, hearing loss, and pulmonary manifestations. Patients are initially treated with enzyme replacement therapy to enable partial immunological reconstitution. Hematopoietic stem cell transplant is the treatment of choice, but in many cases, no suitable donor is identified. By contrast, gene therapy can correct the defect in autologous hematopoietic stem cells and has demonstrated immunological and clinical efficacy [28]. This was the first European Union–approved gene therapy utilizing a retroviral vector. In some cases, the vector nonrandomly integrated near a proto-oncogene and activated cell proliferation, resulting in leukemia [72]. For this reason, this type of approach has now been substituted with a different type of virus and less powerful promoters.

Betibeglogene autotemcel was conditionally approved in Europe in 2019 to treat the anemia produced by beta-thalassemia. Therapy added the beta-globin gene within a lentivirus to correct patient's blood cells and reduced or eliminated the need for long-term red-cell transfusions [73]. As in the case of adenosine deaminase deficiency, there is the possibility of insertional mutagenesis and longer-term studies are necessary to establish safety of this treatment.

8.8 Clinical Trials in Inborn Errors of Metabolism (Listed in clinicaltrials.gov)

The last few years have seen an explosion in the number of clinical trials using gene therapy for inborn errors of metabolism (Table 8.4). Among the therapies listed, only the one for lipoprotein lipase deficiency was at some point approved in Europe to treat hypertriglyceridemia in this condition, but was subsequently withdrawn [74]. Most of these trials are backed by extensive preclinical data in animal models supporting efficacy of gene therapy.

Table 8.4 Clinical trials of gene therapy in inborn errors of metabolism. Clinical trials were obtained from clinicaltrials.gov on 20 March 2021

Condition	Vector/Name/Modality	Start date	Identifier
Aromatic L-amino acid decarboxylase deficiency	AAV2-hAADC/Intrastriatal	2016-07	NCT02852213
CLN2 lipofuscinosis	AAV2/ AAVrh. 10CUhCLN2/ intracerebral	2010-08-19	NCT01161576
CLN3 lipofuscinosis	AAV9/ AT-GTX-502/intrathecal	2018-11-13	NCT03770572
CLN6 lipofuscinosis	AAV9/AT-GTX-501/intrathecal	2016-03	NCT02725580
Cystinosis	Lentivirus/CTNS-RD-04/ex vivo	2019-07-08	NCT03897361
Fabry disease	AAV/4D-310/in vivo	2020-09-01	NCT04519749
Fabry disease	rAAV2/6 / ST-920/in vivo	2019-07-23	NCT04046224
Fabry disease	AAV/FLT190/in vivo	2019-07-08	NCT04040049
Fabry disease	Lentivirus/AVR-RD-01/ex vivo	2018-02-21	NCT03454893
Familial hypercholesterolemia	AAV/RGX-501/in vivo	2019-09-30	NCT04080050
Familial hypercholesterolemia	AAV/hLDR/in vivo	2016-03	NCT02651675
Gaucher disease	Lentivirus/AVR-RD-02/ex vivo	2019-05-30	NCT04145037
Glycogen storage disease 1A	AAV8/ DTX401/in vivo	2019-07-15	NCT03970278
GM1 gangliosidosis	AAV9/GLB1/in vivo	2019-08-19	NCT03952637
GM1 gangliosidosis	AAVrh10/LYS-GM101/intrathecal	2021-03	NCT04273269
GM1 gangliosidosis	AAVHu68/PBGM01/ intrathecal	2021-02	NCT04713475
GM2 gangliosidosis	AAV9/TSHA101/intrathecal	2021-03-12	NCT04798235
GM2 gangliosidosis	AAVrh8/AXO-AAV-GM2/intrathecal	2021-01-15	NCT04669535
Krabbe disease	AAVrh10/ FBX-101/in vivo	2021-04	NCT04693598
Krabbe disease	AAVHu68/PBKR03/intrathecal	2021-04	NCT04771416
Lipoprotein lipase deficiency	AAV1/AMT-011/in vivo	2009-02	NCT00891306
Metachromatic leukodystrophy	Lentivirus/OTL-200/ex vivo	2010-04-09	NCT01560182
Metachromatic leukodystrophy	Lentivirus/TYF-ARFA/intracerebral in vivo	2018-10-30	NCT03725670
Metachromatic Leukodystrophy/ adrenoleukodystrophy	Lentivirus/ARSA-ADCD1/ex vivo	2015-01	NCT02559830

Table 8.4 (continued)

Condition	Vector/Name/Modality	Start date	Identifier
Methylmalonic acidemia	rAAV-LK03/ hLB-001/in vivo	2021-02-15	NCT04581785
Mucopolysaccharidosis 1	AAV9/RGX-111/intrathecal in vivo	2019-04-03	NCT03580083
Mucopolysaccharidosis 1	Lentivirus/IDUA-LV/ex vivo	2018-05-11	NCT03488394
Mucopolysaccharidosis 2	AAV9/RGX-121/intrathecal in vivo	2018-09-27	NCT03566043
Mucopolysaccharidosis 3A	Lentivirus/ CD11b.SGSH/ex vivo	2020-01-07	NCT04201405
Mucopolysaccharidosis 3A	AAVrh10/SAF301 /intracerebral	2011-08	NCT01474343
Mucopolysaccharidosis 3A	AAVrh10/ LYS-SAF302 / intracerebral	2018-12-17	NCT03612869
Mucopolysaccharidosis 3A	AAV9/ABO-102/in vivo	2019-10-29	NCT04088734
Mucopolysaccharidosis 3B	AAV9/CMV.hNAGLU/in vivo	2017-10-16	NCT03315182
Mucopolysaccharidosis type 6	AAV2/8/TBG.hARSB/in vivo	2017-07-17	NCT03173521
Phenylketonuria	AAV /BMN 307 / in vivo	2020-09-24	NCT04480567
Phenylketonuria	AAVHSC15 /HMI-102/in vivo	2019-06-10	NCT03952156
Pompe disease	AAV/SPK-3006/in vivo	2020-10-01	NCT04093349
Pompe disease	AAV8/AT845/in vivo	2020-10-28	NCT04174105
Pyruvate kinase deficiency	Lentivirus/RP-L301/ex vivo	2020-07-06	NCT04105166
Wilson disease	AAV/VTX-801/in vivo	2021-02	NCT04537377

Only one trial is listed for each product. Modality of administration is in vivo when the site is indicated (intrathecal, intracerebral, intrastriatal). All ex vivo modalities involve the introduction of the defective gene in autologous stem cells prior to reimplantation

The targets of current trial can be divided into disorders of intermediary metabolism, lysosomal disorders, and disorders affecting primarily the brain (Table 8.4). For some of these conditions, there are already approved therapies, but for most others, there is none, indicating the urgency toward their development.

In disorders of intermediary metabolism (familial hypercholesterolemia, glycogen storage disease type 1A, lipoprotein lipase deficiency, methylmalonic acidemia, phenylketonuria), the liver will bind most of the AAV vectors delivered systemically. In some cases, the AAV vectors have been modified to increase their capacity to transduce liver cells. Since the liver is the only organ expressing the enzyme defective in phenylketonuria and the one most affected in GSD1A, its correction should greatly improve these conditions. However, in the case of methylmalonic acidemia, all other organs also produce the organic acid and even with perfect correction, the effect should be similar to that seen with a liver transplant.

In lysosomal disorders (cystinosis, lipofuscinoses, Fabry, gangliosidoses, Krabbe, Gaucher, metachromatic leukodystrophy, the mucopolysaccharidoses, and Pompe disease), undigested materials accumulate inside affected organs, causing their dysfunction. In many cases, these organs are populated by cells of the macrophagic lineage, for which correction of hematopoietic stem cells with the defective gene and autologous reimplantation has the potential of correcting the disease process. This also applies to pyruvate kinase deficiency, a disease mostly affecting red cells whose progenitors would be corrected by a bone marrow transplant or autologous reimplantation of hematopoietic stem cells after gene correction.

At the same time, the systemic administration of the virus could reach multiple organs affected by lysosomal disorders, correcting them as well. AAV vectors are constantly being redesigned to reach different organs, targeting those more affected by a certain disease.

Diseases affecting the brain cause more problems since each genetic condition might only affect some brain cells (neurons or glia) and, in some cases, only in specific areas of the brain. Gene therapy administered systemically usually does not reach the brain in significant concentrations unless AAV9 (an adenovirus targeting the brain) is used and it is given very early in life such as in spinal muscular atrophy [75]. For most other conditions, especially if diagnosed symptomatically, gene replacement therapy needs to be delivered directly into the brain or intrathecally (aromatic L-amino acid decarboxylase deficiency, lipofuscinoses, gangliosidoses, Krabbe, metachromatic leukodystrophy, and mucopolysaccharidoses affecting the brain). It is hoped that further development of brain-specific viral vectors will allow them not only to enter the brain, but also to correct specific cell types that are more affected by the disease.

8.9 Limitations, Complications, Challenges, and Future of Gene-Based Therapy

For standard gene replacement therapies, unwanted insertional mutations, inadvertent germline transmission, and immune responses to the vector or the replaced gene products are some of the concerns. Some of these complications, however, have been overcome with innovative vector designs and strategies (Table 8.5). At the same time, many of the strategies described require more patient data and longer time intervals to determine whether they are effective or not.

Compared to gene replacement therapy, somatic genome editing based upon CRISPR-Cas9 nucleases remains translational. The concerns for "off-target" mutations due to nuclease-mediated nonhomologous end-joining and homology-directed repair remain. To address these concerns, new approaches to design nucleases or CRISPR gRNAs to avoid off-target cutting and how to predict, screen for, and detect on- versus off-target genome alterations before or during clinical applications have been established [76]. Notably, high-fidelity CRISPR-Cas9 nuclease variants with no or very few detectable off-target effects have recently been developed [76–78]. But like the gene transfer vectors used in standard gene transfer, concerns for immunogenicity of nucleases for in vivo genome editing [79] and ensuring targeted delivery of editing machinery to the desired target tissue remain.

The rapid advances in genome editing have made heritable germline editing a realistic possibility. Just a few years ago, scientists in China conducted experiments using CRISPR-Cas9 to modify the hemoglobin gene in "nonviable" preimplantation human embryos, demonstrating low efficiency and reportedly frequent off-target mutations [77]. The incident prompted statements of concern from professional societies around the world [78] and a series of meetings sponsored by the U.S. National Academies of Sciences, Engineering, and Medicine that brought together an international group of scientists, clinicians, ethicists, patient advocates, and government officials that outlined principles of governance and oversight for human genome editing, and presented a possible pathway for eventual use of genome editing technologies to correct germline mutations for certain serious diseases [79]. In the United States, federal funds

Table 8.5 Potential complications and their remedies for gene-based therapy

Potential complications	Mitigation strategies
Gene silencing—repression of promoter	Use endogenous cellular promoters, avoid viral-derived regulatory sequences
Genotoxicity—complications arising from insertional mutagenesis	Use vectors with safer integration profile (e.g., self-inactivating lentiviral vectors) Sequence-specific integration (i.e., genome editing)
Phenotoxicity—complications arising from overexpression or ectopic expression of the transgene	Control transgene expression spatially (e.g., endogenous, tissue-specific promoters) and temporally (on/off switch)
Immunotoxicity—harmful immune response to either the vector or transgene	Carefully monitor T-cell reactivity to the vector and transgene to initiate immune suppression if needed
Risk of horizontal transmission—shedding of infectious vector into the environment	Monitor vector shedding in preclinical models when developing novel vectors
Risk of vertical transmission—germline transmission of donated DNA	Use of barrier contraceptive methods until vector shedding is negative

cannot be used for research on germline editing and clinical trials cannot be considered for approval by the FDA. The same restrictions are also adopted in many other countries.

References

1. High KA, Roncarolo MG. Gene therapy. N Engl J Med. 2019;381(5):455–64.
2. Dunbar CE, High KA, Joung JK, Kohn DB, Ozawa K, Sadelain M. Gene therapy comes of age. Science. 2018;359:6372.
3. Raper SE, Chirmule N, Lee FS, Wivel NA, Bagg A, Gao GP, et al. Fatal systemic inflammatory response syndrome in a ornithine transcarbamylase deficient patient following adenoviral gene transfer. Mol Genet Metab. 2003;80(1–2):148–58.
4. Naldini L. Genetic engineering of hematopoiesis: current stage of clinical translation and future perspectives. EMBO Mol Med. 2019;11(3):e9958.
5. Naldini L. Gene therapy returns to centre stage. Nature. 2015;526(7573):351–60.
6. Bushman FD. Retroviral insertional mutagenesis in humans: evidence for four genetic mechanisms promoting expansion of cell clones. Mol Ther. 2020;28(2):352–6.
7. Pasqauli M, Longo N. Newborn screening and inborn errors of metabolism. In: Rifai N, Horvath A, Wittwer C, editors. Fundamentals of clinical chemistry 8th edition. 8th ed. USA: Elsevier; 2020. p. 882–97.
8. Yuzyuk T, Viau K, Andrews A, Pasquali M, Longo N. Biochemical changes and clinical outcomes in 34 patients with classic galactosemia. J Inherit Metab Dis. 2018;41(2):197–208.
9. Jameson E, Remmington T. Dietary interventions for phenylketonuria. Cochrane Database Syst Rev. 2020;7:CD001304.
10. Pearl PL. Amenable treatable severe pediatric epilepsies. Semin Pediatr Neurol. 2016;23(2):158–66.
11. Rahman S. Emerging aspects of treatment in mitochondrial disorders. J Inherit Metab Dis. 2015;38(4):641–53.
12. Manzoni F, Salvatici E, Burlina A, Andrews A, Pasquali M, Longo N. Retrospective analysis of 19 patients with 6-pyruvoyl tetrahydropterin synthase deficiency: prolactin levels inversely correlate with growth. Mol Genet Metab. 2020;131(4):380–9.
13. Trefz FK, Burton BK, Longo N, Casanova MM, Gruskin DJ, Dorenbaum A, et al. Efficacy of sapropterin dihydrochloride in increasing phenylalanine tolerance in children with phenylketonuria: a phase III, randomized, double-blind, placebo-controlled study. J Pediatr. 2009;154(5):700–7.
14. Clayton PT. The effectiveness of correcting abnormal metabolic profiles. J Inherit Metab Dis. 2020;43(1):2–13.
15. Koto Y, Ueki S, Yamakawa M, Sakai N. Experiences of patients with lysosomal storage disorders treated with enzyme replacement therapy: a qualitative systematic review protocol. JBI Evid Synth. 2020;19(3):702–8.
16. Sheth J, Nair A. Treatment for lysosomal storage disorders. Curr Pharm Des. 2020;26(40):5110–8.
17. Sardh E, Harper P, Balwani M, Stein P, Rees D, Bissell DM, et al. Phase 1 trial of an RNA interference therapy for acute intermittent porphyria. N Engl J Med. 2019;380(6):549–58.
18. Baranello G, Darras BT, Day JW, Deconinck N, Klein A, Masson R, et al. Risdiplam in type 1 spinal muscular atrophy. N Engl J Med. 2021;384(10):915–23.
19. Finkel RS, Chiriboga CA, Vajsar J, Day JW, Montes J, De Vivo DC, et al. Treatment of infantile-onset spinal muscular atrophy with nusinersen: a phase 2, open-label, dose-escalation study. Lancet. 2016;388(10063):3017–26.
20. Hacein-Bey-Abina S, Le Deist F, Carlier F, Bouneaud C, Hue C, De Villartay JP, et al. Sustained correction of X-linked severe combined immunodeficiency by ex vivo gene therapy. N Engl J Med. 2002;346(16):1185–93.
21. Aiuti A, Slavin S, Aker M, Ficara F, Deola S, Mortellaro A, et al. Correction of ADA-SCID by stem cell gene therapy combined with nonmyeloablative conditioning. Science. 2002;296(5577):2410–3.
22. Hacein-Bey-Abina S, Von Kalle C, Schmidt M, McCormack MP, Wulffraat N, Leboulch P, et al. LMO2-associated clonal T cell proliferation in two patients after gene therapy for SCID-X1. Science. 2003;302(5644):415–9.
23. Stein S, Ott MG, Schultze-Strasser S, Jauch A, Burwinkel B, Kinner A, et al. Genomic instability and myelodysplasia with monosomy 7 consequent to EVI1 activation after gene therapy for chronic granulomatous disease. Nat Med. 2010;16(2):198–204.
24. Braun CJ, Boztug K, Paruzynski A, Witzel M, Schwarzer A, Rothe M, et al. Gene therapy for Wiskott-Aldrich syndrome--long-term efficacy and genotoxicity. Sci Transl Med. 2014;6(227):227ra33.
25. Wu X, Li Y, Crise B, Burgess SM. Transcription start regions in the human genome are favored targets for MLV integration. Science. 2003;300(5626):1749–51.
26. Aiuti A, Biasco L, Scaramuzza S, Ferrua F, Cicalese MP, Baricordi C, et al. Lentiviral hematopoietic stem cell gene therapy in patients with Wiskott-Aldrich syndrome. Science. 2013;341(6148):1233151.
27. Hacein-Bey-Abina S, Pai SY, Gaspar HB, Armant M, Berry CC, Blanche S, et al. A modified gamma-retrovirus vector for X-linked severe combined immunodeficiency. N Engl J Med. 2014;371(15):1407–17.
28. Aiuti A, Cattaneo F, Galimberti S, Benninghoff U, Cassani B, Callegaro L, et al. Gene therapy for immunodeficiency due to adenosine deaminase deficiency. N Engl J Med. 2009;360(5):447–58.
29. Mount JD, Herzog RW, Tillson DM, Goodman SA, Robinson N, McCleland ML, et al. Sustained pheno-

typic correction of hemophilia B dogs with a factor IX null mutation by liver-directed gene therapy. Blood. 2002;99(8):2670–6.
30. Manno CS, Pierce GF, Arruda VR, Glader B, Ragni M, Rasko JJ, et al. Successful transduction of liver in hemophilia by AAV-factor IX and limitations imposed by the host immune response. Nat Med. 2006;12(3):342–7.
31. Nguyen GN, Everett JK, Kafle S, Roche AM, Raymond HE, Leiby J, et al. A long-term study of AAV gene therapy in dogs with hemophilia A identifies clonal expansions of transduced liver cells. Nat Biotechnol. 2021;39(1):47–55.
32. French RA, Samelson-Jones BJ, Niemeyer GP, Lothrop CD Jr, Merricks EP, Nichols TC, et al. Complete correction of hemophilia B phenotype by FIX-Padua skeletal muscle gene therapy in an inhibitor-prone dog model. Blood Adv. 2018;2(5):505–8.
33. Bennett J, Wellman J, Marshall KA, McCague S, Ashtari M, DiStefano-Pappas J, et al. Safety and durability of effect of contralateral-eye administration of AAV2 gene therapy in patients with childhood-onset blindness caused by RPE65 mutations: a follow-on phase 1 trial. Lancet. 2016;388(10045):661–72.
34. Russell S, Bennett J, Wellman JA, Chung DC, Yu ZF, Tillman A, et al. Efficacy and safety of voretigene neparvovec (AAV2-hRPE65v2) in patients with RPE65-mediated inherited retinal dystrophy: a randomised, controlled, open-label, phase 3 trial. Lancet. 2017;390(10097):849–60.
35. Hwu WL, Muramatsu S, Tseng SH, Tzen KY, Lee NC, Chien YH, et al. Gene therapy for aromatic L-amino acid decarboxylase deficiency. Sci Transl Med. 2012;4(134):134ra61.
36. Mendell JR, Al-Zaidy S, Shell R, Arnold WD, Rodino-Klapac LR, Prior TW, et al. Single-dose gene-replacement therapy for spinal muscular atrophy. N Engl J Med. 2017;377(18):1713–22.
37. Muramatsu S, Fujimoto K, Ikeguchi K, Shizuma N, Kawasaki K, Ono F, et al. Behavioral recovery in a primate model of Parkinson's disease by triple transduction of striatal cells with adeno-associated viral vectors expressing dopamine-synthesizing enzymes. Hum Gene Ther. 2002;13(3):345–54.
38. Sung YK, Kim SW. Recent advances in the development of bio-reducible polymers for efficient cancer gene delivery systems. Cancer Med J. 2019;2(1):6–13.
39. Roberts TC, Langer R, Wood MJA. Advances in oligonucleotide drug delivery. Nat Rev Drug Discov. 2020;19(10):673–94.
40. de Smet MD, Meenken CJ, van den Horn GJ. Fomivirsen - a phosphorothioate oligonucleotide for the treatment of CMV retinitis. Ocul Immunol Inflamm. 1999;7(3–4):189–98.
41. Santos RD, Raal FJ, Catapano AL, Witztum JL, Steinhagen-Thiessen E, Tsimikas S. Mipomersen, an antisense oligonucleotide to apolipoprotein B-100, reduces lipoprotein(a) in various populations with hypercholesterolemia: results of 4 phase III trials. Arterioscler Thromb Vasc Biol. 2015;35(3):689–99.
42. Brannagan TH, Wang AK, Coelho T, Waddington Cruz M, Polydefkis MJ, Dyck PJ, et al. Early data on long-term efficacy and safety of inotersen in patients with hereditary transthyretin amyloidosis: a 2-year update from the open-label extension of the NEURO-TTR trial. Eur J Neurol. 2020;27(8):1374–81.
43. Dowling JJ. Eteplirsen therapy for Duchenne muscular dystrophy: skipping to the front of the line. Nat Rev Neurol. 2016;12(12):675–6.
44. Frank DE, Schnell FJ, Akana C, El-Husayni SH, Desjardins CA, Morgan J, et al. Increased dystrophin production with golodirsen in patients with Duchenne muscular dystrophy. Neurology. 2020;94(21):e2270–e82.
45. de Holanda MR, Jorge Polido G, Ciro M, Jorge Fontoura Solla D, Conti Reed U, Zanoteli E. Clinical outcomes in patients with spinal muscular atrophy type 1 treated with nusinersen. J Neuromuscul Dis. 2021;8(2):217–24.
46. Yuan YR, Pei Y, Chen HY, Tuschl T, Patel DJ. A potential protein-RNA recognition event along the RISC-loading pathway from the structure of A. aeolicus Argonaute with externally bound siRNA. Structure. 2006;14(10):1557–65.
47. de Paula Brandao PR, Titze-de-Almeida SS, Titze-de-Almeida R. Leading RNA interference therapeutics part 2: silencing delta-aminolevulinic acid synthase 1, with a focus on givosiran. Mol Diagn Ther. 2020;24(1):61–8.
48. Milani P, Mussinelli R, Perlini S, Palladini G, Obici L. An evaluation of patisiran: a viable treatment option for transthyretin-related hereditary amyloidosis. Expert Opin Pharmacother. 2019;20(18):2223–8.
49. Schneller JL, Lee CM, Bao G, Venditti CP. Genome editing for inborn errors of metabolism: advancing towards the clinic. BMC Med. 2017;15(1):43.
50. Richards DY, Winn SR, Dudley S, Nygaard S, Mighell TL, Grompe M, et al. AAV-mediated CRISPR/Cas9 gene editing in murine phenylketonuria. Mol Ther Methods Clin Dev. 2020;17:234–45.
51. Callaway E. COVID vaccine excitement builds as Moderna reports third positive result. Nature. 2020;587(7834):337–8.
52. Lu J, Lu G, Tan S, Xia J, Xiong H, Yu X, et al. A COVID-19 mRNA vaccine encoding SARS-CoV-2 virus-like particles induces a strong antiviral-like immune response in mice. Cell Res. 2020;30(10):936–9.
53. Mahase E. Covid-19: Moderna applies for US and EU approval as vaccine trial reports 94.1% efficacy. BMJ. 2020;371:m4709.
54. Polack FP, Thomas SJ, Kitchin N, Absalon J, Gurtman A, Lockhart S, et al. Safety and efficacy of the BNT162b2 mRNA Covid-19 vaccine. N Engl J Med. 2020;383(27):2603–15.
55. An D, Frassetto A, Jacquinet E, Eybye M, Milano J, DeAntonis C, et al. Long-term efficacy and safety of

mRNA therapy in two murine models of methylmalonic acidemia. EBioMedicine. 2019;45:519–28.
56. Balakrishnan B, An D, Nguyen V, DeAntonis C, Martini PGV, Lai K. Novel mRNA-based therapy reduces toxic galactose metabolites and overcomes galactose sensitivity in a mouse model of classic galactosemia. Mol Ther. 2020;28(1):304–12.
57. Truong B, Allegri G, Liu XB, Burke KE, Zhu X, Cederbaum SD, et al. Lipid nanoparticle-targeted mRNA therapy as a treatment for the inherited metabolic liver disorder arginase deficiency. Proc Natl Acad Sci U S A. 2019;116(42):21150–9.
58. Cao J, An D, Galduroz M, Zhuo J, Liang S, Eybye M, et al. mRNA therapy improves metabolic and behavioral abnormalities in a murine model of citrin deficiency. Mol Ther. 2019;27(7):1242–51.
59. Jiang L, Park JS, Yin L, Laureano R, Jacquinet E, Yang J, et al. Dual mRNA therapy restores metabolic function in long-term studies in mice with propionic acidemia. Nat Commun. 2020;11(1):5339.
60. Jiang L, Berraondo P, Jerico D, Guey LT, Sampedro A, Frassetto A, et al. Systemic messenger RNA as an etiological treatment for acute intermittent porphyria. Nat Med. 2018;24(12):1899–909.
61. Zhu X, Yin L, Theisen M, Zhuo J, Siddiqui S, Levy B, et al. Systemic mRNA therapy for the treatment of Fabry disease: preclinical studies in wild-type mice, Fabry mouse model, and wild-type non-human primates. Am J Hum Genet. 2019;104(4):625–37.
62. Tang X, Zhang S, Fu R, Zhang L, Huang K, Peng H, et al. Therapeutic prospects of mRNA-based gene therapy for glioblastoma. Front Oncol. 2019;9:1208.
63. Kauffman KJ, Mir FF, Jhunjhunwala S, Kaczmarek JC, Hurtado JE, Yang JH, et al. Efficacy and immunogenicity of unmodified and pseudouridine-modified mRNA delivered systemically with lipid nanoparticles in vivo. Biomaterials. 2016;109:78–87.
64. Pardi N, Tuyishime S, Muramatsu H, Kariko K, Mui BL, Tam YK, et al. Expression kinetics of nucleoside-modified mRNA delivered in lipid nanoparticles to mice by various routes. J Control Release. 2015;217:345–51.
65. Weissman D, Kariko K. mRNA: fulfilling the promise of gene therapy. Mol Ther. 2015;23(9):1416–7.
66. Kaczmarek JC, Patel AK, Kauffman KJ, Fenton OS, Webber MJ, Heartlein MW, et al. Polymer-lipid nanoparticles for systemic delivery of mRNA to the lungs. Angew Chem Int Ed Engl. 2016;55(44):13808–12.
67. Moderna's Clinical Trials 2021. Available from: https://www.modernatx.com/pipeline/modernas-mrna-clinical-trials-cmv-mma-zika-several-types-cancer-and-other-diseases.
68. Sabnis S, Kumarasinghe ES, Salerno T, Mihai C, Ketova T, Senn JJ, et al. A novel amino lipid series for mRNA delivery: improved endosomal escape and sustained pharmacology and safety in non-human primates. Mol Ther. 2018;26(6):1509–19.
69. An D, Schneller JL, Frassetto A, Liang S, Zhu X, Park JS, et al. Systemic messenger RNA therapy as a treatment for methylmalonic acidemia. Cell Rep. 2017;21(12):3548–58.
70. Wierzbicki AS, Viljoen A. Alipogene tiparvovec: gene therapy for lipoprotein lipase deficiency. Expert Opin Biol Ther. 2013;13(1):7–10.
71. Day JW, Finkel RS, Chiriboga CA, Connolly AM, Crawford TO, Darras BT, et al. Onasemnogene abeparvovec gene therapy for symptomatic infantile-onset spinal muscular atrophy in patients with two copies of SMN2 (STR1VE): an open-label, single-arm, multicentre, phase 3 trial. Lancet Neurol. 2021;20(4):284–93.
72. Fischer A, Hacein-Bey-Abina S, Cavazzana-Calvo M. 20 years of gene therapy for SCID. Nat Immunol. 2010;11(6):457–60.
73. Thompson AA, Walters MC, Kwiatkowski J, Rasko JEJ, Ribeil JA, Hongeng S, et al. Gene therapy in patients with transfusion-dependent beta-thalassemia. N Engl J Med. 2018;378(16):1479–93.
74. Bryant LM, Christopher DM, Giles AR, Hinderer C, Rodriguez JL, Smith JB, et al. Lessons learned from the clinical development and market authorization of Glybera. Hum Gene Ther Clin Dev. 2013;24(2):55–64.
75. Al-Zaidy SA, Mendell JR. From clinical trials to clinical practice: practical considerations for gene replacement therapy in SMA type 1. Pediatr Neurol. 2019;100:3–11.
76. Tsai SQ, Joung JK. Defining and improving the genome-wide specificities of CRISPR-Cas9 nucleases. Nat Rev Genet. 2016;17(5):300–12.
77. Liang P, Xu Y, Zhang X, Ding C, Huang R, Zhang Z, et al. CRISPR/Cas9-mediated gene editing in human tripronuclear zygotes. Protein Cell. 2015;6(5):363–72.
78. Friedmann T, Jonlin EC, King NMP, Torbett BE, Wivel NA, Kaneda Y, et al. ASGCT and JSGT joint position statement on human genomic editing. Mol Ther. 2015;23(8):1282.
79. Human genome editing: science, ethics, and governance. Washington, DC; 2017.

Part II

Aminoacidopathies

9 Phenylketonuria: Phenylalanine Neurotoxicity

Maria Giżewska

Contents

M. Giżewska (✉)
Department of Pediatrics, Endocrinology,
Diabetology, Metabolic Diseases and Cardiology,
Pomeranian Medical University, Szczecin, Poland

L. E. Bernstein et al. (eds.), *Nutrition Management of Inherited Metabolic Diseases*,
https://doi.org/10.1007/978-3-030-94510-7_9

Core Messages

- Phenylketonuria (PKU) was the first inherited metabolic disease identified by newborn screening and treated with diet to prevent the development of intellectual disability.
- Classification of the severity of phenylketonuria is based on the type of the variants in phenylalanine hydroxylase (PAH) gene, dietary phenylalanine tolerance, pretreatment blood phenylalanine concentrations, and the necessity to introduce treatment to achieve target blood phenylalanine concentrations.
- The etiology of brain damage in PKU has not been fully elucidated; however, high blood phenylalanine concentrations are associated with impaired transport of large neutral amino acids into the brain, decreased neurotransmitters synthesis, changes in brain morphology (gray and white matter), and impact on many enzymes involved in brain metabolism.

9.1 Background

Phenylketonuria (PKU) is the most common inherited autosomal-recessive inborn error of amino acid metabolism characterized by decreased activity of the enzyme phenylalanine hydroxylase (PAH) [1, 2]. The Norwegian biochemist and physician, Asbjorn Fölling, discovered PKU in 1934 by detecting phenylketones in the urine of siblings with intellectual disabilities, with subsequent identification of altered phenylalanine metabolism as the cause of this disease [3, 4]. PAH is the enzyme that converts phenylalanine to tyrosine in the presence of the cofactor tetrahydrobiopterin (BH_4), molecular oxygen, and nonheme iron [5] (Fig. 9.1). Loss of PAH activity results in elevated blood phenylalanine concentrations and is referred to as hyperphenylalaninemia (HPA) or phenylketonuria (PKU).

PKU is the exemplar of the effectiveness of newborn screening as it was the first inherited metabolic disease in which infants were identified by newborn screening and treated with diet before the development of intellectual disability

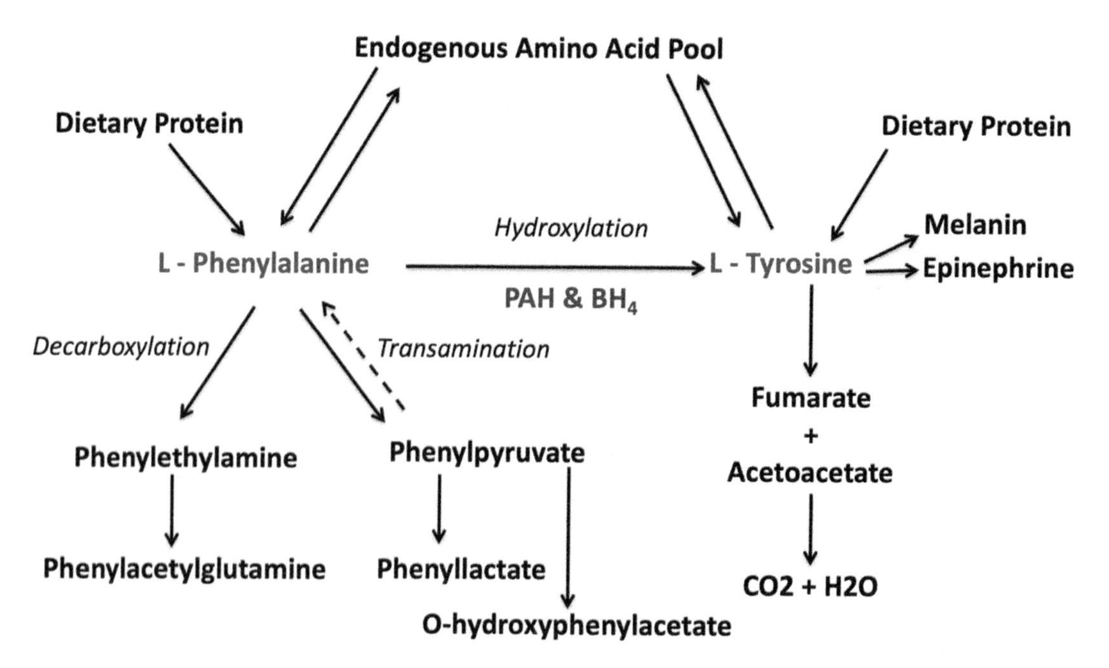

Fig. 9.1 Phenylalanine hydroxylase (PAH) and tetrahydrobiopterin (BH_4) in the presence of molecular oxygen (O_2) and nonheme iron converts phenylalanine to tyrosine. The alternate pathway of phenylalanine metabolism results in the accumulation of phenylalanine as well as phenylpyruvic acid and other phenylketones that are excreted in the urine. (Adapted from Acosta [1] and Donlon J et al. [5])

associated with untreated PKU. If left untreated or ineffectively managed, PKU can cause severe intellectual disability, as well as complex neurological and behavioral disorders. Severely affected patients are unable to live independently, often requiring specialized and continuous supervised care. Conversely, early and continuously treated patients typically have normal or nearly normal cognitive development. [6–8]

9.2 Biochemistry

Phenylalanine is an indispensable amino acid that cannot be synthesized by humans (Chap. 6). It comprises 3–7% of all dietary protein. After protein ingestion and digestion, phenylalanine is absorbed from the gastrointestinal tract to the liver via the portal vein. Phenylalanine is either hydroxylated into tyrosine via PAH in the liver or is incorporated into new proteins in tissues [5]. Hyperphenylalaninemia due to decreased activity of PAH manifests as a spectrum of disorders (severe, moderate, or mild PKU and non-PKU hyperphenylalaninemia). Deficiencies in the activity of PAH cofactor – tetrahydrobiopterin (BH_4) – represent a group of inherited metabolic diseases that result not only in hyperphenylalaninemia but also in alterations in tyrosine and tryptophan metabolism. BH_4 is also a cofactor for tyrosine hydroxylase and tryptophan hydroxylase, as well as three isoforms of nitric oxide synthase. Therefore, proper functioning of BH_4 is essential for the synthesis of dopamine, catecholamines, serotonin, melanin, and nitric oxide [9]. Phenylalanine can also be transaminated to phenylpyruvic acid as an alternative to hydroxylation by PAH. Phenylpyruvic acid, along with other ketones, is excreted in the urine as phenylacetic acid, phenylacetylglutamine, and phenyllactic acid. This pathway of phenylalanine metabolism is much less effective than hydroxylation [1, 5] (Fig. 9.1).

Phenylalanine hydroxylase (PAH) and BH_4 in the presence of molecular oxygen (O_2) and non-heme iron convert phenylalanine to tyrosine. The alternate pathway of phenylalanine metabolism results in the accumulation of phenylalanine as well as phenylpyruvic acid and other phenylketones that are excreted in the urine (Adapted from Acosta [1] and Donlon J et al. [5]).

The enzyme PAH has a complex structure consisting of three domains: regulatory, catalytic, and C-terminal domains. The regulatory domain contains a serine residue that is involved in activation by phosphorylation. The catalytic domain is responsible for cofactor and ferric iron binding, while the C-terminal domain is associated with inter-subunit binding [10]. The liver is the primary site of PAH activity, but it is also synthesized in the kidneys, pancreas, and brain.

9.3 Genetics

Phenylketonuria is an autosomal-recessive disorder. The majority (98%) of genetic variants associated with PKU occur at the phenylalanine hydroxylase locus [5], on the long arm of chromosome 12, in the region of q22-q24.1 [11]. Almost 1291 variants in the PAH locus have been described thus far, with 60% being missense mutations [12]. It is estimated that globally 450,000 individuals have PKU, with global prevalence of 1:23,930 live births [2]. Globally, the incidence in screened populations is estimated at 1:12,000 with a carrier frequency of 1:55 [13] (Box 9.1).

Box 9.1: Global Incidence of PKU [2]

Country	Incidence
Italy	1:4000
Ireland	1:4545
Iran, Jordan	1:5000
Turkey	1:6667
Germany	1:5360
Austria	1:5764
Estonia	1:7143
Poland	1:8039
France	1:9091
United Kingdom	1:10,000
Saudi Arabia	1:14,245
Canada	1:15,000
China	1:15,924
United States of America	1:25,000
Mexico	1:27,778
Peru	1:46,970
Japan	1:125,000
Thailand	1:227,273

Table 9.1 Classification of phenylketonuria, hyperphenylalaninemia, and tetrahydrobiopterin diagnoses

Classification of phenylketonuria	Pretreatment blood phenylalanine concentrations	Percentage of residual PAH activity
Unaffected	50–100 μmol/L (0.50–1.8 mg/dL)	Not applicable
Tetrahydrobiopterin deficiencies	120–2120 μmol/L (2–35 mg/dL)[a]	Varies
Mild hyperphenylalaninemia	120–360 μmol/L (2–6 mg/dL)	>5%
Mild phenlketonuria	360–900 μmol/L (6–15 mg/dL)	1–5%
Moderate phenylketonuria	900–1200 μmol/L (6–20 mg/dL)	1–5%
Severe (classical) phenylketonuria	>1200 μmol/L (>20 mg/dL)	<1%

Adapted from Camp et al. [15]

[a]In some patients with BH_4 deficiencies (e.g., dominant form of GTPCH deficiency and sepiapterin reductase deficiency), pretreatment blood phenylalanine concentrations are <120 μmol/L [14]

Initiation of dietary treatment depends on baseline phenylalanine concentrations; disagreement exists regarding the need for treatment

The prevalence of PKU varies widely among ethnic groups and geographical regions. It is highest in European and some Middle European countries.

The correlation between genotypes and biochemical phenotype, pretreatment phenylalanine concentrations, and phenylalanine tolerance is well established; however, the correlation between genotype and clinical phenotype, including neurological, intellectual, and behavioral outcomes, is weak [13].

9.4 Diagnosis

In most developed countries, PKU is identified by newborn screening by the presence of elevated phenylalanine and/or phenylalanine to tyrosine (Phe:Tyr) ratio in the dry blood spot collected in the first days to week of life (Chap. 2). Tandem mass spectrometry (MS/MS) is the method of choice to analyze the blood spots; however, other methods such as enzymatic techniques or high-pressure liquid chromatography (HPLC) are also used in some laboratories. After a positive newborn screening result, the patient is evaluated at a metabolic center for confirmatory testing and to rule out BH_4 deficiency by the analysis of pterin, as well as dihydropteridine (DHPR) activity. In many centers, a BH_4 loading test is often performed to identify patients with BH_4-responsive variants of PKU, as well as BH_4 deficiencies caused by the disturbance in the production and/or recycling of BH_4 [14]. Table 9.1 describes classifications of PAH deficiency.

9.5 Clinical Presentation

Untreated, late-treated, or poorly controlled patients have chronically elevated blood phenylalanine concentrations that lead to progressive and irreversible neurological, psychological, behavioral, as well as physical impairments that significantly impact quality of life. The degree of impairment depends on the blood concentration of phenylalanine with the most severe symptoms observed in untreated patients with the severe (classical) form of the disease. Although severe intellectual disability (with IQ scores often below 50) is the most typical presentation, untreated patients may demonstrate many other symptoms of persistent hyperphenylalaninemia (Box 9.2).

Box 9.2: Symptoms of Untreated Classical PKU

- "Musty" odor (urine and body)
- Hypopigmentation of the skin, hair, and iris
- Eczema
- Intellectual disability
- Neurological (seizures, tremor)
- Behavioral (hyperactivity, self-injury)
- Psychological (depression, anxiety, agoraphobia)

The outcome of early detected and treated PKU is generally favorable; however, even with good metabolic control, some individuals may demonstrate a higher prevalence of neuropsychological complications, including decreased executive function, internalizing disorders, and low self-esteem. Some patients, especially adults with PKU, are at higher risk of developing mood, anxiety, and attentional disorders across the lifespan [16–18].

9.6 Nutrition Management

The cornerstone of dietary management in PKU is limiting consumption of the offending amino acid, phenylalanine. In general, the diet is restricted in all high protein foods and includes medical foods that contain little or no phenylalanine but supply other amino acids in the diet (Chap. 10).

The amount of phenylalanine a patient can consume daily depends on the residual activity of PAH and other factors including the patient's age and growth rate [19, 20]. The concept of limiting dietary phenylalanine was first demonstrated in the early 1950s by Bickel et al. as they showed positive effects on behavior in a young patient with PKU [6]. The development of medical foods that were low in phenylalanine but contained other amino acids made the dietary treatment of PKU possible. During the early years of PKU treatment, it was generally believed that a low phenylalanine diet could be discontinued at around 6 years of age with no adverse effects [21–23]; however, "treatment for life" is the optimal mode of treatment [24–27]. According to recommendations from the National Institute of Health in 2014 and the first European PKU Guidelines in 2017, treatment should be started in all patients with hyperphenylalaninemia with blood phenylalanine concentrations greater than or equal to 360 μmol/L [14, 15]. Target phenylalanine concentrations used for the long-term follow-up in many centers are age-specific. European countries/centers follow recommendations from European PKU Guidelines suggesting optimal phenylalanine levels between 120 and 360 μmol/L for children up to the age of 12 years with higher values (up to 600 μmol/L) acceptable in older patients [14, 15]. In the United States, the goal is to maintain plasma phenylalanine concentrations below 360 μmol/L [15, 24, 28] across all age groups.

9.7 Phenylalanine Neurotoxicity

Eighty years after the discovery of PKU, the pathogenesis of brain dysfunction and the exact mechanisms of phenylalanine neurotoxicity are yet to be elucidated. Although there is a common agreement about the relationship between blood phenylalanine concentration and cognitive outcome in PKU, the concentration of phenylalanine and a deficiency of other large neutral amino acids in the brain are believed to be the main factors causing neurotoxicity. The impact of elevated blood phenylalanine concentrations, which is especially harmful during early infancy, is complex and multidirectional [11, 18, 29–36] (Box 9.3).

Box 9.3: The Main Theories of the Pathogenesis of PKU

- Impairment of large neutral amino acid (LNAA) transport across the blood-brain barrier (BBB) with disturbances in neurotransmitter metabolism [11, 29, 32–35, 37].
- Impairment in cholesterol synthesis and disturbances in myelin metabolism [29, 32, 34, 38, 39].
- Altered brain protein synthesis [11, 33, 37].
- Interference with the glutamatergic system directly involved in brain development [30, 33, 37, 40, 41].
- Altered glycolysis via inhibition of pyruvate kinase and other enzymes involved in brain energy metabolism [31, 33].
- Damage to cellular DNA, protein, and lipid, as well as decreased antioxidant defenses [33].

The typical symptoms of untreated individuals with PKU are the manifestation of the neurotoxic effect of phenylalanine on the central nervous system. A morphological change in the brain in patients with PKU affects both white and gray matters. Microcephaly, where the brain mass can be only 80% of that of a healthy individual, is a characteristic feature for many untreated PKU patients [37]. This symptom is caused by myelin structure anomalies that result in a loss of myelin volume, disturbances in cortical neuronal development, diffuse cortical atrophy, and general abnormalities in protein synthesis [33, 37–42].

Phenylalanine neurotoxicity affects the brain and related structures during critical windows of growth and development. Periods of particularly rapid growth make neuronal cells especially vulnerable to excessive amounts of toxic factors (e.g., phenylalanine) or a lack of substances needed for optimal development [43].

In PKU, similarly as in the other inherited disorders of amino acid metabolism, the fast-growing brain of the fetus is protected by the mother's enzymatic activity. The disturbances appear after birth, and the central nervous system is at risk of damage until the brain is fully developed and matured [44]. Despite the fact that the increase in brain mass and the creation of synaptic connections occur mainly during the first year of life, the full development of some areas (e.g., prefrontal cortex or white matter myelination) is not complete until adulthood (Box 9.4).

The last region to mature in the prefrontal cortex is the dorso-lateral area responsible for cognitive functions [45]. During the first few years of life, patients with PKU, which are inappropriately treated and have poorly controlled blood phenylalanine concentrations, suffer from inhibited growth of the cortex and a disrupted myelination process. For example, visuospatial speed deficits that result from structural myelin damage, which occurs early in life, followed by poor metabolic control in subsequent years, are difficult to improve despite tight phenylalanine control in adulthood [46]. Therefore, the risk of progressive neuropsychiatric manifestations of PKU in adulthood is higher in patients with poor metabolic control in infancy and early childhood. Of note, the neurotoxic influence of phenylalanine is present throughout life; this is why all patients with PKU require life-long, multidisciplinary care and maintenance of blood phenylalanine concentrations within the treatment range. For example, for complex executive functions, current and adult phenylalanine concentrations are stronger predictors of performance than metabolic control in childhood, demonstrating the importance of strict treatment and follow-up even in adulthood. Additionally, maintaining stable phenylalanine concentrations and minimizing blood phenylalanine fluctuations is of significant importance [46, 47].

High concentrations of blood phenylalanine result in increased uptake of phenylalanine into the brain and concomitant decrease in the uptake of other large neutral amino acids (LNAAs). Phenylalanine is transported into the brain by one of the LNAA carriers, the L-amino acid transporter 1 (LAT-1) [18, 32, 48–51]. This transporter also selectively transports the amino acids valine, isoleucine, methionine, threonine, tryptophan, tyrosine, and histidine. The binding of the LNAA to the LAT-1 transporter is a competitive process; the rate of transport is proportionate to the blood concentration of all the transported amino acids [52]. This system has the highest affinity for phenylalanine. With high blood phenylalanine, there is a significant decrease in the transport of other LNAAs as more phenylalanine is transported into the brain. Elevated brain phenylalanine concentrations also negatively impact the synthesis of catecholamines and serotonin in the brain due to the altered uptake of tyrosine and tryptophan and metabolism of tyrosine and tryptophan hydroxylases [5, 18, 54].

Box 9.4: Brain Development

- The increase in brain mass and the creation of synaptic connections occurs mainly during the first year of life.
- Full development of some areas (e.g., prefrontal cortex and white matter myelination) is not complete until adulthood.

The distribution of dopamine synthesis significantly alters activity of dopaminergic neurons of the prefrontal cortex, especially the dorsolateral area, which receives a large dopamine projection and is characterized by very high dopamine turnover [49]. It has been established that dopamine deficiency and disturbances in neurotransmitter balance may be responsible for cognitive and executive function deficits, as well as emotional problems, even in early-treated patients. The intensity of these dysfunctions is related to the degree of hyperphenylalaninemia. These observations form basic assumptions for the tyrosine-dopamine theory, which explains the complex abnormalities of neuropsychological function resulting from the intra-cerebral decrease of dopamine, secondary to tyrosine deficiency [18, 43, 53, 55].

Despite the significance for the clinical presentation of dopamine depletion, Pilotto et al. showed that serotonin depletion is also of great importance and may occur at much lower cerebral phenylalanine concentrations than the levels influencing dopamine synthesis. Based on the study of 10 adults with early-treated PKU, the authors postulated that the serotonergic axis is more vulnerable to high phenylalanine concentrations and that both serotonin and dopamine deficits are common in adult PKU patients. Additionally, the brain structural 3 T MRI study of these patients showed that decreased syntheses of dopamine and serotonin were correlated with specific gray matter atrophy patterns. These findings support the need for stricter metabolic control in adults to prevent neurotransmitter depletion and accelerated brain damage due to aging [32].

9.8 White Matter Pathology

PKU is associated with a diffuse brain pathology, including white matter changes that can be observed in both early and continuously treated patients [44]. As an integral part of the neuronal network, white matter has a crucial role in brain functioning. It is fundamental for proper motor and sensory functions, as well as sensory organ activity. White matter damage causes complex neurobehavioral syndromes, even if cortical and subcortical regions of gray matter remain intact [56]. The brains of individuals exposed to high blood phenylalanine from early childhood present with hypomyelination and astrocytic gliosis [44]. In addition, foci of segmental demyelination and areas of status spongiosis may occur [37, 39, 40, 49]. In histopathological research in mice, Malamud et al. described the above-mentioned phenomenon as diffuse vacuole formations occurring alongside the nerve fibers or in proximity of oligodendrocytes and stratifying myelin layers [57]. Complex disturbances of myelin metabolism in patients with PKU were coined with the term dysmyelination [58, 59]. The main function of the myelin sheath surrounding an axon is to facilitate the rapid conduction of action potentials along the axons for signal transmission and neurotransmitter synthesis [60]. The myelin takes part in axon maturation and, therefore, its damage causes disturbances in nervous system function. This means that altered myelin synthesis itself is the primary cause of secondary neuronal dysfunction and neurotransmitter synthesis abnormalities, including disturbances in the synthesis of dopamine (myelin-dopamine theory). Myelin-induced maturation of axons is also necessary for proper branching of dendrites during brain development, which is essential for the formation of the brain network [18, 34, 40, 60, 61].

Elevated brain phenylalanine concentrations influence the functioning of oligodendrocytes (glial cells responsible for myelin production) and thus proper axon functioning. Two types of oligodendrocytes are present in the central nervous system. The first type, phenylalanine-sensitive oligodendrocytes, is found in close proximity to neuronal networks that are myelinated after birth. With the exception of the cerebellum, these pathways are localized in frontal brain structures (optic tract, corpus callosum, subcortical white matter, and periventricular white matter). This group of oligodendrocytes is sensitive to phenylalanine concentrations, even in early-treated patients, and therefore, when the brain is exposed to high phenylalanine concentrations, myelin synthesis is disrupted. This leads to axons lacking proper myelin sheathing, further reducing the number of dendritic connections, decreas-

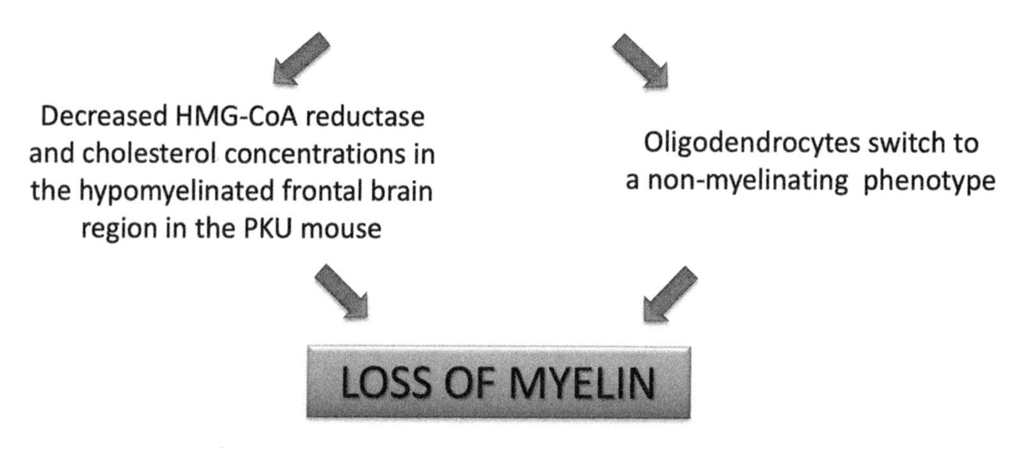

Fig. 9.2 Inhibition of HMG-CoA reductase results in the loss of myelin formation due to elevated phenylalanine concentrations in the brain [18, 60]

ing nervous conductivity and neurotransmitter production in presynaptic areas. The second type of oligodendrocyte cells are phenylalanine non-sensitive oligodendrocytes. These cells myelinate the axon before birth and are situated primarily in hindbrain structures (internal capsule and brainstem) and in spinal cord [18, 53, 60].

Phenylalanine and related metabolites inhibit activity of 3-hydroxy-3-methylglutaryl coenzyme-A (HMG-CoA) reductase (Fig. 9.2). This enzyme is critical for proper synthesis of cholesterol in phenylalanine-sensitive oligodendrocytes located in the frontal brain, especially in the prefrontal cortex. Locally synthesized cholesterol makes up approximately 30% of all myelin lipids of the brain tissue. The function of cholesterol is not only structural but is also required for proper neuronal signal transmission [18, 60]. Inhibition of HMG-CoA reductase by phenylalanine is partially reversible in some individuals. This explains the improvement in myelination observed in MRI scans of poorly controlled patients who have returned to diet and have reduced their blood phenylalanine concentrations. The reduction in phenylalanine allows for proper myelin production in the phenylalanine sensitive oligodendrocyte population [18, 53, 60, 62] (Fig. 9.3).

Phenylalanine neurotoxicity also includes the impact of elevated phenylalanine concentrations on the oligodendroglial enzyme, phenylalanine-sensitive ATP-sulfurylase. This enzyme is involved in the synthesis of cerebrosulphatides that protect the myelin base protein responsible for preventing myelin degradation. A lack of cerebrosulphatides results in an increase in the process of myelin degradation and, if not compensated for by proper synthesis, leads to complex dysmyelination changes [42, 49] (Fig. 9.4).

According to Dyer et al., white matter pathology in untreated PKU is a developmental process in which elevated phenylalanine concentrations arrest the myelination process, causing reduced myelin formation and hypomyelination. In early treated patients, myelin lesions reflect demyelination or dysmyelination and represent loss or impairment of previously assembled myelin [60] (Box 9.5).

The diffuse character of white matter pathology in PKU may compromise multiple pathways, resulting in different deficits in motor

Box 9.5: Dysmyelination Changes in PKU [40, 44, 58]
White matter abnormalities are a result of the following features:

- *Demyelination* (loss of formed myelin) in treated individuals
- *Hypomyelination* (lack of myelin formation) in untreated individuals

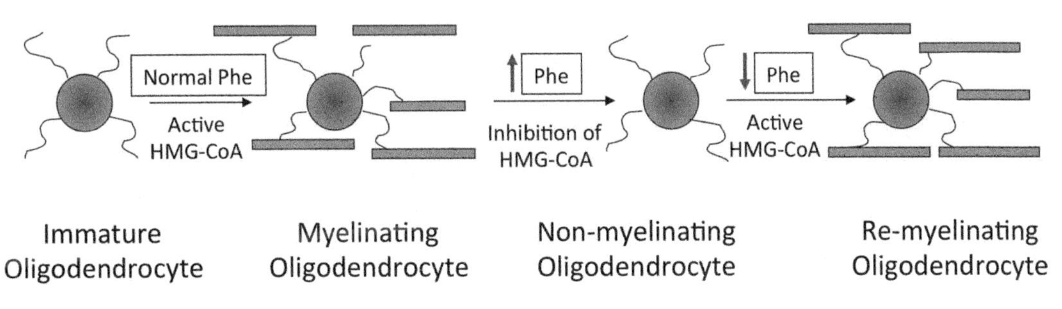

Fig. 9.3 Hypothesized effect of elevated phenylalanine concentrations on Phe-sensitive oligodendrocyte phenotypes in the forebrain [18, 60]

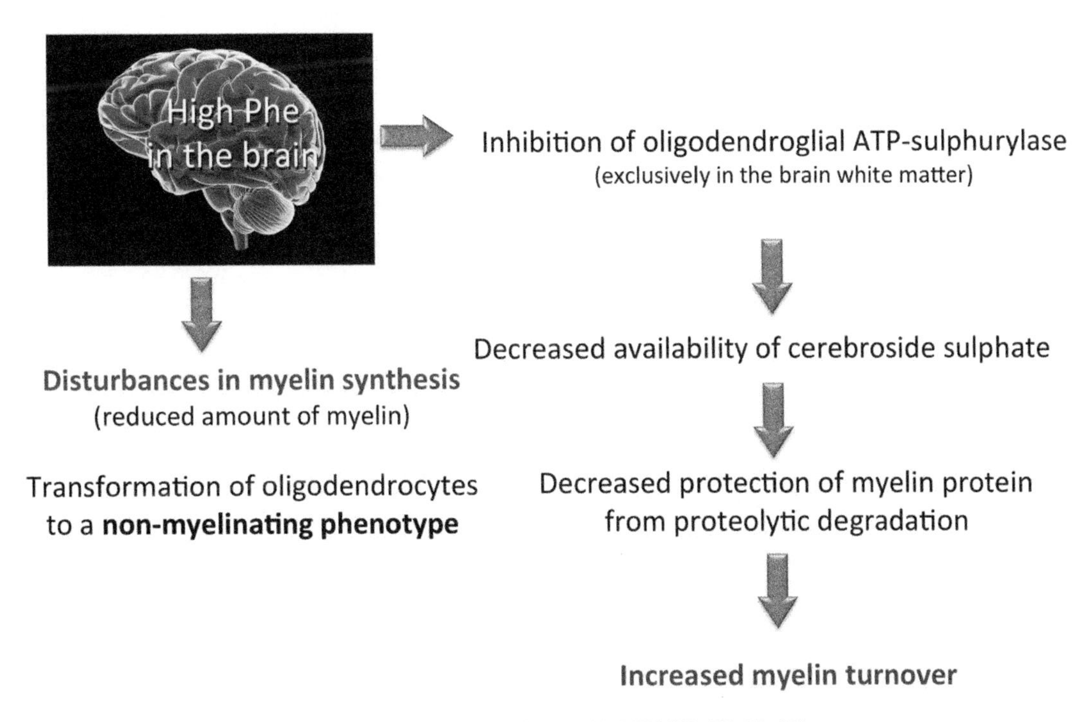

Fig. 9.4 Disturbances in myelination in the brain of patients with PKU [49, 57, 63–65]

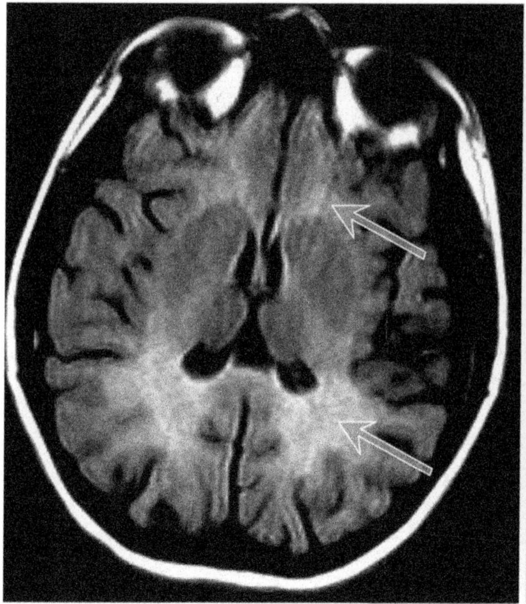

Fig. 9.5 Magnetic resonance imaging (MRI) of the brain: T2-weighted images using FLAIR (*fluid attenuated inversion recovery*) and FSE (*fast spin echo*) reveal enhanced signal intensity representing white matter abnormalities (WMA) in all lobes (arrows) of a female (MM) aged 27 years on low-phenylalanine diet from 3 to 8 years of age with a DQ of 32. Blood phenylalanine concentration at MRI was 1571 μmol/L

skills, coordination, visual functioning, processing speed, language, memory, and learning as well as attention and executive functioning [44].

White matter abnormalities (WMAs) of the brain were first reported in patients with PKU at the end of the 1990s [66, 67]. Dysmyelination in white matter is revealed with MRI as intense lesions and cortico-subcortical atrophy on T2-weighted images with specifically high-signal intensity in periventricular white matter. WMA may be explained by cytotoxic edema and dysmyelination changes with an increase in free water trapped in myelin sheaths [47]. The size and distribution of WMA vary between patients with localization in the white matter primarily in the temporal and occipital lobes [39, 44] (Figs. 9.5 and 9.6).

9.9 Gray Matter Pathology

Phenylalanine also influences the gray matter, with the greatest effect in the neocortex. A state of chronic hyperphenylalaninemia, especially in the neonate, profoundly affects the neocortex on multiple levels (Box 9.6).

Box 9.6: Effects of Hyperphenylalaninemia on Gray Matter [37, 41]

- Inhibition of growth process of the pyramidal pathways
- Disrupted dendritic growth resulting in formation of fewer connections
- Increased cell density of prefrontal cortex
- Inadequate synaptogenesis resulting in decreased synaptic density

The primary location of this effect is the posterior brain (parietal and occipital cortex), and it is strongly correlated with blood phenylalanine concentrations [38].

9.10 Summary

If untreated or poorly controlled, especially in early childhood, PKU can result in severe intellectual disability, neurological deficits, and/or

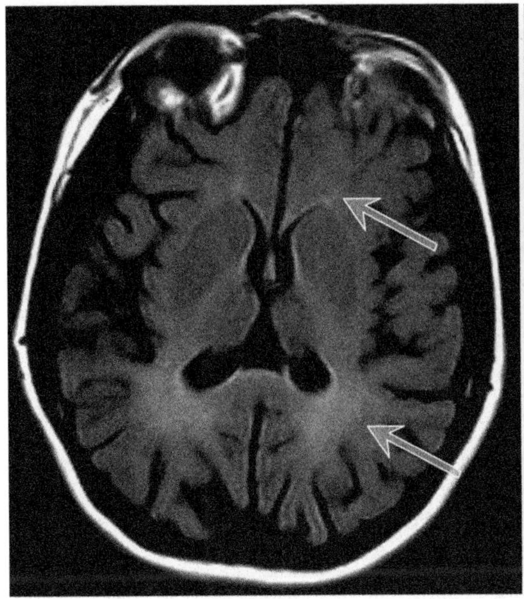

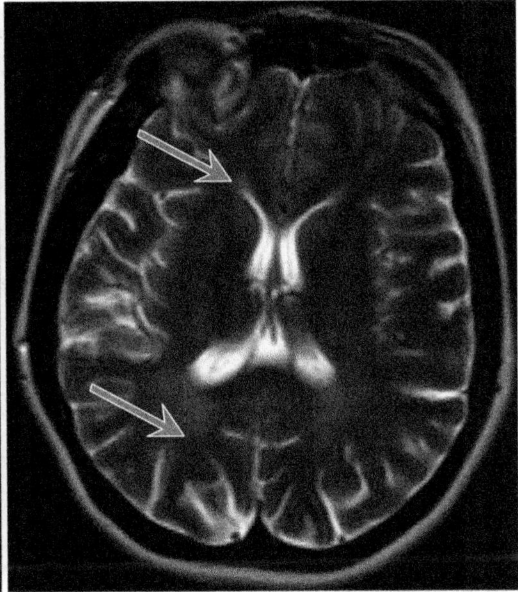

Fig. 9.6 MRI of the head (T2-weighted images, FLAIR and FSE) in the same patient (Fig. 9.5) shows regression of hyperintense lesions in white matter (WMA) of all lobes (arrows) after 7 months of treatment with a low-phenylalanine diet. Mean blood phenylalanine concentration was 724 μmol/L, blood phenylalanine concentration at MRI was 690 μmol/L

psychological/psychiatric manifestations. Early diagnosis with early and continuous treatment allows patients with PKU to achieve normal intellectual development; however, they still may exhibit a variety of neuropsychological difficulties. The pathogenesis of phenylalanine neurotoxicity in PKU is very complex and still far from being fully understood. It consists of both white and gray matter pathologies related to high brain phenylalanine concentrations. One of the main mechanisms of neurotoxicity is the impairment of brain neurotransmitter metabolism, especially in the prefrontal cortex. It is difficult to predict the outcome of discontinuing treatment in adults with early treated PKU; however, given the multidirectional effects of high blood phenylalanine on brain function, it is recommended that patients with PKU continue to be monitored and remain in metabolic control for life.

References

1. Acosta PB. Nutrition management of patients with inherited metabolic disorders. Sudbury: Jones and Bartlett Publishers, LLC; 2010.
2. Hillert A, Anikster Y, Belanger-Quintana A, Burlina A, Burton BK, Carducci C, et al. The genetic landscape and epidemiology of phenylketonuria. Am J Hum Genet. 2020;107(2):234–50.
3. Christ SE. Asbjorn Folling and the discovery of phenylketonuria. J Hist Neurosci. 2003;12(1):44–54.
4. Scriver CR. The PAH gene, phenylketonuria, and a paradigm shift. Hum Mutat. 2007;28(9):831–45.
5. Donlon J, Sarkissian C, Levy H, Scriver C. Hyperphenylalaninemia: phenylalanine hydroxylase deficiency. The online metabolic & molecular bases of inherited disease. McGraw Hill; 2021.
6. Bickel H, Gerrard AJ, Hickman EM. Influence of phenylalanine intake on phenylketonuria. Lancet. 1953;2:812–9.
7. Guthrie R, Susi A. A simple phenylalanine method for detecting phenylketonuria in large populations of newborn infants. Pediatrics. 1963;32:338–43.
8. Chace DH, Millington D, Terada N, Kahler SG, Roe CR, Lindsay FH. Rapid diagnosis of phenylketonuria by quantitative analysis for phenylalanine and tyrosine in neonatal blood spots by tandem mass spec trometry. Clin Chem. 1993;39(1):66–71.
9. Gibson M, Duran M. Simple tests. In: Blau N, editor. Physician's guide to the diagnosis, treatment, and follow-up of inherited metabolic diseases. New York: Springer; 2014.
10. Williams RA, Mamotte CD, Burnett JR. Phenylketonuria: an inborn error of phenylalanine metabolism. Clin Biochem Rev. 2008;29(1):31–41.
11. Blau N, van Spronsen FJ, Levy HL. Phenylketonuria. Lancet. 2010;376(9750):1417–27.

12. http://www.biopku.org/home/home.asp as of March 21, 2021.
13. Burgard P, Lachmann RH, Walter J. Hyperphenylalaninemia: 251–263, In: Saudubray JM, Baumgartner MR, Walter J, editors. Inborn metabolic diseases. Diagnosis and treatment. 6th edn. New York: Springer Medizin; 2016.
14. van Wegberg AMJ, MacDonald A, Ahring K, Belanger-Quintana A, Blau N, Bosch AM, et al. The complete European guidelines on phenylketonuria: diagnosis and treatment. Orphanet J Rare Dis. 2017;12(1):162.
15. Camp KM, Parisi MA, Acosta PB, Berry GT, Bilder DA, Blau N, et al. Phenylketonuria Scientific Review Conference: state of the science and future research needs. Mol Genet Metab. 2014;112(2):87–122.
16. Janos AL, Grange DK, Steiner RD, White DA. Processing speed and executive abilities in children with phenylketonuria. Neuropsychology. 2012;26(6):735–43.
17. Brumm VL, Bilder D, Waisbren SE. Psychiatric symptoms and disorders in phenylketonuria. Mol Genet Metab. 2010;99(Suppl 1):S59–63.
18. Ashe K, Kelso W, Farrand S, Panetta J, Fazio T, De Jong G, et al. Psychiatric and cognitive aspects of phenylketonuria: the limitations of diet and promise of new treatments. Front Psych. 2019;10:561.
19. MacDonald A, van Wegberg AMJ, Ahring K, Beblo S, Belanger-Quintana A, Burlina A, et al. PKU dietary handbook to accompany PKU guidelines. Orphanet J Rare Dis. 2020;15(1):171.
20. Cleary M, et al. Fluctuations in phenylalanine concentrations in phenylketonuria: a review of possible relationships with outcomes. Mol Genet Metab. 2013;110(4):418–23.
21. Horner FA, Streamer CW, Alejandrino LL, Reed LH, Ibbott F. Termination of dietary treatment of phenylketonuria. N Engl J Med. 1962;266:79–81.
22. Vandeman P. Termination of dietary treatment for phenylketonuria. Arch J Dis Child. 1963;106:492–5.
23. Hudson FP. Termination of dietary treatment of phenylketonuria. Arch J Dis Child. 1967;42:198–200.
24. Singh RH, et al. Recommendations for the nutrition management of phenylalanine hydroxylase deficiency. Genet Med. 2014;16(2):121–31.
25. Cerone R, et al. Phenylketonuria: diet for life or not? Acta Paediatr. 1999;88(6):664–6.
26. Smith I, et al. Effect of stopping low-phenylalanine diet on intellectual progress of children with phenylketonuria. Br Med J. 1978;2(6139):723–6.
27. Seashore MR, et al. Loss of intellectual function in children with phenylketonuria after relaxation of dietary phenylalanine restriction. Pediatrics. 1985;75(2):226–32.
28. Vockley J, Andersson HC, Antshel KM, Braverman NE, Burton BK, Frazier DM, et al. Phenylalanine hydroxylase deficiency: diagnosis and management guideline. Genet Med. 2014;16(2):188–200.
29. van Spronsen FJ, Hoeksma M, Reijngoud DJ. Brain dysfunction in phenylketonuria: is phenylalanine toxicity the only possible cause? J Inherit Metab Dis. 2009;32(1):46–51.
30. Martynyuk AE, et al. Impaired glutamatergic synaptic transmission in PKU brain. Mol Genet Metab. 2005;86(Suppl 1):434–42.
31. Feksa LR, et al. Characterization of the inhibition of pyruvate kinase caused by phenylalanine and phenylpyruvate in rat brain cortex. Brain Res. 2003;968(2):199–205.
32. Pilotto A, Blau N, Leks E, Schulte C, Deuschl C, Zipser C, et al. Cerebrospinal fluid biogenic amines depletion and brain atrophy in adult patients with phenylketonuria. J Inherit Metab Dis. 2019;42(3):398–406.
33. Schuck PF, Malgarin F, Cararo JH, Cardoso F, Streck EL, Ferreira GC. Phenylketonuria pathophysiology: on the role of metabolic alterations. Aging Dis. 2015;6(5):390–9.
34. Schlegel G, Scholz R, Ullrich K, Santer R, Rune GM. Phenylketonuria: direct and indirect effects of phenylalanine. Exp Neurol. 2016;281:28–36.
35. Pilotto A, Zipser CM, Leks E, Haas D, Gramer G, Freisinger P, et al. Phenylalanine effects on brain function in adult phenylketonuria. Neurology. 2021;96(3):e399–411.
36. van Spronsen FJ, van Wegberg AM, Ahring K, Belanger-Quintana A, Blau N, Bosch AM, et al. Key European guidelines for the diagnosis and management of patients with phenylketonuria. Lancet Diabetes Endocrinol. 2017;5(9):743–56.
37. Huttenlocher PR. The neuropathology of phenylketonuria: human and animal studies. Eur J Pediatr. 2000;159(Suppl 2):S102–6.
38. Christ SE, Price MH, Bodner KE, Saville C, Moffitt AJ, Peck D. Morphometric analysis of gray matter integrity in individuals with early-treated phenylketonuria. Mol Genet Metab. 2016;118(1):3–8.
39. Clocksin HE, Hawks ZW, White DA, Christ SE. Inter- and intra-tract analysis of white matter abnormalities in individuals with early-treated phenylketonuria (PKU). Mol Genet Metab. 2021;132(1):11–8.
40. Joseph B, Dyer CA. Relationship between myelin production and dopamine synthesis in the PKU mouse brain. J Neurochem. 2003;86(3):615–26.
41. Hartwig C, Gal A, Santer R, Ullrich K, Finckh U, Kreienkamp HJ. Elevated phenylalanine levels interfere with neurite outgrowth stimulated by the neuronal cell adhesion molecule L1 in vitro. FEBS Lett. 2006;580(14):3489–92.
42. Brenton DP, Pietz J. Adult care in phenylketonuria and hyperphenylalaninaemia: the relevance of neurological abnormalities. Eur J Pediatr. 2000;159(Suppl 2):S114–20.
43. Antshel KM, Waisbren SE. Timing is everything: executive functions in children exposed to elevated levels of phenylalanine. Neuropsychology. 2003;17(3):458–68.

44. Anderson PJ, Leuzzi V. White matter pathology in phenylketonuria. Mol Genet Metab. 2010;99(Suppl 1):S3–9.
45. Sijens PE, Oudkerk M, Reijngoud DJ, Leenders KL, de Valk HW, van Spronsen FJ. 1H MR chemical shift imaging detection of phenylalanine in patients suffering from phenylketonuria (PKU). Eur Radiol. 2004;14(10):1895–900.
46. Romani C, Palermo L, MacDonald A, Limback E, Hall SK, Geberhiwot T. The impact of phenylalanine levels on cognitive outcomes in adults with phenylketonuria: effects across tasks and developmental stages. Neuropsychology. 2017;31(3):242–54.
47. Daelman L, Sedel F, Tourbah A. Progressive neuropsychiatric manifestations of phenylketonuria in adulthood. Rev Neurol (Paris). 2014;170(4):280–7.63.
48. de Groot MJ, Hoeksma M, Blau N, Reijngoud DJ, van Spronsen FJ. Pathogenesis of cognitive dysfunction in phenylketonuria: review of hypotheses. Mol Genet Metab. 2010;99(Suppl 1):S86–9.
49. Surtees R, Blau N. The neurochemistry of phenylketonuria. Eur J Pediatr. 2000;159(S2):109–13.
50. van Spronsen FJ, et al. Large neutral amino acids in the treatment of PKU. From theory to practice. J Inherit Metab Dis. 2010;33(6):671–6.
51. Pardridge WM. Blood-brain barrier carrier-mediated transport and brain metabolism of amino acids. Neurochem Res. 1998;23(5):635–44.
52. Smith QR. Glutamate and Glutamine in the Brain. J Nutr. 2000;130:1016S–22S.
53. Dyer CA. Comments on the neuropathology of phenylketonuria. Eur J Pediatr. 2000;159(Suppl 2):S107–8.
54. Christ SE, Huijbregts SC, de Sonneville LM, White DA. Executive function in early-treated phenylketonuria: profile and underlying mechanisms. Mol Genet Metab. 2010;99(Suppl 1):S22–32.
55. Diamond A, Prevor MB, Callender G, Druin DP. Prefrontal cortex cognitive deficits in children treated early and continuously for PKU. Monogr Soc Res Child Dev. 1997;62(4):i–v, 1–208.
56. Filley CM. The behavioral neurology of cerebral white matter. Neurology. 1998;50(6):1535–40.
57. Malamud N. Neuropathology of phenylketonuria. J Neuropathol Exp Neurol. 1966;25(2):254–68.
58. Pietz J. Neurological aspects of adult phenylketonuria. Curr Opin Neurol. 1998;11(6):679–88.
59. Pearsen KD, Gean-Marton AD, Levy HL, Davis KR. Phenylketonuria: MR imaging of the brain with clinical correlation. Radiology. 1990;177(2):437–40.
60. Dyer CA. Pathophysiology of phenylketonuria. Ment Retard Dev Disabil Res Rev. 1999;5:104.
61. Kirkpatrick LL, Brady ST. Modulation in the axonal microtubule cytoskeleton by myelinating Schwann cells. J Neurosci. 1994;14(12):7440–50.
62. Cleary MA, Walter JH, Wraith JE, White F, Tyler K, Jenkins JP. Magnetic resonance imaging in phenylketonuria: reversal of cerebral white matter change. J Pediatr. 1995;127(2):251–5.
63. Shah SN, Peterson NA, McKean CM. Cerebral lipid metabolism in experimental hyperphenylalaninaemia: incorporation of 14C-labelled glucose into total lipids. J Neurochem. 1970;17(2):279–84.
64. Dyer CA, Kendler A, Philibotte T, Gardiner P, Cruz J, Levy HL. Evidence for central nervous system glial cell plasticity in phenylketonuria. J Neuropathol Exp Neurol. 1996;55(7):795–814.
65. Hommes FA. Amino acidaemias and brain maturation: interference with sulphate activation and myelin metabolism. J Inherit Metab Dis. 1985;8(Suppl 2):121–2.
66. Villasana D, Butler IJ, Williams JC, Roongta SM. Neurological deterioration in adult phenylketonuria. J Inherit Metab Dis. 1989;12(4):451–7.
67. Shaw DW, Weinberger E, Maravilla KR. Cranial MR in phenylketonuria. J Comput Assist Tomogr. 1990;14(3):458–60.

Nutrition Management of Phenylketonuria

10

Sandy van Calcar

Contents

S. van Calcar (✉)
Oregon Health & Science University, Molecular and Medical Genetics, Portland, OR, USA
e-mail: vancalca@ohsu.edu

L. E. Bernstein et al. (eds.), *Nutrition Management of Inherited Metabolic Diseases*,
https://doi.org/10.1007/978-3-030-94510-7_10

Core Messages

- The goal of nutrition management of phenylketonuria (PKU) is to maintain blood phenylalanine concentrations between 120 and 360 µmol/L (2–6 mg/dL).
- The diet for PKU includes medical foods low in or devoid of phenylalanine and limited quantities of phenylalanine from intact protein sources.
- Frequent monitoring of blood phenylalanine concentrations is key to successful diet management.
- Frequent diet adjustments are needed to achieve desired blood phenylalanine concentrations, as well as to promote normal growth and feeding development.
- A variety of PKU medical foods and modified low protein foods are available to accommodate different nutrient needs and taste preferences throughout the lifespan.
- Maintaining the diet is challenging for many patients with PKU; alternative therapies are available that may increase phenylalanine tolerance and diet sustainability.

10.1 Background

Phenylketonuria (PKU) is an inborn error in phenylalanine metabolism caused by a deficiency of the phenylalanine hydroxylase (PAH) enzyme (Fig. 10.1). The cofactor for phenylalanine hydroxylase is tetrahydrobiopterin (BH_4). In PKU, blood and brain concentrations of phenylalanine accumulate, affecting myelin and neurotransmitter production (Box 10.1) [1] (Chap. 9).

Box 10.1: Principles of Nutrition Management for Phenylketonuria

- *Restrict:* Phenylalanine
- *Supplement:* Tyrosine
- *Toxic metabolite:* Phenylalanine

With the genetic defect in PAH, phenylalanine is not converted to tyrosine; thus, tyrosine becomes a conditionally essential amino acid and must be supplemented in the diet. The incidence of PKU in those of Northern European descent is approximately 1 in 10,000 births with varying incidence in other populations [2, 3]. PKU is inherited in an autosomal-recessive pattern. Both parents are carriers for PKU but do not show any signs of the disorder. With each pregnancy, there is a 25% chance of having a child affected by PKU. Over 1200 variants have been described in the PAH gene (http://www.biopku.org).

The untreated PKU phenotype was first described in 1934 by Asbjorn Fölling in two siblings with severe cognitive and developmental delays [4]. Other signs and symptoms of untreated PKU may include seizures and autistic-like behavior. Eczema, light hair, and light complexion can also be seen and are caused by the deficiency of tyrosine, a precursor in melanin production [5]. The screening test for PKU was developed by Robert Guthrie, and newborn screening for PKU first started in Massachusetts in 1961 [6]. This public health initiative has allowed for early diagnosis and initiation of diet treatment and has ameliorated the untreated phenotype (Chap. 2).

The options for diet management of PKU have expanded greatly since the initiation of newborn screening with a wide range of available medical foods, including those made from L-amino acids and glycomacropeptide (GMP) as the primary source of protein equivalents. Supplemental large neutral amino acids (LNAAs) can provide an alternative to traditional medical foods. Pharmaceutical treatment includes synthetic tetrahydrobiopterin (BH4) as the cofactor for PAH (Kuvan®, BioMarin Pharmaceutical Inc., Novato, CA). Both LNAAs and pharmaceutical BH4 are addressed later in this chapter. The newest medication for treatment of PKU is pegvaliase (Palynziq®, BioMarin Pharmaceutical Inc., Novato, CA), an enzyme substitution therapy addressed in Chap. 11.

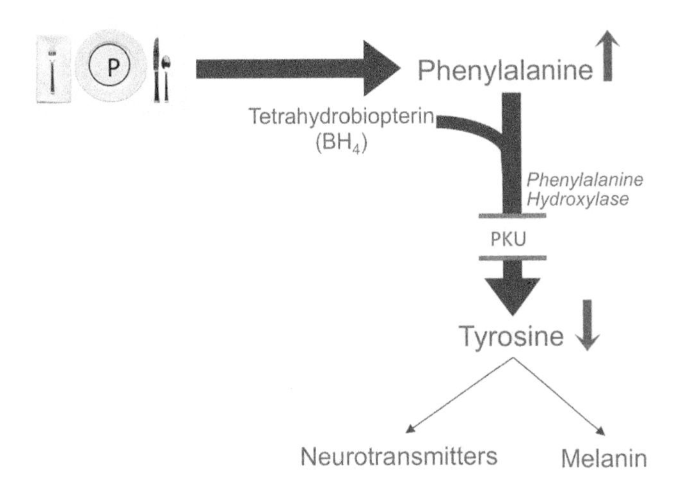

Fig. 10.1 Metabolic pathway of the conversion of phenylalanine to tyrosine

10.2 Nutrition Management of an Infant with PKU

10.2.1 Overview of Nutrition Management

Diet treatment for PKU traditionally includes a diet restricted in phenylalanine and an amino acid–based medical food devoid of phenylalanine. The majority of medical foods for PKU provide all other indispensable amino acids, tyrosine as a conditionally indispensable amino acid, fat, carbohydrate, and micronutrients. The protein equivalents from medical foods often provide the majority of total protein requirements for patients with PKU. (The term protein equivalents applies to the protein provided by an incomplete protein source, such as a PKU medical food that provides all amino acids except phenylalanine.) Especially for those with severe PKU, the amount of intact protein required to meet phenylalanine needs is often so limited that without use of a medical food, protein deficiency could develop [7]. Medical foods also supply the majority of energy, especially in the diets of infants and toddlers.

When an infant is referred to a metabolic clinic with a positive newborn screen for PKU and the diagnosis is confirmed, the first step is to reduce the blood phenylalanine concentration into the treatment range of 120–360 μmol/L (2–6 mg/dL [8]. Once blood phenylalanine decreases into the treatment range, a source of intact protein is added to meet the infant's phenylalanine needs. The goal is to provide sufficient phenylalanine to promote adequate growth and protein nutriture but prevent excessive phenylalanine intake that will increase the blood concentration above the treatment range. The amount of phenylalanine required in the diet depends on the severity of the disease as well as other factors, such as the infant's growth rate. Frequent monitoring of blood phenylalanine concentrations is crucial for successful management of PKU [9].

10.2.2 Initiating Diet for a Newly Diagnosed Neonate

There are several ways to initiate the diet depending on the initial blood phenylalanine concentra-

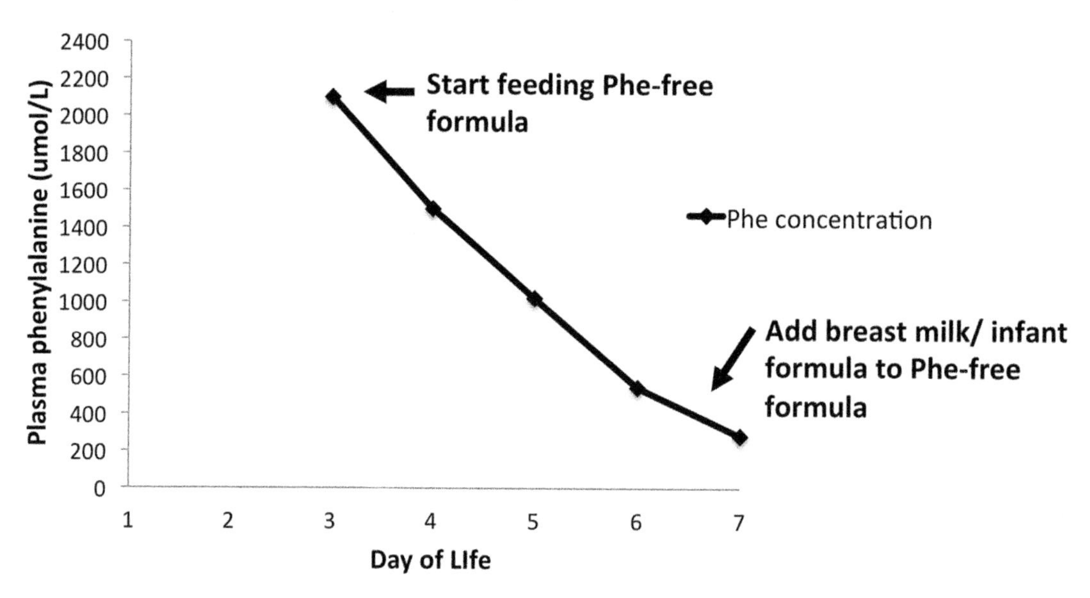

Fig. 10.2 Example of decreasing blood phenylalanine concentration in a neonate started on a phenylalanine-free diet at day of life 3

tion from newborn screening and confirmatory plasma amino acids (Fig. 10.2). The blood phenylalanine concentration can be quickly reduced by completely removing dietary phenylalanine and offering only a phenylalanine-free medical food for a prescribed amount of time; this is often referred to as a "wash-out" period [10]. The higher the initial blood phenylalanine, the longer the time required to reduce the concentration of phenylalanine into treatment range (Box 10.2). The time it takes to obtain blood phenylalanine results from a laboratory can influence the decision to remove phenylalanine entirely from the diet. If results will not be available before the phenylalanine concentration is expected to decrease into the recommended range, a source of phenylalanine should be added to the medical food to prevent excessively low blood concentrations. For those with lower initial phenylalanine concentrations, it may be prudent to initially prescribe 25–50% of estimated phenylalanine needs from an intact protein source to avoid decreasing the blood concentration below the treatment range.

Box 10.2: Suggested Time Frame for Initial Removal of Phenylalanine (PHE) from the Diet

Diagnostic PHE concentration	Remove dietary PHE for
360–600 μmol/L (6–10 mg/dL)	24 hours
600–1200 μmol/L (10–20 mg/dL)	48 hours
1200–2400 μmol/L (20–40 mg/dL)	72 hours
> 2400 μmol/L (> 40 mg/dL)	96 hours

Once the blood phenylalanine concentration is close to or within the treatment range, the next step is to add a calculated amount of standard proprietary infant formula or breastmilk to the medical food to provide the estimated phenylalanine needs of the infant [9, 10]. This diet calculation is somewhat different depending on whether infant formula or breastmilk is used (Boxes 10.3 and 10.4).

The range of dietary phenylalanine required by an infant is 25–70 mg/kg/day [10] or 130–

Box 10.3: Initiating Diet for an Infant with PKU Using Standard Infant Formula as the Source of Phenylalanine

Goal: Reduce plasma phenylalanine concentrations to 120–360 μmol/L (2–6 mg/dL).

Step by step:

1. Establish intake goals based on the infant's diagnostic blood phenylalanine, clinical status, and laboratory values.
2. Determine amount of standard infant formula required to provide the amount of phenylalanine to meet the infant's needs. Determine the amount of protein and energy that will be provided by this amount of standard formula.
3. Subtract the protein provided by the standard infant formula from the infant's total protein needs. Calculate amount of medical food required to meet the remaining protein needs.
4. Determine the number of calories provided by both the infant formula and phenylalanine-free medical food. Provide the remaining calories from a phenylalanine-free medical food.
5. Calculate amount of tyrosine provided by both the infant formula and phenylalanine-free medical food.
6. Determine the amount of fluid required to provide a caloric density of 20–25 kcal/ounce.
7. Divide this volume of medical food into feedings for a 24-hour period. (Diet calculation examples are provided at the end of this chapter.)

Box 10.4: Initiating Diet for an Infant with PKU Using Breastmilk as the Source of Phenylalanine

Goal: Reduce plasma phenylalanine concentrations to 120–360 μmol/L (2–6 mg/dL).

Step by step:

1. Establish intake goals based on the infant's diagnostic blood phenylalanine, clinical status, and laboratory values.
2. Note: In breast-fed infants, the lower end of the protein goal is usually sufficient since breastmilk contains less protein than infant formula, but it is of high biological value.
3. Determine amount of breastmilk required to provide the infant's estimated phenylalanine needs. Determine the amount of protein and energy that will be provided by this volume of breastmilk.
4. Subtract the protein provided by the breastmilk from the infant's total protein needs. Calculate amount of phenylalanine-free medical food required to meet the remaining protein requirement.
5. Determine the number of calories provided by both the breastmilk and phenylalanine-free medical food. Provide the remaining calories from additional phenylalanine-free medical food.
6. Calculate amount of tyrosine provided by both the breastmilk and phenylalanine-free medical food.
7. Determine the amount of fluid required to make a medical food formula with a 20 kcal/ounce concentration.

430 mg/day [9]. Exactly how much phenylalanine to prescribe after the initial wash-out is a matter of judgment – often those with higher blood phenylalanine concentrations prior to introducing phenylalanine into the diet require less phenylalanine to meet their needs. For example, an infant with an initial blood phenylalanine concentration of 1600 μmol/L may be prescribed 45 mg phenylalanine/kg body weight after the recommended 72-hour wash-out, whereas an infant with an initial blood phenylalanine concentration of 900 μmol/L may be prescribed 55 mg phenylalanine/kg after the suggested wash-out of 48 hours. The following table can

Table 10.1 Suggested guidelines to establish the amount of dietary phenylalanine introduced into the diet prescription after the removal of phenylalanine from the diet (wash-out)

Nutrient	Diagnostic blood phenylalanine concentration	Amount of phenylalanine to prescribe after washout period (mg/kg)
Phenylalanine	< 600 µmol/L (< 10 mg/dL)	70
	600–1200 µmol/L (10–20 mg/dL)	55
	1200–1800 µmol/L (20–30 mg/dL)	45
	1800–2400 µmol/L (30–40 mg/dL)	35

serve as a guideline to establish the amount of dietary phenylalanine to introduce into the diet prescription after the washout [10] (Table 10.1).

However, since results from newborn screening are often available more quickly now than in the past, very high phenylalanine concentrations are not seen as often and it may be difficult to determine how much dietary phenylalanine to initially prescribe. In this case, it is appropriate to estimate phenylalanine needs in the middle of the recommended range (45–50 mg/kg/day) as a starting point for calculation. Additionally, premature infants will require a higher initial phenylalanine intake than term infants given their higher protein needs for growth [11].

Infants with PKU consume a similar volume of formula or breastmilk as any typically developing infant. Thus, the caloric density of the initial medical food prescription should be approximately 20 kcal/ounce unless other factors necessitate a higher caloric concentration. Osmolarity and renal solute load should be determined if the formula concentration is greater than 24 kcal/ounce. Caregivers should be instructed to feed infants ad lib as they should be able to self-regulate the frequency of feeding and volume of formula consumed.

If standard infant formula is used as the source of phenylalanine, it is best to provide a recipe that mixes both the standard infant formula with the PKU medical food to assure even distribution of phenylalanine throughout each 24-hour period. Ask the parents to record how often and how much of the formula the infant is consuming for several days. If the total amount of formula consumed is typically greater than the amount anticipated in your calculations, then adjust the formula prescription to include more PKU medical food. If the amount of formula that the infant is consuming is less than the amount anticipated, then adjust the formula prescription by reducing the amount of PKU medical food that is added to the formula. The goal is to make sure that the infant is consuming the entire volume of the standard infant formula over a 24-hour period to meet phenylalanine needs. Additionally, caregivers can be given a recipe for "straight" PKU formula that does not include any standard infant formula. (This is the same recipe used in the washout.) This can be given at the end of the 24 hours if the infant has consumed the anticipated volume but wants additional feedings before the next 24-hour period starts.

If a mother is breastfeeding her infant, it is possible to design a PKU diet to allow her to continue feeding from the breast. Mature breastmilk contains less protein, and thus less phenylalanine, than an equivalent amount of standard infant formula (Table 10.2). The goal is to provide an appropriate amount of breastmilk to meet the infant's phenylalanine requirement and to maintain blood phenylalanine concentrations within the treatment range. This is accomplished by providing a combination of breast feedings and PKU medical food from the bottle.

There are several approaches to designing a diet that uses breastmilk as the source of phenylalanine (Box 10.4). First, the estimated volume of breastmilk to meet the infant's phenylalanine needs is determined. Then the amount of PKU medical food to prescribe can be determined using the estimated caloric needs [12] or total protein needs of the infant (Sect. 10.9).

When feeding the infant, it is best if the medical food is provided by itself and not in combination with a breastfeeding. This allows the mother to completely empty her breast during breastfeeding sessions. One approach is to prescribe a volume of PKU medical food that the infant will consume during the 24 hours, divided into a specified number of feedings. Then, allow ad lib breastfeeding for all other feedings during the 24-hour period. Often the feeding schedule can allow for alternating breast and formula feedings or a breastfeeding followed by two PKU formula feedings.

Alternatively, the volume of phenylalanine-free medical food can be distributed in smaller volumes (e.g. 1–2 ounces) over more feedings throughout a 24-hour period. After consuming the phenylalanine-free medical food, the infant is allowed to breastfeed until he/she is full. This method may not work if a relatively large volume of medical food is required as the mother may find it more difficult to maintain her breastmilk supply. For a mother electing to breastfeed her infant, it is important that she express or pump breastmilk to maintain an adequate milk supply.

Table 10.2 Comparison of nutrients in a typical standard infant formula and mature breastmilk

In 100 ml (standard dilution)	Infant formula	Breastmilk – mature
Phenylalanine	60 mg	47 mg
Tyrosine	58 mg	54 mg
Protein	1.4 g	1.06 g
Energy	68 kcal	72 kcal

10.2.3 Monitoring Blood Phenylalanine to Adjust the Diet Prescription

The only way to know if a diet prescription needs to be adjusted is to measure blood or plasma phenylalanine concentrations. The recommended frequency of monitoring is provided in guidelines developed by Genetic Metabolic Dietitians International (GMDI) [9, 13]. Figure 10.3 shows the diet adjustments that will need to be made whether the infant is receiving phenylalanine from infant formula or from breastfeeding. If the infant is consuming a standard infant formula as the source of phenylalanine, the amount of standard infant formula will be increased if blood phenylalanine is too low or decreased if blood phenylalanine is too high. For an infant consuming breastmilk as the source of phenylalanine, the volume of PKU medical food will be increased if blood phenylalanine is too high or decreased if blood phenylalanine is too low. These adjustments in the volume of PKU medical food effectively increase or decrease the infant's consumption of breastmilk.

Expect to adjust the diet prescription frequently, especially during the first two months of life. How much to adjust a phenylalanine pre-

Adjusting the Diet Prescription
Too High:
Above 6 mg/dL
(360 µmol/L)
If infant formula is the source of phenylalanine, adjust infant formula volume:
Decrease with high levels
Increase with low levels
Optimal:
2-6 mg/dL
120 – 360 µmol/L

If breast milk is the source of phenylalanine, adjust PKU medical food volume:
Increase with high levels
Decrease with low levels
Too Low:
Below 2 mg/dL
(120 µmol/L)

Fig. 10.3 Blood phenylalanine concentrations and recommended diet adjustments

scription depends on the blood phenylalanine concentration. Increasing or decreasing phenylalanine intake in 10% increments is typical, but the percent change can be greater if blood phenylalanine concentrations are <60 μmol/L (<1 mg/dL) or greater than 480 μmol/L (8 mg/dL). However, adjustments need to be individualized for each patient.

10.2.4 Initiating Complementary Feedings

The American Academy of Pediatrics recommends that infants start solid foods between 4 and 6 months of age [14]. At this time, the phenylalanine provided by the infant formula or breastmilk will be decreased and replaced with phenylalanine from solids. A transition plan is developed with reduction in either the ounces of standard infant formula or the number of breastmilk feedings over a 24-hour period. For mothers who are breastfeeding, it may become more difficult to maintain an adequate milk supply as solids are introduced.

When starting solids for an infant with PKU, many clinics recommend introducing low-phenylalanine fruits and vegetables first, especially if using a simplified diet approach for tracking phenylalanine intake (Sect. 10.2.5). Before solid foods are introduced, caregivers need to learn how to track the amount of phenylalanine from foods. Phenylalanine can be counted as milligrams of phenylalanine in all foods or only in higher phenylalanine foods when using the simplified diet (Sect. 10.2.5). Web-based applications, such as How Much Phe® (www.howmuchphe.org), are available to provide accurate phenylalanine and protein content of various foods, including modified low protein products. During the first year, initiating the transition from a bottle to a cup should be encouraged. To avoid struggles with this transition, only medical food or water should be given by cup. At least initially, juice or other sweetened beverages should not be offered from the cup to assure better acceptance of medical food and reduce the risk of excessive weight gain [14].

10.2.5 Simplified Diet

For many patients with PKU, the "simplified diet" is an easier strategy to monitor phenylalanine intake compared to the more traditional methods of counting exchanges (1 exchange = 15 mg phenylalanine) or counting milligrams of phenylalanine in all foods consumed during a day. First described by MacDonald et al., the simplified diet allows for a portion of a patient's phenylalanine requirement to be reserved for foods that are low enough in phenylalanine that they can be eaten in unrestricted amounts and do not need to be "counted" as part of a patient's daily phenylalanine prescription [15–18]. The method has been used in Europe and Australia and, more recently, widely adopted by clinics in the United States [15].

While this dietary management approach is simplified, it is not liberalized as a patient's phenylalanine prescription remains unchanged. While the logistics of the diet can vary, the most common method is to reserve 30% of a patient's total phenylalanine prescription for "free" or "uncounted" foods. Foods in this category include those that contain less than 75 mg phenylalanine/100 g of food. This includes all fruit (except for some dried fruit) and many vegetables with a lower phenylalanine content. The majority of modified low protein foods are also considered "free" or "uncounted" if they contain <20 mg phenylalanine/serving (Appendix G). These foods have traditionally been classified as "free" foods, but the great majority do contain some phenylalanine and the "free" designation can be confusing to caregivers and patients. Thus, "uncounted" may be a more appropriate term for these foods [15].

The remaining 70% of a patient's phenylalanine prescription includes higher phenylalanine foods that need to be measured or weighed and counted as is required with traditional diet methods. Foods in this category include higher phenylalanine vegetables (especially starchy vegetables) and all legumes, as well as breads, cereals, pasta, rice, and snack foods made from grains, corn, and other carbohydrate-based ingredients. These foods can be counted with milligrams of phenylalanine or grams of protein (Box 10.5).

Box 10.5: Implementing the Simplified Diet

What is a patient's recommended phenylalanine (PHE) intake for good control?

- "Hold back" 30% of PHE prescription for fruits and uncounted vegetables.
- Foods with PHE < 75 mg/100 g are "uncounted."
- Low protein products with PHE < 20 mg/serving are "uncounted."
- The remaining 70% of PHE prescription is for "counted" foods.
- If counting protein, convert to protein using 50 mg PHE = 1 g protein.
- Example:
  - Usual intake: 300 mg PHE from food
  - Determine 30% of usual PHE intake = 90 mg PHE
  - Subtract 90 mg from usual PHE intake
  - New Rx = 210 mg PHE counted foods
  - No limits in intake of "uncounted" foods
  - If counting protein: 4 g of protein per day from counted foods
- See Appendix G for simplified diet lists.

The simplified diet approach is now frequently initiated with the introduction of solid foods at 4–6 months of age and continued as the preferred method of tracking phenylalanine for all ages [15]. Counting protein rather than phenylalanine (50 mg phenylalanine = 1 g protein) is often not used during infancy, but reserved for older ages, especially when teaching children to monitor their own intake. Counting protein can be easier for some patients since it allows for the use of food labels for foods found in grocery stores. The author's clinic routinely introduces protein counting when introducing solids foods in infancy and has not observed any differences in the ability to maintain metabolic control with this method versus counting milligrams of phenylalanine.

10.3 Nutrition Management of PKU Beyond Infancy

After infancy, a patient's diet will continue to include naturally low protein foods such as fruits, most vegetables, and foods with a moderate amount of protein such as starchy vegetables and, depending on phenylalanine tolerance, regular grain products. It is often easy for those with PKU to overconsume foods with a moderate amount of protein since small quantities can provide a significant amount of phenylalanine. These foods need to be weighed or measured to maintain good metabolic control [9, 13].

The PKU diet often includes modified low protein products, such as low protein pasta, breads, and baking mixes that are made from wheat or other starch, thus reducing the phenylalanine content. These products are usually ordered from specialty food companies, although some may be available in grocery stores carrying gluten-free foods, as some gluten-free products are also low in protein. The benefit of using modified low protein products is that they increase the energy content and the variety of foods in the diet, yet most are very low in phenylalanine [19]. There are several print and online resources for low protein cooking that can help families provide variety in the diet and learn to use modified low protein foods [20–22]. The diet can also include "free foods," which are carbohydrate- and/or fat-based foods with very little or no phenylalanine. Aside from adding extra energy to the diet, these foods are often of poor nutritional value and need to be used in moderation or in combination with healthier choices. Aspartame (Nutrasweet®/Equal®) is made from the amino acids aspartate and phenylalanine. Patients with PKU should avoid products containing aspartame.

Historically, the phenylalanine tolerance of individuals with PKU was felt to remain consistent during the lifespan, especially after early childhood. Van Spronsen et al. found that phenylalanine tolerance at age 2 or 3 years can reliably predict phenylalanine needs at age 10 years [23] (Table 10.3).

Table 10.3 Recommended intake for a patient with PKU [9, 10]

Age	Protein (g/kg)	Phenylalanine[a] (mg/kg)	Phenylalanine[a] (mg/day)	Tyrosine[a] (mg/day)
Birth to 3 months	2.5–3.0	25–70	130–430	1000–1300
3 to <6 months	2.0–3.0	20–45	135–400	1400–2100
6 to <9 months	2.0–2.5	15–35	145–370	2500–3000
9 to <12 months	2.0–2.5	10–35	135–330	2500–3000
1 to 4 years	1.5–2.0	–	200–320	2800–3500
4 years to adult	120–140% DRI	–	200–1100	4000–6000

[a] Values represent intake recommendations for those with more severe forms of PKU. Those with milder forms of PKU and/or are treated with sapropterin will likely tolerate additional phenylalanine and tyrosine
Energy, vitamin, and mineral intakes should meet the DRI and normal fluid requirements [24, 25] (Appendix D)

However, phenylalanine tolerance may increase as body mass changes with age [26]. A recent study challenged 40 individuals with PKU (age range 12–29 yr) who were maintaining good metabolic control and found that 65% of these patients were able to increase intact protein intake, yet still maintain phenylalanine concentrations in the treatment range, even in those with severe PKU [27]. These results suggest that some patients with PKU may tolerate additional intact protein and periodic re-evaluation of phenylalanine needs should be considered.

Like other chronic disorders, maintaining diet treatment becomes more difficult for adolescents and adults with PKU [28]. However, maintenance of good metabolic control is correlated with improved long-term cognitive outcomes [29]. Studies have also suggested that the variability of phenylalanine concentrations over time may also be a significant predictor of long-term outcome [30, 31]. Thus, efforts need to be made to support and motivate individuals in these age groups to continue diet therapy. To reduce the burden of diet adherence, utilizing a simplified diet approach and counting grams of protein rather than milligrams of phenylalanine may help [16].

Box 10.6: Returning to Diet

Recommended Steps to Restart the PKU Diet:

1. Reintroduce medical food
2. Remove any high protein foods from diet
3. Consider a trial of BH_4 supplementation
4. Reintroduce counting/limiting foods with moderate protein content
5. Consider introducing a "Simplified Diet" plan
6. Reintroduce modified low protein products
7. Establish connections with other adults on diet

(See National PKU Alliance (NPKUA) website, adultswithpku.org, for more information)

10.3.1 Returning to Diet

Adults with PKU who were previously treated but are not currently following the PKU diet often consume little or no medical food, while avoiding most high protein foods and beverages and/or foods containing aspartame. This increases the risk for developing micronutrient deficiencies, and supplementation may be required [32–34]. Adolescents and adults who have discontinued diet may return to their metabolic clinics to restart the diet. This requires several steps, outlined in Box 10.6.

10.3.2 Acute Management

During illness or other catabolic stress (teething, surgery, fractures, etc.), patients with PKU often have elevated blood phenylalanine concentrations. Unlike other inherited metabolic diseases such as organic acidemias or urea cycle disorders that require a decrease in intact protein intake during illness, the diet is generally not modified during illness for patients with PKU. Patients are encouraged to follow medical advice in treating the illness. Some medications contain aspartame; these should be avoided if an equivalent medication without aspartame is available, but if not, treating the illness takes priority over avoiding the phenylalanine in the medication.

10.4 Medical Foods for PKU[c]

After infancy, medical food continues to be the mainstay of the diet for PKU. Medical food provides almost all of an individual's protein and tyrosine needs and, often, a majority of energy needs, especially for those with severe PKU.

A wide variety of medical foods are available for those over age 2 years. At this age, most clinics transition from a complete medical food designed for infants to one designed for toddlers and children; however, there are many factors to consider in this decision, including the child's acceptance of medical food, interest in solids, phenylalanine tolerance, and energy needs. Medical foods designed for these younger age groups provide carbohydrate, fat, and a complete micronutrient profile, in addition to protein equivalents from L-amino acids or glycomacropeptide (GMP).

There are numerous medical foods for older age groups. Many are designed to reduce the amount of medical food that an individual needs to consume to meet their needs for protein equivalents, increase convenience, and/or provide alternative taste profiles. Many contain little or no fat, and others are concentrated in protein with little fat and carbohydrate. These medical foods can meet protein needs with a smaller volume and are often used for those requiring a lower-energy formula. However, use of these lower-energy options can also lead to excessive phenylalanine intake from foods. Various convenience forms of medical food such as bars, tablets, and ready-to-drink products are available as well. Table 10.4 provides an overview of the medical foods available to patients with PKU in the United States (as of April 2021).

Table 10.4 Selected medical foods for the treatment of PKU

		Older Child/Adult (Incomplete[b])	
Infant/Toddler (Complete[a])	Older Child/Adult (Complete [a])	Powder	Liquid, Tablet, and Other Forms
PKU Periflex Early Years[c] PKU Periflex Junior Plus[c] Phenex-1[d] Phenyl-Free 1[e]	Glytactin BetterMilk[f,g] Glytactin RTD and RTD Lite[f,g] Glytactin Swirl[f,g] Phenex-2[d] Phenyl-Free 2[e] Phenyl-Free 2HP[e] PhenylAde Essential[c] PhenylAde GMP Ready[c,g] PhenylAde GMP Drink Mix[c,g] Periflex Advance[c] PKU Trio[h]	Glytactin Restore Powder[f,g] Glytactin Restore Lite Powder[f,g] Glytactin Build 10[f,g] Glytactin Build 20/20[f,g] Lanaflex[c,i] Lophlex Powder[c] PhenylAde Drink Mix 40 and 60[c] Phlexy 10 Drink Mix[c] PhenylAde MTE Amino Acid Blend[c] PhenylAde PheBLOC[c,i] PhenylAde GMP Mix-Ins[c,g] XPhe Maxamum[c] PKU Express[h] PKU Sphere 15 and 20[g,h]	CaminoPro Drinks[f] Glytactin Restore[f,g] Glytactin Restore Lite[f,g] Glytactin Complete 10 and 15 Bar[f,g] Phenactin AA Plus[f] Lophlex LQ[c] Periflex LQ[c] PKU Coolers[h] PKU Air[h] Phlexy 10 Tablets[c] PKU Sphere Liquid[g,h]

[a] Contains L-amino acids (minus phenylalanine) as protein source unless noted, as well as fat, carbohydrate, vitamins, and minerals
[b] Contains L-amino acids (minus phenylalanine) as protein source unless noted. Low in or devoid of fat, carbohydrate, vitamins, or minerals. See company websites for specific nutrient composition
[c] Nutricia North America (Rockville MD; medicalfood.com)
[d] Abbott Nutrition (Columbus OH; abbottnutrition.com)
[e] Mead Johnson Nutrition (Evansville IN; meadjohnson.com)
[f] Cambrooke Therapeutics (Ayer, MA; cambrooke.com)
[g] Contains glycomacropeptide (GMP) as the protein source
[h] Vitaflo USA (Alexandria, VA; nestlehealthscience.us.com)
[i] Contains large neutral amino acids as the protein source

10.4.1 Glycomacropetide (GMP)-Based Medical Foods

The whey protein glycomacropeptide (GMP) is a by-product of cheese production and purified GMP contains no aromatic amino acids, including phenylalanine, which makes this intact protein suitable for medical foods designed for PKU. However, isolation of GMP from cheese whey results in contamination from other whey proteins; thus, commercially available GMP contains approximately 1.8 mg phe/g protein equivalent [35]. Additionally, GMP does not contain a complete profile of amino acids and some amino acids, including L-tyrosine, need to be added to GMP-based medical foods [35, 36].

Various medical food options using GMP are available, often with improved subjective markers of acceptability (i.e., taste, texture) and an improved feeling of satiety compared to a subject's usual amino acid–based medical food [37, 38]. Both inpatient and outpatient clinical trials have noted benefits of GMP compared to L-amino acid based medical foods for treatment of PKU, including improved markers of phenylalanine utilization and satiety [36, 39].

A meta-analysis of studies primarily with adolescent and adult subjects found no significant differences in blood phenylalanine control with GMP compared to L-amino acid based medical foods, despite the additional intake of phenylalanine from the GMP [40]. However, trials in a younger patient population (ages 5–16 years) did find significantly higher blood phenylalanine concentrations when subjects consumed GMP versus amino acid–based medical foods [41, 42]. This may reflect that younger patients tend to maintain better control of blood phenylalanine concentrations than older patients, and the additional phenylalanine in GMP may have a greater impact on metabolic control when added to the diet of patients who are maintaining strict phenylalanine intake and/or who have a lower phenylalanine tolerance. Thus, the need to "count" the phenylalanine in GMP as part of the overall dietary phenylalanine prescription must be evaluated on an individual basis.

10.5 Metabolic and Nutrition Monitoring

Monitoring is key to successful management of patients with PKU. Particularly important is the frequent monitoring of blood phenylalanine and tyrosine. These values are needed to adjust the diet to ensure that blood phenylalanine remains in the treatment range of 120–360 μmol/dL (2–6 mg/L) [8]. In many clinics, phenylalanine is monitored between clinic visits by analysis of blood that has been collected at home on a filter paper card. These specimens are often tested by the newborn screening (NBS) laboratory. There can be differences between the phenylalanine results obtained from blood on filter paper compared to phenylalanine analyzed as part of an amino acid profile of plasma. One study found that phenylalanine concentrations from filter paper blood spots was, on average, 26% lower than plasma concentrations obtained from the amino acid analyzer [43], although this difference may vary in other labs and with different collection tubes and methods [44]. Anthropometric measurements, nutritional intake, biochemical data, and neurocognitive development should be assessed periodically [8, 9, 13] (Box 10.7).

10.6 Large Neutral Amino Acids as an Alternative Diet Treatment for PKU

Large neutral amino acids (LNAAs) are comprised of the aromatic amino acids phenylalanine, tyrosine and tryptophan; the branched chain amino acids leucine, valine and isoleucine; as well as methionine, histidine and threonine (Box 10.8). All LNAAs are essential amino acids except tyrosine, which is conditionally essential in PKU. Each of these amino acids share the same transporters at the blood-brain barrier and intestinal mucosal cells. At the blood-brain barrier, the LAT-1 transporter is responsible for transport of LNAA from the blood into the brain [45, 46]. The LAT-1 transporter has selective affinity for phenylalanine, resulting in more effi-

Box 10.7: Nutrition Monitoring of a Patient with Phenylketonuria[a]

- Routine assessments including anthropometrics, dietary intake, physical findings
- Laboratory Monitoring
  - Diagnosis specific
    Plasma amino acids
    - Phenylalanine
    - Tyrosine
  - Nutrition-related laboratory monitoring of patients on protein-restricted diets may include markers of
    - Protein sufficiency (plasma amino acids, prealbumin)
    - Nutritional anemia (hemoglobin, hematocrit, MCV, serum vitamin B12 and/or methylmalonic acid, total homocysteine, ferritin, iron, folate, total iron-binding capacity)
    - Vitamin and mineral status (25-hydroxyvitamin D, zinc, trace minerals)
    - Essential fatty acid sufficiency: plasma or erythrocyte fatty acid profile
    - Others, as clinically indicated

[a] See GMDI/SERN PKU Guideline for suggested frequency of monitoring [9].

Box 10.8: Large Neutral Amino Acids

- Histidine (HIS)
- Isoleucine (ILE)
- Leucine (LEU)
- Methionine (MET)
- Phenylalanine (PHE)
- Threonine (THR)
- Tryptophan (TRP)
- Tyrosine (TYR)
- Valine (VAL)

cient transport of phenylalanine at the expense of other LNAAs [46]. This reduces the production of serotonin and dopamine from tryptophan and tyrosine and decreases protein synthesis in the central nervous system, thus contributing to the adverse neuropsychological phenotype associated with poorly controlled PKU (Fig. 10.4).

The basic principles of LNAA supplementation are to competitively inhibit the uptake of phenylalanine at the blood-brain barrier and improve the uptake of other LNAA for neurotransmitter and protein synthesis [47] (Fig. 10.5). While the main function of LNAA supplementation is to reduce phenylalanine uptake at the brain, a modest reduction in blood phenylalanine may occur with reduced phenylalanine absorption through the intestinal mucosa [49, 50]. In a double-blind crossover clinical trial, Schindeler et al. reported a positive effect of LNAA supplementation on executive function skills in 16 subjects with treated PKU [51]. Similar improvements in executive function, attention, and vigilance scores were measured in 10 patients with poorly controlled PKU treated with LNAA for 12 months [52].

Supplementation with LNAA is not recommended for young children or pregnant women with PKU (or those planning pregnancy) but may be a helpful option for adults with PKU who are not maintaining metabolic control and do not adhere to other treatment options [13] (Box 10.9).

The LNAA diet limits total protein to the DRI for adults (0.8 g/kg) [24] with approximately 70% to 80% of total protein from intact sources and 20% to 30% of total protein from LNAA. Another option is to dose LNAA from 0.25 to 0.5 g LNAA/kg/day [50, 51, 53] with the

Box 10.9: Contraindications for LNAA Use

- Individuals who are considered in "good" metabolic control
- Pregnant women or women planning pregnancy
- Infants and young children

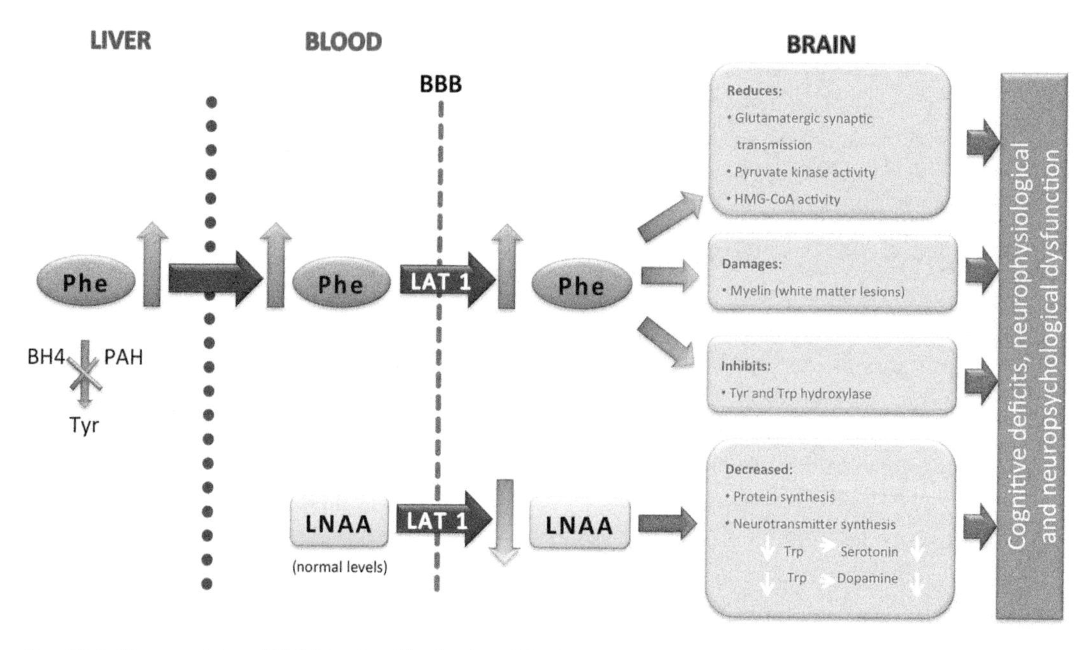

Fig. 10.4 Neurotoxicity of high blood and brain phenylalanine [48]

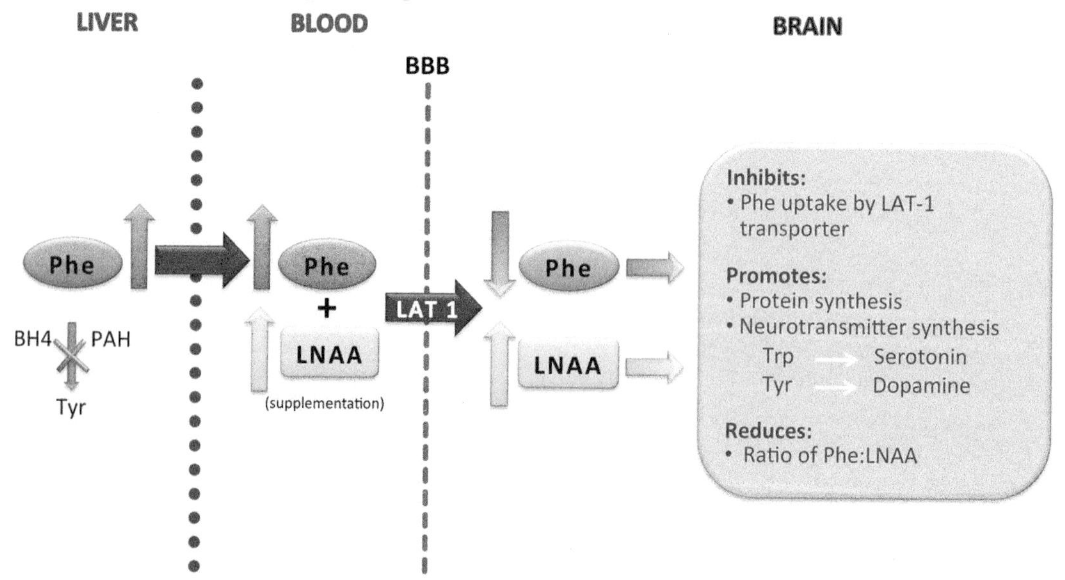

Fig. 10.5 Effect of LNAA supplementation on the transport of phenylalanine into the brain [48]

Box 10.10: Initiating diet with a LNAA supplement

Calculation based on providing 0.25 g LNAA/kg body weight

1. Obtain actual body weight of patient (e.g., 60 kg)
2. Calculate grams of LNAA required each day

$60\ \text{kg} \times 0.25\ \text{g} = 15\ \text{g LNAA per day}^{a}$

Calculation based on using a ratio of 70–80% intact protein to 20–30% from LNAA

1. 60 kg × 0.8 g protein/kg = 48 g protein per day
2. 80% of protein from intact protein = 38 g
3. 20% of protein equivalents from LNAA = 10 g LNAA[a]

[a]Divide the total grams of LNAA by the number of meals

remainder of total protein from intact sources (Box 10.10). The LNAA dose is divided into protein-containing meals throughout the day.

Blood or plasma phenylalanine concentrations do not accurately reflect brain phenylalanine concentrations and monitoring phenylalanine in patients taking LNAA is not useful as phenylalanine will remain elevated, despite LNAA treatment. Using standard questionnaires to assess depression, anxiety, and/or behavior prior to and after initiating an LNAA diet can be beneficial to detect changes in neuropsychological functioning on this treatment. Additionally, Yano et al. suggested that measurement of serum melatonin may be a potential surrogate marker to quantify the effect of LNAA, since melatonin is synthesized in the brain from serotonin and may reflect effects of diet intervention [54, 55].

10.7 Tetrahydrobiopterin Treatment for PKU

The pharmaceutical form of tetrahydrobiopterin (BH4), sapropterin hydrochloride (Kuvan®, BioMarin Pharmaceutical, Novato CA), was approved for treating individuals with PKU by the Food and Drug Administration (FDA) in 2007 and by the European Medicines Agency in 2008. Sapropterin can activate residual PAH activity, resulting in significant reductions in blood phenylalanine concentrations [56] and improved phenylalanine tolerance in approximately 30% to 50% of patients with PKU [57, 58]. Sapropterin treatment can also reduce fluctuations in blood phenylalanine concentrations [59], reduce symptoms of attention deficit, and improve executive function skills [60]. Potential responsiveness may be predicted by PAH genotype for some patients [61]. Waisbren et al. followed 65 infants and young children who started sapropterin before age six for a 7-year period and found that 60% of the patients maintained mean blood phenylalanine concentrations in the treatment range over the entire study. For this cohort, intellectual function was preserved, mean full scale IQ (FSIQ) scores remained at or above the norm expected for the general population, and expected growth patterns were maintained [62].

A trial is required to determine if a patient responds to sapropterin. Those with milder forms of PKU are more likely to respond to sapropterin than those with severe PKU [63]; however, guidelines from the American College of Medical Genetics (ACMG) suggest completing a response trial for all patients with PKU, regardless of severity, unless two null variants are present [8]. Protocols to determine response vary between different countries and, often, within clinics in a specific country. An international committee evaluated current practices to determine the best approach to complete a response trial and recommended a 24-hour loading test with blood collection every 4 hours for infants [64]. For older infants and children, a loading test for >48 hours or a 4-week trial is suggested. For pregnant women who are unable to reduce blood phenylalanine <360 μmol/L with diet treatment alone, a 48-hour response trial of sapropterin may be considered [64]. The recommended sapropterin dose for a trial is 20 mg/kg, and response is traditionally defined as a reduction of blood phenylalanine of ≥30% [56, 64]. However, some patients may respond to sapropterin with lower, but still significant

Box 10.11: Recommendations for Sapropterin (Kuvan®) Trials

- Every individual should be offered a sapropterin response trial except those with two null mutations for PAH[a].
  - Start with dose of 20 mg/kg/day
  - Trial for at least 4 weeks
  - Collect a baseline PHE level and repeat weekly
- Responsiveness
  - Lower blood PHE
    - Traditional definition: ≥ 30% reduction
  - Increased dietary PHE tolerance
  - Improved neuropsychological and behavioral outcomes

[a]Recommendations from American College of Medical Genetics and Genomics, 2014 [8]

reductions in phenylalanine concentrations and/or improved behavioral or cognitive outcomes [9, 57] (Box 10.11).

In the United States, the most common protocol for a response trial is 4 weeks with a baseline blood phenylalanine collected just before starting the trial. Phenylalanine concentrations are then collected at a minimum of once a week throughout the trial. For some, response can be detected as soon as 24 hours, other may not see reduction in blood phenylalanine until 2–4 weeks after initiation of the trial [57]. For those who enter a trial in good metabolic control, a significant decrease in blood phenylalanine may not be detected. In this case, response can be determined by gradual introduction of additional dietary phenylalanine while still maintaining phenylalanine concentrations in the treatment range [57, 64]. In general, a stepwise increase of approximately 20% in phenylalanine intake with similar reductions in protein equivalents from medical food is suggested. An additional increase in intact protein can be considered if three consecutive phenylalanine concentrations continue to remain in the treatment range. When phenylalanine concentrations exceed the recommended range, stepwise decreases of 10–30% are recommended [63]. Adding dried milk powder to the medical food is a way to increase phenylalanine intake without making major changes to a patient's dietary pattern. Once a patient's new phenylalanine tolerance is determined, then the powdered milk can be removed and replaced with higher phenylalanine foods [57].

In a recent meta-analysis of 18 studies representing 306 patients who were treated with sapropterin on a long-term basis, a 1.5- to 4.3-fold increase in dietary phenylalanine tolerance compared to pre-sapropterin tolerance was noted. Of all responders, 51% were able to discontinue use of a medical food, while 49% continued to need some medical food. In those requiring continued medical food, patients were still able to reduce their medical food intake by 40–80% of their pre-sapropterin needs [63].

It may be of benefit for some patients, especially infants and young children, to continue some medical food even if their tolerance for intact protein meets recommendations for age given the difficulty returning to a medical formula once it has been discontinued [9, 57, 63]. With the reduction or elimination of medical food, patients are at increased risk of developing micronutrient deficiencies, especially if they do not fully liberalize their diets and include some nutrient-dense protein sources. With a reduction of medical food of at least 50%, significantly decreased intakes of vitamin D, vitamin B12, folic acid, iron, zinc, and calcium were noted, although reduced serum concentrations of these various nutrients were not routinely detected [65]. A complete multivitamin and mineral supplement and/or targeted micronutrient supplements should be considered in these cases.

10.8 Summary

Early diagnosis and treatment of PKU is a well-known example of the success of newborn screening and diet treatment in preventing intellectual disability that is associated with the untreated disorder. The goal of management of PKU is to maintain blood phenylalanine concentrations of 120–360 μmol/L (2–6 mg/dL) throughout the lifespan while providing adequate nutrition. The diet is based on medical foods that are low in or devoid of phenylalanine, as well as limited quantities of intact protein-containing foods. The diet is highly individualized based on the patient's phenylalanine tolerance and food preferences. Frequent monitoring of blood phenylalanine and tyrosine, as well as nutrition assessment of growth and biochemical parameters to ensure nutrient adequacy of the restricted diet is necessary. The diet is challenging to follow, and alternative therapies may increase dietary phenylalanine tolerance in some patients with PKU.

10.9 Diet Calculation Examples for an Infant with PKU

Example 1.
PKU Diet Calculation Example Using Standard Infant Formula as the Source of Intact Protein
Patient History:

A newborn infant tested positive for PKU upon the newborn screen. Plasma phenylalanine collected on day 6 of life was 1800 µmol/L (30 mg/dL). Based on this result, all phenylalanine was removed from the diet for 72 hours. The infant is now 10 days old, and the most recent blood phenylalanine concentration is 310 µmol/L (5.1 mg/dL) and phenylalanine needs to be introduced into the diet. Based on the blood phenylalanine concentration collected prior to initiating diet (1800 µmol/L), the recommended amount of phenylalanine to introduce into the diet is 45 mg/kg.

Patient Information and Nutrient Intake Goals
Weight: 4.0 kg
Age: 10 days; post 72 hours of phenylalanine removal from diet (washout period)
Currently drinking 22 oz. of PKU medical food per day
PHE Goal: 45 mg/kg (range 25–70 mg/kg or 130–430 mg/d)
Protein Goal: 3.0 g/kg (range 2.5–3.0 g/kg)
Energy Goal: 100–120 kcal/kg
TYR Goal: 300–350 mg/kg (Table 10.5)

Table 10.5 Select nutrient composition of formulas for PKU diet calculation example (using standard infant formula as the source of intact protein)

Medical food	Amount	PHE (mg)	TYR (mg)	Protein (g)	Energy (kcal)
PKU Periflex® Early Years powder[a]	100 g	0	1400	13.5	473
Enfamil® Premium Newborn powder[b]	100 g	430	500	10.8	510

[a]Nutricia North America (Rockville, MD; Medicalfood.com)
[b]Mead Johnson Nutrition (Evansville IN; meadjohnson.com)
Note: Check manufacturer's website for the most up-to-date nutrient composition

Step-by-Step Calculation

Step 1 Calculate the amount of PHE required each day.

$$PHE\,\text{Goal} \times \text{Infant Weight} = \text{mg}\,PHE\,\text{per day}$$

$$45\ \text{mg}\ PHE \times 4\,\text{kg} = 180\ \text{mg}\,PHE\,/\,\text{day}$$

Step 2 Calculate amount of standard infant formula needed to meet daily PHE requirement.

Amount of PHE required per day ÷ Amount of PHE in 100 g of standard formula

$$180\ \text{mg}\ PHE \div 430\,\text{mg}\,PHE\,\text{in}\,100\,\text{g Enfamil®} = 0.42$$

$$0.42 \times 100 = 42\,\text{g Enfamil®Premium needed to meet daily}\ PHE\ \text{requirement.}$$

Step 3 Calculate protein and energy provided from standard infant formula

Amount of standard formula × protein provided in 100 g of standard formula

$$0.42 \times 10.8 \text{ g protein} = 4.5 \text{ g protein from Enfamil}^{®}$$

Amount of standard formula × energy provided in 100 g standard formula

$$0.42 \times 510 \text{ kcal} = 214 \text{ kcal from Enfamil}^{®}$$

Step 4 Calculate amount of remaining protein needed to fill the diet prescription.

Protein goal × Infant weight

$$3.0 \text{ g protein} \times 4 \text{ kg} = 12 \text{ g daily protein requirement}$$

Infant's total protein needs - protein provided by standard infant formula

$$12 \text{ g} - 4.5 \text{ g} = 7.5 \text{ g protein needed to fill in the diet prescription}$$

Step 5 Calculate amount of PHE-free medical food needed to meet remaining protein needs.

Protein needed to fill diet prescription ÷ protein provided in 100 g of medical food

$$7.5 \text{ g protein needed} \div 13.5 \text{ g protein in Periflex}^{®} PKU \text{ Early Years} = 0.55$$

$$0.55 \times 100 = 55 \text{ g Periflex}^{®} PKU \text{ Early Years required in the diet prescription}$$

Step 6 Calculate amount of tyrosine provided from standard infant formula and PHE-free medical food.

Amount of standard formula × TYR in 100 g of standard formula

$$0.42\left(\text{Enfamil}^{®} \text{ Premium}\right) \times 500 \text{ mg } TYR = 210 \text{ mg } TYR$$

Amount of PHE-free medical food × TYR in 100 g of PHE-free medical food

$$0.55\left(\text{Periflex}^{®} PKU \text{ Early Years}\right) \times 1400 \text{ mg } TYR = 770 \text{ mg } TYR$$

Add TYR from standard formula + PHE-free medical food for total TYR provided in diet prescription.

$$210 \text{ mg from Enfamil}^{®} + 770 \text{ mg from Periflex}^{®} = 980 \text{ mg}$$

$$980 \text{ mg} / 4 \text{ kg} = 245 \text{ mg } TYR / \text{kg}$$

Step 7 Calculate total energy provided from standard infant formula and PHE-free medical food.

Amount of standard infant formula × kcal in 100 g of standard formula.

$$0.42\left(\text{Enfamil}^{®}\right) \times 510 \text{ kcal} = 214 \text{ kcal}$$

Amount of PHE-free medical food × kcal in 100g of PHE-free medical food.

$$0.55\left(\text{Periflex}^{®} PKU \text{ Early Years}\right) \times 473 \text{ kcal} = 260 \text{ kcal}$$

Add energy from standard formula + PHE-free medical food for total kcal provided in diet prescription.

$$214\,\text{kcal from Enfamil}^{\circledR} + 260\,\text{kcal from Periflex}^{\circledR} = 474\,\text{kcal}$$

$$474\,\text{kcal} / 4\,\text{kg} = 118\,\text{kcal} / \text{kg}$$

Step 8 Calculate the final volume of formula to make a concentration of 20 kcal per ounce.
Amount of total calories provided by diet prescription ÷ 20 kcal/ounce = number of ounces of formula needed to provide concentration of 20 kcal/ounce (Table 10.6)

$$473\,\text{kcal} \div 20\,\text{kcal} / \text{ounce} = 24\,\text{ounces of formula}$$

Table 10.6 Diet prescription summary for sample calculation of PKU diet using standard infant formula as the source of intact protein[a]

Medical food	Amount	PHE (mg)	TYR (mg)	Protein (g)	Energy (kcal)
PKU Periflex® Early Years powder[b]	55 g	0	770	7.4	260
Enfamil® Premium Newborn powder[c]	42 g	180	210	4.5	214
Total per day		180	980	11.9	474
Total per kg		45 mg/kg	245 mg/kg	3.0 g/kg	118 kcal/kg

[a]Rounded to nearest whole number for amount of formula powders, phenylalanine and energy and rounded to the nearest 0.1 g for protein
[b]Nutricia North America (Rockville, MD; Medicalfood.com)
[c]Mead Johnson Nutrition (Evansville IN; meadjohnson.com)

Example 2. PKU Diet Calculation Example Using Breastmilk as the Source of Intact Protein

Patient Information and Nutrient Intake Goals
Weight: 4.0 kg
Age: 10 days; post 72-hour removal of phenylalanine from diet (wash-out period)
PHE Goal: 45 mg/kg (range 25–70 mg/kg or 130–430 mg/day)
Protein Goal: 2.5 g/kg (range 2.5–3.0 g/kg)
Energy Goal: 100–120 kcal/kg
TYR Goal: 300–350 mg/kg (Table 10.7)

Table 10.7 Select nutrient composition of formula and breastmilk for sample PKU diet calculation using breastmilk as the source of intact protein

Medical food	Amount	PHE (mg)	TYR (mg)	Protein (g)	Energy (kcal)
PKU Periflex® Early Years powder[a]	100 g	0	1400	13.5	473
Breastmilk	100 mL	47	54	1.06	72

[a]Nutricia North America (Rockville, MD; Medicalfood.com)

Step-by-Step Calculation

Step 1 Calculate the amount of PHE required each day.

$$PHE\,\text{Goal} \times \text{Infant Weight} = \text{mg}\,PHE\,\text{per day}$$

$$45\,\text{mg}\ \ PHE \times 4\,\text{kg} = 180\,\text{mg / day}\,PHE$$

Step 2 Calculate amount of breastmilk needed to meet daily PHE requirement.

Amount of PHE required per day ÷ Amount of PHE in 100 mL of breastmilk

$$180\,\text{mg}\ \ PHE \div 47\,\text{mg}\,PHE\,/\,100\,\text{mL} = 3.8$$

$$3.8 \times 100 = 380\,\text{mL breastmilk needed to meet daily}\,PHE\,\text{requirement.}$$

Step 3 Calculate the amount of protein provided by 380 ml breastmilk

$$380\ \text{ml breastmilk} \times 1.06\ \text{g protein / 100 ml}$$
$$= 4.0\ \text{g protein from breastmilk}$$

Step 4 Calculate grams of PHE-free medical food needed to meet total protein needs.

Protein goal × infant's weight = total protein needs

$$2.5\ \text{g / kg} \times 4\ \text{kg} = 10\ \text{g protein needs}$$

Total protein needs – protein provided by breastmilk = protein needed from PHE-free medical food

10 g protein needs-4.0 g protein from breastmilk = 6 g protein needed from Periflex® PKU Early Years

Protein needed from PHE-free medical food ÷ Protein provided by PHE-free medical food

$$6\,\text{g}\ \ \text{protein needs} \div 13.5\,\text{g protein / 100 g Periflex}^{\circledR}\ \text{PKU Early Years} =$$

$$0.44 \times 100 = 44\,\text{g Periflex}^{\circledR}\ PKU\ \text{Early Years needed to meet total protein needs}$$

Step 5 Calculate amount of TYR provided by breastmilk and PHE-free medical food

Volume of breastmilk × TYR in 100 ml breastmilk

$$3.8(\text{breastmilk}) \times 54\,\text{mg}\,TYR\,\text{in 100 ml breastmilk} = 205\,\text{mg}\,TYR$$

Amount of PHE-Free medical food × TYR in 100 g PHE-free medical food

$$0.44(\text{Periflex}^{\circledR}) \times 1400\,\text{mg}\,TYR\,\text{in 100 g Periflex}^{\circledR}\ PKU\ \text{Early Years} = 616\,\text{mg}\,TYR$$

Total TYR = 205 mg from breastmilk +616 mg from Periflex® = 821 mg TYR

Step 6 Calculate energy provided by breastmilk and PHE-free medical food

Volume of breastmilk × energy in 100 ml breastmilk

$$3.8(\text{breastmilk}) \times 72\,\text{kcal in}\,100\,\text{g breastmilk} = 274\,\text{kcals}$$

Amount of PHE-Free medical food × energy in 100 g PHE-free medical food

$$0.44(\text{Periflex}^{\circledR}) \times 473\,\text{kcal in}\,100\,\text{g Periflex}^{\circledR}\,\textit{PKU}\,\text{Early Years} = 208\,\text{kcals}$$

Total kcals = 274 kcal from breastmilk +208 kcals from Periflex® = 482 kcals (Table 10.8)
380 ml (13 oz) of breastmilk, and 44 g Periflex® in 10 oz. volume (20 kcal/oz)

The diet could be provided in two different ways:

Option 1. Limit the Periflex® feedings to 10 ounces per day and ask mother to adlib breastfeed at other times. With this option, the mother has a goal (and a limit) on the amount of Periflex® to provide over 24 hours. Bottle feedings should be 2–3 ounces per day at this age. One potential scenario would be to alternate breast and bottle feedings. Once all 10 ounces of Periflex has been consumed by the baby, all remaining feedings during the 24 hours can be breastfeedings.

Option 2. Mother can express breastmilk and add 13 ounces to 10 ounces of Periflex® (using recipe above) to make one 23-ounce mixture of formula/breastmilk and feed the infant from a bottle. Use this method only if mother chooses NOT to feed the infant from the breast but prefers to pump and feed from bottle.

Table 10.8 Diet prescription summary for sample calculation of PKU diet using breastmilk as the source of intact protein[a]

Medical Food	Amount	PHE (mg)	TYR (mg)	Protein (g)	Calories
Breastmilk	380 mL	180	205	4.0	274
PKU Periflex® Early Years powder[b]	44 g	0	616	5.9	208
Total per day		180	821	9.9	482
Total per kg		45 mg/kg	205 mg/kg[c]	2.5 g/kg	120 kcal/kg

[a]Values rounded to nearest whole number for amount of formula powders, phenylalanine and energy and rounded to the nearest 0.1 g for protein

[b]Nutricia North America (Rockville, MD; Medicalfood.com)

[c]Tyrosine/kg is lower than recommended. Monitor blood tyrosine results, but it is unnecessary to add supplemental L-tyrosine to this diet prescription unless blood tyrosine is consistently low

Acknowledgments Thank you to Steven Yannicelli of Nutricia North America and Elaina Jurecki of BioMarin Pharmaceutical for their contributions to this chapter's content in the first Edition of Nutrition Management of Inherited Metabolic Diseases.

References

1. Anderson PJ, Leuzzi V. White matter pathology in phenylketonuria. Mol Genet Metab. 2010;99(Suppl 1):S3–9.
2. Hillert A, Anikster Y, Belanger-Quintana A, Burlina A, Burton BK, Carducci C, et al. The genetic landscape and epidemiology of phenylketonuria. Am J Hum Genet. 2020;107(2):234–50.
3. Regier DS, Greene CL. Phenylalanine hydroxylase deficiency. In: Adam MP, Ardinger HH, Pagon RA, Wallace SE, Bean LJH, Mirzaa G, et al., editors. GeneReviews. Seattle (WA)1993–2021, updated 2017 Jan 5.
4. Christ SE. Asbjorn Folling and the discovery of phenylketonuria. J Hist Neurosci. 2003;12(1):44–54.
5. van Spronsen FJ, Reijngoud DJ, Smit GP, Nagel GT, Stellaard F, Berger R, et al. Phenylketonuria. The in vivo hydroxylation rate of phenylalanine into tyrosine is decreased. J Clin Invest. 1998;101(12):2875–80.
6. Guthrie R. The introduction of newborn screening for phenylketonuria. A personal history. Eur J Pediatr. 1996;155 Suppl 1:S4–5.
7. MacDonald A, Rocha JC, van Rijn M, Feillet F. Nutrition in phenylketonuria. Mol Genet Metab. 2011;104(Suppl):S10–18.
8. Vockley J, Andersson HC, Antshel KM, Braverman NE, Burton BK, Frazier DM, et al. Phenylalanine hydroxylase deficiency: diagnosis and management guideline. Genet Med. 2014;16(2):188–200.
9. Singh RH, Cunningham AC, Mofidi S, Douglas TD, Frazier DM, Hook DG, et al. Updated, web-based nutrition management guideline for PKU: an evidence and consensus based approach. Mol Genet Metab. 2016;118(2):72–83.
10. Acosta PB, Yannicelli S. Nutrition protocols updated for the US. 4th ed. Abbott Laboratories: Columbus OH; 2001.
11. Weiss K, Lotz-Havla A, Dokoupil K, Maier EM. Management of three preterm infants with phenylketonuria. Nutrition. 2020;71:110619.
12. Greve LC, Wheeler MD, Green-Burgeson DK, Zorn EM. Breast-feeding in the management of the newborn with phenylketonuria: a practical approach to dietary therapy. J Am Diet Assoc. 1994;94(3):305–9.
13. Singh RH, Rohr F, Frazier D, Cunningham A, Mofidi S, Ogata B, et al. Recommendations for the nutrition management of phenylalanine hydroxylase deficiency. Genet Med. 2014;16(2):121–31.
14. American Academy of Pediatrics, Section on Breastfeeding. Breastfeeding and the use of human milk. Pediatrics. 2012;129(3):e827–41.
15. Hansen J, Hollander S, Drilias N, Van Calcar S, Rohr F, Bernstein L. Simplified diet for nutrition management of phenylketonuria: a survey of U.S. metabolic dietitians. JIMD Rep. 2020;53(1):83–9.
16. MacDonald A, Rylance G, Davies P, Asplin D, Hall SK, Booth IW. Free use of fruits and vegetables in phenylketonuria. J Inherit Metab Dis. 2003;26(4):327–38.
17. Bernstein L, Burns C, Sailer-Hammons M, Kurtz A, Rohr F. Multi-clinic observations on the simplified diet in PKU. J Nutr Metab. 2017;2017:4083293.
18. Rohde C, Mutze U, Weigel JF, Ceglarek U, Thiery J, Kiess W, et al. Unrestricted consumption of fruits and vegetables in phenylketonuria: no major impact on metabolic control. Eur J Clin Nutr. 2012;66(5):633–8.
19. Daly A, Evans S, Pinto A, Ashmore C, Rocha JC, MacDonald A. A three year longitudinal prospective review examining the dietary profile and contribution made by special low protein foods to energy and macronutrient intake in children with phenylketonuria. Nutrients. 2020;12(10):3153.
20. Schuett VE. Low protein cookery for phenylketonuria, 3rd ed. Madison: University of Wisconsin Press; 1997.
21. Schuett VE, Corry D. Apples to Zucchini. A collection of favorite low protein recipes: National PKU News; 2005.
22. Winiarska B. Cook for love- low protein recipes. Available from: https://cookforlove.org.
23. van Spronsen FJ, van Rijn M, Dorgelo B, Hoeksma M, Bosch AM, Mulder MF, et al. Phenylalanine tolerance can already reliably be assessed at the age of 2 years in patients with PKU. J Inherit Metab Dis. 2009;32(1):27–31.
24. Institute of Medicine (U.S.) Panel on Macronutrients. Standing Committee on the Scientific Evaluation of Dietary Reference Intakes. Dietary reference intakes for energy, carbohydrate, fiber, fat, fatty acids, cholesterol, protein, and amino acids. Washington, D.C.: National Academies Press; 2005. xxv, 1331 p.
25. Holliday MA, Segar WE. The maintenance need for water in parenteral fluid therapy. Pediatrics. 1957;19(5):823–32.
26. MacLeod EL, Gleason ST, van Calcar SC, Ney DM. Reassessment of phenylalanine tolerance in adults with phenylketonuria is needed as body mass changes. Mol Genet Metab. 2009;98(4):331–7.
27. Pinto A, Almeida MF, MacDonald A, Ramos PC, Rocha S, Guimas A, et al. Over restriction of dietary protein allowance: the importance of ongoing reassessment of natural protein tolerance in phenylketonuria. Nutrients. 2019;11(5):995-1005.

28. Jurecki ER, Cederbaum S, Kopesky J, Perry K, Rohr F, Sanchez-Valle A, et al. Adherence to clinic recommendations among patients with phenylketonuria in the United States. Mol Genet Metab. 2017;120(3):190–7.
29. Camp KM, Parisi MA, Acosta PB, Berry GT, Bilder DA, Blau N, et al. Phenylketonuria scientific review conference: state of the science and future research needs. Mol Genet Metab. 2014;112(2):87–122.
30. Anastasoaie V, Kurzius L, Forbes P, Waisbren S. Stability of blood phenylalanine levels and IQ in children with phenylketonuria. Mol Genet Metab. 2008;95(1-2):17–20.
31. Hood A, Grange DK, Christ SE, Steiner R, White DA. Variability in phenylalanine control predicts IQ and executive abilities in children with phenylketonuria. Mol Genet Metab. 2014;111(4):445–51.
32. Montoya Parra GA, Singh RH, Cetinyurek-Yavuz A, Kuhn M, MacDonald A. Status of nutrients important in brain function in phenylketonuria: a systematic review and meta-analysis. Orphanet J Rare Dis. 2018;13(1):101.
33. Hochuli M, Bollhalder S, Thierer C, Refardt J, Gerber P, Baumgartner MR. Effects of inadequate amino acid mixture intake on nutrient supply of adult patients with phenylketonuria. Ann Nutr Metab. 2017;71(3–4):129–35.
34. Rohde C, von Teeffelen-Heithoff A, Thiele AG, Arelin M, Mutze U, Kiener C, et al. PKU patients on a relaxed diet may be at risk for micronutrient deficiencies. Eur J Clin Nutr. 2014;68(1):119–24.
35. van Calcar SC, Ney DM. Food products made with glycomacropeptide, a low-phenylalanine whey protein, provide a new alternative to amino acid-based medical foods for nutrition management of phenylketonuria. J Acad Nutr Diet. 2012;112(8):1201–10.
36. van Calcar SC, MacLeod EL, Gleason ST, Etzel MR, Clayton MK, Wolff JA, et al. Improved nutritional management of phenylketonuria by using a diet containing glycomacropeptide compared with amino acids. Am J Clin Nutr. 2009;89(4):1068–77.
37. Lim K, van Calcar SC, Nelson KL, Gleason ST, Ney DM. Acceptable low-phenylalanine foods and beverages can be made with glycomacropeptide from cheese whey for individuals with PKU. Mol Genet Metab. 2007;92(1–2):176–8.
38. Ney DM, Stroup BM, Clayton MK, Murali SG, Rice GM, Rohr F, et al. Glycomacropeptide for nutritional management of phenylketonuria: a randomized, controlled, crossover trial. Am J Clin Nutr. 2016;104(2):334–45.
39. MacLeod EL, Clayton MK, van Calcar SC, Ney DM. Breakfast with glycomacropeptide compared with amino acids suppresses plasma ghrelin levels in individuals with phenylketonuria. Mol Genet Metab. 2010;100(4):303–8.
40. Pena MJ, Pinto A, Daly A, MacDonald A, Azevedo L, Rocha JC, et al. The use of glycomacropeptide in patients with phenylketonuria: a systematic review and meta-analysis. Nutrients. 2018;10(11):1794–1809.
41. Daly A, Evans S, Chahal S, Santra S, Pinto A, Jackson R, et al. Glycomacropeptide: long-term use and impact on blood phenylalanine, growth and nutritional status in children with PKU. Orphanet J Rare Dis. 2019;14(1):44.
42. Daly A, Evans S, Pinto A, Jackson R, Ashmore C, Rocha JC, et al. The impact of the use of glycomacropeptide on satiety and dietary intake in phenylketonuria. Nutrients. 2020;12(9):2443–56.
43. Groselj U, Murko S, Zerjav Tansek M, Kovac J, Trampus Bakija A, Repic Lampret B, et al. Comparison of tandem mass spectrometry and amino acid analyzer for phenylalanine and tyrosine monitoring--implications for clinical management of patients with hyperphenylalaninemia. Clin Biochem. 2015;48(1–2):14–18.
44. van Vliet K, van Ginkel WG, van Dam E, de Blaauw P, Koehorst M, Kingma HA, et al. Dried blood spot versus venous blood sampling for phenylalanine and tyrosine. Orphanet J Rare Dis. 2020;15(1):82.
45. Hawkins RA, O'Kane RL, Simpson IA, Vina JR. Structure of the blood-brain barrier and its role in the transport of amino acids. J Nutr. 2006;136(1 Suppl):218S–26S.
46. Pardridge WM. Blood-brain barrier biology and methodology. J Neurovirol. 1999;5(6):556–69.
47. Hoeksma M, Reijngoud DJ, Pruim J, de Valk HW, Paans AM, van Spronsen FJ. Phenylketonuria: high plasma phenylalanine decreases cerebral protein synthesis. Mol Genet Metab. 2009;96(4):177–82.
48. Feillet F, van Spronson FJ, MacDonald A, Trefz FK, Demirkol M, et al. Challenges and pitfalls in the management of phenylketonuria. Pediatrics. 2010;126(2):333–41.
49. Sanjurjo P, Aldamiz L, Georgi G, Jelinek J, Ruiz JI, Boehm G. Dietary threonine reduces plasma phenylalanine levels in patients with hyperphenylalaninemia. J Pediatr Gastroenterol Nutr. 2003;36(1):23–6.
50. Matalon R, Michals-Matalon K, Bhatia G, Burlina AB, Burlina AP, Braga C, et al. Double blind placebo control trial of large neutral amino acids in treatment of PKU: effect on blood phenylalanine. J Inherit Metab Dis. 2007;30(2):153–8.
51. Schindeler S, Ghosh-Jerath S, Thompson S, Rocca A, Joy P, Kemp A, et al. The effects of large neutral amino acid supplements in PKU: an MRS and neuropsychological study. Mol Genet Metab. 2007;91(1):48–54.
52. Scala I, Riccio MP, Marino M, Bravaccio C, Parenti G, Strisciuglio P. Large neutral amino acids (LNAAs) supplementation improves neuropsychological performances in adult patients with phenylketonuria. Nutrients. 2020;12(4):1092.
53. Koch R, Moseley KD, Yano S, Nelson M Jr, Moats RA. Large neutral amino acid therapy and phenylketonuria: a promising approach to treatment. Mol Genet Metab. 2003;79(2):110–3.
54. Yano S, Moseley K, Azen C. Large neutral amino acid supplementation increases melatonin synthe-

sis in phenylketonuria: a new biomarker. J Pediatr. 2013;162(5):999–1003.
55. Yano S, Moseley K, Fu X, Azen C. Evaluation of tetrahydrobiopterin therapy with large neutral amino acid supplementation in phenylketonuria: effects on potential peripheral biomarkers, melatonin and dopamine, for brain monoamine neurotransmitters. PLoS One. 2016;11(8):e0160892.
56. Levy HL, Milanowski A, Chakrapani A, Cleary M, Lee P, Trefz FK, et al. Efficacy of sapropterin dihydrochloride (tetrahydrobiopterin, 6R-BH4) for reduction of phenylalanine concentration in patients with phenylketonuria: a phase III randomised placebo-controlled study. Lancet. 2007;370(9586):504–10.
57. Singh RH, Quirk ME. Using change in plasma phenylalanine concentrations and ability to liberalize diet to classify responsiveness to tetrahydrobiopterin therapy in patients with phenylketonuria. Mol Genet Metab. 2011;104(4):485–91.
58. Trefz FK, Burton BK, Longo N, Casanova MM, Gruskin DJ, Dorenbaum A, et al. Efficacy of sapropterin dihydrochloride in increasing phenylalanine tolerance in children with phenylketonuria: a phase III, randomized, double-blind, placebo-controlled study. J Pediatr. 2009;154(5):700–7.
59. Burton BK, Bausell H, Katz R, Laduca H, Sullivan C. Sapropterin therapy increases stability of blood phenylalanine levels in patients with BH4-responsive phenylketonuria (PKU). Mol Genet Metab. 2010;101(2–3):110–4.
60. Burton B, Grant M, Feigenbaum A, Singh R, Hendren R, Siriwardena K, et al. A randomized, placebo-controlled, double-blind study of sapropterin to treat ADHD symptoms and executive function impairment in children and adults with sapropterin-responsive phenylketonuria. Mol Genet Metab. 2015;114(3):415–24.
61. Anjema K, van Rijn M, Hofstede FC, Bosch AM, Hollak CE, Rubio-Gozalbo E, et al. Tetrahydrobiopterin responsiveness in phenylketonuria: prediction with the 48-hour loading test and genotype. Orphanet J Rare Dis. 2013;8:103.
62. Waisbren S, Burton BK, Feigenbaum A, Konczal LL, Lilienstein J, McCandless SE, et al. Long-term preservation of intellectual functioning in sapropterin-treated infants and young children with phenylketonuria: a seven-year analysis. Mol Genet Metab. 2021;132(2):119–27.
63. Ilgaz F, Marsaux C, Pinto A, Singh R, Rohde C, Karabulut E, et al. Protein substitute requirements of patients with phenylketonuria on tetrahydrobiopterin treatment: a systematic review and meta-analysis. Nutrients. 2021;13(3):1040.
64. Muntau AC, Adams DJ, Belanger-Quintana A, Bushueva TV, Cerone R, Chien YH, et al. International best practice for the evaluation of responsiveness to sapropterin dihydrochloride in patients with phenylketonuria. Mol Genet Metab. 2019;127(1):1–11.
65. Thiele AG, Rohde C, Mutze U, Arelin M, Ceglarek U, Thiery J, et al. The challenge of long-term tetrahydrobiopterin (BH4) therapy in phenylketonuria: effects on metabolic control, nutritional habits and nutrient supply. Mol Genet Metab Rep. 2015;4:62–7.

Medical and Nutrition Management of Phenylketonuria: Pegvaliase

11

Nicola Longo, Ashley Andrews, and Fran Rohr

Contents

N. Longo (✉) · A. Andrews
Division of Medical Genetics, University of Utah School of Medicine, University of Utah Hospital, Salt Lake City, UT, USA
e-mail: Nicola.Longo@hsc.utah.edu; Ashley.Andrews@hsc.utah.edu

F. Rohr
Met Ed Co, Boulder, CO, USA
e-mail: fran.rohr@met-ed.net

L. E. Bernstein et al. (eds.), *Nutrition Management of Inherited Metabolic Diseases*,
https://doi.org/10.1007/978-3-030-94510-7_11

Core Messages

- Phenylalanine ammonia lyase (PAL) converts phenylalanine to ammonia and trans-cinnamic acid and can reduce phenylalanine concentrations in individuals with phenylketonuria (PKU).
- Injectable pegvaliase (recombinant *Anabaena variabilis* PAL produced in *E. coli* conjugated with polyethylene glycol [PEG] to reduce immunogenicity (marketed as Palynziq®) has been shown to reduce blood phenylalanine concentrations in the majority of subjects with PKU in Phase 1, 2 and 3 clinical trials.
- The most frequently reported adverse events are injection-site reactions, arthralgia, dizziness, and skin reactions. There is a risk of anaphylaxis. This requires premedication with histamine-receptor blockers and anti-inflammatory drugs and to have epinephrine available.
- Long-term use of pegvaliase causes a persistent reduction of blood phenylalanine concentrations and a continued improvement of executive function measures.
- Nutrition management of patients treated with pegvaliase focuses on increasing intact protein once blood phenylalanine is in the treatment range. This diet transition can be challenging for some patients.

11.1 Background

Standard therapy for phenylketonuria (PKU) consists of a protein and phenylalanine-restricted diet for life [1]. If consistent adherence to this stringent dietary regimen decreases as a patient gets older, this will cause an increase in phenylalanine concentrations that can result in cognitive and executive dysfunction and psychiatric issues in the long term [2, 3]. Sapropterin, a synthetic form of tetrahydrobiopterin, can increase residual phenylalanine hydroxylase activity and decreases phenylalanine concentrations in about one-third of all patients with PKU when used in conjunction with diet [4, 5]. Individuals with the most severe forms of PKU usually do not respond to sapropterin and struggle to maintain a strict diet once they approach adult age. For this reason, additional therapies are being developed to treat PKU [4].

Pegvaliase (PEGylated recombinant [*Anabaena variabilis*] phenylalanine ammonia lyase [PAL]; marketed in the United States as PALYNZIQ™) is a novel enzyme substitution therapy administered via subcutaneous injection that lowers blood phenylalanine independently of diet [6, 7]. PAL (EC 4.3.1.24) is an enzyme not present in mammals that converts phenylalanine to ammonia and trans-cinnamic acid (Fig. 11.1) [8].

Ammonia is removed by the urea cycle while trans-cinnamic acid is converted to benzoic acid by an unknown mechanism and, after conjugation with glycine by glycine N-acyltransferase, produces hippuric acid that can be excreted in urine [9]. Initial trials of oral PAL in humans yielded a modest decrease in blood phenylalanine concentrations [10]. Subsequent studies in animal models led to the development of a recombinant *Anabaena variabilis* PAL genetically modified to improve protease resistance and PEGylated to reduce immunogenicity (rAvPAL-PEG; pegvaliase) [11]. In a murine model of PKU deficient in PAH activity (BTBRPahenu2 [ENU2]), weekly subcutaneous administration of rAvPAL-PEG and, to a lesser extent, oral administration of PEGylated PAL, reduced blood phenylalanine concentrations over 3 months [11, 12]. Pegylation was essential to mask the bacterial protein and to allow persistent enzymatic activity.

11.2 Human Clinical Trials

Phase 3 trials for pegvaliase as enzyme substitution therapy for PKU began in 2013 and pegvaliase was FDA-approved on May 24, 2018 to reduce blood phenylalanine concentrations in adult patients with PKU with phenylalanine concentrations >600 μmol/L on existing management.

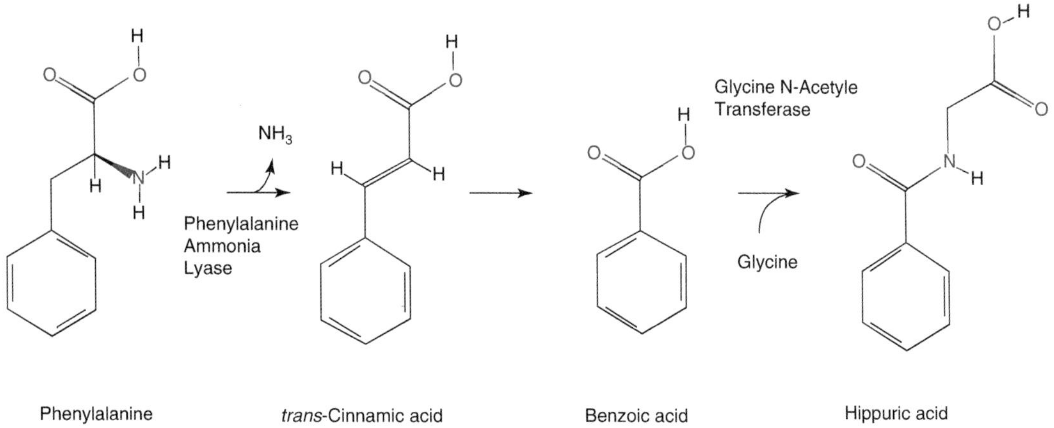

NH_3

Phenylalanine Ammonia Lyase

Glycine N-Acetyle Transferase

Glycine

Phenylalanine *trans*-Cinnamic acid Benzoic acid Hippuric acid

Fig. 11.1 Degradation of phenylalanine to trans-cinnamic acid and ammonia by the enzyme PAL. Ammonia generated by PAL is converted to urea in the liver by the urea cycle. Trans-cinnamic acid is converted to benzoic acid by unknown processes. Benzoic acid is conjugated with glycine to form hippuric acid and excreted in urine [8]

Phase 1 clinical trials in adult patients with PKU started in 2008 and demonstrated that a single subcutaneous dose of 0.1 mg/kg of pegvaliase reduced plasma phenylalanine concentrations [13]. Adverse events included injection-site reactions, dizziness, and rashes (local or generalized). No significant changes in safety laboratory tests were observed, but all patients developed antidrug antibodies. Blood PAL levels peaked about 5 days after drug administration with a mean 54% reduction in blood phenylalanine concentrations, with a nadir approximately 6 days after injection (Fig. 11.2a). There was an inverse correlation between drug and phenylalanine concentrations in plasma (Fig. 11.2b) [9]. Phenylalanine concentrations returned to near-baseline concentrations approximately 21 days after the single injection of rAvPAL-PEG.

11.3 Efficacy and Safety

Multiple Phase 2 studies examined the effects of repeated administration of pegvaliase to subjects with PKU (Table 11.1). The objective of these trials was to define the best way to progressively increase pegvaliase dosing, identifying the regimen producing the most rapid decrease in phenylalanine concentrations, while minimizing side effects. The three Phase 2 studies increased pegvaliase dosing very slowly (PAL-002) [7], then very rapidly (PAL-004) [7, 14] until an interme-

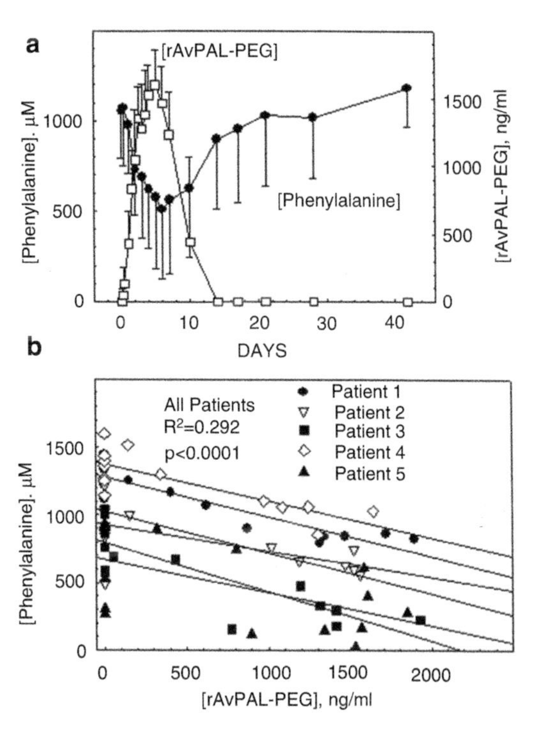

Fig. 11.2 Panel (**a**) Concentrations of plasma phenylalanine (filled circle) and rAvPAL-PEG (open squares) in subjects with phenylketonuria after one dose (time zero) of 0•1 mg/kg of rAvPAL-PEG. Points are averages with the SD indicated in one direction. Panel (**b**) Correlation between plasma concentrations of rAvPAL-PEG and phenylalanine. Note the significant inverse correlation between plasma rAvPAL-PEG and phenylalanine concentrations in subjects with phenylketonuria who received a single dose of 0•1 mg/kg of rAvPAL-PEG. The thick line represents the regression using all points with the parameters indicated. The lines are regression to individual subjects. These were all highly significant ($p < 0•01$) except in Subject 5 where the regression was statistically significant ($p < 0•05$). rAvPAL-PEG = pegvaliase [13]

Table 11.1 Clinical trials with pegvaliase

Phase	Identifier	Duration (w)	Design	Dates	Objective	Results
I	NCT00634660 (PAL-001)	6	Single dose 0.001–0.1 mg/kg	5/2008–4/2009	Safety, reduction of Phe concentrations	Fairly safe, development of antibodies against PEG and PAL, reduction of Phe concentrations with 0.1 mg/kg
II	NCT00925054 (PAL-002)	22	Repeat dose 0.001–1 mg/kg/week	9/2009–12/2012	Reduction of Phe concentrations, safety, antibody response, pharmacokinetics	All Phase 2 studies combined indicated reduction of Phe concentrations from baseline,
II	NCT01212744 (PAL-004)	16	Repeat dose 0.06–0.8 mg/kg/day	3/2011–1/2013	Reduction of Phe concentrations, safety, antibody response, pharmacokinetics	Generally well-tolerated, but requiring slow titration to full dose
II	NCT01560286 (165–205)	24	Repeat dose 2.5–375 mg/week divided 1–5 times/week	5/2012–1/2014	Reduction of Phe concentrations, safety, antibody response, pharmacokinetics	Due to adverse reactions, hypersensitivity-type reactions are the most frequent
II	NCT00924703 (PAL-003)	261	Stable dosing up to 5 mg/kg/week	1/2010–1/2019	Reduction of Phe concentrations, safety, antibody response, pharmacokinetics	Long-term therapy with pegvaliase (20–40 mg/day) can maintain Phe concentrations in the therapeutic range without
III	NCT01819727 (165–301; Prism-1)	15–44	Repeat dose 20, 40 mg/day	5/2013–11/2015	Safety, reduction of Phe concentrations, dietary protein intake	the need of diet with improvement of executive function over time
III	NCT01889862 (165–302; Prism-2)	172	Repeat dose 20, 40 mg/day or placebo, randomized discontinuation	7/2013–1/2016	Safety, cognitive and mood symptoms, reduction of Phe concentrations Dietary protein intake	Randomized discontinuation of pegvaliase causes Phe concentrations to increase again, no changes in neurocognitive function during discontinuation
III	NCT02468570 (165–303; Prism-3)	63	Repeat dose 20, 40 mg/day or placebo	7/2015–2/2017	Evaluation of changes in executive function	
III	NCT03694353 (165–304)	37	Repeat dose, >40–60 mg/day	9/2018–present	Safety, reduction of Phe concentrations with higher drug dose	Pegvaliase at >40 mg per day can decrease Phe concentrations in previously unresponsive patients

diate rate of dose increase was found acceptable (165–205) [15]. Most patients continued into a Phase 2 extension study (PAL-003) [15] to determine efficacy and safety over time [7]. Patients maintained consistent diets (many of them had unrestricted diets) with mean pretreatment baseline blood phenylalanine concentrations >1200 μmol/L (Fig. 11.3). There was a progressive decrease in plasma phenylalanine levels with time as the dosage of pegvaliase was increased (independent of whether the patients were initially started on a low dose (PAL-002, Fig. 11.3a) or high dose (PAL-004, Fig. 11.3b) of pegvaliase. In both cases, significant reductions of blood phenylalanine were seen once the weekly pegvaliase dose was increased to >80 mg per week and phenylalanine concentrations of <600 μmol/L were observed at a dose of 140–280 mg per week

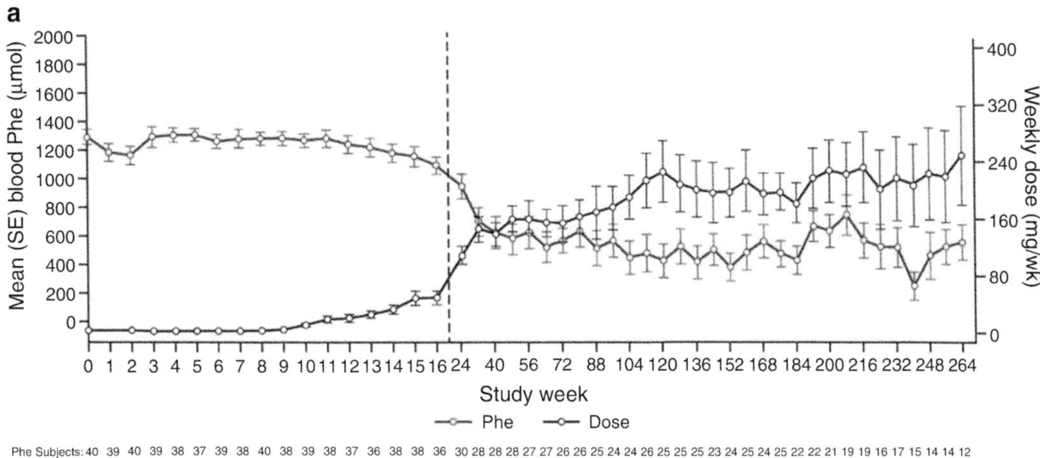

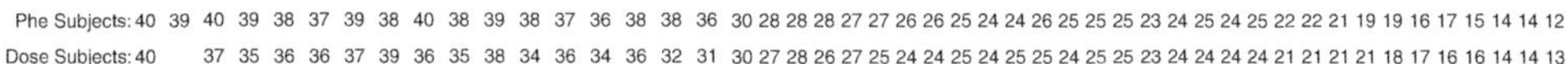

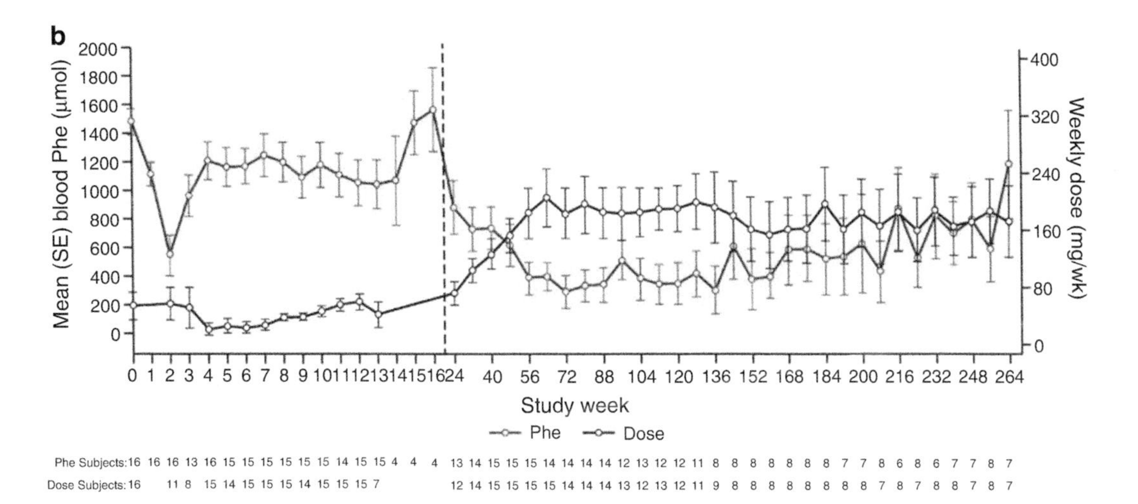

SE. standard error

Fig. 11.3 Mean blood phenylalanine concentration and pegvaliase dose over time in (**a**) PAL-002 and (**b**) PAL-004 continuing through PAL-003. Data are presented as mean (SE). Dotted line indicates transition of participants from the PAL-002 or PAL-004 studies to the PAL-003 study. Sample size reflects the participants with data available at the indicated time point and who had reached the time point at the time of the data cut; the study was ongoing at the time of this analysis [7]

(Fig. 11.3). The Phase 2 data indicated that the dose of pegvaliase needs to be increased gradually to avoid severe reactions and that the majority of patients who continue dosing can expect a meaningful reduction of plasma phenylalanine concentrations with doses of 20 mg or 40 mg of pegvaliase per day. All patients developed antibodies against pegvaliase and the reduction in plasma phenylalanine was dependent on the individual immune response, the dose of drug, and the duration of therapy. The majority (81%) of Phase 2 subjects entering the long-term extension study achieved at least two consecutive blood phenylalanine concentrations ≤600 μmol/L after an average of 26 weeks of therapy [15, 16].

Three Phase 3 studies evaluated the efficacy and safety of self-injection of pegvaliase in adults with PKU (165–301 [Prism301] and

165–302 [Prism302]), including a sub-study aimed at identifying changes in executive functioning caused by reduction of phenylalanine concentrations in adults (Prism003). A more recent trial (165–304) is evaluating the effect of higher doses of pegvaliase (up to 60 mg/day) on reduction of phenylalanine concentrations.

Since it was not possible to predict which patients would respond to pegvaliase with a reduction of phenylalanine concentrations without dose-limiting side effects, the pivotal trial was an 8-week double-blind, placebo-controlled randomized discontinuation trial in which subjects who had reduction of phenylalanine concentrations with proper induction therapy were randomly assigned to receive placebo, 20 mg or 40 mg per day of pegvaliase [6]. The administration of placebo and discontinuation of pegvaliase caused a significant increase of plasma phenylalanine concentrations (Fig. 11.4) from 504–564 μmol/L to 1173–1513 μmol/L in patients assigned to the placebo arm, but no significant increase in plasma phenylalanine was noted in patients receiving 20 or 40 mg per day of pegvaliase (Fig. 11.4) [6]. No significant changes in psychometric measures were observed in the 8 weeks of the randomized discontinuation trial [6].

Continuation of therapy with pegvaliase further reduced phenylalanine concentrations in patients with PKU, with more than 60% of participants maintaining plasma phenylalanine concentrations <360 μmol/L after 24 months of therapy [16]. The reduction in phenylalanine concentrations was associated with a progressive improvement in ADHD scores in patients who displayed elevated scores at baseline (Fig. 11.5) [16]. Even though this part of the study was open label, the consistency of the continued improvement and the descriptions provided by patients were suggestive of a true effect.

In terms of safety, the Phase 3 study (165–205) demonstrated that weekly, low-dose intro-

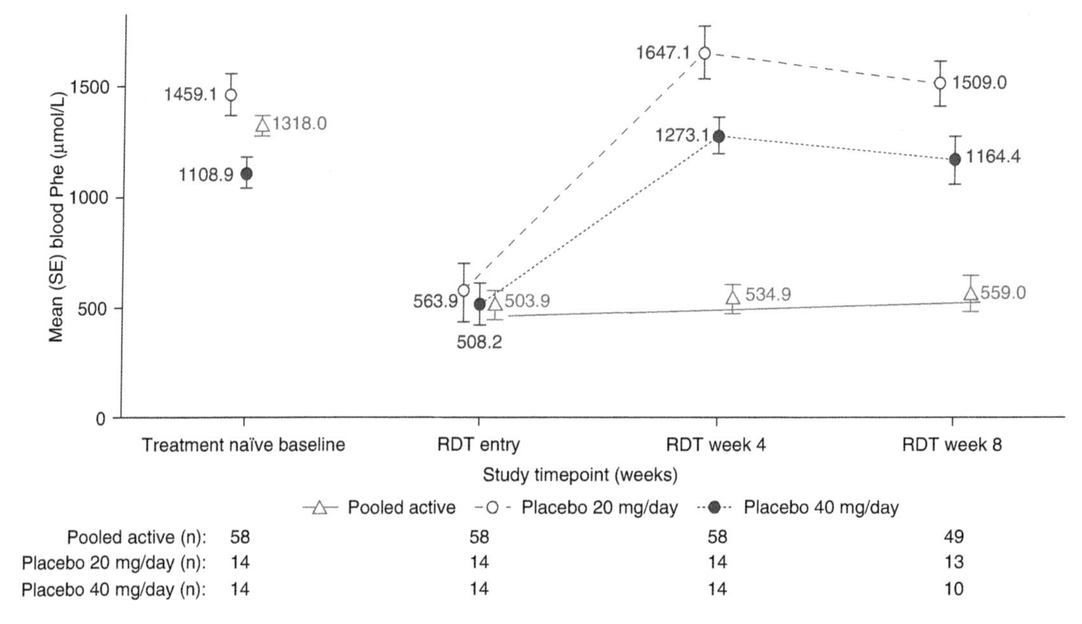

Fig. 11.4 Plasma phenylalanine concentrations in patients with phenylketonuria undergoing randomized discontinuation (RDT) of pegvaliase treatment. Baseline phenylalanine concentration ranged from 1109 to 1459 μmol/L in the different groups. Phenylalanine concentrations decreased to 504–564 μmol/L with open-label pegvaliase therapy. Discontinuation of pegvaliase and administration of placebo instead increased phenylalanine concentrations to 1164–1509 μmol/L after 8 weeks whereas continuation of pegvaliase at either 20 or 40 mg per day maintained phenylalanine concentrations at 559 μmol/L. Points represent the average of the patient population and are shown ± standard errors [6]

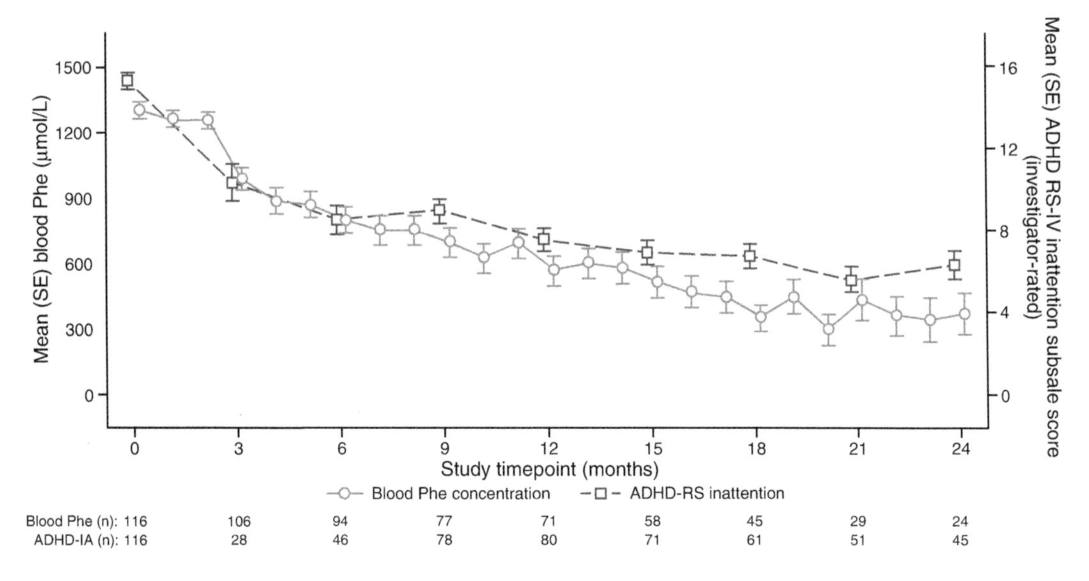

Fig. 11.5 Plasma phenylalanine concentration (continuous line) and investigator-rated ADHD RS-IV IA scores (dashed line) in participants with baseline scores >9 (inattention subgroup, N = 116). Sample size reflects participants with data available at study timepoint and who have reached study timepoint at data cut; study is ongoing. ADHD RS-IV IA Attention Deficit Hyperactivity Disorder Rating Scale IV inattention subscale, SE standard error [16]

duction of treatment, followed by gradual dosage and frequency increases, was well tolerated, with hypersensitivity events limited to mild or moderate severity. The most common adverse events included hypersensitivity-type reactions consisting of injection-site reactions, skin reactions, and/or joint pains (Table 11.2) [14].

While hypersensitivity-type reactions were observed in nearly all subjects during initial drug administration, the reactions were generally mild to moderate and self-limited. The majority of subjects with these reactions were all successfully re-treated. The most common adverse events in long-term extension studies were injection-site reaction (72.5%), injection-site erythema (67.5%), headache (67.5%), and arthralgia (65.0%) [15]. Acute systemic hypersensitivity events, including potential events of anaphylaxis, were not associated with immunoglobulin E, and all events resolved without sequelae.

Adverse events were more frequent with initiation of therapy and dose escalation and were associated with anti-PEG antibodies in the first 24 weeks of therapy (Fig. 11.6) [15]. As antibody concentrations decreased, the frequency and severity of side effects improved. The use of premedications and the development of specific guidelines to deal with these side-effects improved the drug tolerability by subjects [17].

11.4 Hypophenylalaninemia

The majority of subjects in PAL-003 had at least one blood sample where pegvaliase reduced phenylalanine concentrations below the normal range (≤30 µmol/L). No consistent association was found between these low concentrations and adverse effects. An increase in dietary protein and/or a reduction in the weekly dose of pegvaliase were found to be effective to normalize phenylalanine concentrations. Detailed studies about hypophenylalaninemia have not yet been published.

11.5 Immunogenicity

All subjects treated with pegvaliase developed antibodies against PAL and polyethylene glycol (PEG). Antidrug antibodies against PAL peaked

Table 11.2 Most frequent adverse events related to pegvaliase in any group reported by incidence (*n*), event rate (events/person-years), and total number of events

	Early treatment (≤24 weeks)		Long-term treatment (>24 weeks)	
	Group A (*n* = 11)	Group B (*n* = 13)	Group A (*n* = 10)	Group B (*n* = 10)
Exposure, person-years	5.16	5.42	22.96	27.16
Incidence, event rate (total number of events)				
Adverse event	*n* = 10 24.40 (126)	*n* = 13 59.38 (322)	*n* = 10 9.15 (210)	*n* = 10 13.92 (378)
Arthralgia	*n* = 7 5.23 (27)	*n* = 11 9.59 (52)	*n* = 4 0.91 (21)	*n* = 5 0.81 (22)
Injection-site reaction	*n* = 5 3.49 (18)	*n* = 13 19.36 (105)	*n* = 3 0.13 (3)	*n* = 5 0.26 (7)
Injection-site erythema	*n* = 2 1.94 (10)	*n* = 11 5.53 (30)	*n* = 4 0.39 (9)	*n* = 2 0.15 (4)
Rash	*n* = 3 1.16 (6)	*n* = 5 0.92 (5)	*n* = 5 1.00 (23)	*n* = 3 0.37 (10)
Urticaria	0	*n* = 3 1.11 (6)	*n* = 5 3.05 (70)	*n* = 5 4.79 (130)
Pruritus	*n* = 1 0.39 (2)	*n* = 4 0.74 (4)	*n* = 3 0.30 (7)	*n* = 2 0.15 (4)
Injection-site pruritus	*n* = 3 1.36 (7)	*n* = 2 0.74 (4)	*n* = 4 0.44 (10)	0
Injection-site rash	*n* = 4 2.13 (11)	*n* = 4 0.92 (5)	0	0
Rash generalized	*n* = 2 1.16 (6)	*n* = 3 0.74 (4)	0	*n* = 1 0.11 (3)

Group A: achieved maintenance dose in the first 24 weeks of treatment; Group B: did not achieve maintenance dose in the first 24 weeks of treatment. Event rate was calculated as total number of events divided by person-years of exposure [14]

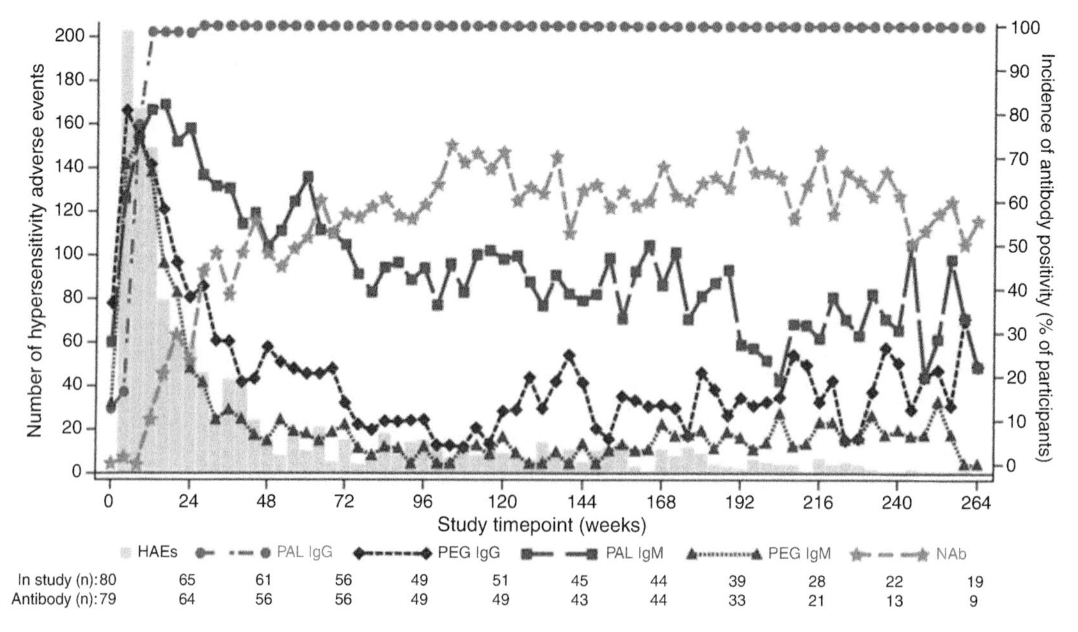

Fig. 11.6 Frequency of hypersensitivity events (pink bars) and incidence of antibody positivity over time. Antibody positivity is calculated as the number of participants testing positive divided by the total number of participants at each study visit. All Phase 2 data are included. Sample size reflects participants with data available at study timepoint; study is ongoing. *Abbreviations*: IgG immunoglobulin G, IgM immunoglobulin M, PAL phenylalanine ammonia lyase, PEG polyethylene glycol, NAb neutralizing antibody [15]

by 6 months and then stabilized (Fig. 11.6). Most patients developed transient antibody responses against PEG, peaking by 3 months, then returning to baseline by 9 months (Fig. 11.6). Pegvaliase bound to antidrug antibodies formed circulating immunocomplexes that caused complement activation, with reduction of serum complement concentrations [18]. Complement activation was highest during early treatment and decreased with time. Plasma phenylalanine concentrations decreased with time as circulating immune complex concentrations and complement activation declined and pegvaliase dosage increased [18, 19]. Hypersensitivity adverse events were most frequent at the beginning of treatment and declined over time (Fig. 11.6). No subject with acute systemic hypersensitivity events tested positive for pegvaliase-specific IgE near the time of the event. IgE could not be detected even after depleting the IgG and IgM, immunoglobulins that could have prevented detection of IgE [20]. Laboratory evidence was consistent with immune complex-mediated type III hypersensitivity. There was no evidence of pegvaliase-associated immune complex-mediated end organ damage [19].

11.6 Practical Use of Pegvaliase in Phenylketonuria

Since commercial therapy with pegvaliase is relatively new, there is variation in the practice from clinic to clinic. This section describes the management of patients receiving pegvaliase therapy at University of Utah Metabolic Clinic.

Therapy for patients with PKU is individualized. Typically, pegvaliase therapy is reserved for adults with PKU who cannot maintain phenylalanine concentrations <600 μmol/L with available therapies. However, given the considerable constraints of the long-term PKU diet, more and more adults, including those responsive to sapropterin and those able to achieve consistent phenylalanine concentrations <360 μmol/L with diet, are attracted to pegvaliase therapy. Pegvaliase therapy requires education about its risks, proper drug administration, administration of premedications and rescue medications as necessary. Educational videos have been developed for patients and those living with them to explain proper procedures [17].

Based on the available immunogenicity data, pegvaliase induces a Type III hypersensitivity reaction, causing hypersensitivity adverse events that peak during induction/titration and decline over time as therapy is continued [18]. An induction, titration, and maintenance dosing regimen has been developed in our clinic with a schedule of events that patients need to understand and follow (Table 11.3).

At each clinic visit, the patient brings a 3-day diet record that is discussed with the dietitian, medical history is reviewed, and the patient is observed to self-inject the drug. Visits may be done virtually, including initial visits, if they are completed with the assistance of a home health nurse observing the injection and monitoring the patient for at least 60 minutes for severe reactions. The dose of pegvaliase is progressively increased until a response is observed. Levels of phenylalanine and tyrosine are monitored by plasma amino acids during clinic visits or by filter paper testing as per standard of care (at least once a month). The highest dose (60 mg per day) is usually necessary in patients with very elevated diagnostic phenylalanine concentrations (>3000 μmol/L) or with high antidrug antibody titers.

Because adverse events are common, patients are educated about possible side-effects, the need to have a responsible adult present for at least 1 hour after dosing in the first 16 weeks, and the requirement to carry auto-injectable adrenaline (epinephrine) [17, 18]. Risk mitigation strategies include premedication with H1-receptor antagonists (cetirizine 10 mg per day or fexofenadine 180 mg per day), H2-receptor antagonists (famotidine 20 mg per day), anti-inflammatory drugs (ibuprofen 600 mg per day with food). Premedications can typically be discontinued once the patient is on maintenance therapy and is free of reactions. Patients require close monitoring of adverse events and extending the titration period if hypersensitivity adverse events occur.

All patients are given contact information for the clinic with the number to call in case they suf-

Table 11.3 Sample dosing and clinic schedule for naïve patients

Week	Pegvaliase dose (mg)	Frequency	Clinic/telemedicine	Representative visit	Laboratory
Baseline	0		X	X	PAA, nutritional labs**
Week 1	2.5	1 per week	X	X (in clinic)	PAA, nutritional labs**
Week 2	2.5	1 per week		X virtual	
Week 3	2.5	1 per week		X virtual	
Week 4	2.5	1 per week			
Week 5	2.5	2 per week		X virtual (2nd)	Filter paper
Week 6	10	1 per week	X		PAA
Week 7	10	2 per week		X virtual (2nd)	Filter paper
Week 8	10	4 per week		X virtual (4th)	Filter paper
Week 9	10	Daily			Filter paper
Week 10	20	Daily	X		PAA
Week 14	20	Daily			Filter paper
Week 18	20	Daily			Filter paper
Week 20	20	Daily			Filter paper
Week 26	20	Daily			Filter paper
Week 30	20	Daily			Filter paper
Week 34	40	Daily	X		PAA
Week 38	40	Daily			Filter paper
Week 40	40	Daily			Filter paper
Week 46	40	Daily			Filter paper
Week 52	40	Daily	X		PAA, nutritional lab

After 52 weeks, clinic visits every 6 months
PAA plasma amino acids. Nutritional labs: CMP prealbumin, plasma iron, TIBC, ferritin, vitamin B12, 25-OH vitamin D, zinc

fer an adverse event. After hours, they are instructed to contact the geneticist/fellow on call. Adverse events should be promptly communicated with the clinic and summarized during in-person or remote visits. Hypersensitivity adverse events are usually managed by telemedicine using Benadryl or, rarely, steroids. In case of severe reactions, the patient is instructed to proceed to the closest emergency room.

If hypophenylalaninemia (phenylalanine <30 μmol/L) is observed, natural protein is increased by 10–20 g/day each week with a concurrent decrease in protein from medical food by 10–20 g/day, until reaching a goal protein intake with appropriate blood phenylalanine concentrations. Once diet is liberalized, but phenylalanine concentrations remain <30 μmol/L, the pegvaliase dose is decreased by 10%. Phenylalanine concentrations are measured about 2 weeks after each dose reduction until an increase of phenylalanine concentrations into the therapeutic range (45–360 μmol/L) is observed. Patients who continue therapy for a long time (>5 years) sometimes require dose reduction to maintain phenylalanine concentrations >0 μmol/L.

All patients are offered a neuropsychological assessment within 30 days of starting pegvaliase. Testing is repeated at approximately 12 months after starting therapy or after the patient reaches efficacy (phenylalanine concentrations <360 μmol/L), whichever comes first Current guidance suggests that pegvaliase is not to be used during pregnancy [17]; the label states that there is no data in humans and that the drug may cause fetal harm [21]. Despite this, the teratogenic effects of elevated blood phenylalanine on the fetus are well known [22] and the risks of the use of pegvaliase should be weighed against the risk of elevated phenylalanine concentrations. There is one case report of a successful outcome in a woman who continued pegvaliase during pregnancy [23]. Several women have discontinued pegvaliase prior to pregnancy, and with extensive education and support, were able to restart a phenylalanine-restricted diet and achieve blood phenylalanine in the treatment range for maternal

PKU with successful pregnancy outcomes. It is unlikely that pegvaliase passes into breastmilk [24] and limited evidence from one case supports this [25]. If a woman is treated with pegvaliase during lactation, it is important to monitor maternal blood phenylalanine closely and avoid hypophenylalaninemia to ensure that the infant receives adequate phenylalanine for growth [21].

The safety and efficacy of pegvaliase has not been studied in the children younger than 16 years or in individuals over 65 years of age.

11.7 Nutrition Management of Patients with PKU Treated with Pegvaliase

Approved in 2018, Palynziq® (BioMarin, Novato, CA) or pegvaliase pqpz (pegvaliase) is an injectable enzyme substitution therapy for treating adults with PKU who have blood phenylalanine concentrations over 600 μmol/L while on other therapies [21], including diet and/or sapropterin dihydrochloride. While a phenylalanine-restricted diet has long been the primary mode of therapy for individuals with PKU, there is a shift to medical management that offers adults with PKU the possibility of attaining blood phenylalanine concentrations <360 μmol/L while consuming a "normal" diet (one that contains at least the recommended amount of protein from food sources). Nutrition management of patients on pegvaliase remains an important component of treatment, especially during the transition from a phenylalanine-restricted diet to a normal diet, and approaches to the nutrition management of these patients can be thought of in stages.

11.7.1 Nutrition Management During Pegvaliase Initiation and Titration

All patients starting pegvaliase should undergo a thorough nutrition assessment at baseline to establish the patient's usual phenylalanine intake and nutrition status prior to a pegvaliase trial [17]. Nutrition assessment includes anthropometrics, nutrient analysis of dietary intake, as well as laboratory monitoring for patients with PKU as described in Chap. 10. Bone density and body composition assessments are recommended by some, as well as measures of food phobias and quality of life [26]. Measurements of inflammatory markers such as C-reactive protein and erythrocyte sedimentation rate may also be performed [27].

Detailed attention to the patient's protein intake at baseline is especially important, including assessment of the amount and sources of protein in the diet. Adults with PKU may fall anywhere on the PKU diet spectrum, ranging from those who are taking medical food and restricting intact protein to those who have gone "off diet" and are eating a wide variety of foods. In the clinical trials, 15.7% of subjects were considered to be "on diet," defined as taking at least 75 percent of protein from medical food [16]. However, most (57%) reported consuming some medical food in their diets, indicating that they were not on unrestricted diets [16]. Protein intake from medical food and/or intact sources should meet the DRI of 0.8 g/kg/d [28], and for patients consuming a vegan diet (without medical food), the requirement is slightly higher (0.9 g/kg/d) [17]. If protein intake goals are not met, nutrition counseling about the addition of medical food or high-quality sources of protein to the patient's diet should be considered prior to commencing drug therapy.

Once it is established that the patient's protein intake is adequate, the metabolic dietitian counsels them to maintain a consistent intake while the drug is initiated and titrated up to the target dose. This ensures that changes in blood phenylalanine can be attributed to the drug and not to a change in diet or lifestyle. Maintaining a consistent diet means avoiding drastic changes in food intake, such as adding high protein foods before being advised to or starting a weight reduction diet. Some clinics require patients to keep food records along with blood phenylalanine monitoring in order to verify that protein intake remains within 10% of baseline, as was required in the clinical trials [16], but the reliability of food records in assessing intake is limited [29].

Patients are counseled not to adjust their diets until the blood phenylalanine reaches the target range and the dietitian recommends a diet change. During the clinical trials, there was an increase over time in subjects' mean protein intake [16, 25]; and while some of the increase was due to recommended changes, some was due to a tendency for subjects to add protein-containing foods before being counseled to do so.

Since pegvaliase therapy may take a year or longer before a reduction in blood phenylalanine is seen, the drug titration period is a good time to explore what the patient's wishes are for the new diet, including food groups they wish to try or avoid, weight goals, interest in cooking, and any financial constraints.

The titration period is also a good time to discuss whether the patient has any food aversions or fears about adding new foods [17]. There are several tools available to assess food neophobias [30]. In a study of pegvaliase-treated patients who had been on a normal diet for at least 6 months, most reported low to moderate food neophobia, which correlated with increased enjoyment of food [31]. More research is needed to assess the degree of food phobias in this population as well as nutrition counseling approaches that address the emotional aspects of eating that may accompany a drastic change in diet.

During the initiation and titration phase, blood phenylalanine is monitored every 1–4 weeks [17]. Clinic approaches vary; monitoring too frequently can be discouraging if the time to respond to the drug is long, yet it is important to monitor blood frequently enough to capture a reduction in blood phenylalanine. Blood tyrosine is monitored with the same frequency and L-tyrosine is supplemented if postprandial blood phenylalanine is consistently low [17].

11.7.2 Nutrition Management During Diet Normalization

The goal of pegvaliase therapy is to allow a patient to maintain blood phenylalanine in the treatment range while consuming a normal diet [17]. A normal diet is considered to be one that meets or exceeds the DRI for protein [28] and does not contain medical food. For patients who have been restricting protein and/or are consuming a medical food, once the blood phenylalanine reaches the target range, intact protein is added to the diet and protein from medical food is decreased. Current guidance is to add intact protein once blood phenylalanine is 120 μmol/L or below [17]; however, some clinics counsel their patients to add intact protein to their diets when blood phenylalanine is under 240–360 μmol/L, especially if the drop in blood phenylalanine is abrupt, in order to prevent low blood phenylalanine.

Protein is added in increments of 10–20 g with monitoring of blood phenylalanine and subsequent increases in protein if blood phenylalanine remains in the treatment range or below [17]. Nutrition counseling about diet adjustments is highly individualized and depends on the patient's blood phenylalanine concentration, clinic policy and patient preferences. Some dietitians counsel patients to add intact protein in larger increments (i.e., 40 g) if blood phenylalanine has dropped quickly, and for others, a slower approach is taken, especially if the patient's blood phenylalanine does not fall below the physiologically normal blood phenylalanine concentration of 30 μmol/L [32].

Adding intact protein to the diet is challenging for some patients who have no or limited experience with eating high protein foods. Extensive nutrition counseling is crucial to help the patient transition to a new way of eating and includes individualized education about higher protein food options, counting protein to reach intake goals, food preparation and safety, grocery shopping and budgeting, and incorporating more protein in a healthy manner, to name a few. Also, some patients find it emotionally challenging to eat foods that were previously forbidden and may require more intensive counseling. Educational resources for teaching patients to increase protein in the diet are available at www.met-ed.net and www.gmdi.org.

For patients consuming medical food, an equal amount of protein from medical food is removed from the diet as intact protein is added [17]. For many with PKU, adherence to consuming the recommended amount of medical food has been a struggle during adulthood [33] and not having to consume it is a welcome change. But for others, medical food intake is associated with feeling full and well, and discontinuing it is not an easy transition. Moreover, medical food is a source of many nutrients other than protein equivalents, such as energy, tyrosine, vitamins and minerals, and a full assessment of nutrient intake is imperative as medical food is decreased. In addition, periodic monitoring of nutrition status is recommended (Chap. 10). Supplementation of vitamins and minerals may be necessary [17].

Supplementation of L-tyrosine is recommended if a patient's postprandial blood tyrosine is consistently below 30 μmol/L. Blood tyrosine concentrations fluctuate diurnally, and a fasting blood tyrosine is more likely to be lower than a postprandial one [34]. During the pegvaliase clinical trials, supplementation with 1500 mg of L-tyrosine (500 mg tablets taken 3 times daily) was recommended [16]. Mean blood tyrosine remained normal throughout the study. It is expected that once a patient is consuming a high protein diet, tyrosine intake will be adequate. During commercial use of pegvaliase, one study indicated that 56 percent of patients had low fasting blood tyrosine, even after normalization of protein intake [31].

Hypophenylalaninemia, or low blood phenylalanine, defined as 2 or more blood phenylalanine concentrations below 30 μmol/L, was experienced by 35% of subjects in the Phase 3 pegvaliase clinical trials. Compared to the group of subjects who did not have low blood phenylalanine, subjects with low blood phenylalanine had a more rapid response to pegvaliase, experienced fewer adverse events, and discontinued the drug less frequently [35]. The only adverse event experienced more frequently in patients with low blood phenylalanine was alopecia [35]. However, alopecia occurred in both groups and patients with alopecia had new hair growth even when blood phenylalanine was low. The recommendation for patients whose blood phenylalanine falls below 30 μmol/L is first to normalize the diet with intact protein and then to lower the pegvaliase dose [17].

11.7.3 Nutrition Management After Diet Normalization

Nutrition counseling of a patient who is no longer on a restricted diet for PKU becomes less frequent and focuses on monitoring the patient's intake and nutrition status. After a patient has normalized their diet, nutrition counseling is helpful, at least in the short term, to ensure that the patient's protein intake continues to meet the DRI, weight status is appropriate and vitamin/mineral status is adequate. Guidance regarding healthful eating may be necessary; preliminary evidence shows that the diets of patients on pegvaliase do not meet healthy eating goals [31]. In the long term, the role of the metabolic dietitian for patients managed with pegvaliase remains to be seen.

References

1. Camp KM, Parisi MA, Acosta PB, Berry GT, Bilder DA, Blau N, et al. Phenylketonuria scientific review conference: state of the science and future research needs. Mol Genet Metab. 2014;112(2):87–122.
2. Bilder DA, Burton BK, Coon H, Leviton L, Ashworth J, Lundy BD, et al. Psychiatric symptoms in adults with phenylketonuria. Mol Genet Metab. 2013;108(3):155–60.
3. Viau KS, Wengreen HJ, Ernst SL, Cantor NL, Furtado LV, Longo N. Correlation of age-specific phenylalanine levels with intellectual outcome in patients with phenylketonuria. J Inherit Metab Dis. 2011;34(4):963–71.
4. Blau N, Longo N. Alternative therapies to address the unmet medical needs of patients with phenylketonuria. Expert Opin Pharmacother. 2015;16(6):791–800.
5. Blau N. Sapropterin dihydrochloride for the treatment of hyperphenylalaninemias. Expert Opin Drug Metab Toxicol. 2013;9(9):1207–18.
6. Harding CO, Amato RS, Stuy M, Longo N, Burton BK, Posner J, et al. Pegvaliase for the treatment of phenylketonuria: a pivotal, double-blind randomized discontinuation phase 3 clinical trial. Mol Genet Metab. 2018;124(1):20–6.

7. Burton BK, Longo N, Vockley J, Grange DK, Harding CO, Decker C, et al. Pegvaliase for the treatment of phenylketonuria: results of the phase 2 dose-finding studies with long-term follow-up. Mol Genet Metab. 2020;130(4):239–46.
8. Sarkissian CN, Gamez A. Phenylalanine ammonia lyase, enzyme substitution therapy for phenylketonuria, where are we now? Mol Genet Metab. 2005;86(Suppl 1):S22–6.
9. Hoskins JA, Holliday SB, Greenway AM. The metabolism of cinnamic acid by healthy and phenylketonuric adults: a kinetic study. Biomed Mass Spectrom. 1984;11(6):296–300.
10. Hoskins JA, Jack G, Wade HE, Peiris RJ, Wright EC, Starr DJ, et al. Enzymatic control of phenylalanine intake in phenylketonuria. Lancet. 1980;1(8165):392–4.
11. Sarkissian CN, Gamez A, Wang L, Charbonneau M, Fitzpatrick P, Lemontt JF, et al. Preclinical evaluation of multiple species of PEGylated recombinant phenylalanine ammonia lyase for the treatment of phenylketonuria. Proc Natl Acad Sci U S A. 2008;105(52):20894–9.
12. Sarkissian CN, Kang TS, Gamez A, Scriver CR, Stevens RC. Evaluation of orally administered PEGylated phenylalanine ammonia lyase in mice for the treatment of phenylketonuria. Mol Genet Metab. 2011;104(3):249–54.
13. Longo N, Harding CO, Burton BK, Grange DK, Vockley J, Wasserstein M, et al. Single-dose, subcutaneous recombinant phenylalanine ammonia lyase conjugated with polyethylene glycol in adult patients with phenylketonuria: an open-label, multicentre, phase 1 dose-escalation trial. Lancet. 2014;384(9937):37–44.
14. Zori R, Thomas JA, Shur N, Rizzo WB, Decker C, Rosen O, et al. Induction, titration, and maintenance dosing regimen in a phase 2 study of pegvaliase for control of blood phenylalanine in adults with phenylketonuria. Mol Genet Metab. 2018;125(3):217–27.
15. Longo N, Zori R, Wasserstein MP, Vockley J, Burton BK, Decker C, et al. Long-term safety and efficacy of pegvaliase for the treatment of phenylketonuria in adults: combined phase 2 outcomes through PAL-003 extension study. Orphanet J Rare Dis. 2018;13(1):108.
16. Thomas J, Levy H, Amato S, Vockley J, Zori R, Dimmock D, et al. Pegvaliase for the treatment of phenylketonuria: results of a long-term phase 3 clinical trial program (PRISM). Mol Genet Metab. 2018;124(1):27–38.
17. Longo N, Dimmock D, Levy H, Viau K, Bausell H, Bilder DA, et al. Evidence- and consensus-based recommendations for the use of pegvaliase in adults with phenylketonuria. Genet Med. 2019;21(8):1851–67.
18. Hausmann O, Daha M, Longo N, Knol E, Muller I, Northrup H, et al. Pegvaliase: immunological profile and recommendations for the clinical management of hypersensitivity reactions in patients with phenylketonuria treated with this enzyme substitution therapy. Mol Genet Metab. 2019;128(1–2):84–91.
19. Gupta S, Lau K, Harding CO, Shepherd G, Boyer R, Atkinson JP, et al. Association of immune response with efficacy and safety outcomes in adults with phenylketonuria administered pegvaliase in phase 3 clinical trials. EBioMedicine. 2018; 37:366–73.
20. Larimore K, Nguyen T, Badillo B, Lau K, Zori R, Shepherd G, et al. Depletion of interfering IgG and IgM is critical to determine the role of IgE in pegvaliase-associated hypersensitivity. J Immunol Methods. 2019;468:20–8.
21. FDA. PALYNZIQ (pegvaliase-pqpz) injection, for subcutaneous use. Initial U.S. Approval 2018. Available from: https://www.accessdata.fda.gov/drugsatfda_docs/label/2018/761079s000lbl.pdf.
22. Lenke RR, Levy HL. Maternal phenylketonuria and hyperphenylalaninemia. An international survey of the outcome of untreated and treated pregnancies. N Engl J Med. 1980;303(21):1202–8.
23. Boyer M, Skaar J, Sowa M, Tureson JR, Chapel-Crespo CC, Chang R. Continuation of pegvaliase treatment during pregnancy: a case report. Mol Genet Metab Rep. 2021;26:100713.
24. Pegvaliase [Internet]. Drugs and lactation database.
25. Rohr F, Burton BK, Longo N, Thomas J, Harding C, Rosen O, et al. Evaluating change in diet with Pegvaliase treatment in adults with phenylketonuria: results from phase 2 and 3 clinical trials. American College of Medical Genetics and Genomics Annual Meeting 2020.
26. Rocha JC, Bausell H, Belanger-Quintana A, Bernstein LB, Gokmen-Ozel H, Jung A, et al. Practical dietitian road map for the nutritional management of phenylketonuria (PKU) patients on pegvaliase treatment. Mol Genet Metab Rep. 2021;28:100771. https://doi.org/10.1016/j.ymgmr.2021.100771. PMID: 34094869; PMCID: PMC8167196.
27. Sacharow S, Papaleo C, Almeida K, Goodlett B, Kritzer A, Levy H, et al. First 1.5 years of pegvaliase clinic: experiences and outcomes. Mol Genet Metab Rep. 2020;24:100603.
28. Institute of Medicine (U.S.). Panel on Macronutrients., Institute of Medicine (U.S.). Standing Committee on the Scientific Evaluation of Dietary Reference Intakes. Dietary reference intakes for energy, carbohydrate, fiber, fat, fatty acids, cholesterol, protein, and amino acids. Washington, D.C.: National Academies Press; 2005. xxv, 1331 p. p.
29. Shim JS, Oh K, Kim HC. Dietary assessment methods in epidemiologic studies. Epidemiol Health. 2014;36:e2014009.
30. Damsbo-Svendsen M, Frost MB, Olsen A. A review of instruments developed to measure food neophobia. Appetite. 2017;113:358–67.

31. Viau K, Wessel A, Martell L, Sacharow S, Rohr F. Nutrition status of adults with phenylketonuria treated with pegvaliase. Mol Genet Metab. 2021;133(4):345–51.
32. Bernstein LB, Rohr F. Palynziq in practice: one year after FDA approval (Survey) 2019.
33. Jurecki ER, Cederbaum S, Kopesky J, Perry K, Rohr F, Sanchez-Valle A, et al. Adherence to clinic recommendations among patients with phenylketonuria in the United States. Mol Genet Metab. 2017;120(3):190–7.
34. van Spronsen FJ, van Rijn M, Bekhof J, Koch R, Smit PG. Phenylketonuria: tyrosine supplementation in phenylalanine-restricted diets. Am J Clin Nutr. 2001;73(2):153–7.
35. Thomas J, Jurecki E, Lane P, Olbertz J, Wang B, Longo N, et al. Dietary intakes and adverse events in pegvaliase-treated phenylketonuria adults who had low blood phenylalanine levels. American College of Medical Genetics and Genomics Annual Meeting. 2020.

Nutrition Management of Maternal Metabolic Disorders

12

Fran Rohr and Sandy van Calcar

Contents

F. Rohr (✉)
Met Ed Co, Boulder, CO, USA
e-mail: fran.rohr@met-ed.net

S. van Calcar
Oregon Health & Science University, Molecular and Medical Genetics, Portland, OR, USA
e-mail: vancalca@ohsu.edu

L. E. Bernstein et al. (eds.), *Nutrition Management of Inherited Metabolic Diseases*,
https://doi.org/10.1007/978-3-030-94510-7_12

Core Messages

- Children born to mothers with phenylketonuria (PKU) who have high blood phenylalanine during pregnancy are at risk of developing intellectual disability, microcephaly, congenital heart defects, low birth weight and facial dysmorphism.
- Women with PKU should maintain blood phenylalanine below 360 μmol/L before and during pregnancy for optimal pregnancy outcomes.
- In inherited metabolic disorders other than PKU, the fetus does not appear to be at risk; however, the mother is at risk of metabolic crises associated with catabolism during pregnancy or in the post-partum period unless energy intake is sufficient.
- The maternal diet for amino- and organic acidopathies typically includes a disease-specific medical food as the main source of protein, a limited amount of intact protein, and sufficient energy, fat, vitamins and minerals to support fetal growth.

12.1 Background

The nutrition management of inherited metabolic disorders during pregnancy runs the spectrum from maternal phenylketonuria (PKU) that has been studied for decades to case reports for rarer metabolic diseases. More women with urea cycle disorders, maple syrup urine disease and organic acidemias have been well-treated from birth and are now of childbearing age. The impact of metabolic disease on pregnancies differs according to the specific disorder. In PKU, it is well understood that high maternal blood phenylalanine concentrations can affect the developing fetus, whereas in other inherited metabolic disorders it is the mother who is at greater risk, especially during the postpartum period when protein catabolism is greatest. Unlike in PKU, it appears that in these disorders, the infant is not at increased risk of adverse outcomes. Regardless of the metabolic disorder, proper nutrition management and monitoring is important to assure positive pregnancy outcomes.

12.2 Maternal Phenylketonuria

Maternal PKU (MPKU) refers to pregnancy and childbearing in a woman with PKU. Phenylalanine is teratogenic to the developing fetus and therefore, in MPKU, the infant is at risk because of the metabolic disorder of the mother. Children born to mothers with PKU whose blood phenylalanine is not controlled before and during pregnancy may be born with intellectual disability, microcephaly, congenital heart defects (CHD), low birth weight and facial dysmorphism [1, 2]. The incidence of adverse outcomes in MPKU is related to maternal blood phenylalanine concentration, and is highest in children born to mothers who did not have blood phenylalanine in the recommended treatment range during their pregnancies. The recommended maternal blood phenylalanine concentration throughout pregnancy is 120–360 μmol/L. [3–6] This recommendation is based on the MPKU Collaborative Study, a 12-year study of 413 pregnancies which showed lower intelligence in offspring of mothers whose average blood phenylalanine concentration exceeded 360 μmol/L. [7]

The British Registry of 228 live births found a negative correlation between intellectual outcomes of the offspring and maternal blood phenylalanine concentrations exceeding 300 μmol/L; therefore, in the United Kingdom, it is recommended that blood phenylalanine be maintained between 100 and 250 μmol/L for optimal outcomes [8]. In Australia, even lower blood phenylalanine concentrations of 60–120 μmol/L are recommended during pregnancy [9]. Many centers in the United States also counsel women to maintain blood phenylalanine under 240 μmol/L [5]. However, there is some evidence that low (<120 μmol/L) blood phenylalanine concentrations may be associated with poor fetal growth [10] and suggests that low blood phenylalanine should be avoided. With the advent of medical management for PKU, the potential for a woman to have a sustained low blood phenylalanine during pregnancy is greater than with diet management alone. Care must be taken to ensure that adequate amounts of phenylalanine are available to support normal fetal growth.

Stability of blood phenylalanine throughout pregnancy was associated with better development in the offspring of MPKU in one study [11], which showed that the variability in maternal blood phenylalanine concentration had an impact on intellectual outcome at 1, 8 and 14 years, even in women who had good metabolic control. Variability of blood phenylalanine may be a marker for the severity of PKU; women who have severe PKU are less able to tolerate day-to-day changes in dietary phenylalanine intake and, therefore, have greater variation in blood phenylalanine concentrations. In the MPKU Collaborative Study, women were given a severity score (based on genotype, untreated blood phenylalanine concentration and dietary phenylalanine tolerance) and the score was the strongest predictor of both maternal blood phenylalanine during pregnancy and of variability in maternal blood phenylalanine concentrations [12].

In addition to phenylalanine, other nutrients are of importance in MPKU outcomes, including protein, fat, energy and vitamin B_{12}. Maternal protein, fat and energy intake are negatively correlated with blood phenylalanine concentration [13]. Inadequate energy intake was associated with poor maternal weight gain and lower birth measurements. A higher incidence of congenital heart defects was seen in children born to women with lower total protein intakes (intact and medical food), especially when both low vitamin B_{12} and folate intake were also observed [14].

12.3 Nutrition Management of MPKU

The principles of nutrition management in MPKU are to maintain blood phenylalanine concentrations in the target range, support normal weight gain for pregnancy (Table 12.1) and provide adequate nutrients for pregnancy. Other than phenylalanine, protein and tyrosine, the nutrient needs of a pregnant woman with PKU do not differ from the Dietary Reference Intakes (Table 12.2) [15]; however, obtaining adequate nutrition for pregnancy while on a phenylalanine-restricted diet can be a challenge.

Table 12.1 Recommendations for total and rate of weight gain during pregnancy by prepregnancy BMI [22]

Prepregnancy BMI	BMI[a] (kg/m²)	Total weight gain (pounds)	Rates of weight gain in second and third trimesters[b] (pounds/week)
Underweight	<18.5	28–40	1 (1–1.3)
Normal weight	18.5–24.9	25–35	1 (0.8–1)
Overweight	25.0–29.9	15–25	0.6 (0.5–0.7)
Obese (includes all classes)	>30.0	11–20	0.5 (0.4–0.6)

[a] To calculate BMI go to www.nhlbisupport.com/bmi/
[b] Calculations assume a 0.5–2 kg (1.1–4.4 lbs) weight gain in the first trimester [74–76]

Table 12.2 Recommended daily intake of phenylalanine, tyrosine and protein in pregnancy and lactation for women with MPKU [13]

	Phenylalanine (mg)	Tyrosine (mg)	Protein (g)
Trimester 1	265–770	6000–7600	≥70
Trimester 2	400–1650	6000–7600	≥70
Trimester 3	700–2275	6000–7600	≥70
Lactation	700–2275	6000–7600	≥70

Box 12.1: Points to Consider if Blood Phenylalanine Is Too High
- Is medical food intake sufficient?
- Is phenylalanine intake excessive?
- Is energy intake sufficient?
- Has there been adequate weight gain?
- Has there been an illness?

12.3.1 Phenylalanine and Tyrosine

Phenylalanine should be provided in the amount needed to maintain blood phenylalanine in the target range. For a woman with PKU who comes to the attention of the clinic during pregnancy, it is important to reduce phenylalanine intake as soon as possible. Some centers suggest a "washout" period where only medical food, fruits, low phenylalanine vegetables, and low protein foods are included in the diet until the blood phenylalanine concentration decreases to within the desired range. In severe PKU, the average phenylalanine intake is 250–300 mg/day; if a patient's phenylalanine tolerance is not known, this is a reasonable goal, to begin with. Phenylalanine intake in the first trimester ranges from 265 to 770 mg/day [5].

With frequent monitoring of blood phenylalanine and food intake records, dietary phenylalanine can be adjusted until the target range is reached. If blood phenylalanine concentrations are not in good control within a few days, consider whether the woman is getting enough protein (medical food) and/or energy (Box 12.1). Morning sickness or hyperemesis gravida can also be a cause of high blood phenylalanine. Prolonged morning sickness can be treated with antiemetics. In cases where metabolic control is compromised due to hyperemesis gravida, hospitalization may be necessary in order to reverse catabolism and reduce blood phenylalanine concentrations. Hospitalization may also be necessary for intensive diet education.

If the blood phenylalanine concentration becomes too low, 10–25% more phenylalanine is added to the diet. As pregnancy progresses and the woman gains weight, phenylalanine tolerance will increase. This is especially true in the second and third trimesters when the fetus is growing rapidly and phenylalanine intake doubles or triples over prepregnancy intake [5].

Tyrosine is a conditionally essential amino acid in the MPKU diet. Medical food is the major source of dietary tyrosine; therefore, if a woman has low blood tyrosine, check to make sure that she is consuming all of her medical food. Blood tyrosine fluctuates diurnally and is lowest after an overnight fast. Before adding a tyrosine supplement, monitor non-fasting blood tyrosine concentrations to assess whether supplementation is necessary [16].

12.3.2 Protein

The Dietary Recommended Intake (DRI) for protein in pregnancy is 71 g/day [15]. This is an additional 21 grams over non-pregnancy protein recommendations in order to support the growth of the placenta and fetal tissue. Medical food is the major source of protein for individuals with PKU treated with diet alone. When protein is supplied as medical food containing L-amino acids, it is oxidized more rapidly than intact protein and, therefore, the amount of protein needed is greater than normal (1.2 times the DRI or 85 g/day). In severe PKU, medical food provides about 80% of the protein or about 68 g protein/day. A simple way to assure that adequate protein is being provided during pregnancy is to meet the DRI for protein from amino acid-based medical food alone.

The nutrient content of medical foods varies widely. If high-protein, lower-calorie medical foods are used, the volume of medical food required is lower, but fat and energy content are also lower and sufficient energy must be supplied elsewhere in the diet. Conversely, when lower-protein, higher-fat medical foods are used, a higher volume of medical food is necessary to meet protein requirements. The choice of medical food is made on an individual basis depending on the needs and preferences of the pregnant woman, and sometimes a combination of medical foods is best. Additional medical food or intact protein is often needed as the pregnancy progresses and should be added if plasma prealbumin or plasma amino acid concentrations are low for pregnancy (Table 12.3).

Medical foods containing glycomacropeptide (GMP) (Chap. 10) have been used successfully in MPKU pregnancies. While GMP-medical foods contain a small amount of phenylalanine (less than 2 mg per gram of protein equivalent) [17], the amount provided is usually well tolerated, especially during periods of anabolism such as pregnancy. In case reports, reduction in phenylalanine from food has not been needed to account for the phenylalanine provided in the medical food [18]. However, for women with very low prepregnancy phenylalanine tolerance, the additional phenylalanine from GMP may need to be counted in the dietary prescription. Ideally, the effect of the additional phenylalanine in medical food on blood phenylalanine concentrations would be determined during the prepregnancy period.

Large neutral amino acids (LNAA) are contraindicated as a sole source of protein in women with MPKU because LNAA do not sufficiently lower blood phenylalanine to within the desired treatment range of 120–360 μmol/L. [19] The proposed mechanism of action of LNAA is to block uptake of phenylalanine into the brain by supplementing other amino acids that share the LAT-1 transport system across the blood-brain barrier. Some reduction in blood phenylalanine has been seen with LNAA use, but not to the degree necessary to protect the fetus [20].

Table 12.3 Amino acid concentrations during pregnancy (in women without PKU; [Mean +/– SD (μmol/L) [77]

	<20 weeks	20–30 weeks	>30 weeks
Isoleucine	53 ± 23	53 ± 15	46 ± 15
Leucine	114 ± 38	107 ± 30	91 ± 23
Methionine	34 ± 54	20 ± 7	27 ± 7
Phenylalanine	67 ± 30	60 ± 18	54 ± 12
Threonine	118 ± 34	168 ± 42	193 ± 50
Tyrosine	55 ± 22	50 ± 11	50 ± 17
Valine	196 ± 60	179 ± 43	162 ± 43

12.3.3 Energy

Energy requirements in pregnancy are the same for women with PKU as other individuals [21]. Sufficient energy is especially important in MPKU to prevent protein from being used as an energy source, thereby increasing blood phenylalanine concentrations. Energy intake is sufficient if the woman with PKU is gaining weight appropriately (Table 12.1) [22].

12.3.4 Fat and Essential Fatty Acids

Fat is needed in pregnancy to supply sufficient energy as well as the precursors for essential fatty acids that are needed for fetal brain development. In pregnancy, about 30–35% of calories should come from fat [15]. For a 2400-calorie diet, this translates to 93 grams of fat, the equivalent to approximately 6 tablespoons of fat. For expectant mothers on a fat-free or low-fat medical food,

Box 12.2: Facts About Fat in the MPKU Diet

- Provide 30–35% of energy as fat.
- DRI for essential fatty acids [15]:
  - Linoleic acid (omega-6) – 13 g/day
  - α-linolenic acid (omega-3) – 1.4 g/day
- Soybean and canola oils are readily available essential fatty acid sources.
- DHA intake of 300 mg/day is recommended.

special attention must be paid to providing other sources of dietary fat.

The type of fat is also important in order to ensure that the requirements for the essential fatty acids, linoleic and α-linolenic acid are met (Box 12.2). Essential fatty acids compete for the same desaturase enzymes and omega-6 and omega-3 fatty acids must be provided in the proper ratio of approximately 5:1, or synthesis of docosahexaenoic acid (DHA) and eicosapentaenoic acid (EPA) from the omega-3 fatty acids may be inadequate. In order to ensure that sufficient DHA is provided, 650 mg of omega-3 fatty acids, of which 300 mg is DHA, is recommended [2].

12.3.5 Vitamins and Minerals

The DRI for pregnancy should be met for all vitamins and minerals. Medical food is the source of many vitamins and minerals in the MPKU diet; however, if not taken as prescribed or if the medical food does not contain a full complement of vitamins and minerals, intakes may be low. Vitamins and minerals that are of particular concern in MPKU are vitamin B_{12} and folate [14] as low maternal intakes have been correlated with increased risk of congenital heart defects in the offspring. Women with PKU are also at risk for deficiencies in zinc, iron and vitamin B6 as these nutrients are most often found in high protein foods that individuals with PKU do not usually consume. Prenatal supplements or specific vitamins and mineral supplementation may be necessary if monitoring of intake and/or if nutritional biomarkers indicate a problem.

Excessive intake of vitamin A intake leads to hypervitaminosis A that has been associated with birth defects, including malformations of the eye, skull, lungs, and heart [23]. High intakes are possible in the diet for MPKU if a medical food containing vitamin A is taken along with a prenatal supplement or fish oil. The upper safe limit for vitamin A intake during pregnancy is 2800–3000 μg/day, or approximately 10,000 IU (1 μg Retinol Activity Equivalent is equal to 3.3 IU) [24]. Vitamin A from animal sources (fish oil, or vitamin A palmitate, retinol and acetate) is of concern, but vitamin A supplied as carotenoids does not cause hypervitaminosis A because the conversion of beta-carotene to the active form of vitamin A is highly regulated by the body. Prenatal vitamin supplements often specify the source of Vitamin A.

12.4 Nutrition Management in Lactation and the Postpartum Period

Women with PKU are counseled to be on diet for life including in the postpartum period. It is possible for the woman with PKU to breastfeed her infant. If the woman chooses not to be on diet after pregnancy yet is breastfeeding, there will be a slightly higher phenylalanine content in her breast milk, but this has no effect on the infant's blood phenylalanine concentration, as long as the infant does not have PKU. Even then, limited amounts of breast milk would be allowed in combination with a phenylalanine-free infant formula. While staying on the phenylalanine-restricted diet is not necessary for breastfeeding, it is encouraged in order to maintain optimal neuropsychological functioning, which is important for coping with the demands of caring for an infant [25].

The nutrient requirements for breastfeeding are the same as in the third trimester of pregnancy due to the high protein, phenylalanine and energy demands of producing breast milk. Monitoring of blood phenylalanine and continued support of the woman with PKU is needed but this is often difficult to accomplish once the mother's attention turns from her diet and pregnancy to caring for an infant.

12.5 Medical Management in Maternal PKU

12.5.1 Sapropterin Dihydrocloride

Medical management for PKU includes sapropterin dihydrochloride (Kuvan®) and pegvaliase-pqpz (Palynziq®). Gene therapy trials are underway (Chap. 8). Because of the well-known adverse effects of high blood phenylalanine on the developing fetus, the imperative is great for health care providers to consider all treatment options for women who are not able to keep blood phenylalanine within treatment range on diet alone. Yet, information on the use of medical therapies in pregnant women is gained gradually with commercial use over time.

Evidence about sapropterin dihydrochloride from a registry of women who have been on sapropterin during pregnancy shows that they tolerated the drug well, maintained blood phenylalanine in good control during pregnancy, and had normal birth outcomes [25]. The typical sapropterin dose was 20 mg/kg at the start of pregnancy and was not adjusted for weight gain during pregnancy. Likewise, a European study of pregnant women treated with sapropterin concluded that its use was safe and effective [26]. Consensus is that sapropterin should be used in women with PKU who are planning pregnancy if they are known responders, or if they are unable to attain good metabolic control. If a woman with PKU presents during pregnancy, sapropterin can be tried as long as it does not delay the onset of other therapies [27]. There is no evidence regarding the safety of sapropterin dihydrochloride use during lactation [3].

12.5.2 Pegvaliase

Per the pegvaliase label in the US, pegvaliase is not contraindicated during pregnancy and lactation; therefore, the decision about its use is left to the medical provider's clinical judgement. Consideration should be given on a case-by-case basis to the benefits–risks of continuing pegvaliase therapy versus the teratogenic effects of hyperphenylalaninemia [28]. There is very limited evidence about the use of pegvaliase during pregnancy. In one case study, a pregnant woman who continued pegvaliase during pregnancy had a positive outcome [29]. Close monitoring and diet adjustment are needed to prevent low maternal phenylalanine concentrations in order to support normal fetal growth.

Should the decision be made to discontinue pegvaliase for a planned pregnancy, women should be advised to stop pegvaliase at least 4 weeks prior to pregnancy as pharmacological data shows that this is sufficient time to washout the drug [28]. Resuming a low phenylalanine diet for a planned pregnancy after being on a normal diet is possible, but difficult [30]. Pegvaliase treatment can be reintroduced successfully in the post-partum period [30].

Information on the presence of pegvaliase in breast milk is limited; one case study reported that pegvaliase was not present in a single breast milk sample. Therefore, the decision to allow breastfeeding while on pegvaliase should include the benefit to the mother (lower blood phe) and the infant (optimal nutrition) as well as psychological factors. Although no study data are available, there is no evidence to suggest that pegvaliase is contraindicated in men anticipating fatherhood.

12.6 Monitoring

Box 12.3: Nutrition Monitoring of a Patient with Maternal PKU[a]

- Routine assessments including anthropometrics, dietary intake, physical findings
- Laboratory Monitoring
  - Diagnosis-Specific
    Plasma amino acids
    - Phenylalanine
    - Tyrosine
  - Nutrition laboratory monitoring of patients on phenylalanine-restricted diets may include markers of:
    Protein sufficiency (plasma amino acids, prealbumin, albumin)
    Nutritional anemia (hemoglobin, hematocrit, MCV, serum vitamin B_{12} and/or methylmalonic acid, total homocysteine, ferritin, iron, folate, total iron binding capacity)
    Vitamin and mineral status: 25-hydroxy vitamin D, zinc, trace minerals, folic acid
    Essential fatty acid sufficiency: plasma or erythrocyte fatty acids.
    Others as clinically indicated

[a] For suggested frequency of monitoring: www.southeastgenetics.org/ngp

Careful metabolic and nutritional monitoring of a pregnant woman with PKU is important to ensure that the fetus is not exposed to high blood phenylalanine and sufficient nutrition is provided for proper fetal development. Frequent (once or twice weekly) monitoring of blood phenylalanine is especially important, as is routine monitoring of protein status including plasma amino acids and prealbumin levels (Box 12.3). The reference ranges for many laboratory tests, including amino acids, differ for pregnancy. The laboratory monitoring can be completed by the metabolic clinic or by the obstetrician if the woman lives far from the clinic or if traveling becomes difficult later in pregnancy, as long as communication between providers occurs. Weight gain should be monitored regularly, and ultrasounds performed twice during pregnancy, once early in pregnancy to establish that the fetus is viable, and once at 18 weeks' gestation to rule out cardiac and other anomalies [22].

12.7 Pregnancy in Maple Syrup Urine Disease

Pregnancies in women with classical maple syrup urine disease (MSUD) require close monitoring throughout pregnancy, delivery and the postpartum period. There are eight publications that describe maternal MSUD cases [31–38], and other successful pregnancies are known to the MSUD Family Support Group as well [39]. Significantly increased tolerance of leucine is reported (2–3 times prepregnancy leucine needs), especially during the second and third trimesters as additional leucine is required for maternal and fetal growth. In all cases, additional caloric support (oral and/or IV) was provided during delivery. Elevated leucine concentrations were noted in the postpartum period as protein catabolism increases after delivery with the rapid involution of the uterus [40]. Plasma leucine concentrations >1000 μmol/L were reported in three women on day 9 or 10 postpartum [31, 32, 35]; one of these women did not adhere to post-pregnancy recommendations and died 51 days after delivery [33], emphasizing the importance of continued monitoring and treatment after delivery in these women. In all cases, normal infant outcomes were reported, even for an infant born to a woman with poor leucine control throughout pregnancy [33]. Successful breastfeeding while maintaining maternal metabolic control is possible [34, 38].

12.8 Pregnancy in Propionic Acidemia

There are four published reports of successful pregnancy in women with propionic acidemia [31, 41–43] and additional pregnancies in women with mild propionic acidemia (7% and 9% residual propionyl-CoA carboxylase activity) are known to the author. Frequent monitoring to adjust both diet treatment and carnitine supplementation was necessary throughout the pregnancies and additional caloric support (oral and/or IV dextrose) was provided during delivery and the immediate postpartum period. Complications included placenta previa [41], preeclampsia (Case Report 2), hypothyroidism and gestational diabetes [44]. One woman developed heart failure symptoms two days after delivery but responded to aggressive treatment that included IV dextrose and insulin [44]. None of the infants showed congenital anomalies and normal developmental outcomes in infancy were reported.

12.9 Pregnancy in Methylmalonic Acidemia

There have been several reports in the literature of pregnancies in women with various forms of methylmalonic acidemia (MMA), including mutase, cobalamin A and mild cobalamin C defects; both cobalamin responsive and unresponsive phenotypes are included in these reports [41, 45–51]. A summary of ten pregnancies in women with MMA found a wide range of treatment regimens including diet, L-carnitine supplementation and/or intramuscular (IM) hydroxocobalamin injection [50]. Half of the completed pregnancies resulted in preterm deliveries (32 to 36 weeks' gestation) with 7 of 10 pregnancies requiring Cesarean section delivery, often because of fetal distress [50]. At delivery, all women were treated with IV dextrose (+/-IV carnitine) for up to 8 days postpartum. No adverse outcomes for the infants were reported, despite elevated serum methylmalonic acid concentrations throughout pregnancy.

12.10 Pregnancy in Urea Cycle Disorders

Numerous cases in the literature describe pregnancy and fetal outcome in women with various urea cycle disorders (UCD) [52–60]. Similar to pregnancies in MSUD and organic acidemias, women with UCD are especially at risk for metabolic decompensation during the first trimester when poor energy intake is common, during any intercurrent illness, with prolonged delivery, and in the postpartum period. Women are especially vulnerable to hyperammonemia during the postpartum period when severe mental status changes, coma and death have been reported after delivery in UCD, even in women with mild forms of the disorder [52, 53, 60]. In some reports, the patient was not diagnosed with a UCD until she developed symptoms during the postpartum period [53, 54, 60].

During pregnancies in women with UCD, frequent monitoring is needed to prevent essential amino acid (EAA) deficiency and reintroduction of an EAA-based medical food may be necessary [56]. During delivery, initiating IV dextrose with or without oral supplements (i.e. glucose polymer solutions) is typical. To prevent increasing ammonia concentrations following delivery, additional energy support, increased nitrogen scavenger medications and L-arginine with gradual reintroduction of protein sources may be necessary [56, 60]. Initiation of IV nitrogen scavenger medications and L-arginine throughout delivery in two women who were carriers of ornithine transcarbamylase deficiency (OTC) prevented initial hyperammonemia for their male neonates who were prenatally diagnosed with severe OTC deficiency [61].

12.11 Overview of Recommendations for the Nutrition Management for Pregnancies in Women with Disorders of Protein Metabolism

Based on published cases and the author's experience, there are some general recommendations that apply to all pregnancies in women with disorders of protein metabolism:

12.11.1 Maintain Normal Maternal Weight Gain During Pregnancy

Generally, weight gain goals are the same for pregnancies in women with inherited metabolic disease as for the general population (Table 12.1).

Weight loss should be avoided to prevent protein catabolism and elevations in amino acids, ammonia and other associated metabolites. Energy needs increase as pregnancy progresses, especially in late pregnancy when fetal growth is the greatest [24].

12.11.2 Maintain Adequate Energy and Protein Nutriture Throughout Pregnancy

Both energy and protein needs increase as pregnancy progresses to allow for increased maternal requirements and adequate fetal growth [24] (Fig. 12.1). To prevent protein deficiency, any woman requiring a medical food prior to pregnancy will need to continue this throughout pregnancy. Even if a woman has a milder form of a disorder and has not required medical food as an adult, reintroduction of a medical food may be necessary during pregnancy [43]. Protein needs are also higher when consuming an amino acid-based medical food compared with a diet exclusively of intact protein sources (Chap. 6).

12.11.3 Maintain Plasma Amino acid Concentrations Within the Reference Range and Anticipate a Higher Intact Protein Tolerance as Pregnancy Progresses

Blood concentrations of many amino acids decrease as pregnancy progresses with the increases in maternal plasma volume, urinary protein excretion and fetal utilization during pregnancy [62]. This needs to be considered in the interpretation of plasma amino acid profiles (Table 12.3).

As with total protein, the needs for individual amino acids increase as pregnancy progresses, especially in the late second and third trimesters when fetal growth is the greatest [22, 31]. Even for patients with classical phenotypes, higher protein foods may be needed towards the end of pregnancy to maintain normal plasma amino acid concentrations. Adding milk to the medical food, if tolerated, is an easy option.

Over restriction of amino acids may have contributed to the poor fetal growth detected in the second and third trimester in MSUD and MMA pregnancies [31, 50]. If a single amino acid is supplemented as part of treatment, additional supplementation may be required to prevent low plasma concentrations, even with the increase in intact protein intake as pregnancy progresses.

In the author's experience with MSUD pregnancies, supplementation of valine and isoleucine may be needed, even for women who did not require supplementation to maintain normal plasma concentrations before pregnancy. If the plasma leucine concentration is in the goal range, but elevated valine and/or isoleucine are noted, the amount of the supplements should be decreased rather than reducing intake of intact protein. Although the teratogenicity of the branched-chain amino acids (BCAA) remains uncertain, limited experience suggests that moderate elevations in valine and isoleucine may not pose harm to the mother or fetus.

$EER_{nonpregnant}$ + additional energy for pregnancy + energy deposition

	Energy	Protein
Trimester 1:	EER + 0 + 0 kcals	No additional
Trimester 2:	EER + 160 + 180 kcals	+14.7 g/day
Trimester 3:	EER + 272 + 180 kcals	+27.3 g/day

DRI = 0.88 g/kg/d or +21 g/d
RDA = 1.1 g/kg/d or +25 g/d

Fig. 12.1 Estimated energy and protein requirements for each trimester of pregnancy [24]

12.11.4 Plan Ahead for Intercurrent Illness and Complications Affecting Dietary Intake

As with any pregnancy, persistent nausea and vomiting and intercurrent illness can occur. For women with intoxication disorders, these catabolic events need to be aggressively addressed to prevent increasing concentrations of amino acids and associated toxic metabolites. Antiemetics can be prescribed. For women who have a difficult time consuming medical food, a gastrostomy tube may need to be considered [63]. A plan for any needed admissions should be established ahead of time and emergency protocols updated [64].

12.11.5 Refer to an Obstetric Clinic Specializing in High-Risk Pregnancy

Given the risk of metabolic decompensation during pregnancy and the postpartum period, women with amino acidopathies, organic acidemias or urea cycle defects should be followed by an obstetric clinic specializing in high-risk pregnancies [31]. Frequent assessment of fetal growth is often needed. For successful maternal and fetal outcomes, a multidisciplinary approach is required with input from both the obstetric and metabolic teams [34, 56, 59].

Box 12.4: Nutrition Interventions for Pregnancy in Women with Disorders of Protein Metabolism

- Promote normal maternal weight gain during pregnancy.
- Provide adequate energy and protein nutriture throughout pregnancy.
- Maintain plasma amino acid concentrations within the reference range.
- Anticipate a higher intact protein tolerance as pregnancy progresses.
- Plan ahead for intercurrent illness and complications affecting dietary intake.
- Refer to an obstetric clinic specializing in high-risk pregnancy.
- Anticipate postpartum catabolism and plan to provide adequate nutrition.

12.11.6 Anticipate Postpartum Catabolism

Delivery and the postpartum period are catabolic processes and women with amino acidopathies, organic acidemias or UCD are at high risk for metabolic decompensation during these times. The risk may be greatest for women with classical forms of these disorders, although severe decompensation has been reported in women considered to have milder phenotypes [52, 57]. The risk for decompensation increases if delivery is prolonged and/or a sufficient source of energy and protein equivalents is not provided during delivery and the postpartum period.

Postpartum catabolism is caused by rapid protein turnover associated with hormonal changes and the involution of the uterus. Uterine mass decreases approximately 50% during the first 10 days after delivery [40]. In the author's experience with MSUD pregnancies, the greatest risk for decompensation occurred between 3 and 14 days after delivery. Many of the cases reported in the literature note an increase in concentrations of amino acids or associated metabolites during this time frame. Even after discharge, frequent monitoring and contact with the mother are needed to assure adequate energy intake and to assess for signs of decompensation. Catabolism gradually slows, but it may take 6–8 weeks after delivery for protein metabolism to return to a prepregnancy state [40, 64] (Box 12.4).

12.12 Pregnancy in Fatty Acid Oxidation Disorders

The metabolic changes and energy demands of pregnancy, delivery, and the postpartum period present challenges for a woman with a disorder in long-chain fatty acid oxidation (LC-FAOD) and can be influenced by the severity of the disorder. The course of pregnancy and the postpartum period has been reported for 12 pregnancies among 8 women with very-long-chain acyl-CoA dehydrogenase deficiency (VLCAD) [65–68] and one woman with long-chain 3-hydroxyacyl-CoA dehydrogenase deficiency (LCHAD) [69] although a few other women with LCHAD and trifunctional protein deficiency (TFP) who experienced successful pregnancy are known [70]. Pregnancy-related nausea and vomiting leading to catabolism is a concern. Elevated creatine kinase (CK) concentrations with myalgia and rhabdomyolysis are commonly reported complications [65, 67, 68] that resolve with IV dextrose support and bed rest [68]. Nutrition management guidance during pregnancy includes minimizing fasting, adhering to restrictions of dietary long-chain fat intake and supplementation with medium-chain triglycerides (MCT), use of L-carnitine, and providing additional energy from carbohydrate and protein sources in the second and third trimesters of pregnancy [65, 67–69, 71]. Additionally, supplementation with omega-3-fatty acids and use of nocturnal cornstarch was included in LCHAD pregnancy management [69, 71]. Laboratory monitoring during pregnancy can include CK, plasma carnitine, and plasma acylcarnitine profile [65–69] Reports documented reductions of CK and acylcarnitine concentrations in the second and third trimester attributed to fatty acid oxidation by the placenta [65, 67, 68]. Higher concentrations of these metabolites returned following delivery [67, 68]. Both vaginal and Cesarean deliveries with successful infant outcomes are reported [65–67, 69]. Planning for labor and delivery included the use of continuous IV dextrose along with oral energy sources to meet metabolic demands and prevent catabolism, rhabdomyolysis, and renal insufficiency [67, 68].

Women with LC-FAOD are also at risk for rhabdomyolysis and abnormal laboratory findings in the postpartum period due to inadequate energy intake and catabolism associated with tissue breakdown during the puerperium period, the period of about 6 weeks after childbirth when the mother's reproductive organs return to their original nonpregnant condition [67, 68]. Acute heart failure due to cardiomyopathy was reported after delivery in a woman with VLCAD who had hyperemesis gravidarum with severe metabolic decompensation at gestation week 14 [66] and unresolved tachycardia requiring Cesarean section delivery at 34 weeks' gestation in a woman with LCHAD [69].

Breastfeeding is not contraindicated; however, it can contribute to catabolism if maternal energy needs are not met [68]. Close monitoring of the woman's nutritional intake and laboratory markers should continue through at least 8 weeks postpartum and as long as the woman is breastfeeding [68].

12.13 Pregnancy in Disorders of Carbohydrate Metabolism

Successful pregnancy and infant outcomes have been documented in women with GSD type Ia, type 1b and type III [72, 73]. Carbohydrate requirements increase during pregnancy, especially during the first trimester. An increase in frequency and severity of hypoglycemia has been noted during pregnancy in some women. Close glucose monitoring, increased cornstarch doses and/or overnight enteral feedings have been utilized during pregnancy to maintain euglycemia. A goal of preventing maternal hypoglycemia is paramount as intrauterine growth retardation and low birth weight has been reported in inadequately controlled pregnancies [73]. Close monitoring of preexisting maternal complications (such as hepatic adenomas, cardiac dysfunction) is necessary as these can be exacerbated during pregnancy [72, 73]. Intravenous dextrose has been administered during delivery and the postpartum period to reduce the risk of hypoglycemia during these times. With optimal metabolic control during gestation, infant outcomes have been positive [72].

Another disorder in carbohydrate metabolism requiring medical nutrition therapy is galactosemia due to deficiency of galactose-1-phosphate uridyltransferase. Primary ovarian insufficiency affects >90% of women with classical forms of this disorder resulting in infertility for the majority [71]. However, as more treated women are reaching child-bearing age, an increase in viable pregnancies has been reported [71]. This needs to be considered in the treatment and counseling for women with this disorder.

12.14 Summary

Maternal PKU Women with PKU must maintain blood phenylalanine below 360 μmol/L before and during pregnancy to prevent the MPKU Syndrome. Because of the teratogenic effect of phenylalanine on the fetus, all treatment options to control blood phenylalanine including a phenylalanine-restricted diet, sapropterin and pegvaliase should be considered. The phenylalanine-restricted diet must provide sufficient protein, energy, fat and micronutrients to support a developing fetus. Medical food for PKU provides protein equivalents with limited or no phenylalanine and, depending on the nutrient profile of the medical food, supplemental energy, fat, essential fatty acids, vitamins and minerals may be needed. Insufficient protein and vitamin B_{12} in the diets of women with PKU are associated with fetal congenital heart defects. Close monitoring of blood phenylalanine and other laboratory values, as well as assessment of weight gain and nutrient intake is recommended. Women with PKU are encouraged to breastfeed their infants and to stay on the diet in the postpartum period. More data on medical therapy in pregnancy is needed.

Other IMD Although experience is still limited, it appears that women with inherited metabolic disorders that pose a risk for metabolic decompensation are at greater risk for adverse outcomes than are their infants. The postpartum period is of particular concern for metabolic decompensation in these women. Infant outcomes are often reported as normal, although in most cases reports, the children were not followed beyond toddler years and formal developmental testing was not completed. However, despite overall poor control in some of the reported pregnancies, the infants do not have the dysmorphology, microcephaly, cardiac defects or developmental delays that have been described in infants born to women with poorly controlled PKU. Systematic collection of data from additional pregnancies is needed before definitive conclusions and standardized recommendations can be provided.

Additional information about pregnancy in other inherited metabolic diseases includes classical homocystinuria (Chap. 14) and hereditary tyrosinemia (Chap. 13).

12.15 Case Reports

To illustrate the recommendations described in this chapter, the following case reports of pregnancy in a woman with classical MSUD and a woman with mild propionic acidemia are discussed.

Case Report 1: Pregnancy in Maple Syrup Urine Disease

A 22-year-old woman homozygous for the classical variant Y393N found in the Mennonite population presented to the metabolic clinic at approximately 4 weeks gestation in good metabolic control. Her history included a severe neonatal presentation at 4 days of age with numerous admissions for illness as a child. However, as an adolescent and adult, she was able to manage the majority of illnesses at home. She maintained excellent metabolic control throughout her life and had no evidence of cognitive delay or other complications associated with poorly treated MSUD.

Plasma amino acid concentrations were monitored one to two times per week. Goals for the pregnancy included maintaining leucine and isoleucine concentrations between 100 and 300 μmol/L and valine concentrations between 200 and 400 μmol/L. Prealbumin, albumin and other nutrition markers were monitored monthly. She was referred to a high-risk obstetrics clinic and a fetal ultrasound was completed monthly after the first trimester. Maternal weight gain and fetal growth were normal throughout pregnancy.

During the first trimester, the patient struggled with morning sickness and required antiemetic medication. Her leucine tolerance remained essentially unchanged during the first trimester but increased rapidly during the second and third trimesters (Fig. 12.2b). Her initial leucine tolerance was 550 mg/day and increased to 3400 mg/day prior to delivery. Weekly increases of >100 mg leucine/day were required to prevent low leucine concentrations after 25 weeks' gestation (Fig. 12.2a, b).

A vaginal delivery was planned, but the fetus was in a breech position and a Cesarean section was performed at 39 weeks' gestation. Since delivery and the postpartum period are catabolic processes, a central PICC line was placed prior to delivery to administer BCAA-free parenteral solution with dextrose and lipid for energy. Isoleucine and valine supplements were given orally. To reduce postpartum catabolism, her treatment plan included maintaining the same

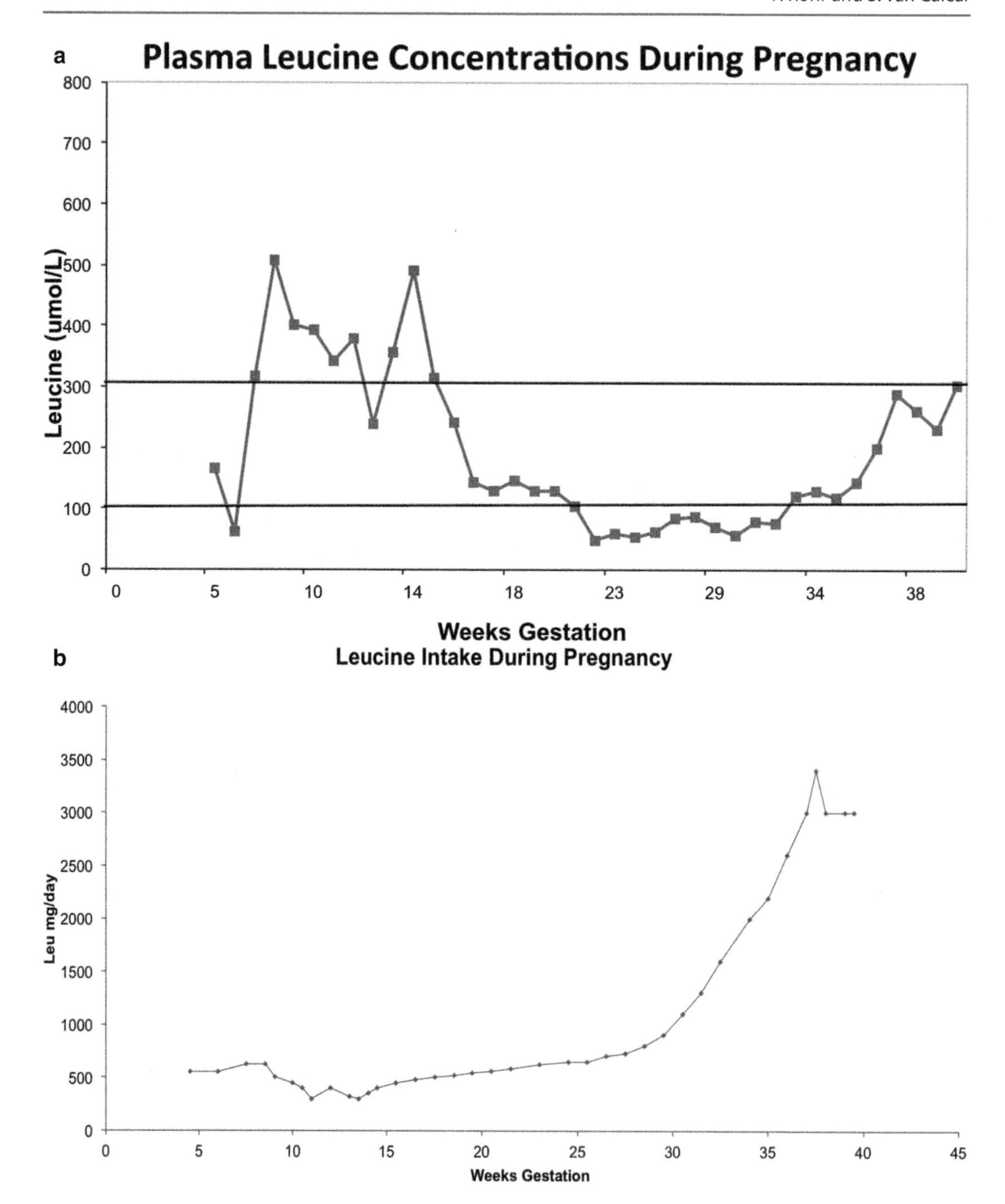

Fig. 12.2 (**a**, **b**) A marked increase in dietary leucine prescription was required to maintain plasma leucine concentrations between 100 and 300 μmol/L after 25 weeks' gestation in a woman with classical MSUD

energy and protein intake that she tolerated at the end of pregnancy. Plasma amino acids were measured daily, and reintroduction of dietary leucine was based on the plasma leucine concentration.

The patient was able to restart medical food by 12 hours after delivery and by postpartum day 2, she was consuming as much medical food as she consumed at the end of pregnancy. Leucine concentrations remained within the normal range.

Thus, she was weaned off of parenteral solutions over a two-day period, and her oral leucine prescription was incrementally increased to her prepregnancy leucine requirement of 550 mg/day. However, her leucine concentration began to increase on Day 5 after delivery so intact protein sources were removed from the diet and additional energy was provided by reintroduction of IV glucose and lipid solutions. However, the plasma leucine continued to increase, and it was only after reintroduction of protein equivalents from the BCAA-free parenteral amino acid solution that the plasma leucine concentration decreased. On Day 6, she was consuming 3.0 g/kg protein equivalents (50% formula, 50% IV) and 4500 kcals from both oral and IV sources. The leucine concentration decreased rapidly on this regimen.

To prevent another spike in plasma leucine, IV energy and amino acid sources were reduced gradually over a four-day period. She was discharged on Day 11 after delivery. After discharge, plasma amino acids were checked two times/week for 2 weeks and then weekly. Her dietary leucine tolerance increased slowly, and it was not until 30 days after delivery that she tolerated her prepregnancy leucine intake of 550 mg/day.

The infant had normal APGAR scores at birth with weight at 25%ile and length at 50%ile. The mother attempted to breastfeed, but her milk production remained poor even with pumping. It is unclear if MSUD contributed to this; however, a subsequent report describes a woman with MSUD who was able to breastfeed successfully [34]. At the age of 3 years, the child was developing and growing without concern.

This woman's second pregnancy progressed similarly to her first with a dramatic increase in BCAA tolerance as the pregnancy progressed. To avoid the increase in leucine concentrations during the postpartum period as seen in her first pregnancy, the reduction in energy and protein from parenteral sources was reduced gradually over 7 days and leucine from oral sources was introduced more gradually. At her discharge 10 days after delivery, her leucine prescription was only 60% of her prepregnancy prescription. Her leucine tolerance did not reach her prepregnancy tolerance until 6 weeks after delivery.

Case Report 2: Pregnancy in Propionic Acidemia

This is the second pregnancy for a 28-year-old woman with variants in the β-subunit of the gene for propionyl-CoA carboxylase. She was diagnosed at 4 years of age in a metabolic coma. She had a history of seizures and a cardiac complication of long-QT syndrome. As an adult, she did not consume a medical food, but self-restricted her protein intake to 0.6–0.8 g/kg prior to pregnancy. Her first pregnancy was complicated by preeclampsia requiring a Cesarean delivery at 31 weeks' gestation with slowed fetal growth by ultrasound. Despite complications of prematurity, the child showed no cognitive or growth delays at 10 years of age.

Unlike her first pregnancy when a medical food was not started until 14 weeks gestation, a medical food was started prior to pregnancy to assure better protein nutriture during her second pregnancy. Maternal weight gain was normal. To maintain normal plasma concentrations of valine, isoleucine, methionine and threonine, her intake of intact protein increased as pregnancy progressed. Even with the increased intake of intact protein, valine and isoleucine supplements were added later in pregnancy to achieve normal concentrations of these two amino acids. She continued biotin (10 mg/day) and L-carnitine supplementation throughout pregnancy. Plasma carnitine concentrations were frequently monitored, and her L-carnitine dose was gradually increased from 50 to 150 mg/kg prepregnancy weight to maintain low normal free carnitine concentrations for pregnancy.

Ultrasounds showed improved fetal growth during her second pregnancy. Despite more aggressive treatment, she again developed preeclampsia and delivered at 32 weeks' gestation by Cesarean section. A 10% dextrose solution was provided by peripheral line during delivery and for 3 days postpartum. Despite prematurity complications, the child showed no cognitive or growth delays at 7 years of age. Improved energy and protein nutriture may have played a role in better fetal growth during the second pregnancy. Figure 12.3

	1st Pregnancy (◆)	2nd Pregnancy (■)
Pre-Pregnancy Total Protein intake	0.7 g/kg	1.0 g/kg
Total Protein intake @ 20 weeks	1.1 g/kg	1.3 g/kg
Total Protein intake at Delivery	1.4 g/kg	1.6 g/kg
Initiation of medical food	14 weeks	Pre-Pregnancy
Total maternal weight gain	15 kg (33 lbs)	13 kg (28 lbs)
Carnitine dose at Delivery	150 mg/kg	100 mg/kg
Gestational age at delivery	31 1/7 weeks	32 0/7 weeks
Birth Weight	1170 g	1826 g

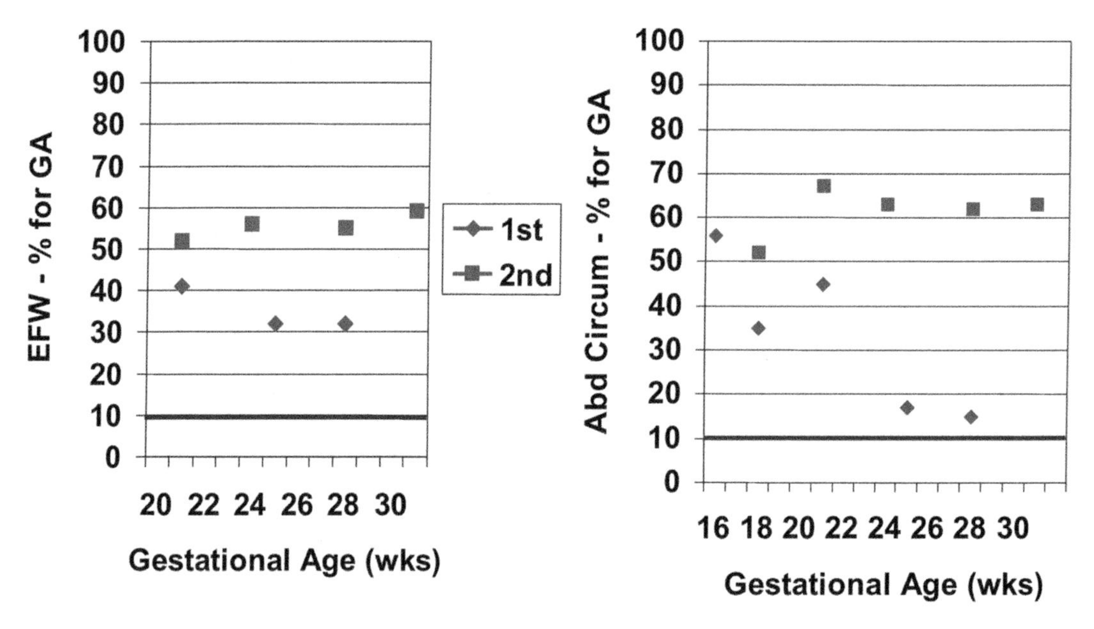

Fig. 12.3 Comparison of energy and protein intake and estimated fetal weight (EFW) and abdominal circumference (Abd Circum) measured by ultrasound in two pregnancies in a woman with mild propionic acidemia. Ultrasound measurements are reported as percentiles based on gestational age

shows total protein intake, maternal weight gain and fetal growth measurements during both pregnancies.

It is unknown if propionic acidemia played a role in the development of preeclampsia for this woman. The other 3 pregnancies to women with propionic acidemia known to the author delivered at term. In all 5 pregnancies, there were no cognitive delays or other complications reported in the children.

12.16 Diet Example for a Pregnant Woman with PKU

Patient Information	The following are the intake goals for this woman
29-year-old woman with severe PKU 4 weeks gestation Blood phenylalanine concentration: 960 μmol/L (16 mg/dL)	Protein from medical food: at least 70 g/day Phenylalanine (protein) from intact sources: washout; as low as possible Energy: at least 2200 kcal/day Fat: 73 g/day (30% of total energy) Supplements: prenatal supplement with 300 mg DHA, per day

Initially, counsel the pregnant woman to avoid all "counted foods" until her blood phenylalanine is in treatment range. During the washout, she should consume low protein foods and uncounted foods (Appendix G).

Table 12.4 is an example of a diet that contains 2300 kcal and 80 g of protein. Amounts are shown for the dietitian's use; the patient is counseled to include unlimited "Uncounted Foods" from the Simplified Diet (Appendix G). According to the diet analysis (MetabolicPro®), this diet contains 220 mg of phenylalanine.

Table 12.4 Example diet for pregnant woman with PKU

Diet plan	Amount
Lophlex LQ, tropical	4 pouches
Uncounted foods	
Breakfast	
Low protein bread	2 slices
Butter	2 pats
Jelly	2 Tbsp
Coffee, decaf	1cup
Nondairy coffee creamer	1 oz
Grapes	10
Lunch	
Low protein cheese	1 slice
Low protein bread	2 slices
Butter for grilling	2 tsp
Baby carrots	10
French dressing	1 Tbsp
Dinner	
Tomatoes, cherry	10
Lettuce	1 cup
Celery	1 stalk
Salad dressing, Italian	2 Tbsp
Low protein pasta	2 cups
Olive oil	2 tbsp
Garlic	2 cloves
Snacks	
Low protein cookies	2
Sorbet	1 cup

Acknowledgement The author, Sandy van Calcar, wishes to thank the metabolic team at the University of Wisconsin-Madison and the patients followed by this clinic for allowing publication of their experiences.

References

1. Lenke RR, Levy HL. Maternal phenylketonuria and hyperphenylalaninemia. An international survey of the outcome of untreated and treated pregnancies. N Engl J Med. 1980;303(21):1202–8.
2. Rouse B, Azen C. Effect of high maternal blood phenylalanine on offspring congenital anomalies and developmental outcome at ages 4 and 6 years: the importance of strict dietary control preconception and throughout pregnancy. J Pediatr. 2004;144(2):235–9.
3. Camp KM, Parisi MA, Acosta PB, Berry GT, Bilder DA, Blau N, et al. Phenylketonuria scientific review conference: state of the science and future research needs. Mol Genet Metab. 2014;112(2):87–122.
4. Vockley J, Andersson HC, Antshel KM, Braverman NE, Burton BK, Frazier DM, et al. Phenylalanine hydroxylase deficiency: diagnosis and management guideline. Genet Med. 2014;16(2):188–200.
5. Singh RH, Rohr F, Frazier D, Cunningham A, Mofidi S, Ogata B, et al. Recommendations for the nutrition management of phenylalanine hydroxylase deficiency. Genet Med. 2014;16(2):121–31.
6. van Spronsen FJ, van Wegberg AM, Ahring K, Belanger-Quintana A, Blau N, Bosch AM, et al. Key European guidelines for the diagnosis and management of patients with phenylketonuria. Lancet Diabetes Endocrinol. 2017;5(9):743–56.
7. Koch R, Hanley W, Levy H, Matalon K, Matalon R, Rouse B, et al. The maternal phenylketonuria international study: 1984–2002. Pediatrics. 2003;112(6 Pt 2):1523–9.
8. Lee PJ, Ridout D, Walter JH, Cockburn F. Maternal phenylketonuria: report from the United Kingdom Registry 1978–97. Arch Dis Child. 2005;90(2):143–6.
9. Ng TW, Rae A, Wright H, Gurry D, Wray J. Maternal phenylketonuria in Western Australia: pregnancy outcomes and developmental outcomes in offspring. J Paediatr Child Health. 2003;39(5):358–63.
10. Teissier R, Nowak E, Assoun M, Mention K, Cano A, Fouilhoux A, et al. Maternal phenylketonuria: low phenylalaninemia might increase the risk of intrauterine growth retardation. J Inherit Metab Dis. 2012;35(6):993–9.
11. Maillot F, Lilburn M, Baudin J, Morley DW, Lee PJ. Factors influencing outcomes in the offspring of mothers with phenylketonuria during pregnancy: the importance of variation in maternal blood phenylalanine. Am J Clin Nutr. 2008;88(3):700–5.
12. Widaman KF, Azen C. Relation of prenatal phenylalanine exposure to infant and childhood cognitive outcomes: results from the International Maternal PKU Collaborative Study. Pediatrics. 2003;112(6 Pt 2):1537–43.
13. Acosta PB, Matalon K, Castiglioni L, Rohr FJ, Wenz E, Austin V, et al. Intake of major nutrients by women in the Maternal Phenylketonuria (MPKU) Study and effects on plasma phenylalanine concentrations. Am J Clin Nutr. 2001;73(4):792–6.
14. Matalon KM, Acosta PB, Azen C. Role of nutrition in pregnancy with phenylketonuria and birth defects. Pediatrics. 2003;112(6 Pt 2):1534–6.
15. USDA. Dietary reference intakes: recommended intakes for individuals by age, size, sex and life stage. 2014. Available from: http://fnic.nal.usda.gov/dietary-guidance/dietary-reference-intakes/dri-tables.
16. van Spronsen FJ, van Rijn M, Bekhof J, Koch R, Smit PG. Phenylketonuria: tyrosine supplementation in phenylalanine-restricted diets. Am J Clin Nutr. 2001;73(2):153–7.
17. Lim K, van Calcar SC, Nelson KL, Gleason ST, Ney DM. Acceptable low-phenylalanine foods and beverages can be made with glycomacropeptide from cheese whey for individuals with PKU. Mol Genet Metab. 2007;92(1–2):176–8.
18. Pinto A, Almeida MF, Cunha A, Carmona C, Rocha S, Guimas A, et al. Dietary management of maternal phenylketonuria with glycomacropeptide and amino acids supplements: a case report. Mol Genet Metab Rep. 2017;13:105–10.
19. Lindegren ML, Krishaswami S, Fonnesbeck C, Reimschisel T, Fisher J, Jackson K, et al. Adjuvant treatment for Phenylketonuria (PKU). Rockville: Agency for Healthcare Research and Quality; 2012.
20. Matalon R, Michals-Matalon K, Bhatia G, Burlina AB, Burlina AP, Braga C, et al. Double blind placebo control trial of large neutral amino acids in treatment of PKU: effect on blood phenylalanine. J Inherit Metab Dis. 2007;30(2):153–8.
21. Butte NF, Wong WW, Treuth MS, Ellis KJ, O'Brian SE. Energy requirements during pregnancy based on total energy expenditure and energy deposition. Am J Clin Nutr. 2004;79(6):1078–87.
22. Institute of Medicine. Weight gain during pregnancy: re-examining the guidelines. 2014. Available from: http://iom.edu/Reports/2009/Weight-Gain-During-Pregnancy-Reexamining-the-Guidelines.aspx.
23. Simopoulos AP, Leaf A, Salem N Jr. Essentiality of and recommended dietary intakes for omega-6 and omega-3 fatty acids. Ann Nutr Metab. 1999;43(2):127–30.
24. Institute of Medicine (U.S.). Standing Committee on the Scientific Evaluation of Dietary Reference Intakes. Dietary reference intakes for energy, carbohydrate, fiber, fat, fatty acids, cholesterol, protein, and amino acids, vol. xxv. Washington, D.C.: National Academies Press; 2005. p. 1331.
25. Waisbren S. Maternal Phenylketonuria: Long-term outcomes in offspring and post-pregnancy maternal characteristics. JIMD Ref. 2014;21:23.
26. Feillet F, Muntau AC, Debray FG, Lotz-Havla AS, Puchwein-Schwepcke A, Fofou-Caillierez MB, et al.

Use of sapropterin dihydrochloride in maternal phenylketonuria. A European experience of eight cases. J Inherit Metab Dis. 2014;37(5):753–62.
27. Muntau AC, Adams DJ, Belanger-Quintana A, Bushueva TV, Cerone R, Chien YH, et al. International best practice for the evaluation of responsiveness to sapropterin dihydrochloride in patients with phenylketonuria. Mol Genet Metab. 2019;127(1):1–11.
28. Longo N, Dimmock D, Levy H, Viau K, Bausell H, Bilder DA, et al. Evidence- and consensus-based recommendations for the use of pegvaliase in adults with phenylketonuria. Genet Med. 2019;21(8):1851–67.
29. Boyer M, Skaar J, Sowa M, Tureson JR, Chapel-Crespo CC, Chang R. Continuation of pegvaliase treatment during pregnancy: a case report. Mol Genet Metab Rep. 2021;26:100713.
30. Rohr F, Kritzer A, Harding CO, Viau K, Levy HL. Discontinuation of Pegvaliase therapy during maternal PKU pregnancy and postnatal breastfeeding: a case report. Mol Genet Metab Rep. 2020;22:100555.
31. Van Calcar SC, Harding CO, Davidson SR, Barness LA, Wolff JA. Case reports of successful pregnancy in women with maple syrup urine disease and propionic acidemia. Am J Med Genet. 1992;44(5):641–6.
32. Grunewald S, Hinrichs F, Wendel U. Pregnancy in a woman with maple syrup urine disease. J Inherit Metab Dis. 1998;21(2):89–94.
33. Yoshida S, Tanaka T. Postpartum death with maple syrup urine disease. Int J Gynaecol Obstet. 2003;81(1):57–8.
34. Wessel AE, Mogensen KM, Rohr F, Erick M, Neilan EG, Chopra S, et al. Management of a woman with maple syrup urine disease during pregnancy, delivery, and lactation. JPEN J Parenter Enteral Nutr. 2015;39(7):875–9.
35. Tchan M, Westbrook M, Wilcox G, Cutler R, Smith N, Penman R, et al. The management of pregnancy in maple syrup urine disease: experience with two patients. JIMD Rep. 2013;10:113–7.
36. Heiber S, Zulewski H, Zaugg M, Kiss C, Baumgartner M. Successful pregnancy in a woman with maple syrup urine disease: case report. JIMD Rep. 2015;21:103–7.
37. Brown J, Tchan M, Nayyar R. Maple syrup urine disease: tailoring a plan for pregnancy. J Matern Fetal Neonatal Med. 2018;31(12):1663–6.
38. Grunert SC, Rosenbaum-Fabian S, Schumann A, Schwab KO, Mingirulli N, Spiekerkoetter U. Successful pregnancy in maple syrup urine disease: a case report and review of the literature. Nutr J. 2018;17(1):51.
39. Bulcher S. MSUD Family Support Group. Personal Communication, 2020.
40. Berens P. Overview of the postpartum period: normal physiology and routine maternal care. UpToDate Website 2019. Available from: https://www-uptodate-com.liboff.ohsu.edu/contents/overview-of-the-postpartum-period-normal-physiology-and-routine-maternal-care.
41. Langendonk JG, Roos JC, Angus L, Williams M, Karstens FP, de Klerk JB, et al. A series of pregnancies in women with inherited metabolic disease. J Inherit Metab Dis. 2012;35(3):419–24.
42. Scott Schwoerer J, van Calcar S, Rice GM, Deline J. Successful pregnancy and delivery in a woman with propionic acidemia from the Amish community. Mol Genet Metab Rep. 2016;8:4–7.
43. Mungan NO, Kor D, Buyukkurt S, Atmis A, Gulec U, Satar M. Propionic acidemia: a Turkish case report of a successful pregnancy, labor and lactation. J Pediatr Endocrinol Metab. 2016;29(7):863–6.
44. Wojtowicz A, Hill M, Strobel S, Gillett G, Kiec-Wilk B. Successful in vitro fertilization, twin pregnancy and labor in a woman with inherited propionic acidemia. Ginekol Pol. 2019;90(11):667.
45. Wasserstein MP, Gaddipati S, Snyderman SE, Eddleman K, Desnick RJ, Sansaricq C. Successful pregnancy in severe methylmalonic acidaemia. J Inherit Metab Dis. 1999;22(7):788–94.
46. Lubrano R, Bellelli E, Gentile I, Paoli S, Carducci C, Carducci C, et al. Pregnancy in a methylmalonic acidemia patient with kidney transplantation: a case report. Am J Transplant. 2013;13(7):1918–22.
47. Boneh A, Greaves RF, Garra G, Pitt JJ. Metabolic treatment of pregnancy and post delivery period in a patient with cobalamin A disease. Am J Obstet Gynecol. 2002;187(1):225–6.
48. Deodato F, Rizzo C, Boenzi S, Baiocco F, Sabetta G, Dionisi-Vici C. Successful pregnancy in a woman with mut- methylmalonic acidaemia. J Inherit Metab Dis. 2002;25(2):133–4.
49. Brunel-Guitton C, Costa T, Mitchell GA, Lambert M. Treatment of cobalamin C (cblC) deficiency during pregnancy. J Inherit Metab Dis. 2010;33(Suppl 3):S409–12.
50. Raval DB, Merideth M, Sloan JL, Braverman NE, Conway RL, Manoli I, et al. Methylmalonic acidemia (MMA) in pregnancy: a case series and literature review. J Inherit Metab Dis. 2015;38(5):839–46.
51. Grandone E, Martinelli P, Villani M, Vecchione G, Fischetti L, Leccese A, et al. Prospective evaluation of pregnancy outcome in an Italian woman with late-onset combined homocystinuria and methylmalonic aciduria. BMC Pregnancy Childbirth. 2019;19(1):318.
52. Enns GM, O'Brien WE, Kobayashi K, Shinzawa H, Pellegrino JE. Postpartum "psychosis" in mild argininosuccinate synthetase deficiency. Obstet Gynecol. 2005;105(5 Pt 2):1244–6.
53. Peterson DE. Acute postpartum mental status change and coma caused by previously undiagnosed ornithine transcarbamylase deficiency. Obstet Gynecol. 2003;102(5 Pt 2):1212–5.
54. Eather G, Coman D, Lander C, McGill J. Carbamyl phosphate synthase deficiency: diagnosed during pregnancy in a 41-year-old. J Clin Neurosci. 2006;13(6):702–6.
55. Potter MA, Zeesman S, Brennan B, Kobayashi K, Gao HZ, Tabata A, et al. Pregnancy in a healthy woman with untreated citrullinemia. Am J Med Genet A. 2004;129A(1):77–82.
56. Lamb S, Aye CY, Murphy E, Mackillop L. Multidisciplinary management of ornithine transcarbamylase (OTC) deficiency in pregnancy: essen-

tial to prevent hyperammonemic complications. BMJ Case Rep. 2013;2013
57. Arn PH, Hauser ER, Thomas GH, Herman G, Hess D, Brusilow SW. Hyperammonemia in women with a mutation at the ornithine carbamoyltransferase locus. A cause of postpartum coma. N Engl J Med. 1990;322(23):1652–5.
58. Kotani Y, Shiota M, Umemoto M, Tsuritani M, Hoshiai H. Carbamyl phosphate synthetase deficiency and postpartum hyperammonemia. Am J Obstet Gynecol. 2010;203(1):e10–1.
59. Mendez-Figueroa H, Lamance K, Sutton VR, Aagaard-Tillery K, Van den Veyver I. Management of ornithine transcarbamylase deficiency in pregnancy. Am J Perinatol. 2010;27(10):775–84.
60. Torkzaban M, Haddad A, Baxter JK, Berghella V, Gahl WA, Al-Kouatly HB. Maternal ornithine transcarbamylase deficiency, a genetic condition associated with high maternal and neonatal mortality every clinician should know: a systematic review. Am J Med Genet A. 2019;179(10):2091–100.
61. Wilnai Y, Blumenfeld YJ, Cusmano K, Hintz SR, Alcorn D, Benitz WE, et al. Prenatal treatment of ornithine transcarbamylase deficiency. Mol Genet Metab. 2018;123(3):297–300.
62. Herrera E. Metabolic adaptations in pregnancy and their implications for the availability of substrates to the fetus. Eur J Clin Nutr. 2000;54(Suppl 1): S47–51.
63. Schwoerer JA, Obernolte L, Van Calcar S, Heighway S, Bankowski H, Williams P, et al. Use of gastrostomy tube to prevent maternal PKU syndrome. JIMD Rep. 2012;6:15–20.
64. Lee PJ. Pregnancy issues in inherited metabolic disorders. J Inherit Metab Dis. 2006;29(2–3):311–6.
65. Laforet P, Acquaviva-Bourdain C, Rigal O, Brivet M, Penisson-Besnier I, Chabrol B, et al. Diagnostic assessment and long-term follow-up of 13 patients with Very Long-Chain Acyl-Coenzyme A dehydrogenase (VLCAD) deficiency. Neuromuscul Disord. 2009;19(5):324–9.
66. Murata KY, Sugie H, Nishino I, Kondo T, Ito H. A primigravida with very-long-chain acyl-CoA dehydrogenase deficiency. Muscle Nerve. 2014;49(2): 295–6.
67. Mendez-Figueroa H, Shchelochkov OA, Shaibani A, Aagaard-Tillery K, Shinawi MS. Clinical and biochemical improvement of very long-chain acyl-CoA dehydrogenase deficiency in pregnancy. J Perinatol. 2010;30(8):558–62.
68. Yamamoto H, Tachibana D, Tajima G, Shigematsu Y, Hamasaki T, Tanaka A, et al. Successful management of pregnancy with very-long-chain acyl-coenzyme A dehydrogenase deficiency. J Obstet Gynaecol Res. 2015;41(7):1126–8.
69. van Eerd DC, Brusse IA, Adriaens VF, Mankowski RT, Praet SF, Michels M, et al. Management of an LCHADD patient during pregnancy and high intensity exercise. JIMD Rep. 2017;32:95–100.
70. Vockley J. Pittsburgh Children's Hospital. Personal Communication, 2018.
71. Van Erven B, Berry GT, Cassiman D, Voss R, Wortmann SB, Rubio-Gozalbo E. Fertility in adult women with classic galactosemia and primary ovarian insufficiency. Fertil Steril. 2017;108(1):168–74.
72. Ferrecchia IA, Guenette G, Potocik EA, Weinstein DA. Pregnancy in women with glycogen storage disease Ia and Ib. J Perinat Neonatal Nurs. 2014;28(1):26–31.
73. Ramachandran R, Wedatilake Y, Coats C, Walker F, Elliott P, Lee PJ, et al. Pregnancy and its management in women with GSD type III – a single centre experience. J Inherit Metab Dis. 2012;35(2):245–51.
74. Siega-Riz AM, Evenson KR, Dole N. Pregnancy-related weight gain–a link to obesity? Nutr Rev. 2004;62(7 Pt 2):S105–11.
75. Abrams B, Carmichael S, Selvin S. Factors associated with the pattern of maternal weight gain during pregnancy. Obstet Gynecol. 1995;86(2):170–6.
76. Carmichael S, Abrams B, Selvin S. The pattern of maternal weight gain in women with good pregnancy outcomes. Am J Public Health. 1997;87(12):1984–8.
77. Acosta PB, Evaluation of nutrition status. In: Acosta PB, editor. Nutrition management of patients with inherited metabolic disorders. boston: Jones and Bartlett Publishers; c2010. p. 87.

13 Hereditary Tyrosinemia

Austin Larson

Contents

A. Larson (✉)
Clinical Genetics and Metabolism, Children's Hospital Colorado, University of Colorado Denver – Anschutz Medical Campus, Aurora, CO, USA
e-mail: Austin.Larson@childrenscolorado.org

L. E. Bernstein et al. (eds.), *Nutrition Management of Inherited Metabolic Diseases*,
https://doi.org/10.1007/978-3-030-94510-7_13

Core Messages

- Tyrosinemia type 1 causes liver failure, liver cancer, renal tubular dysfunction, and recurrent episodes of peripheral neuropathy when untreated, resulting in significantly shortened life expectancy.
- Treatment with NTBC prevents the severe manifestations of disease but results in hypertyrosinemia.
- Dietary treatment of tyrosinemia type 1 with limitation of phenylalanine and tyrosine intake is indicated to prevent severe hypertyrosinemia and the associated complications in patients treated with NTBC as well as in those with type 2.

13.1 Background

Disorders resulting from enzyme deficiencies in the tyrosine catabolism pathway have widely variable phenotypes depending on the specific location of the enzymatic block in the pathway and the resultant perturbation of biochemistry. This chapter will focus primarily on tyrosinemia type 1, including both the treated and untreated phenotypes, and will also discuss tyrosinemias type 2 and 3. Other disorders of tyrosine catabolism such as alkaptonuria and hawkinsinuria will not be addressed.

13.2 Biochemistry

Tyrosinemia type 1 is caused by a deficiency in fumarylacetoacetate hydrolase (FAH), which is the final step in the phenylalanine/tyrosine catabolic pathway (Fig. 13.1). The enzyme deficiency results in the accumulation of fumarylacetoacetate, maleylacetoacetate, succinylacetoacetate and succinylacetone. The accumulation of these molecules results in direct toxicity to cells in the liver and kidneys [1]. Additionally, succinylacetone is an inhibitor of porphobilinogen synthase, which can result in both a biochemical and clinical phenocopy of an acute porphyria neurological crisis due to accumulation of neurotoxic heme

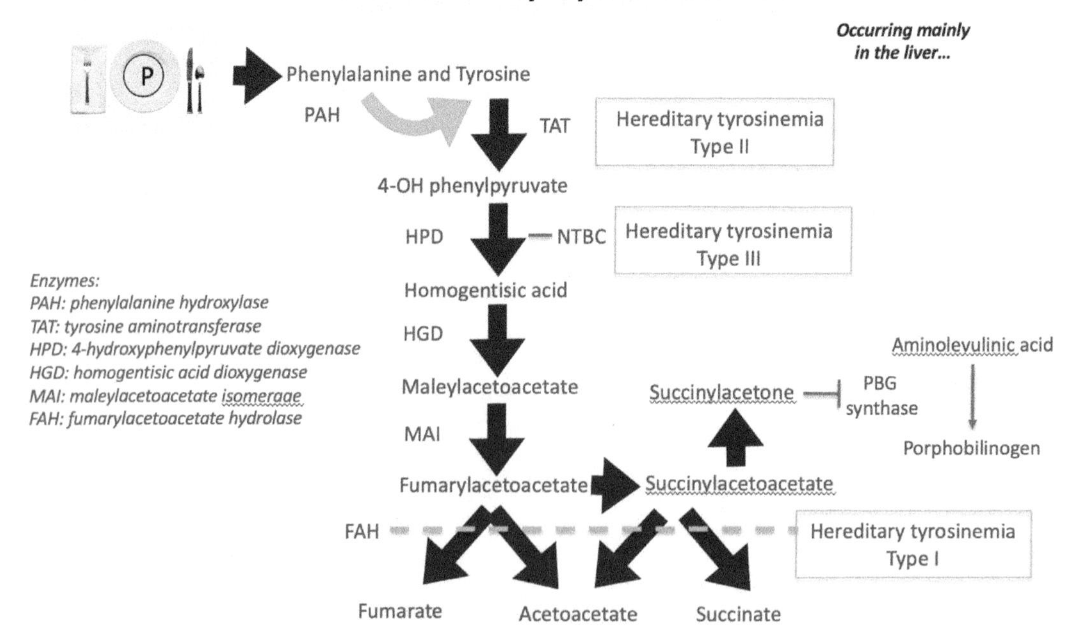

Fig. 13.1 Hereditary tyrosinemia. Enzymes: PAH phenylalanine hydroxylase, TAT tyrosine aminotransferase, HPD 4-hdroxyphenylpyruvate dioxygenase, HGD homogentisic acid dioxygenase, MAI maleylacetoacetate isomeraae, FAH fumarylacetaacetate hydrolase

precursors in some patients [2]. Despite the name, tyrosinemia type 1 does not typically result in clinically significant elevations in tyrosine because the causative enzyme block is several reactions removed from tyrosine, though there may be mildly elevated tyrosine concentrations as a secondary phenomenon.

In contrast, tyrosinemia type 2 (tyrosine aminotransferase (TAT) deficiency) and tyrosinemia type 3 (4-hydroxyphenylpyruvate dioxygenase (HPD) deficiency) do cause significant tyrosine elevations since these two reactions are more proximal in the tyrosine catabolism pathway. Unlike untreated tyrosinemia type 1, the toxic metabolite responsible for most of the manifestations of tyrosinemias type 2 and 3 is tyrosine itself.

13.3 Diagnosis

Tyrosinemia type 1 is on the Recommended Uniform Screening Panel and is now typically diagnosed via newborn screening. Succinylacetone and tyrosine are both detectable in dried blood spot samples. Succinylacetone is a much more sensitive and specific diagnostic metabolite for tyrosinemia type 1 than tyrosine and is the preferred test [3]. Until recent years, many U.S. states did not assess succinylacetone concentration as part of NBS and as a result, many patients were diagnosed only after the development of symptoms. Succinylacetone has been used as a diagnostic metabolite on NBS in Quebec for much longer than in other regions because the prevalence of tyrosinemia type 1 is much higher due to the prevalence of an *FAH* variant (c.1065 + 5 G > A) in the population [4]. Much of the initial literature highlighting the differences in natural history between presymptomatic diagnosis and treatment versus ascertainment only of symptomatic patients is derived from the experience in Quebec.

Tyrosinemias type 2 and 3 are considered secondary conditions for NBS. Tyrosine itself is the diagnostic metabolite for identification of risk for these two conditions on NBS. However, significantly elevated tyrosine may have other etiologies as well. Transient tyrosinemia is a relatively common and benign condition that has increased prevalence in premature infants and typically resolves without intervention in the first few months of life. Tyrosine may also be elevated in those with liver disease of any etiology [5]. When liver disease is the etiology of elevated tyrosine, methionine and phenylalanine are often also elevated concurrently.

All the tyrosinemias are autosomal recessive conditions and molecular genetic testing demonstrating biallelic pathogenic (or likely pathogenic) variants can confirm a suspected diagnosis based on biochemical and clinical features. Tyrosinemia type 1 is caused by biallelic variants in *FAH,* type 2 by variants in *TAT* and type 3 by variants in *HPD*.

Repeatedly elevated measurements of succinylacetone in blood should be considered a presumed diagnosis of tyrosinemia type 1 and treated accordingly even prior to confirmatory testing. Succinylacetone measurement in blood is preferred to measurement in urine due to increased sensitivity [6].

13.4 Clinical Presentation and Natural History

Most individuals with tyrosinemia type 1 who are not diagnosed and treated presymptomatically will develop liver disease in the first year of life. There may be acute liver failure requiring liver transplantation or chronic hepatopathy. The acute liver failure may be fatal if not successfully managed with liver transplantation. Hepatocellular carcinoma is common in untreated tyrosinemia type 1, with a peak incidence at age 4–5 years and is a frequent cause of death in untreated tyrosinemia type 1 [7]. Significantly elevated alpha-fetoprotein is a nonspecific biomarker of tyrosinemia-associated hepatopathy. It is important to interpret alpha-fetoprotein concentrations using expected values for age since the normal concentrations of alpha-fetoprotein change by orders of magnitude over the first months of life [8].

The patients that do not have symptoms of hepatopathy as their primary manifestation may come to clinical attention due to renal disease. These individuals likely have some residual FAH enzyme activity resulting in slower progression of disease. Renal tubular dysfunction results in acidosis and phosphate wasting. The renal tubular acidosis contributes to growth restriction. Hypophosphatemia leads to rickets, which also causes decreased linear growth. Urine studies for patients with renal manifestations of tyrosinemia type 1 include generalized aminoaciduria and impaired tubular resorption of phosphorus [9].

About 40% of individuals with tyrosinemia type 1 develop neurological crises that are often recurrent. The pathogenesis of the neurological symptoms is the same as in acute intermittent porphyria and results from the inhibition of porphobilinogen synthase by succinylacetone. The resultant lack of flux through the heme synthesis pathway results in accumulation of heme precursors that are toxic to both the central and peripheral nervous system. Patients with tyrosinemia-related neurological crises develop acute-onset neuropathy resulting in hypotonia, gastrointestinal dysmotility and weakness that may affect the diaphragm and require intubation and mechanical ventilation [10]. The neurological crises may be fatal in some patients.

Tyrosinemia type 2 is associated with keratopathy, manifesting as photophobia, lacrimation, and ulceration of the cornea. These symptoms are a direct manifestation of hypertyrosinemia and are largely reversible if tyrosine levels are decreased with treatment [11]. Hyperkeratosis and blistering of the palms and soles are also associated with hypertyrosinemia. Individuals with both types 2 and 3 tyrosinemia have increased prevalence of developmental delay and intellectual disability, which may be a direct effect of increased tyrosine in the brain interfering with neurotransmitter metabolism [12].

13.5 Pharmaceutical Treatment of Tyrosinemia Type 1

Prior to the advent of pharmaceutical therapy, physicians had determined that dietary restriction of phenylalanine and tyrosine did not sufficiently decrease the production of toxic metabolites for patients with tyrosinemia type 1 to alter the natural history of the disease. Treatment consisted of close monitoring for hepatopathy, hepatocellular carcinoma or neurological crises and then liver transplantation upon occurrence of one or more of those outcomes. Liver transplantation significantly reduces but does not eliminate the production of succinylacetone. Patients that underwent liver transplantation for tyrosinemia type 1 had 90% 5-year survival and did not have recurrence of hepatocellular carcinoma in the graft [13]. Despite liver transplantation, there may be some ongoing risk of renal disease related to ongoing low-level production of succinylacetone [14].

The discovery that 2-(2-nitro-4-trifluoromethylbenzyol)-1,3 cyclohexanedione (NTBC), also known as nitisinone, inhibits 4-hydroxyphenylpyruvate dioxygenase led to its development as a treatment for tyrosinemia type 1 and it was approved by regulatory agencies for that indication in the early 1990s [15]. By blocking flux through the tyrosine catabolism pathway at a more proximal step, NTBC treatment prevents the accumulation of fumarylacetoacetate and succinylacetone [16]. The natural history of tyrosinemia type 1 has changed dramatically due to pre-symptomatic diagnosis and treatment with NTBC. Patients that maintain therapeutic concentrations of NTBC and sufficiently block the production of succinylacetone have extremely low rates of hepatopathy, hepatocellular carcinoma, renal disease and acute neurological crises. Those few occurrences of these complications in treated patients are likely related to nonadherence to therapy.

While NTBC has proven to be a highly effective therapy, treatment does cause significant hypertyrosinemia and resultant symptoms unless dietary restriction of phenylalanine and tyrosine is implemented concurrently with initiation of NTBC. Patients treated with NTBC are at risk for keratopathy and palmoplantar hyperkeratosis if tyrosine concentrations remain significantly elevated without intervention. A slit lamp evaluation by an ophthalmologist is indicated at the onset of any ocular symptoms, particularly photophobia, pain, or excessive lacrimation. For patients on NTBC, the goal of nutrition management is to maintain a plasma tyrosine concentration between 200 and 600 μmol/L [6]. Individuals with plasma tyrosine levels below 600 μmol/L are extremely unlikely to have ocular or cutaneous symptoms related to hypertyrosinemia.

Long-term follow-up of patients treated with NTBC shows a reduction in full-scale intelligence quotient (FSIQ) for many treated patients as well as attentional or behavioral concerns [17–19]. Some patients have had a progressive decrease of FSIQ with time [20]. The pathogenesis of the cognitive and behavioral effects of NTBC treatment is not known for certain, but the probable role of hypertyrosinemia itself provides additional justification for close monitoring and attention to nutrition management even for those patients without any ocular or cutaneous symptoms. The neurocognitive phenotype of tyrosinemia type 3 provides additional evidence that hypertyrosinemia is likely the primary driver of the behavioral, developmental and intellectual symptoms seen in NTBC-treated patients.

Intellectual disability is not typically associated with tyrosinemia type 1 in the absence of treatment with NTBC but with the extremely high level of morbidity and mortality due to liver failure and cancer for those with untreated tyrosinemia type 1, the risk to benefit ratio favors the use of NTBC for most, if not all, patients.

The NTBC dose required by the patient may vary based on genotype, age, and other factors. NTBC therapy should be initiated as soon as possible after diagnosis of tyrosinemia type 1. Typical dosing is 1 mg/kg/day given in two daily doses [6]. NTBC has a relatively long half-life and once-daily dosing may be appropriate after the first year of life. The primary goal of NTBC treatment is to suppress succinylacetone production. If the succinylacetone concentration in blood is above the reference range, then a higher dose of NTBC should be considered. If succinylacetone concentration is normal then a lower dose of NTBC should be considered, especially if plasma tyrosine concentrations are above 600 μmol/L despite appropriate nutrition management. In addition to using succinylacetone and tyrosine concentrations to guide dosing, blood levels of NTBC itself can be measured in commercial laboratories and can provide valuable guidance. While NTBC levels of 30–70 μmol/L are recommended, the suppression of succinylacetone should be the primary determinant of dose changes [6].

There have been three reported pregnancies for women taking NTBC with plasma tyrosine concentrations of up to 800 μmol/L during pregnancy. The children born to these women have been reported to be healthy and to have typical development. NTBC is classified as a category C medication with regards to safety during pregnancy. Based on animal models, hypertyrosinemia induced by NTBC may have teratogenic effects and so close monitoring and strict attention to nutrition management is warranted during pregnancy. Given the potential risk of cessation of NTBC, there is not currently a consensus on whether or not it should be continued during pregnancy [6, 21].

13.6 Nutrition Management

Nutrition management of patients on NTBC treatment for tyrosinemia type 1 is implemented to maintain plasma tyrosine concentration within the goal range (200–600 μmol/L). Since most dietary phenylalanine is converted to tyrosine, restriction of both phenylalanine and tyrosine intake is required. For most patients, medical foods are needed to meet overall protein and energy requirements and still achieve sufficient restriction of phenylalanine and tyrosine. Medical foods with amino acid composition lacking in phenylalanine and tyrosine are commercially available from multiple manufacturers.

For infants diagnosed via newborn screening and started on NTBC therapy, a typical initial approach includes provision of intact protein via either breast milk or infant formula with the addition of medical foods to meet overall protein requirements. The relative quantity of intact protein versus medical food required by the patient is determined by frequent assessments of plasma amino acid concentrations, though typical ranges of intake at initiation of diet are 185–550 mg/day of phenylalanine and 95–275 mg/day of tyrosine [22]. Tyrosine concentrations above 600 μmol/L indicate the need to further restrict intact protein in the diet (or decreasing the NTBC dose if possible). Conversely, plasma concentrations of phenylalanine below the reference range may indicate a need to increase the intake of intact protein or to supplement with L-phenylalanine [6].

Unlike other conditions discussed in this textbook, the patient's tolerance for intake of tyrosine and phenylalanine is not only a function of their specific gene variants and the resultant degree of residual enzyme activity. Rather, the intolerance of dietary tyrosine and phenylalanine is iatrogenic and is directly correlated with the dose of NTBC that the patient is taking. The avoidance of severe hypertyrosinemia in patients with tyrosinemia type 1 taking NTBC requires attention to both the dose of NTBC and resultant concentrations of the drug in blood as well as the dietary intake of phenylalanine and tyrosine. The patient should be prescribed the lowest effective dose of NTBC with their nutrition management adjusted accordingly.

The nutrition management of tyrosinemia type 2 and type 3 is identical to that of individuals undergoing NTBC treatment for tyrosinemia type 1.

13.7 Monitoring

Frequent monitoring of plasma amino acids, blood succinylacetone concentration and blood NTBC concentration are needed to determine the appropriate dose of NTBC, as well as dietary tyrosine and phenylalanine tolerance for the patient. Current recommendations are to assess these labs monthly for the first year of life, every 3 months until age 5 and then every 6 months after that time. Additionally, patients should have hepatic and renal function assessed with alpha-fetoprotein, coagulation studies, transaminases, electrolytes, calcium and phosphate concentrations. Patients should have annual imaging of the liver to assess for tumors [6].

13.8 Summary

Tyrosinemia type 1 is caused by a distal enzymatic block in tyrosine catabolism. The resultant accumulation of succinylacetone and other metabolites causes liver failure, liver cancer and renal tubular dysfunction. Succinylacetone also inhibits the heme synthesis pathway and causes an accumulation of toxic heme precursors that mimic acute porphyria both clinically and biochemically. The drug NTBC is a targeted inhibitor of a more proximal enzyme in tyrosine catabolism, which prevents the accumulation of succinylacetone and the resultant clinical sequela. Given the dramatic reduction in the incidence of life-limiting complications of disease, NTBC treatment is considered standard of care for patients with tyrosinemia type 1.

Administration of NTBC results in a biochemical and clinical phenocopy of tyrosinemia type 3 with severe hypertyrosinemia in the absence of dietary therapy. Severe and sustained hypertyrosinemia causes corneal and dermatological disease and likely causes developmental delay and cognitive impairment. Whether caused by type 2 tyrosinemia, type 3 tyrosinemia or by NTBC treatment, elevated tyrosine levels can be treated with reduction of dietary tyrosine and phenylalanine intake. Patients typically use medical foods in combination with reduced intake of intact protein to lower serum tyrosine levels.

Tyrosinemia type 1 is usually diagnosed via detection of succinylacetone in dried blood spots as part of newborn screening. Optimal care includes initiation of NTBC therapy early in life with regular monitoring of succinylacetone and tyrosine levels to ensure that the patient is on the lowest dose of NTBC that effectively suppresses accumulation of succinylacetone. Maintaining the lowest effective NTBC dose, in conjunction with dietary therapy, can prevent many of the manifestations of hypertyrosinemia. While patients that maintain therapeutic levels of NTBC levels are extremely unlikely to have renal and hepatic disease, ongoing monitoring for these complications is recommended.

References

1. Endo F, Sun MS. Tyrosinaemia type I and apoptosis of hepatocytes and renal tubular cells. J Inherit Metab Dis. 2002;25(3):227–34.
2. Lindblad B, Lindstedt S, Steen G. On the enzymic defects in hereditary tyrosinemia. Proc Natl Acad Sci U S A. 1977;74(10):4641–5.

3. Grenier A, Lescault A, Laberge C, Gagne R, Mamer O. Detection of succinylacetone and the use of its measurement in mass screening for hereditary tyrosinemia. Clin Chim Acta. 1982;123(1–2):93–9.
4. Giguere Y, Berthier MT. Newborn screening for hereditary tyrosinemia type I in Quebec: update. Adv Exp Med Biol. 2017;959:139–46.
5. Morgan MY, Marshall AW, Milsom JP, Sherlock S. Plasma amino-acid patterns in liver disease. Gut. 1982;23(5):362–70.
6. Chinsky JM, Singh R, Ficicioglu C, van Karnebeek CDM, Grompe M, Mitchell G, et al. Diagnosis and treatment of tyrosinemia type I: a US and Canadian consensus group review and recommendations. Genet Med. 2017;19(12):1380.
7. van Ginkel WG, Pennings JP, van Spronsen FJ. Liver cancer in tyrosinemia type 1. Adv Exp Med Biol. 2017;959:101–9.
8. Wu JT, Book L, Sudar K. Serum alpha fetoprotein (AFP) levels in normal infants. Pediatr Res. 1981;15(1):50–2.
9. Morrow G, Tanguay RM. Biochemical and clinical aspects of hereditary tyrosinemia type 1. Adv Exp Med Biol. 2017;959:9–21.
10. Mitchell G, Larochelle J, Lambert M, Michaud J, Grenier A, Ogier H, et al. Neurologic crises in hereditary tyrosinemia. N Engl J Med. 1990;322(7):432–7.
11. Macsai MS, Schwartz TL, Hinkle D, Hummel MB, Mulhern MG, Rootman D. Tyrosinemia type II: nine cases of ocular signs and symptoms. Am J Ophthalmol. 2001;132(4):522–7.
12. Thimm E, Herebian D, Assmann B, Klee D, Mayatepek E, Spiekerkoetter U. Increase of CSF tyrosine and impaired serotonin turnover in tyrosinemia type I. Mol Genet Metab. 2011;102(2):122–5.
13. Arnon R, Annunziato R, Miloh T, Wasserstein M, Sogawa H, Wilson M, et al. Liver transplantation for hereditary tyrosinemia type I: analysis of the UNOS database. Pediatr Transplant. 2011;15(4):400–5.
14. Pierik LJ, van Spronsen FJ, Bijleveld CM, van Dael CM. Renal function in tyrosinaemia type I after liver transplantation: a long-term follow-up. J Inherit Metab Dis. 2005;28(6):871–6.
15. Lindstedt S, Holme E, Lock EA, Hjalmarson O, Strandvik B. Treatment of hereditary tyrosinaemia type I by inhibition of 4-hydroxyphenylpyruvate dioxygenase. Lancet. 1992;340(8823):813–7.
16. van Ginkel WG, Rodenburg IL, Harding CO, Hollak CEM, Heiner-Fokkema MR, van Spronsen FJ. Long-term outcomes and practical considerations in the pharmacological management of tyrosinemia type 1. Paediatr Drugs. 2019;21(6):413–26.
17. Thimm E, Richter-Werkle R, Kamp G, Molke B, Herebian D, Klee D, et al. Neurocognitive outcome in patients with hypertyrosinemia type I after long-term treatment with NTBC. J Inherit Metab Dis. 2012;35(2):263–8.
18. van Ginkel WG, Jahja R, Huijbregts SCJ, van Spronsen FJ. Neurological and neuropsychological problems in tyrosinemia type I patients. Adv Exp Med Biol. 2017;959:111–22.
19. van Ginkel WG, Jahja R, Huijbregts SC, Daly A, MacDonald A, De Laet C, et al. Neurocognitive outcome in tyrosinemia type 1 patients compared to healthy controls. Orphanet J Rare Dis. 2016;11(1):87.
20. Garcia MI, de la Parra A, Arias C, Arredondo M, Cabello JF. Long-term cognitive functioning in individuals with tyrosinemia type 1 treated with nitisinone and protein-restricted diet. Mol Genet Metab Rep. 2017;11:12–6.
21. Mitchell GA, Yang H. Remaining challenges in the treatment of tyrosinemia from the clinician's viewpoint. Adv Exp Med Biol. 2017;959:205–13.
22. Acosta PB. Nutrition management of patients with inherited metabolic disorders. Sudbury: Jones and Bartlett Publishers, LLC; 2010.

Homocystinuria and Cobalamin Disorders

14

Janet A. Thomas

Contents

J. A. Thomas (✉)
Department of Pediatrics, Section of Clinical Genetics and Metabolism, University of Colorado School of Medicine, Aurora, CO, USA
e-mail: janet.thomas@childrenscolorado.org

L. E. Bernstein et al. (eds.), *Nutrition Management of Inherited Metabolic Diseases*, https://doi.org/10.1007/978-3-030-94510-7_14

Core Messages

- Homocystinuria is caused by a deficiency in the enzyme, cystathionine-β-synthase (CBS) and results in the accumulation of homocysteine and methionine.
- Homocystinuria is a multisystem disorder with significant morbidity and mortality if untreated.
- The goal of therapy is the reduction of total homocysteine levels.
- Treatment is multifaceted with dietary restriction of methionine and supplementation with betaine, B_6, B_{12}, and folate.
- Outcome is improved with early diagnosis via newborn screening and treatment.
- Disorders of cobalamin metabolism should be considered in patients presenting with hyperhomocysteinemia.

14.1 Homocystinuria Background

Homocystinuria (OMIM# 236200) was first reported in 1962 by Carson, Neill, and colleagues [1]. Two years later, the enzymatic defect was identified [2]. Homocystinuria occurs worldwide, but with variable penetrance depending on ethnicity and methods of ascertainment. The true incidence of homocystinuria is unknown and varies from1 in 1800 (Qatar) to 1 in a million with an overall incidence estimated to be approximately 1 in 200,000 to 300,000 [3–5].

Homocystinuria is an autosomal recessive condition caused by a deficiency of the enzyme, cystathionine-β-synthase (CBS), which results in the accumulation of homocysteine and methionine and a deficiency of cystathionine and cysteine. There are other disorders to consider when an elevated homocysteine concentration is identified.

These disorders include vitamin B_{12} uptake or activation defects, which may or may not have associated elevated methylmalonic acid, severe 5,10-methylenetetrahydrofolate reductase deficiency, and 5-methyl-THF-homocysteine-methyl transferase deficiency. The latter two are typically associated with an elevated homocysteine, but low methionine concentrations, so it is relatively easy to discriminate these conditions from homocystinuria. It is also important to consider that non-genetic causes of hyperhomocysteinemia exist, such as dietary deficiencies, especially folate and vitamin B_{12} deficiency, end-stage renal disease, and administration of several drugs [3, 6]. Pyridoxine (vitamin B_6) is a cofactor for the enzyme, cystathionine-β-synthase. Hence, two forms of homocystinuria are characteristically described: one form in which individuals are responsive to treatment with vitamin B_6 (B_6 responsive homocystinuria) and another form in which individuals are not (B_6 non-responsive homocystinuria). Pyridoxine-responsive patients always have some residual enzyme activity [4].

Homocystinuria may be diagnosed via newborn screening with the detection of elevated methionine on dried blood spots. Although tandem mass spectrometry (MS/MS) is more sensitive for identifying elevated methionine concentrations than past methods, it is estimated that 20–50% of B_6 non-responsive patients may be missed by newborn screening; the majority of B_6-responsive patients are likely missed as well [4, 6, 7]. Consequently, patients diagnosed via newborn screening are seldom B_6-responsive. Specificity of screening is increased by analyzing total homocysteine as a secondary marker and calculating the methionine:total homocysteine ratio [6, 7].

14.2 Biochemistry

Homocysteine is an intermediate metabolite generated during the metabolism of methionine, an essential sulfur-containing amino acid. The biochemical pathways involved in homocystinuria perform two important processes: trans-sulfuration and remethylation (Fig. 14.1).

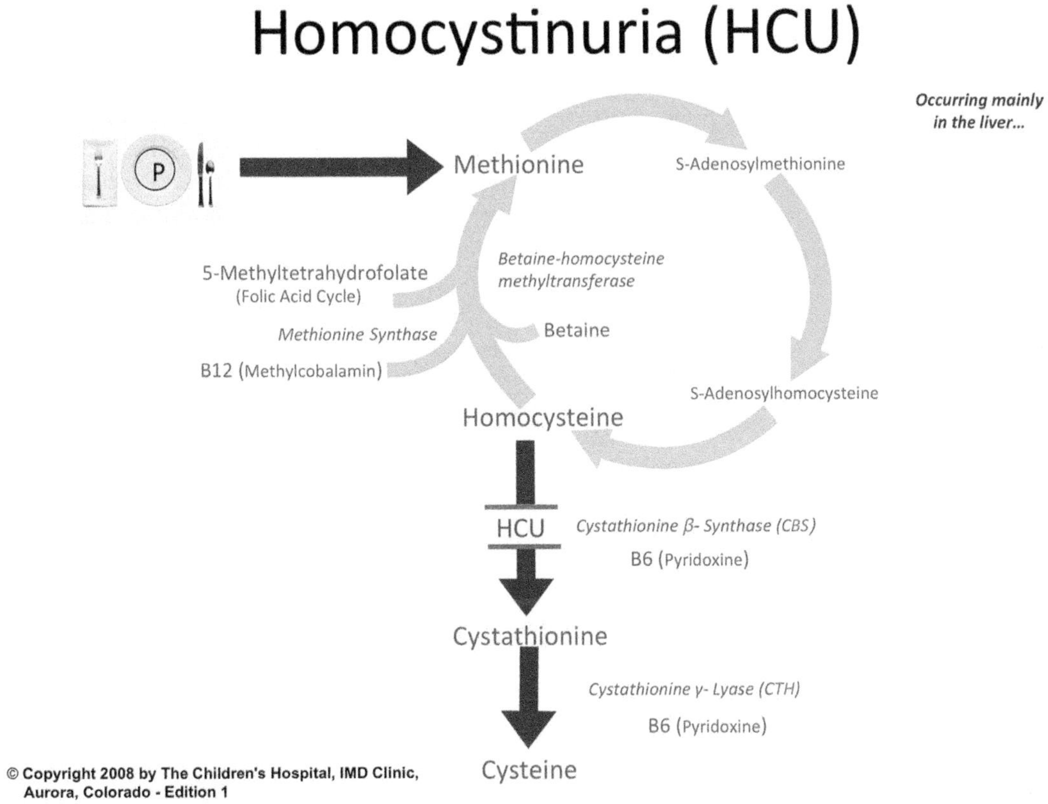

Fig. 14.1 Trans-sulfuration and remethylation in the biochemical pathway of homocystinuria

Trans-sulfuration is facilitated by the action of two vitamin B_6 dependent enzymes, cystathionine-β-synthase (CBS), the enzyme deficient in homocystinuria, and cystathionine-γ-lyase (CTH). CBS catalyzes the condensation of homocysteine and serine to cystathionine and CTH subsequently catalyzes the hydrolysis of cystathionine to cysteine and α-ketobutyrate. Cysteine is important in protein synthesis, taurine synthesis, and is a precursor to glutathione, a strong antioxidant and essential compound in detoxification of many xenobiotics [5, 8, 9].

The remethylation cycle allows the conversion of homocysteine back to methionine by two pathways. The first and major pathway is catalyzed by the enzyme, methionine synthase, and links the folate cycle with homocysteine metabolism. Methionine synthase requires the cofactor, methylcobalamin. The second pathway utilizes the enzyme, betaine-homocysteine methyltransferase [5]. This pathway remethylates homocysteine using a methyl group derived from betaine, formed via oxidation of choline, and is estimated to be responsible for up to 50% of homocysteine remethylation [8]. Both methionine and homocysteine play important roles in protein synthesis, folding, and function.

14.3 Clinical Presentation

Box 14.1: Organ Systems Involved in Homocystinuria

- **Eye**
  Ectopia lentis (lens displacement), myopia, glaucoma, retinal detachment, optic atrophy, cataracts
- **Skeleton**
  Osteoporosis, scoliosis, fractures, tall stature and long extremities, genu valgum, pes cavus, pectus, restricted joint mobility
- **CNS**
  Intellectual disability, seizures, psychiatric disease
- **Vascular**
  Thromboembolic disease, thrombophlebitis, pulmonary embolism, ischemic heart disease

Homocystinuria involves four major organ or body systems (Box 14.1).

14.3.1 Eyes

Ectopia lentis (lens displacement) is often the first sign recognized in an undiagnosed patient and is usually present between 5 and 10 years of age [3, 4]. It may present with severe or rapidly progressive myopia or iridodonesis (quivering of the iris) [6]. Classically, the lens dislocates downwards, in contrast to Marfan syndrome, a condition often considered in the differential diagnosis of homocystinuria, where the lens classically dislocates upwards. Exceptions occur. Lens dislocation may lead to retinal detachment, strabismus, and glaucoma [6]. Other eye findings may include optic atrophy, cataracts, and keratoconus [10].

14.3.2 Skeletal

The skeletal system is also characteristically involved and the features are quite prominent. Individuals with homocystinuria are frequently, but not always, of tall stature with long extremities and long appearing fingers and toes. They are frequently described as having a Marfanoid habitus and hence, homocystinuria should be considered in any individual being evaluated for tall stature and/or Marfan syndrome (NBS Chapter case). Low bone mineral density is a common finding in patients with homocystinuria [11]. Osteoporosis is almost invariably detected after childhood with a tendency to fracture and may lead to vertebral collapse. Other skeletal features include scoliosis, genu valgum (knocked-kneed), pes cavus (high instep), pectus carinatum or excavatum, and restricted joint mobility [4]. Notably, there is a significant connective tissue component in the clinical features of individuals with homocystinuria.

14.3.3 Central Nervous System

Developmental delay affects about 60% of patients to a variable degree [3]. Seizures, EEG abnormalities, and psychiatric disease are also reported. Psychiatric symptoms, such as schizophrenia, depression, and personality disorder, were observed in more than half in one series of 63 patients [12]. In a more recent study, psychological symptoms, especially anxiety and depression, were noted in 64% of the patients (16 of 25 patients) and correlated with lower IQ scores (<85) [13]. There was no correlation with age of diagnosis (NBS and < 2 years of age vs > 2 years of age) or medical complications [13]. Focal neurologic signs may be seen as a consequence of a thromboembolic event [3]. In addition, reversible cerebral white matter lesions, basal ganglia signal abnormalities, and evidence of increased intracranial pressure, as seen on magnetic resonance imaging (MRI), and associated with poor biochemical control has been reported [14, 15].

14.3.4 Vascular System

The largest cause of morbidity and mortality comes from the involvement of the vascular system, particularly from thromboembolic events which can occur in both arteries and veins –

although venous thrombosis is more common than arterial – and in all sizes of vessels [3]. Thrombophlebitis and pulmonary embolism are the most frequent vascular accidents whereas thrombosis of large and medium arteries, especially carotid and renal arteries, are frequent causes of death [4]. Cerebral venous thrombosis may be the presenting feature in both children and adults [6, 16]. Ischemic heart disease is less common. Neuroimaging may demonstrate evidence of infarction or thrombosis. Association with other genotypes linked to increased risk of vascular diseases, such as factor V Leiden and thermolabile methylenetetrahydrofolate reductase, may increase the risk of thrombosis in individuals with homocystinuria [17, 18].

14.3.5 Other

Spontaneous pneumothorax, pancreatitis, lower gastrointestinal bleed, and spontaneous perforation of the small bowel are rare findings reported in homocystinuria [19–21]. In addition, acute liver failure with neurologic involvement has also been reported [22, 23]. A subset of patients may have isolated aortic root dilation similar to that observed in Marfan syndrome [24].

14.4 Natural History

At birth, individuals with homocystinuria appear normal, typically without symptoms in the newborn period or early childhood. This feature makes homocystinuria an excellent candidate condition for newborn screening. Undiagnosed, the condition is progressive with involvement of eyes, skeleton, central nervous system, and vascular system over time. The spectrum of clinical abnormalities is broad as is the age of onset and rate of symptom progression. Treated, however, risks of the complications can be reduced significantly, likely directly related to the reduction in total homocysteine. Good compliance with therapy recommendations may prevent eye disease, osteoporosis, and thromboembolic events and can lead to normal intellectual outcomes [6]. Individuals with B_6 responsive disease generally have milder disease.

Time-to-event curves, based on detailed information on 629 patients, were calculated by Mudd et al. for the main clinical manifestations of homocystinuria [25]. The data demonstrated that the risk for a vascular event was 25% by age 16 years and 50% by age 30 years for both B_6 responsive and B_6 unresponsive forms of homocystinuria (Fig. 14.2). Of the patients in whom events occurred, 51% had peripheral vein thrombosis (with 25% having pulmonary embolism), 32% had cerebral vascular accidents, 11% had peripheral arterial occlusion, 4% had myocardial infarction, and 2% had other ischemic events [25].

The data by Mudd et al. also demonstrated that ectopia lentis occurred by age 6 years in 50% of patients with B_6 unresponsive homocystinuria and by age 10 years in B_6 responsive disease [25]. Eighty-six percent of patients with homocystinuria were ascertained on the basis of ectopia lentis. Finally, the time to event curves demonstrated a $>$ 50% occurrence of radiographic spinal osteoporosis by approximately age 16 years.

It is notable that the aforementioned natural history study that resulted in the data from which the time to event graphs were calculated was published in 1985 and advances in therapy as well as newborn screening have subsequently occurred. Hence, it is likely that the natural history of homocystinuria has changed. New reports suggest that many individuals with homocystinuria may be asymptomatic or may present only with vascular disease later in life [26–28]. Population studies using known common mutations increase the estimate of disease frequency. There are, however, fewer known patients with homocystinuria than would be suggested by known gene mutation rates [26, 27]. This suggests that many patients may be asymptomatic. This also suggests that perhaps the older data represents an ascertainment bias for the natural history of homocystinuria.

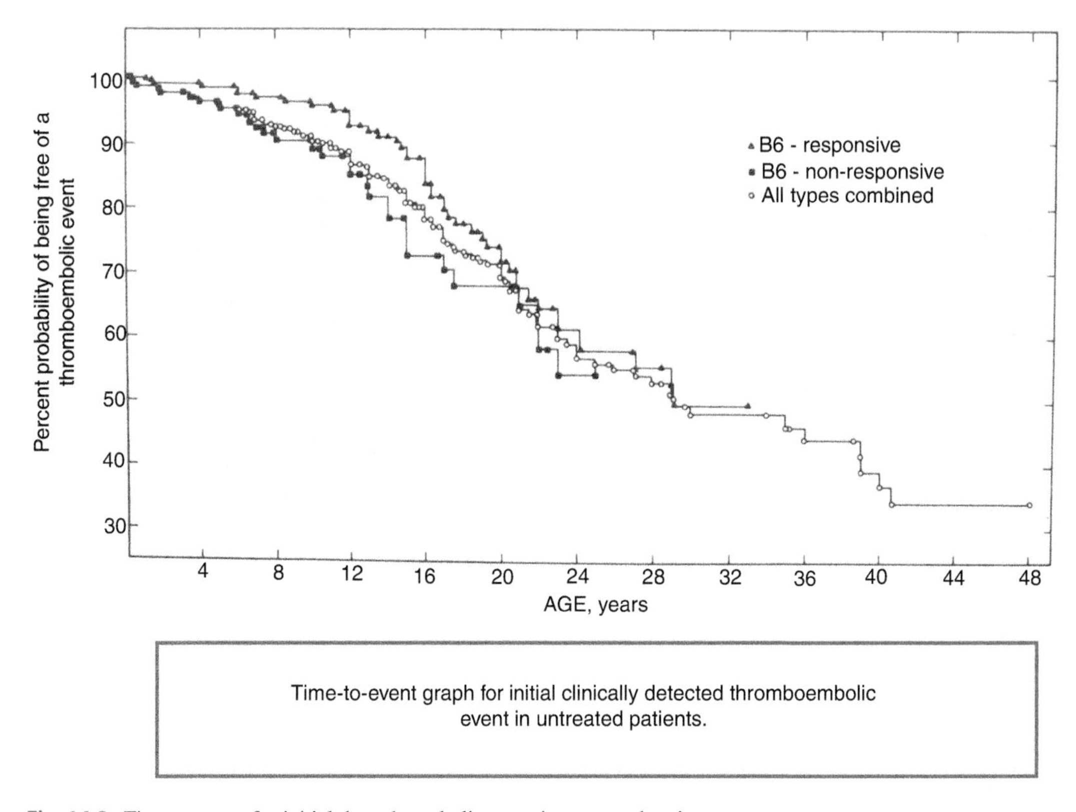

Fig. 14.2 Time-to-event for initial thromboembolic event in untreated patients

14.5 Diagnosis

In 2017, Morris et al. published guidelines for the diagnosis and management of CBS deficiency based on a systematic review of the literature and expert opinion [6]. This article warrants a review. The diagnosis of homocystinuria is based on the recognition of the clinical phenotype in conjunction with the identification of an elevated total plasma homocysteine and elevated (or high normal) plasma methionine concentrations (via quantitative plasma amino acid analysis). Low cystine and low normal to low cystathionine are also seen (Box 14.2). In addition, increased urinary excretion of homocystine as well as cysteine-homocysteine disulfide can be identified on urine amino acid analysis. Notably, the diagnosis can be masked in patients with mild disease who are taking pyridoxine or pyridoxine-fortified multivitamins and foods prior to biochemical testing [6]. Confirmation of the diagnosis can be completed via enzyme assay, typically performed on cultured skin fibroblasts, lymphocytes, or liver tissue, or via molecular studies. Each method may miss the diagnosis and hence, a combination of methods may be needed to confirm the diagnosis in some cases [6]. Molecular analysis is the preferred technique for prenatal diagnosis, although enzyme analysis can be performed on cultured amniocytes, but not in chorionic villi [6].

Box 14.2: Biochemical Features of Untreated Homocystinuria

Disorder	Methionine	L-Cystine	Total homocysteine	Cystathionine
Homocystinuria (CBS deficiency)	↑	↓	↑↑↑	↓

14.6 Pathophysiology

The pathophysiology of homocystinuria appears to be highly complex and is incompletely understood. Much of the pathophysiology is likely due to accumulating homocysteine and it is known that outcomes are improved by lowering homocysteine concentrations. It is known that homocysteine-induced abnormalities of platelets, endothelial cells, and coagulation factors contribute to the hypercoagulable state and/or altered stability of the arterial walls seen in this condition and thus, contribute to the risk for thromboembolic events [3, 29]. Homocysteine is also a known risk factor for early atherosclerosis [29, 30]. Oxidative stress has also been strongly implicated in the vascular injury and remodeling in hyperhomocysteinemia [31]. Elevated homocysteine causes endoplasmic reticulum stress with endothelial dysfunction, glutathione depletion, hydrogen peroxide production, and reactive oxygen species formation with consequent oxidative damage and decreased oxidative antioxidant defenses resulting in protein, lipid, and DNA damage [6, 31–36]. Elevated homocysteine also enhances smooth muscle proliferation and alters intracellular signaling including effects on calcium-activated potassium channel signaling [6, 31].

There is increasing evidence suggesting a role of hydrogen sulfide (H_2S) deficiency in homocystinuria and other cardiovascular diseases [6, 31]. CBS and cystathionine-γ-lyase are key enzymes producing H_2S from homocysteine and/or cysteine [31]. Homocysteine and H_2S have intertwined regulation and patients with homocystinuria demonstrate H_2S deficiency [31]. H_2S is a gasotransmitter molecule also known to regulate bone formation [37]. Experiments in mice models of homocystinuria have demonstrated that normalizing H_2S levels via supplementation can prevent bone loss and improve muscle fatigability seen in the affected mice [37, 38]. Evidence suggests that H_2S inhibits homocysteine-induced oxidative and endoplasmic reticulum stress, mediates endothelial protection, ameliorates homocysteine-induced neurovascular remodeling, and may also function as an antioxidant [31, 38].

In addition, decreased cystathionine and cysteine may also play a role in the pathophysiology of homocystinuria as they are also associated with apoptosis, oxidative stress, and alterations in structural proteins, such as fibrillin and collagen, which may contribute to the connective tissue features of the disorder [6]. A reduction in available cysteine results in weakened collagen and weak collagen likely contributes to the clinical features of lens subluxation, osteoporosis, and skeletal features such as pectus excavatum and marfanoid appearance [39]. Homocysteine is also known to disrupt collagen cross-linking [6]. In addition, disruption of disulfide bonds by the formation of homocysteine-cystine mixed disulfides in fibrillin, a protein important in the lens of the eye, may contribute to the feature of ectopic lentis [40]. Formation of mixed disulfides also contributes to reactive oxygen species formation [36]. Other elements may also play a role in the pathophysiology of homocystinuria. For example, Keating et al. demonstrated evidence of chronic inflammation suggesting that aberrant cytokine expression may be contributing to the pathogenesis of the disease [41] and there is continued controversy as to the role played by altered lipid metabolism [42].

Finally, several hypotheses have been proposed to explain the neurological manifestations seen in individuals with homocystinuria. Orendác et al. proposed a decrease in serine concentration, secondary to an increased remethylation rate, as the cause due to serine's role in the synthesis of myelin [23, 43]. Mudd et al. suggested that the altered S-adenosylmethionine to S-adenosylhomocysteine ratio inhibits transmethylation reactions, including myelin synthesis, contributing to the neurologic manifestations [23, 40].

14.7 Management

The goal of the management of homocystinuria is to reduce or normalize plasma homocysteine concentrations. Management is multifaceted and necessarily individualized and is understandable when one considers the biochemical pathway.

Following diagnosis, all patients with homocystinuria require a trial of vitamin B_6. It is estimated that ~50% of patients with homocystinuria are responsive or partially responsive to B_6 [3]. Responsiveness is chiefly determined by the individual's genotype. Doses of B_6 vary greatly, typically beginning at 10 mg/kg/d or 100 mg/d and progressively increasing to 500 mg/d pending response. Morris and colleagues recommend avoiding doses >500 mg/d [6]. Certainly, doses higher than 1000 mg/d should be avoided due to an association with sensory neuropathy [44, 45]. In responsive patients, the dose of B_6 should be kept at the lowest dose able to achieve adequate metabolic control [8] and plasma total homocysteine levels should be as close to normal as possible or < 50 μmol/L. [6] Total homocysteine concentrations and plasma methionine concentrations can be used to monitor response. Response to B_6 is also influenced by folate depletion, thus, folic acid (5–10 mg/d) or folinic acid (1–5 mg/d) should be given [3, 8]. Low doses of B_6 (50–200 mg/d) are often continued even in those patients determined not to be B_6-responsive due to its role as a cofactor for cystathionine-β-synthase [8, 46]. This latter recommendation is not supported in the recent management guidelines [6].

For individuals who are not fully responsive to B_6, a methionine-restricted diet is necessary as described in Chap. 15.

The other mainstay of therapy is the use of betaine (N,N,N-trimethylglycine) [47]. It is often used in conjunction with a methionine-restricted diet and can improve metabolic control even in individuals with optimal diet control [48, 49]. Betaine is a substrate for the enzyme, betaine-homocysteine methyltransferase, and works to remethylate homocysteine to methionine which consequently lowers homocysteine concentrations but raises methionine concentrations and increases cysteine levels. Betaine may also act as a chemical chaperone and correct partial misfolding of the protein [6]. Moderately elevated methionine concentrations do not appear to have physiological consequences; however, concentrations >1000 nmol/mL have been associated with cerebral edema [50, 51]. Hence, high concentrations of methionine >1000 nmol/mL should be avoided [6]. Betaine is given orally, typically at doses of 150–250 mg/kg/d divided two to three times daily or 6–9 gm/d for children >6 years old and adults; doses up to 20 g/d have been used [3, 8, 52]. For children, the typical starting dose is 50 mg/kg twice daily and for adults 3 gm twice daily. Dose and frequency are adjusted according to biochemical response [6]. There may be limited benefit to utilizing doses higher than 150–200 mg/kg/d [6, 52]. Betaine is well tolerated and has a manageable safety profile [52].

The decision of what modality to begin first, diet vs betaine, is often at the discretion of the treating physician. Unfortunately, achievement of normal total homocysteine concentrations, even with a combination of therapies, is very difficult in most patients. The published guidelines by Morris et al. suggest targeting total homocysteine levels to below 100 μmol/L for optimal control and outcome [6]. Prevention of long-term consequences of homocystinuria requires lifelong therapy. A new therapeutic option, utilizing PEGylated, modified cystathionine-β-synthase enzyme replacement therapy, may prove beneficial and is currently in clinical trials [53–55].

Additional management recommendations vary and remain to be proven. Considerations include a daily aspirin, other antiplatelet aggregation medications (dipyridamole), or anticoagulation therapy, all used to reduce hypercoagulability and thromboembolic risks, and vitamin C supplementation (1 g/d) to ameliorate endothelial dysfunction [3, 9]. Estrogen-containing contraceptives should be avoided due to increased risk of thrombosis [6]. Liver transplantation has been reported as treatment for homocystinuria in two individuals [22, 56]. To further reduce thromboembolic risk, it is important to ensure adequate hydration during times of illness or surgery and to avoid immobilization and long periods of sitting or inactivity. Dehydration and infection increase the risk of venous thrombosis, especially in children [6]. These considerations are most important in individuals with elevated homocysteine concentrations. Management should also include a frequent discussion of the signs and symptoms of potential complications, such as stroke, deep vein thrombosis, and pulmonary embolism, with the patient, family, or care providers.

Further, if surgery is required for an individual with homocystinuria, it is recommended that dextrose-containing intravenous fluids be started preoperatively and continue throughout the procedure to maintain circulating fluid volume and avoid hypoglycemia. Nitrous oxide should be avoided as postoperative cardiac ischemic episodes have been reported after its administration and use may increase the risk of vascular thrombosis and raise homocysteine concentrations [39, 57–59]. Regional anesthetic techniques may be contraindicated: nerve blocks may be complicated by damage to adjacent blood vessels with the potential for vascular thrombosis and spinal or epidural analgesia may lead to vascular stasis [39]. Surgical management may also include elastic stockings, pneumatic leg compression systems, and early mobilization to aid in the prevention of thromboembolism [59, 60]. Low molecular weight heparin is recommended in cases of prolonged immobilization [6].

14.8 Monitoring and Outcome

Monitoring of an individual with homocystinuria includes the responsiveness to therapeutic interventions as well as monitoring for potential complications. Bone mineral density should be monitored via DEXA scans (dual-energy X-ray absorptiometry) every 3–5 years from adolescence onwards and regular ophthalmology evaluations are recommended [6]. Routine neuroimaging or EEG surveillance is not recommended unless clinically indicated [6]. In addition, patients on a methionine-restricted diet should have consistent monitoring of laboratory values (Chap. 15).

The outcome of homocystinuria has improved with current therapeutic regimes and with early diagnosis via newborn screening [61]. The prognosis is directly associated with the occurrence of vascular ischemia since, as noted, the majority of morbidity and mortality is associated with thromboembolic events. Outcome is also determined by B_6 responsiveness with B_6 responsive patients having an improved prognosis [4, 25]. Historically, almost 25% of individuals with homocystinuria died before the age of 30 years, most commonly from thromboembolism. Thrombosis is also a major risk for pregnant women with homocystinuria, especially in the first 6 weeks postpartum [6]. Lowering homocysteine concentrations significantly reduces the risk of vascular events [48, 62]. Therapy with betaine has contributed to the ability to lower homocysteine concentrations and improve prognosis. Early diagnosis and treatment with good biochemical control can reduce the incidence of ocular complications, osteoporosis, seizures, and thromboembolic events and can lead to normal cognitive development [7, 25, 61, 62]. Family and social support is imperative for successful management and optimal outcome.

14.9 Cobalamin Disorders: Background

Cobalamin (Cbl or vitamin B_{12}) is a water-soluble, organometallic vitamin that is synthesized in lower organisms, but not by higher plants and animals. The only source of Cbl in the human diet is animal products [63, 64]. Cbl is only needed for two reactions in man, but its metabolism involves complex absorption and transport systems and multiple intracellular conversions. As methylcobalamin (MeCbl), it is the cofactor for the enzyme methionine synthase, and as adenosylcobalamin (AdoCbl), it is the cofactor for the enzyme methylmalonyl-CoA mutase [63, 64].

Disorders of Cbl metabolism are generally divided into those involved in the absorption and transport of Cbl and disorders of intracellular utilization. The latter group is further divided into disorders with combined deficiencies of both AdoCbl and MeCbl or deficiencies of each individual cofactor alone. Serum Cbl concentrations are usually low in patients with disorders of absorption and transport (transcobalamin II deficiency is the exception) and usually normal in disorders of intracellular utilization (although may be reduced in cblF) [64]. Elevated total homocysteine in blood and urine is found in patients with disorders of absorption and transport as well as in defects of intracellular metabolism affecting the synthesis of MeCbl. Elevated methylmalonic acid in blood and urine is seen in disorders affecting the synthesis of AdoCbl. Defects in the earlier, shared pathway of intracellular metabolism result in both homocystinuria/emia and methylmalonic aciduria/emia. Thus, defects in intracellular metabolism of Cbl must be considered in all patients presenting with elevated homocysteine and/or methylmalonic acid in blood and urine. The plasma methionine concentration helps differentiate between Cbl disorders and homocystinuria caused by CBS deficiency; methionine is low or normal in Cbl disorders. Diagnosis of Cbl disorders is now most often confirmed by molecular analysis.

14.10 Clinical Presentation

Disorders of Cbl absorption and transport are rare. Impaired intestinal uptake of dietary Cbl is characteristic of hereditary intrinsic factor (IF) deficiency and Imerslund-Gräsbeck syndrome, a defect in the IF-Cbl receptor [64]. Both typically present between 1 and 5 years of age with developmental delay, failure to thrive, feeding difficulties, and megaloblastic anemia [63]. Individuals with Imerslund-Gräsbeck may develop proteinuria and neurologic symptoms [64]. Transcobalamin (TC) deficiency presents within the first months of life with failure to thrive, vomiting, diarrhea, weakness, and megaloblastic anemia or pancytopenia [63, 64]. TC deficiency has been misdiagnosed as leukemia due to the presence of immature white cell precursors in an otherwise hypocellular bone marrow [63, 64]. Neurologic features may develop with delayed treatment. Individuals with transcobalamin receptor deficiency have been identified via newborn screening. The individuals had moderate elevations of serum methylmalonic acid and, in most cases, also of homocysteine, but did not have clinical symptoms of Cbl deficiency [64]. Similarly, haptocorrin deficiency is characterized by low serum Cbl concentrations without consistent clinical features [64]. Treatment of these conditions involves provision of parenteral hydroxocobalamin (OHCbl), typically with good biochemical response, with the addition of folic acid or folinic acid in TC deficiency [64].

Disorders of intracellular Cbl metabolism have been classified based on the biochemical phenotype and previously on complementation analysis, but now primarily on molecular analysis. The disorders are labeled cblA-G, cblJ, and cblX. Two disorders affecting AdoCbl alone have been classified – cblA and cblB – and present biochemically with methylmalonic aciduria/emia without homocystinuria/emia. Most patients present with a metabolic crisis in the first year of life, similar to classic methylmalonic acidemia secondary to methylmalonyl-CoA mutase deficiency, but later presentations occur. These disorders are often at least partially responsive to Cbl supplementation (cblA more so than cblB). Prognosis remains guarded with late renal and neurologic complications occurring. Two disorders affecting MeCbl alone have also been classified – cblE and cblG – and present biochemically with homocystinuria/emia and low methionine levels without methylmalonic aciduria/emia. The two disorders are indistinguishable from each other clinically and commonly present with megaloblastic anemia and neurologic and ophthalmologic symptoms [7, 65]. The age of presentation is quite variable, from infancy to adulthood, with the majority presenting before 3 years of age [7]. Treatment with OHCbl and betaine is recommended; methionine supplementation may also be needed [64].

Combined defects of both MeCbl and AdoCbl include cblC, cblD, cblF, and cblJ with cblC being the most frequent inborn error of Cbl metabolism [64, 66, 67]. Biochemically, accumulation of both methylmalonic acid and homocysteine are seen in both blood and urine. CblF and cblC typically present in the first year of life and many cblC patients are acutely ill in the first months of life [64]. Symptoms may include feeding difficulties, failure to thrive, developmental delay, and bone marrow suppression with anemia, neutropenia, and thrombocytopenia. An acutely ill infant may demonstrate progressive neurologic deterioration with abnormalities of tone, movement disorder, seizures, and coma. The clinical presentation varies considerably, and multisystem involvement occurs with liver, renal, pulmonary, and cardiac involvement [64–67]. Focal segmental glomerulorsclerosis, atypical glomerulopathy, and thrombotic microangiopathy leading to hemolytic uremic syndrome and pulmonary hypertension may also occur [7, 65–67]. In addition, patients with cblC develop a pigmentary retinopathy that is progressive over time despite appropriate therapy. CblC is one of the few disorders that can present with infantile maculopathy typically progressing to a "bull's eye" maculopathy by 6–12 months of age and leading to blindness within the first decade of life [65, 67]. Intrauterine growth retardation, mild facial dysmorphism, congenital malformations, most commonly structural congenital heart disease, and fetal cardiomyopathy may be seen suggesting in utero involvement [63, 64, 67]. Further, late-onset forms of cblC, including adult presentations, are well known [64, 66, 67].

Rare individuals with cblJ have been described with a similar infantile presentation as above or a later onset form (4 and 6 years of age) with hyperpigmentation and prematurely grey hair; macrocytic anemia was present in all cases [64]. The presentation of cblD is variable with the first patients described presenting in adolescence with behavioral difficulties, mild cognitive impairment and neurologic symptoms [68]. Rare additional patients have been described. Individuals with cblD may present with combined deficiency of MeCbl and AdoCbl or with isolated defects – homocystinuria in cblD variant 1 and methylmalonic aciduria in cblD variant 2, the variation determined by genotype [64, 65].

Most recently, cblX has been described [69]. This is the only X-linked disorder of Cbl metabolism known, the others being autosomal recessive. CblX involves pathways outside of those of central Cbl synthesis and intracellular transport. Patients present in the first months of life with a similar presentation to cblC patients, but typically develop more severe neurologic disease [64]. The majority of patients (90%) have intractable epilepsy, usually with severe developmental delay and microcephaly (50%) [70]. Cortical malformations and congenital anomalies may be present [71]. All patients described have had a moderate increase in methylmalonic acid concentrations with several patients also having elevated homocysteine [64].

14.11 Management and Outcome

Guidelines for the diagnosis and management of Cbl disorders have been published [65]. Treatment primarily involves provision of parenteral OHCbl (IV, IM, SC), betaine (250 mg/kg/d) with or without folinic acid (5–30 mg daily) and carnitine (50–100 mg/kg/d); the latter two used without clear beneficial effects [64, 65, 67]. Cyanocobalamin (CNCbl) is not as effective as OHCbl in the treatment of these disorders [64, 67]. The beginning dose of OHCbl is typically 0.3 mg/kg/d and is titrated upwards pending biochemical response. This often requires high doses up to 20 mg daily [63, 66, 67]. Patients with cblA and cblB may respond to a protein-restricted diet; however, such diets are not recommended in cblC, particularly with the use of methionine-restricted formulas [65, 67, 72]. Methionine supplementation may be required to maintain normal serum methionine concentrations [65]. Metabolite levels can be improved with treatment, but clinical improvement is variable, and mortality and morbidity remain high [63, 65, 66, 73].

Early treatment is important and appears to improve survival, corrects hematologic abnormalities, and prevents some of the long-term consequences, but has little effect on the eye disease or the neurocognitive outcome [65, 66]. Newborn screening detecting elevated C3 acylcarnitines from methylmalonic acid has increasingly led to the diagnosis of Cbl defects in the newborn period. The positive predictive value can be substantially increased by performing methylmalonic acid or total homocysteine levels as second-tier analytes [65]. Newborn screening for cblD, cblE, and cblG may be feasible by detecting low methionine and methionine to phenylalanine ratio [65].

Second-tier testing with total homocysteine differentiates patients from controls [65]. Prenatal treatment with administration of OHCbl to the mother has been described [64, 67].

References

1. Carson NA, Neill DW. Metabolic abnormalities detected in a survey of mentally backward individuals in Northern Ireland. Arch Dis Child. 1962;37:505–13.
2. Mudd SH, Finkelstein JD, Irreverre F, Laster L. Homocystinuria: an enzymatic defect. Science. 1964;143(3613):1443–5.
3. Andria G, Fowler B, Sebastio G. Disorders of sulfur amino acid metabolism. In: Saudubray JM, Walter JH, editors. Inborn metabolic diseases: diagnosis and treatment. 5th ed. Berlin: Springer-Verlag; 2012.
4. Nyhan WL, Barshop BA, Ozand PT. Homocystinuria. In: Atlas of metabolic diseases. 2nd ed. London: Hodder Arnold; 2005.
5. Blom HJ, Smulders Y. Overview of homocysteine and folate metabolism. With special references to cardiovascular disease and neural tube defects. J Inherit Metab Dis. 2011;34(1):75–81.
6. Morris AA, Kozich V, Santra S, Andria G, Ben-Omran TI, Chakrapani AB, et al. Guidelines for the diagnosis and management of cystathionine beta-synthase deficiency. J Inherit Metab Dis. 2017;40(1):49–74.
7. Huemer M, Burer C, Jesina P, Kozich V, Landolt MA, Suormala T, et al. Clinical onset and course, response to treatment and outcome in 24 patients with the cblE or cblG remethylation defect complemented by genetic and in vitro enzyme study data. J Inherit Metab Dis. 2015;38(5):957–67.
8. Schiff M, Blom HJ. Treatment of inherited homocystinurias. Neuropediatrics. 2012;43(6):295–304.
9. Pullin CH, Bonham JR, McDowell IF, Lee PJ, Powers HJ, Wilson JF, et al. Vitamin C therapy ameliorates vascular endothelial dysfunction in treated patients with homocystinuria. J Inherit Metab Dis. 2002;25(2):107–18.
10. Gus PI, Pilati NP, Schoenardie BO, Marinho DR. Classic homocystinuria and keratoconus: a case report. Arq Bras Oftalmol. 2018;81(4):336–8.
11. Weber DR, Coughlin C, Brodsky JL, Lindstrom K, Ficicioglu C, Kaplan P, et al. Low bone mineral density is a common finding in patients with homocystinuria. Mol Genet Metab. 2016;117(3):351–4.
12. Abbott MH, Folstein SE, Abbey H, Pyeritz RE. Psychiatric manifestations of homocystinuria due to cystathionine beta-synthase deficiency: prevalence, natural history, and relationship to neurologic impairment and vitamin B6-responsiveness. Am J Med Genet. 1987;26(4):959–69.
13. Almuqbil MA, Waisbren SE, Levy HL, Picker JD. Revising the psychiatric phenotype of homocystinuria. Genet Med. 2019;21(8):1827–31.
14. Sasai H, Shimozawa N, Asano T, Kawamoto N, Yamamoto T, Kimura T, et al. Successive MRI findings of reversible cerebral white matter lesions in a patient with cystathionine beta-synthase deficiency. Tohoku J Exp Med. 2015;237(4):323–7.
15. Li CQ, Barshop BA, Feigenbaum A, Khanna PC. Brain magnetic resonance imaging findings in poorly controlled homocystinuria. J Radiol Case Rep. 2018;12(1):1–8.
16. Woods E, Dawson C, Senthil L, Geberhiwot T. Cerebral venous thrombosis as the first presentation of classical homocystinuria in an adult patient. BMJ Case Rep. 2017;2017
17. Mandel H, Brenner B, Berant M, Rosenberg N, Lanir N, Jakobs C, et al. Coexistence of hereditary homocystinuria and factor V Leiden–effect on thrombosis. N Engl J Med. 1996;334(12):763–8.
18. Kluijtmans LA, Boers GH, Verbruggen B, Trijbels FJ, Novakova IR, Blom HJ. Homozygous cystathionine beta-synthase deficiency, combined with factor V Leiden or thermolabile methylenetetrahydrofolate reductase in the risk of venous thrombosis. Blood. 1998;91(6):2015–8.
19. De Franchis R, Sperandeo MP, Sebastio G, Andria G. Clinical aspects of cystathionine beta-synthase deficiency: how wide is the spectrum? The Italian Collaborative Study Group on Homocystinuria. Eur J Pediatr. 1998;157(Suppl 2):S67–70.
20. Muacevic-Katanec D, Kekez T, Fumic K, Baric I, Merkler M, Jakic-Razumovic J, et al. Spontaneous perforation of the small intestine, a novel manifestation of classical homocystinuria in an adult with new cystathionine beta-synthetase gene mutations. Coll Antropol. 2011;35(1):181–5.
21. Al Humaidan M, Al Sharkawy I, Al Sanae A, Al Refaee F. Homocystinuria with lower gastrointestinal bleeding: first case report. Med Princ Pract. 2013;22(5):500–2.
22. Snyderman SE. Liver failure and neurologic disease in a patient with homocystinuria. Mol Genet Metab. 2006;87(3):210–2.
23. Gupta P, Goyal S, Grant PE, Fawaz R, Lok J, Yager P, et al. Acute liver failure and reversible leukoencephalopathy in a pediatric patient with homocystinuria. J Pediatr Gastroenterol Nutr. 2010;51(5):668–71.
24. Lorenzini M, Guha N, Davison JE, Pitcher A, Pandya B, Kemp H, et al. Isolated aortic root dilation in homocystinuria. J Inherit Metab Dis. 2018;41(1):109–15.
25. Mudd SH, Skovby F, Levy HL, Pettigrew KD, Wilcken B, Pyeritz RE, et al. The natural history of homocystinuria due to cystathionine beta-synthase deficiency. Am J Hum Genet. 1985;37(1):1–31.
26. Janosik M, Sokolova J, Janosikova B, Krijt J, Klatovska V, Kozich V. Birth prevalence of homocystinuria in Central Europe: frequency and pathogenicity of mutation c.1105C>T (p.R369C) in the cystathionine beta-synthase gene. J Pediatr. 2009;154(3):431–7.

27. Skovby F, Gaustadnes M. A revisit to the natural history of homocystinuria due to cystathionine beta-synthase deficiency. Mol Genet Metab. 2010;99(1):1–3.
28. Magner M, Krupkova L, Honzik T, Zeman J, Hyanek J, Kozich V. Vascular presentation of cystathionine beta-synthase deficiency in adulthood. J Inherit Metab Dis. 2011;34(1):33–7.
29. Moghadasian MH, McManus BM, Frohlich JJ. Homocyst(e)ine and coronary artery disease. Clinical evidence and genetic and metabolic background. Arch Intern Med. 1997;157(20):2299–308.
30. Boushey CJ, Beresford SA, Omenn GS, Motulsky AG. A quantitative assessment of plasma homocysteine as a risk factor for vascular disease. Probable benefits of increasing folic acid intakes. JAMA. 1995;274(13):1049–57.
31. Yang Q, He GW. Imbalance of homocysteine and H2S: significance, mechanisms, and therapeutic promise in vascular injury. Oxidative Med Cell Longev. 2019;2019:7629673.
32. Tsai JC, Perrella MA, Yoshizumi M, Hsieh CM, Haber E, Schlegel R, et al. Promotion of vascular smooth muscle cell growth by homocysteine: a link to atherosclerosis. Proc Natl Acad Sci U S A. 1994;91(14):6369–73.
33. Loscalzo J. The oxidant stress of hyperhomocyst(e)inemia. J Clin Invest. 1996;98(1):5–7.
34. Vanzin CS, Biancini GB, Sitta A, Wayhs CA, Pereira IN, Rockenbach F, et al. Experimental evidence of oxidative stress in plasma of homocystinuric patients: a possible role for homocysteine. Mol Genet Metab. 2011;104(1–2):112–7.
35. Vanzin CS, Manfredini V, Marinho AE, Biancini GB, Ribas GS, Deon M, et al. Homocysteine contribution to DNA damage in cystathionine beta-synthase-deficient patients. Gene. 2014;539(2):270–4.
36. Richard E, Gallego-Villar L, Rivera-Barahona A, Oyarzabal A, Perez B, Rodriguez-Pombo P, et al. Altered redox homeostasis in branched-chain amino acid disorders, organic acidurias, and homocystinuria. Oxidative Med Cell Longev. 2018;2018:1246069.
37. Behera J, Kelly KE, Voor MJ, Metreveli N, Tyagi SC, Tyagi N. Hydrogen sulfide promotes bone homeostasis by balancing inflammatory cytokine signaling in CBS-deficient mice through an epigenetic mechanism. Sci Rep. 2018;8(1):15226.
38. Majumder A, Singh M, Behera J, Theilen NT, George AK, Tyagi N, et al. Hydrogen sulfide alleviates hyperhomocysteinemia-mediated skeletal muscle atrophy via mitigation of oxidative and endoplasmic reticulum stress injury. Am J Physiol Cell Physiol. 2018;315(5):C609–C22.
39. Bissonnette B, Luginbuehl I, Marciniak B. Homocystinuria in syndromes: rapid recognition and perioperative implications. New York: McGraw Hill Companies; 2006.
40. Mudd SH, Levy HL, Kraus JP. Disorders of transsulferation. Metabolic and molecular basis of inherited disease. New York: McGraw Hill Companies; 2001.
41. Keating AK, Freehauf C, Jiang H, Brodsky GL, Stabler SP, Allen RH, et al. Constitutive induction of pro-inflammatory and chemotactic cytokines in cystathionine beta-synthase deficient homocystinuria. Mol Genet Metab. 2011;103(4):330–7.
42. Poloni S, Schweigert Perry ID, D'Almeida V, Schwartz IV. Does phase angle correlate with hyperhomocysteinemia? A study of patients with classical homocystinuria. Clin Nutr. 2013;32(3):479–80.
43. Orendac M, Zeman J, Stabler SP, Allen RH, Kraus JP, Bodamer O, et al. Homocystinuria due to cystathionine beta-synthase deficiency: novel biochemical findings and treatment efficacy. J Inherit Metab Dis. 2003;26(8):761–73.
44. Echaniz-Laguna A, Mourot-Cottet R, Noel E, Chanson JB. Regressive pyridoxine-induced sensory neuronopathy in a patient with homocystinuria. BMJ Case Rep. 2018;2018
45. Bendich A, Cohen M. Vitamin B6 safety issues. Ann N Y Acad Sci. 1990;585:321–30.
46. Baric I, Fowler B. Sulphur amino acids. In: Blau N, et al., editors. Physician's guide to the diagnosis, treatment, and follow-up of inherited metabolic diseases. Heidelberg: Springer-Verlag; 2014. p. 43.
47. Lawson-Yuen A, Levy HL. The use of betaine in the treatment of elevated homocysteine. Mol Genet Metab. 2006;88(3):201–7.
48. Wilcken DE, Wilcken B. The natural history of vascular disease in homocystinuria and the effects of treatment. J Inherit Metab Dis. 1997;20(2):295–300.
49. Singh RH, Kruger WD, Wang L, Pasquali M, Elsas LJ 2nd. Cystathionine beta-synthase deficiency: effects of betaine supplementation after methionine restriction in B6-nonresponsive homocystinuria. Genet Med. 2004;6(2):90–5.
50. Yaghmai R, Kashani AH, Geraghty MT, Okoh J, Pomper M, Tangerman A, et al. Progressive cerebral edema associated with high methionine levels and betaine therapy in a patient with cystathionine beta-synthase (CBS) deficiency. Am J Med Genet. 2002;108(1):57–63.
51. Devlin AM, Hajipour L, Gholkar A, Fernandes H, Ramesh V, Morris AA. Cerebral edema associated with betaine treatment in classical homocystinuria. J Pediatr. 2004;144(4):545–8.
52. Valayannopoulos V, Schiff M, Guffon N, Nadjar Y, Garcia-Cazorla A, Martinez-Pardo Casanova M, et al. Betaine anhydrous in homocystinuria: results from the RoCH registry. Orphanet J Rare Dis. 2019;14(1):66.
53. Bublil EM, Majtan T, Park I, Carrillo RS, Hulkova H, Krijt J, et al. Enzyme replacement with PEGylated cystathionine beta-synthase ameliorates homocystinuria in murine model. J Clin Invest. 2016;126(6):2372–84.
54. Koeberl DD. Vision of correction for classic homocystinuria. J Clin Invest. 2016;126(6):2043–4.
55. Majtan T, Park I, Cox A, Branchford BR, di Paola J, Bublil EM, et al. Behavior, body composition, and vascular phenotype of homocystinuric mice on

methionine-restricted diet or enzyme replacement therapy. FASEB J. 2019;33(11):12477–86.
56. Lin NC, Niu DM, Loong CC, Hsia CY, Tsai HL, Yeh YC, et al. Liver transplantation for a patient with homocystinuria. Pediatr Transplant. 2012;16(7):E311–4.
57. Koblin DD. Homocystinuria and administration of nitrous oxide. J Clin Anesth. 1995;7(2):176.
58. Badner NH, Beattie WS, Freeman D, Spence JD. Nitrous oxide-induced increased homocysteine concentrations are associated with increased postoperative myocardial ischemia in patients undergoing carotid endarterectomy. Anesth Analg. 2000;91(5):1073–9.
59. Asghar A, Ali FM. Anaesthetic management of a young patient with homocystinuria. J Coll Physicians Surg Pak. 2012;22(11):720–2.
60. Lowe S, Johnson DA, Tobias JD. Anesthetic implications of the child with homocystinuria. J Clin Anesth. 1994;6(2):142–4.
61. Yap S, Naughten E. Homocystinuria due to cystathionine beta-synthase deficiency in Ireland: 25 years' experience of a newborn screened and treated population with reference to clinical outcome and biochemical control. J Inherit Metab Dis. 1998;21(7):738–47.
62. Yap S, Boers GH, Wilcken B, Wilcken DE, Brenton DP, Lee PJ, et al. Vascular outcome in patients with homocystinuria due to cystathionine beta-synthase deficiency treated chronically: a multicenter observational study. Arterioscler Thromb Vasc Biol. 2001;21(12):2080–5.
63. Watkins D, Rosenblatt DS. Inborn errors of cobalamin absorption and metabolism. Am J Med Genet C Semin Med Genet. 2011;157C(1):33–44.
64. Watkins D, Rosenblatt DS, Fowler B. Disorders of cobalamin and folate transport and metabolism. In: Saudubray JM, Baumgartner M, Walter J, editors. Inborn metabolic diseases: diagnosis and treatment. 6th ed. Berlin: Springer-Verlag; 2016. p. 385–99.
65. Huemer M, Diodato D, Schwahn B, Schiff M, Bandeira A, Benoist JF, et al. Guidelines for diagnosis and management of the cobalamin-related remethylation disorders cblC, cblD, cblE, cblF, cblG, cblJ and MTHFR deficiency. J Inherit Metab Dis. 2017;40(1):21–48.
66. Martinelli D, Deodato F, Dionisi-Vici C. Cobalamin C defect: natural history, pathophysiology, and treatment. J Inherit Metab Dis. 2011;34(1):127–35.
67. Carrillo-Carrasco N, Chandler RJ, Venditti CP. Combined methylmalonic acidemia and homocystinuria, cblC type. I. Clinical presentations, diagnosis and management. J Inherit Metab Dis. 2012;35(1):91–102.
68. Goodman SI, Moe PG, Hammond KB, Mudd SH, Uhlendorf BW. Homocystinuria with methylmalonic aciduria: two cases in a sibship. Biochem Med. 1970;4(5):500–15.
69. Yu HC, Sloan JL, Scharer G, Brebner A, Quintana AM, Achilly NP, et al. An X-linked cobalamin disorder caused by mutations in transcriptional coregulator HCFC1. Am J Hum Genet. 2013;93(3):506–14.
70. Scalais E, Osterheld E, Weitzel C, De Meirleir L, Mataigne F, Martens G, et al. X-linked cobalamin disorder (HCFC1) mimicking nonketotic hyperglycinemia with increased both cerebrospinal fluid glycine and methylmalonic acid. Pediatr Neurol. 2017;71:65–9.
71. Gerard M, Morin G, Bourillon A, Colson C, Mathieu S, Rabier D, et al. Multiple congenital anomalies in two boys with mutation in HCFC1 and cobalamin disorder. Eur J Med Genet. 2015;58(3):148–53.
72. Manoli I, Myles JG, Sloan JL, Carrillo-Carrasco N, Morava E, Strauss KA, et al. A critical reappraisal of dietary practices in methylmalonic acidemia raises concerns about the safety of medical foods. Part 2: cobalamin C deficiency. Genet Med. 2016;18(4):396–404.
73. Weisfeld-Adams JD, Bender HA, Miley-Akerstedt A, Frempong T, Schrager NL, Patel K, et al. Neurologic and neurodevelopmental phenotypes in young children with early-treated combined methylmalonic acidemia and homocystinuria, cobalamin C type. Mol Genet Metab. 2013;110(3):241–7.

15

Nutrition Management of Homocystinuria and Cobalamin Disorders

Ann-Marie Roberts

Contents

A.-M. Roberts (✉)
Medical Genetics and Metabolism Department,
Valley Children's Hospital, Madera, CA, USA
e-mail: ARoberts@VALLEYCHILDRENS.ORG

L. E. Bernstein et al. (eds.), *Nutrition Management of Inherited Metabolic Diseases*,
https://doi.org/10.1007/978-3-030-94510-7_15

Core Messages

Homocystinuria

- Cystathionine synthase deficiency is the most common inborn error of sulfur metabolism causing classical homocystinuria (HCU) and is associated with elevated plasma total homocysteine and methionine.
- HCU can be pyridoxine (vitamin B_6) responsive or pyridoxine- nonresponsive.
- In pyridoxine-nonresponsive HCU, management includes dietary restriction of methionine, medical food free of methionine, and supplementation with betaine, Vitamin B_{12} and folate.
- The goal therapy is to maintain total homocysteine less than 50 μmol/L in responsive patients and less than 100 μmol/L in nonresponsive patients.

Cobalamin Disorders

- Cobalamin disorders are associated with elevated total homocysteine low or normal methionine.
- Combined cobalamin disorders are also associated with elevated methylmalonic acid.
- Cobalamin C is the most common inborn error of cobalamin metabolism.
- The goal therapy is to lower total homocysteine and methylmalonic acid concentrations and maintain normal plasma methionine and cysteine concentrations.

15.1 Background

Homocystinuria (homocystinemia) can result from nutritional deficiencies or an inherited metabolic disorder. Classical homocystinuria (HCU) due to cystathionine beta-synthase deficiency and cobalamin C disorder are two of the most common genetic causes of homocystinuria [1]. While both of these disorders present with elevated total homocysteine (tHCY) concentrations, HCU presents with elevated methionine concentrations and disorders of cobalamin metabolism present with decreased or normal methionine. Elevated methylmalonic acid can also be detected in some combined cobalamin disorders but not in HCU. Cobalamin disorders will be reviewed at the end of this chapter.

Classical HCU is a rare genetic disorder of methionine metabolism caused by the deficiency in the enzyme cystathionine beta-synthase (CBS) [2]. Homocysteine is a sulfur amino acid synthesized from the degradation of the essential amino acid methionine. Homocysteine is irreversibly metabolized to cystathionine by CBS. Cystathionine is further metabolized to the nonessential amino acid cysteine. Homocysteine can also be remethylated back to methionine by two remethylation pathways via methionine synthase or betaine-homocysteine methyltransferase [3, 4] (Fig. 15.1). When there is a deficiency of CBS, the concentrations of both homocysteine and methionine increase and the blocked pathway of homocysteine to cystathionine results in a deficiency of cysteine. Thus in HCU, cysteine is a conditionally essential amino acid [5]. CBS is dependent upon the cofactor pyridoxal phosphate, the active form of vitamin B_6. HCU has two phenotypes: vitamin B_6 responsive and vitamin B_6 nonresponsive. Those who are vitamin B_6 responsive tend to have a milder phenotype as compared to those with the vitamin B_6 nonresponsive phenotype [2, 3, 6–8].

HCU can have variable expressions affecting the vascular system, central nervous system, skeleton and eyes [5, 7]. Common characteristics include intellectual disabilities, dislocated lenses, marfanoid habitus and cardiovascular complications [1–3]. Thromboembolic complications are common amongst those with poorly controlled HCU. Decreasing tHCY is the single most important factor in reducing risks of thromboembolic disease [2, 3].

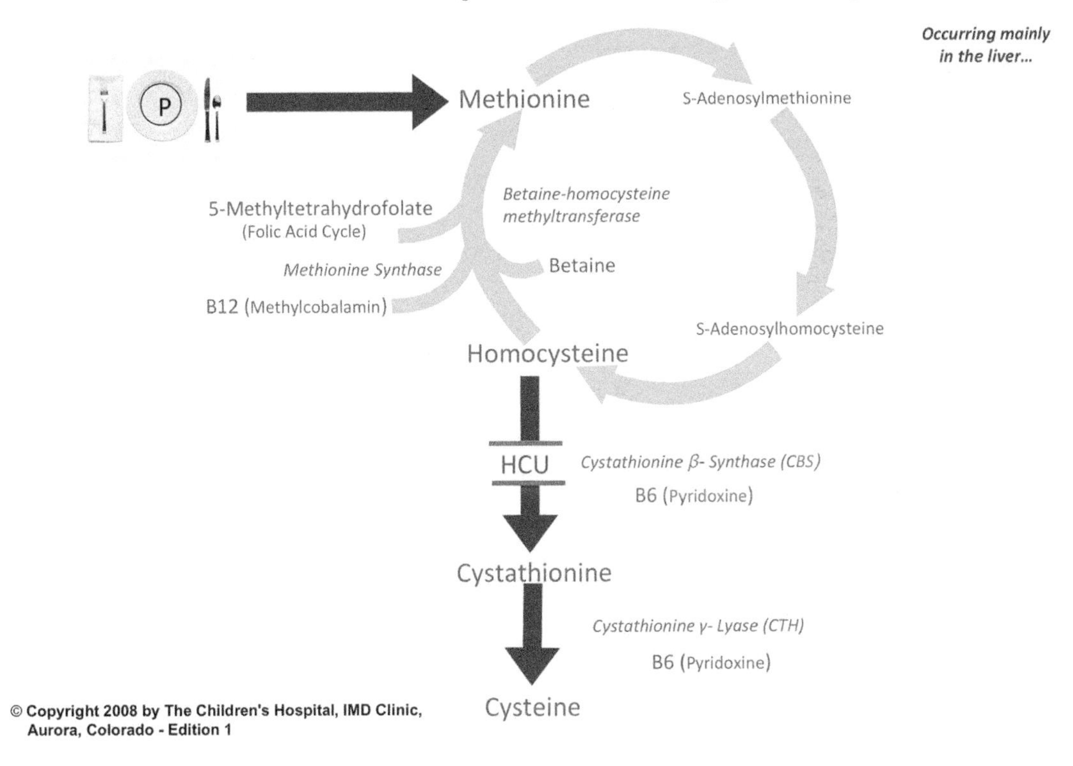

Fig. 15.1 Metabolic pathway of HCU

> **Box 15.1: Principles of Nutrition Management of Classical Homocystinuria**
> *Restrict*: Methionine
> *Supplement*: Vitamin B_6 (Vitamin responsive)
> - [a]Folic acid and vitamin B_{12} as needed to correct deficiency
> - Cystine supplementation as needed
> - [a]Vitamin C
> - Betaine
>
> [a] Clinical practice may vary on administration and dosing

Newborn screening is successful at identifying hypermethioninemia but does not capture all cases of HCU. Unlike many inborn errors of metabolism, HCU does not present with symptoms during the newborn period [4]. Diagnosis can be confirmed with biochemical testing, enzyme assay and gene sequencing [1–3, 5, 7]. HCU) is characterized biochemically with an accumulation of tHCY, decreased synthesis of cystathionine and cysteine and, often, an increase of methionine [2, 3]. A more detailed description of clinical findings and medical management can be found in Chap. 14 (Box 15.1).

15.2 Nutrition Management

15.2.1 Chronic Management of HCU

During diagnosis, supplementation with multivitamins containing vitamin B_6 should be avoided since vitamin B_6 intake may mask the diagnosis of HCU by reducing the tHCY concentration in those who are vitamin B_6 responsive [3]. HCU is treated with diet modification, medication and vitamin supplementation. The goal of management is to reduce or normalize tHCY and methionine concentrations, promote normal growth and development in children, meet macro- and micronutrient needs and prevent disease-causing sequelae. Management depends largely on whether the affected individual is vitamin B_6 responsive or nonresponsive.

All patients diagnosed with HCU should complete a vitamin B_6 trial to determine if they are responsive prior to initiating dietary restrictions [2, 5, 7]. Response to vitamin B_6 is influenced by folate and vitamin B_{12} deficiency, thus folic acid or folinic acid should be provided during the trial [1–3, 5, 8]. Vitamin B_{12} concentrations need to be evaluated and any deficiency treated [9]. Conducting the trial during a catabolic state is not recommended [3].

Consensus guidelines for HCU suggest that dosing for a vitamin B_6 trial varies from 10 mg/kg to a maximum dose of 500 mg/d for 6 weeks [3, 9]. Newborns testing positive for HCU on newborn screening are often started on a vitamin B_6 dose of 100 mg/day for 2 weeks [2, 3, 5, 9]. Monitoring of plasma tHCY concentrations during the trial is necessary as the dose is gradually increased until a maximum dose of 500 mg/d is achieved or response is seen [3]. A decrease in tHCY concentration to <50 μmol/L or a 30% reduction suggests vitamin B_6 responsiveness [3, 5, 7]. Once a response is determined, the lowest possible dose of vitamin B_6 should be used to maintain and achieve metabolic control [2–5, 8, 9].

Management with dietary restriction of methionine is necessary for all patients who do not achieve a tHCY concentration of <50 μmol/L with vitamin B_6 therapy [9]. Vitamin B6 responsive patients who maintain a tHCY concentration < 50 μmol/L may not need dietary intervention [1]. Those who do not respond to vitamin B_6 are often maintained on a low dose of vitamin B_6 (50–200 mg/d) given its role as a cofactor for CBS [2, 5], although this practice has been questioned [3].

As an essential amino acid, methionine cannot be completely eliminated from the diet. Methionine tolerance is largely dependent upon the patient's phenotype. For infants, dietary restriction of methionine can be achieved by utilizing a methionine-free, cysteine supplemented medical food with a limited volume of a standard infant formula or breast milk to meet methionine needs and maintain normal plasma concentrations. Insufficient energy and/or total protein intake can result in catabolism which can increase methionine concentrations. Methionine over-restriction is associated with poor growth [3]. Methionine and cysteine requirements are provided in Table 15.1.

Table 15.1 Estimated energy and protein recommendations

Age	Energy DRI/EER	Intact protein	Total protein
All	80–120% based on growth trend	60–100% based on plasma tHCY and methionine	100–140% DRI 120–140% DRI for those on medical food
Fluid requirements: 100–150% of maintenance			

When determining a medical food prescription for an infant with HCU, the patient's appetite, tHCY and methionine concentrations need to be considered. Intact protein requirements can be as low as 60% of total protein needs or may provide 100% of the DRI depending on the patient's methionine concentration. Total protein requirements may be as high as 120–140% of DRI to optimize nitrogen retention with the use of L-amino acid containing medical foods [10] (Table 15.2) [2, 5].

When calculating a diet prescription, methionine requirements are filled first with an intact protein source and a methionine-free medical food provides the remaining energy, protein and essential nutrients (Box 15.2). Breast milk is a good feeding option as it is naturally lower in protein, and therefore lower in methionine compared to standard infant formula. Despite its low-protein content, breast milk may contain too much methionine to be used as a sole source of nutrition for some infants. In these cases, breastfeeding may be continued by providing a prescribed volume of medical food over 24 hours; this effectively decreases the number of breastfeedings an infant consumes, thus reducing methionine intake [3]. If the mother chooses not to breastfeed, infant formula is an appropriate substitution. Diet prescriptions may need to be

Table 15.2 Estimated methionine and cystine requirements [2, 5]

Age	Methionine mg/kg/day	Cystine mg/kg/day
0–6 months	15–60	85–150
6 months – 1 year	12–43	85–150
1–4 years	9–28	60–100
4–7 years	7–22	50–80
7–11 years	7–22	30–50
Women		
11–15 years	7–21	30–50
15–19 years	6–19	25–40
>19 years	5–19	20–30
Men		
11–15 years	7–22	30–50
15–19 years	7–21	25–40
>19 years	5–19	20–30

adjusted frequently based on laboratory test results and growth trends.

For the first 4–6 months, breast milk or standard infant formula with a HCU medical food is adequate to meet the infant's nutritional needs. Low-protein solid foods are typically introduced between 4 and 6 months of age when the patient is developmentally ready. First foods may include low-protein infant cereal, fruits and lower protein vegetables. High-protein foods such as meat, eggs, nuts, beans and dairy are avoided. Clinics may approach initiation and advancement of diet in many different ways. Counting milligrams of methionine is the most accurate method of tracking methionine intake; however, the methionine content of foods is not widely available. Others may track grams of protein to monitor methionine intake [3, 5]. When using this method there is an estimated 20 mg of methionine per gram of protein. Utilizing the "simplified diet" concept (Appendix G) is another possible approach. As oral intake of foods increase, breastmilk or standard infant formula will need to be adjusted to allow for dietary advancement of solid foods [3]. Soft table foods are typically introduced around 6–9 months of age. This is a good age to introduce modified low-protein foods, such as low-protein pasta and bread (Box 15.2).

Box 15.2: Initiating Nutrition Management of an Infant with Vitamin Nonresponsive Homocystinuria

Goals:

- Reduce or normalize total homocysteine
- Normalize plasma concentrations of methionine and cysteine
- Provide sufficient energy to prevent catabolism and promote normal growth
- Meet macro and micronutrient needs

Step by Step:

1. Establish nutrient goals based on age, phenotype and laboratory values
2. Determine the amount of breastmilk or standard infant formula required to meet methionine needs.
3. Determine the amount of intact protein and energy that will be provided by the breastmilk or formula.
4. Calculate the methionine and cystine provided by the intact formula
5. Determine the amount of methionine-free medical formula required to provide the remainder of the patient's protein needs
6. Calculate the calories provided by the breastmilk or infant formula plus the methionine-free medical formula. Provide the remaining calories as a protein free medical carbohydrate, fat and micronutrients.
7. Calculate the amount of cystine provided by the breastmilk or formula plus the methionine-free medical formula. Determine if additional cystine is required to meet cystine goals.
8. Determine the amount of fluid required to make a formula that provides 20–25 kcal/oz. (depending on the energy needs and volume tolerated).

Table 15.3 Medical foods

	Abbott	Cambrooke	Mead Johnson	Nutricia	Vitaflo
Infant 0–1 year	Hominex-1		HCY-1	HCU Anamix early years	
Toddler & young children	Hominex-2	Homactin AA plus	HCY-1 HCY-2	HCU Anamix next	HCU gel HCU express 15 HCU cooler 15
Older children & adults		Homactin AA plus	HCY-2	HCU Anamix next XMET Maxamum HCU LQ	HCU express 15,20 HCU cooler 15

Methionine-free medical foods are available for infants, young children and adults, and their nutrient profiles differ based on the age group they are designed for. Choosing the appropriate medical food and monitoring its nutrient composition is an important component of meeting the patient's nutrient needs. Medical foods designed for adults tend to be fat-free, low-volume products which are not appropriate for infants and young children. Regardless of age, protein utilization is optimized when medical foods are consumed 3–4 times daily (Table 15.3) [3].

Medical foods are supplemented with the conditional essential amino acid cysteine. Additional supplementation may be needed if plasma cysteine concentrations are low. Cysteine deficiency is more likely in those with poorly controlled tHCY concentrations. As tHCY concentrations decrease, cysteine concentrations will increase [3]. Additional supplementation of L-cysteine can be difficult to consume due to poor solubility and unpleasant taste. Dietary adherence of adolescents and late-diagnosed individuals is challenging. Treatment of HCU must be continued throughout life, as poor metabolic control can be associated with thromboembolism and other serious complications [3, 4, 9].

15.3 Adjunct Treatments for Homocystinuria

Adjunct therapies are often included in a patient's treatment plan to maximize its effectiveness. When diet restriction and vitamin B_6 therapy fail to achieve optimal tHCY concentrations, betaine therapy can be added. Betaine is an oral medication that increases remethylation of homocysteine to methionine via the betaine-homocysteine methyltransferase pathway. By converting homocysteine to methionine, plasma methionine concentrations will increase [6, 9]. Cerebral edema has been reported in individuals on betaine therapy with methionine concentrations >1000 μmol/L and maintaining plasma methionine below this level is recommended [2, 6, 7, 9]. Adherence to betaine therapy can be poor due to its unpleasant taste and large doses required [6, 9]. Betaine can be mixed in medical food, water, juice, milk substitutes or semi-solid foods such as applesauce. In children less than 3 years of age, betaine is prescribed at 100–250 mg/kg divided into two doses. Older children and adults are typically prescribed 6–9 g divided into two doses [1–3, 6–8], but doses of betaine up to 20 g daily have been required for some [2, 6, 8].

Supplementation of various B vitamins is often used in the management of HCU [1, 5]. Folate and vitamin B_{12} optimize the remethylation of homocysteine to methionine by the enzyme methionine synthase, thus helping to reduce the tHCY concentration. Deficiencies of these vitamins may exacerbate elevated tHCY concentrations. Folic acid (5–10 mg/day) or folinic acid (1–5 mg/day) is prescribed to prevent folate depletion [1, 2, 4, 8]. Hydroxocobalamin is the preferred form of vitamin B_{12}; oral doses vary from 1 mg/day to 1 mg/month to achieve normal serum Vitamin B_{12} concentrations [7, 8]. Some clinics prescribe 1 g of vitamin C daily to reduce endothelial damage which may reduce the long term risk of atherothrombotic complications [2, 9] (Box 15.3).

Box 15.3: Management of Patients with Homocystinuria

Vitamin B_6 responsive	Vitamin B_6 nonresponsive
Vitamin B_6 supplementation 200–250 mg/day newborns 400–500 mg/day children < 900 mg/day adults	*Vitamin B_6 supplementation 50–200 mg/day
Folic acid supplementation 5–10 mg/day or folinic acid 1–5 mg/day	Folic acid supplementation 5–10 mg/day or folinic acid 1–5 mg/day
Methionine-restricted diet May not be required based on tHCY concentrations	Methionine-restricted diet With a methionine-free medical food
Betaine therapy May be required if unable to achieve desirable tHCY concentrations	*L-Cystine supplementation *Vitamin B_{12} supplementation *Vitamin C 1 g/day Betaine therapy 100–250 mg/kg/day divided into 2–3 doses for children and 6–20 g/day for adults
Target tHCY concentrations < 50 μmol/L [3] Target methionine concentrations < 1000 μmol/L	Target tHCY concentrations < 100 μmol/L [3] Target methionine concentrations < 1000 μmol/L

* Varies depending on individual clinic practice

15.4 Monitoring

15.4.1 Growth

Routine monitoring of growth parameters is necessary for patients with HCU [9]. Weight, height, head circumference, weight for height and z-score values should be evaluated monthly for infants. Toddlers and young children may need anthropometrics evaluated every 3 months and for older children and adolescents, every 6 months [5]. Body mass index can be evaluated for all patients 2 years and older. Assessing a 3-day diet history prior to lab draws is useful to evaluate adequacy of diet and growth trends. Poor growth can be related to inadequate medical food consumption, over restriction of protein, inadequate energy intake or nutrient deficiencies.

15.4.2 Laboratory Monitoring

Appropriate management of HCU includes assessment of various routine and metabolic labs. Plasma amino acid profiles, including methionine, cysteine and essential amino acid concentrations are important to evaluate the adequacy of the diet and medical formula [5]. Total homocysteine concentrations are a critical indicator of metabolic control and effectiveness of betaine therapy. The frequency of obtaining these labs depends on the severity of HCU, age of the patient and need for dietary restriction. Some suggest weekly monitoring during the newborn period and every 3–6 months after stabilization [4]. Target tHCY concentrations for vitamin B_6 responsive patients are <50 μmol/L and < 100 μmol/L in vitamin B_6 nonresponsive patients [3, 5, 11]. Nutrition labs, including total 25-hydroxyvitamin D, albumin or prealbumin, zinc, CBC and ferritin are recommended at least annually [3] (Box 15.4). Due to the increased risk of osteoporosis, DEXA scans are recommended every 3–5 years starting in adolescence. Selenium and essential fatty acids concentrations can be obtained if there is a concern or a clinical indication [3, 7].

15.5 Acute Nutrition Management

Unlike other inborn errors of metabolism, HCU does not require additional diet modifications during illness. Patients with HCU are encouraged to continue their usual diet, medications and medical food during illness. Hydration is extremely important as dehydration increases the risk of throm-

Box 15.4: Nutrition Monitoring of a Patient with Homocystinuria

- Routine assessments including anthropometrics, dietary intake, physical findings
- Laboratory monitoring
  - Diagnosis-specific
    Plasma amino acids
    Methionine
    Cystine
    Total Homocysteine
  - Nutrition-related laboratory monitoring
    Protein sufficiency (plasma amino acids, prealbumin)
    Nutrition anemia (hemoglobin, hematocrit, MCV, serum vitamin and/or methylmalonic acid, total homocysteine, ferritin, iron, folate, total iron binding capacity)
    Vitamin and mineral (25-hydroxy vitamin D, zinc, trace minerals)
    Others as clinically indicated

botic events [2, 3]. If a patient is unable to tolerate fluids by mouth, IV fluids with 5% dextrose at 1.5 times maintenance may be needed to maintain hydration and prevent catabolism [7]. Elevated tHCY concentrations are expected during illness due to catabolism. Surgery and anesthesia pose an additional risk for thromboembolic events in patients with HCU. Optimization of nutritional status, good metabolic control and adequate hydration are priorities prior to surgery [9] and initiating dextrose-containing IV fluids preoperatively and throughout the surgical procedure is recommended [2, 3, 5].

15.6 Pregnancy

Pregnancy, delivery and the postpartum period pose additional risks of thrombosis for women with HCU [5]. Nausea and vomiting may inhibit consumption of medical food and medication. Methionine requirements increase during pregnancy due to fetal growth, especially in the second and third trimesters. Increased monitoring of plasma amino acids will help identify methionine deficiency, which could result in fetal growth failure. Additional intact protein and medical food may be required to meet increased protein demands of pregnancy. Frequent biochemical monitoring is needed to make appropriate dietary adjustments [7, 9]. Folate supplementation is recommended, with a minimum dose of 400 mcg/day. Dietary adjustment, including use of medical foods and addition of betaine, may be necessary additions for those with vitamin B_6 responsive HCU. Women with vitamin B_6nonresponsive HCU who are routinely prescribed betaine may continue this medication during pregnancy as betaine does not appear to have teratogenic effects on the fetus [4]. Elevated tHCY concentrations during pregnancy do not appear to have major teratogenic effects but dietary adherence is strongly recommended due to risk of thrombotic events for the mother [7, 9]. Zinc and selenium deficiencies have been documented in pregnant women with HCU. Participation in regular physical activity, maintaining a healthy weight in addition to dietary and medication adherence may help reduce risks of blood clots during pregnancy. During the postpartum period, methionine requirements will decrease back to prepregnancy needs [3].

15.7 Homocystinuria Summary

Early identification and treatment with dietary management, adjunct therapies and biochemical monitoring have improved the long-term outcome of patients with HCU. Current management is dependent on whether the patient is vitamin B_6 responsive or vitamin B_6 nonresponsive. Vitamin B_6 responsive patients may not require dietary restriction if they are able to maintain a tHCY of <50 μmol/L. Dietary restriction of methionine is recommended for all patients who are unable to maintain a tHCY <50 μmol/L. Medical food and modified low-protein foods are utilized to meet the nutrient needs of the patient following a low-protein

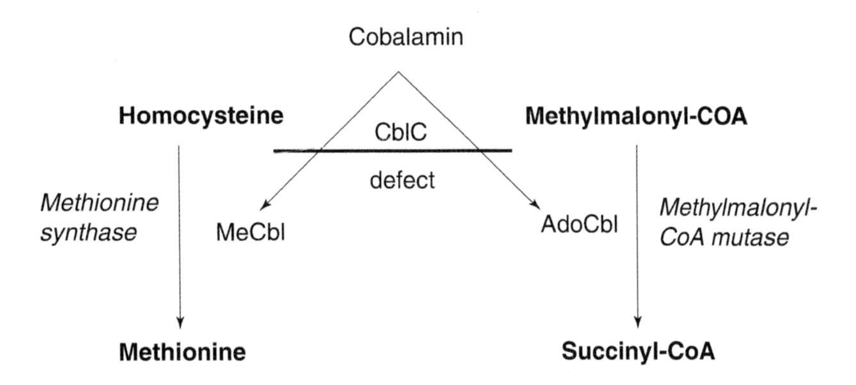

Fig. 15.2 Metabolic pathway of cobalamin

diet. Current treatment presents challenges due to lifelong dietary restriction of methionine, unpalatable adjunct therapies and innate risk factors for thrombotic events. As with all rare diseases, more research is needed to develop better therapies and treatment options for the patients.

15.8 Background Cobalamin Disorders

Cobalamin is an essential cofactor in many metabolic pathways. Cobalamin disorders are caused by an impaired conversion of dietary vitamin B_{12} into its more metabolically active forms methylcobalamin and adenosylcobalamin [1, 12]. Methylcobalamin is the cofactor for the enzyme methionine synthase which is responsible for the remethylation of homocysteine to methionine. Adenosylcobalamin is a cofactor for the mitochondrial enzyme methylmalonyl Co-A mutase which metabolizes methylmalonyl CoA to succinyl CoA [1, 13]. The intracellular conversion of cobalamin to the coenzymes adenosylcobalamin and methylcobalamin are essential for the homeostasis of methylmalonic acid and homocysteine. There are nine described defects of intracellular cobalamin metabolism. Cobalamin C (cblC) is the most common cobalamin disorder and will be the focus of this section [1, 13]. CblC is a combined cobalamin disorder meaning that the enzymatic defect affects the pathway producing adenosylcobalamin and the pathway producing methylcobalamin. This results in the elevation of homocysteine and methylmalonic acid with a decrease in endogenous methionine synthesis [14] (Fig. 15.2).

Common characteristics of cobalamin disorders include intellectual disabilities, feeding difficulties, failure to thrive, hypotonia, nystagmus and seizures [1, 12]. Newborn screening can detect some combined cobalamin disorders with abnormal propionylcarnitine (C3) concentrations on the acylcarnitine profile [1, 14]. Methionine concentrations may be normal or low on the newborn screen; thus, methionine is not a good diagnostic indicator for these disorders. Diagnosis can be confirmed with biochemical testing and gene sequencing. CblC is characterized biochemically with an elevated tHCY, decreased or low normal methionine and elevated methylmalonic acid [13]. A more detailed description of clinical findings and medical management can be found in Chap. 14.

15.9 Nutrition Management

15.9.1 Chronic Management Cobalamin Disorders

Box 15.5: Principles of Nutrition Management of Cobalamin C Disorder

Restrict: No dietary restriction indicated

Supplement:

- Hydroxocobalamin injection
- Folic acid
- Carnitine
- Betaine
- Methionine to correct deficiency

Management goals for cblC includes reducing tHCY and methylmalonic acid concentrations, maintaining or achieving normal plasma methionine [1], meeting macro- and micronutrient needs, preventing catabolism and promoting normal growth and development [13]. Protein-restricted diets were recommended in the past but are no longer indicated for patients with cblC [13–15]. In this disorder, there is an inability to produce adequate methylcobalamin resulting in endogenous methionine deficiency with low or low normal methionine concentrations. Methionine deficiency is associated with poor growth and may contribute to poor neurological and ophthalmological outcomes. Dietary restriction of protein reduces methionine intake, thus increasing the potential for methionine deficiency. A protein-restricted diet is not required to improve methylmalonic acid concentrations in this disorder. Methylmalonic acid will decline if adequate hydroxocobalamin is provided. The goals for energy and protein needs are based on the DRI for age and can be adjusted based on growth trends.

Management of cblC is dependent upon a combined approach of medication and vitamin supplementation. Cyanocobalamin is not an effective form of vitamin B_{12} for these patients. Oral administration of hydroxocobalamin is also not effective. The only form of cobalamin proven to be effective in managing cblC is intramuscular or subcutaneous hydroxocobalamin injections. Dosing of hydroxocobalamin is typically started at 1 mg daily or 0.33 mg/kg/day [1, 13–15]. Utilizing a concentrated dose of hydroxocobalamin of 20–30 mg/mL may promote optimal metabolic control and improve compliance to daily injections. Plasma vitamin B_{12} concentrations >1,000,000 pg/mL are suggested for optimal metabolic response. Potential side effects include injection site reactions and red discoloration of the urine and skin [13, 14].

15.10 Adjunct Therapy for Cobalamin

As with HCU, betaine is also prescribed for cobalamin disorders. Betaine and hydroxocobalamin have synergistic effects. Betaine is a methyl group donor to remethylate homocysteine to methionine via the betaine-homocysteine methyltransferase pathway, thus bypassing the methylcobalamin-dependent methionine synthase pathway [12, 13]. In children less than 3 years of age, betaine is dosed at 100–250 mg/kg divided into two doses [1, 13]. Carnitine conjugates with the toxic acyl-CoA groups produced in combined cobalamin disorders. To prevent carnitine deficiency, L-carnitine supplementation ranging from 50 to 200 mg/kg/day has been prescribed although there is not a clear consensus on a recommended dose [12, 14]. Folate or folinic acid is another adjunct therapy for cobalamin disorders. Folinic acid is preferred due to its ability to cross the blood-brain barrier. Providing folinic acid may help improve tHCY and methionine concentrations by augmenting remethylation. Dosing recommendations for folinic acid range from 5–15 mg/day to 5–30 mg divided 2–3 times per week [13, 14].

15.11 Monitoring

Regular clinic visits during the first year of life are vital for evaluation of growth and feeding difficulties. Feeding dysfunction and failure to thrive are frequently observed in patients with cobalamin disorders. Evaluation of anthropometrics (z score values for weight, height, head circumference, weight for height or BMI) needs to be evaluated at every clinic visit. During the first year, infants may need to be evaluated once or twice a month. Toddlers and older children should be evaluated at least twice annually and adults at least once annually [15]. Evaluation of a 3-day diet history is helpful to determine if a patient is meeting nutritional needs. There is not a clear guideline for frequency of laboratory monitoring. Plasma amino acids, tHCY, methylmalonic acid, carnitine and vitamin B_{12} concentrations are recommended. Hydroxocobalamin, betaine and L-carnitine doses may need to be adjusted based on laboratory results. Therapy goals are to improve biochemical parameters (Box 15.6).

Box 15.6: Nutrition Monitoring for a Patient with Cobalamin Disorder

- Routine assessments including anthropometrics, dietary intake, physical findings
- Laboratory monitoring
  - Diagnosis-specific
    - Plasma amino acids
    - Methionine
    - Total Homocysteine
    - Methylmalonic acid
    - Vitamin B_{12}
  - Nutrition-related laboratory monitoring
    - Protein sufficiency (plasma amino acids, prealbumin)
    - Nutrition anemia (hemoglobin, hematocrit, MCV, serum vitamin B_{12} and/or methylmalonic acid, total homocysteine, ferritin, iron, folate, total iron binding capacity)
    - Vitamin and mineral (25-hydroxy vitamin D, zinc, trace minerals)
    - Carnitine
    - Others as clinically indicated

15.12 Acute Management

Metabolic decompensation is less common in cobalamin disorders as compared to organic acidemias such as propionic or methylmalonic acidemia [15]. Patients are encouraged to continue with their usual diet and medications during illness. Fasting should be avoided to prevent catabolism. If a patient is unable to tolerate fluids, IV fluids containing 10–12.5% dextrose may be needed to reverse catabolism [15]. Dehydration adds additional risk of thrombotic events in the presence of elevated tHCY concentrations. Total homocysteine concentrations are expected to rise during illness due to catabolism.

15.13 Cobalamin Disorders Summary

Early identification and treatment of cobalamin disorders improve survival rate, hematological symptoms and feeding difficulties, but poor neurocognitive and retinopathies often persist [12]. Current management is focused on improving biochemical markers with hydroxocobalamin and betaine therapy. Low-protein diets and medical foods are not recommended for cobalamin disorders as they may lead to methionine deficiency.

15.14 Diet Example Diet Calculation Example for an Infant with Vitamin B6 Nonresponsive Homocystinuria

Patient Information	Nutrient Intake Goals (per day)
Age: Twenty-eight (28) day old male infant Weight: 4.5 kg Diagnosed with HCU based on elevated tHCY and methionine concentrations Asymptomatic and eating well Current intake is 24 oz. of Enfamil Premium per day	Methionine: 30 mg/kg/day (range 15–60 mg/kg/day) Cystine: 95 mg/kg/day (range 85–150 mg/kg/day) Protein: 2.5–3 g/kg Energy: 110–130 kcal/kg Fluid: 100 ml/kg (Tables 15.4 and 15.5)

Table 15.4 Select nutrient composition of products used in HCU diet calculation example (using standard infant formula as the source of intact protein)

Medical food/formula	Amount (g)	Methionine (mg)	Cystine (mg)	Protein (g)	Energy (kcal)
HCU Anamix® Early Years[a]	100	–	410	13.5	473
Enfamil® Premium Infant Powder[b]	100	230	184	10.1	500
Cystine 500™	4 g packet	–	500	--	–

[a]Nutricia North America (Rockville, MD)
[b]Mead Johnson Nutrition (Evansville, IN)
Note: Check manufacturer's website for the most up-to-date nutrient composition

Step-by-Step Diet Calculation

Step 1 Calculate the amount of each nutrient required each day.

$$\text{Nutrient goal} / \text{kg} \times \text{infant weight} = \text{daily requirement}$$
$$\text{Methionine}: 30\,\text{mg} / \text{kg} \times 4.5\,\text{kg} = 135\,\text{mg methionine per day}$$
$$\text{Cystine}: 95\,\text{mg} / \text{kg} \times 4.5 = 428\,\text{mg cystine per day}$$
$$\text{Protein}: 2.5 - 3.0\,\text{g protein} \times 4.5\,\text{kg} = 11.3 - 13.5\,\text{g protein per day}$$
$$\text{Energy}: 110 - 130\,\text{kcal} / \text{kg} \times 4.5\,\text{kg} = 495 - 585\,\text{kcal} / \text{kg per day}$$

Step 2 Calculate the amount of standard infant formula needed to meet the daily methionine requirement

Amount of methionine required per day ÷ mg methionine in standard infant formula

$$135\,\text{mg} / \text{day} \div 230 = 0.59$$

$$0.59 \times 100\,\text{g} = 59\,\text{g standard infant formula needed to meet daily methionine requirements}$$

Step 3 Calculate protein provided from standard infant formula

Amount of standard infant formula × protein provided in 100 g of standard infant formula

$$0.59 \times 10.1\,\text{g} = 6\,\text{g protein from standard infant formula}$$

Step 4 Calculate the amount of protein required to fill diet prescription

Daily protein requirement – protein provided in standard infant formula

$$12.5\,\text{g} - 6\,\text{g} = 6.5\,\text{g protein needed to fill in the diet prescription}$$

Step 5 Calculate the amount of methionine-free metabolic formula required to fill diet prescription

Protein needed to fill diet prescription ÷ protein provided in 100 g of methionine-free formula

$$6.5\,\text{g} \div 13.5\,\text{g} = 0.48$$

$$0.48 \times 100 = 48\,\text{g of methionine free metabolic formula required in the diet prescription}$$

Step 6 Calculate the amount of cystine provided by standard infant formula and methionine-free metabolic formula

Amount of standard infant formula × cystine in 100 g of standard infant formula

$$0.59 \times 184\,\text{mg cystine} = 109\,\text{mg cystine}$$

Amount of methionine-free metabolic formula × cystine in 100 g of methionine-free metabolic formula

$$0.48 \times 410\,\text{mg cystine} = 197\,\text{mg cystine}$$

Step 7 Calculate the amount of cystine that needs to be supplemented by supplemental Cystine in order to meet requirements determined in Step 1

Cystine provided by standard infant formula + cystine provided by methionine-free metabolic formula

$$109\,\text{mg} + 197\,\text{mg} = 306\,\text{mg provided by both formulas}$$

Amount of cystine required in Step 1 – amount provided by both formulas

$$428 - 306 = 122\,\text{mg cystine needed by supplemental cystine to meet requirements}$$

Step 8 Calculate the amount of cystine powder needed to meet cystine requirements

Cystine is available in a premeasured 4 g sachet which provides 500 mg cystine

$500\,\text{mg} \div 4\,\text{g sachet} = 125\,\text{mg cystine per gram of powder}$

$122\,\text{cystine} \div 125\,\text{mg cystine} = 1\,\text{g}$ of cystine powder required to meet cystine requirements

Step 9 Calculate total energy provided from standard infant formula and methionine-free metabolic formula

Amount of standard infant formula × kcal in 100 g of standard infant formula

$$0.59 \times 500\,\text{kcal} = 295\,\text{kcal}$$

Amount of methionine-free metabolic formula × kcal in 100 g of methionine-free metabolic formula

$$0.48 \times 473\,\text{kcal} = 227\,\text{kcal}$$

Add standard infant formula + methionine-free formula kcal to determine total calories provided by prescription

$$295\,\text{kcal} + 227\,\text{kcal} = 522\,\text{kcal total}$$

Step 10 Calculate the final volume of the formula to make a concentration of 20 kcal per ounce

$$522\ \text{kcal} \div 20\ \text{kcal}/\text{oz} = 26\ \text{oz of formula}$$

Table 15.5 Diet prescription summary for diet calculation example (using standard infant formula as the source of intact protein)

Medical food/formula	Amount (g)	Methionine (mg)	Cystine (mg)	Protein (g)	Energy (kcal)
HCU Anamix® early years[a]	48	–	197	6.5	227
Enfamil® Premium powder[b]	59	136	109	6	295
Cystine 500™	1	–	125	–	–
Total per day		136	431	12.5	522
Total per kg		30	96	2.8	116

Values rounded to the nearest whole number for the amount of formula powder, methionine, cystine and energy
Values rounded to the nearest 0.1 g for protein
[a] Nutricia North America (Rockville, MD)
[b] Mead Johnson Nutrition (Evansville, IN)

References

1. Hoss GR, Poloni S, Blom HJ, Schwartz IV. Three main causes of homocystinuria: CBS, cblC and MTHFR deficiency. What do they have in common? J Inborn Errors Metab Screen. 2019;7:e20190007.
2. Thomas J. Nutrition management of inherited metabolic diseases. 1st ed. Cham: Springer International Publishing; 2015.
3. Morris AA, Kozich V, Santra S, Andria G, Ben-Omran TI, Chakrapani AB, et al. Guidelines for the diagnosis and management of cystathionine beta-synthase deficiency. J Inherit Metab Dis. 2017;40(1):49–74.
4. Ekvall S, Ekvall VK. Pediatric nutrition in chronic diseases and developmental disorders: prevention, assessment, and treatment. 2nd ed. Singh R, editor. New York: Oxford University Press; 2005. xxiv, 532 p. p.
5. Acosta PB. Nutrition management of patients with inherited metabolic disorders. 1st ed. Sudbury: Jones & Bartlett Learning; 2009.
6. Valayannopoulos V, Schiff M, Guffon N, Nadjar Y, Garcia-Cazorla A, Martinez-Pardo Casanova M, et al. Betaine anhydrous in homocystinuria: results from the RoCH registry. Orphanet J Rare Dis. 2019;14(1):66.
7. Sacharow SJ, Picker JD, Levy HL. Homocystinuria caused by cystathionine beta-synthase deficiency. In: Adam MP, Ardinger HH, Pagon RA, Wallace SE, Bean LJH, Stephens K, et al., editors. GeneReviews((R)). Seattle (WA); 1993.
8. Schiff M, Blom HJ. Treatment of inherited homocystinurias. Neuropediatrics. 2012;43(6):295–304.
9. Kozich V, Majtan T. Inherited disorders of sulfur amino acid metabolism: recent advances in therapy. Curr Opin Clin Nutr Metab Care. 2021;24(1):62–70.
10. Yannicelli S. Nutrition management of inherited metabolic diseases. Cham: Springer; 2015.
11. Wilcken B. Therapeutic targets in homocystinuria due to cystathionine β-synthase deficiency: new European guidelines. Expert Opin Orphan Drugs. 2016;5(1):1–3.
12. Martinelli D, Deodato F, Dionisi-Vici C. Cobalamin C defect: natural history, pathophysiology, and treatment. J Inherit Metab Dis. 2011;34(1):127–35.
13. Carrillo-Carrasco N, Chandler RJ, Venditti CP. Combined methylmalonic acidemia and homocystinuria, cblC type. I. Clinical presentations, diagnosis and management. J Inherit Metab Dis. 2012;35(1):91–102.
14. Huemer M, Diodato D, Schwahn B, Schiff M, Bandeira A, Benoist JF, et al. Guidelines for diagnosis and management of the cobalamin-related remethylation disorders cblC, cblD, cblE, cblF, cblG, cblJ and MTHFR deficiency. J Inherit Metab Dis. 2017;40(1):21–48.
15. Sloan JL, Carrillo N, Adams D, Venditti CP. Disorders of intracellular cobalamin metabolism. In: Adam MP, Ardinger HH, Pagon RA, Wallace SE, LJH B, Stephens K, et al., editors. GeneReviews((R)). Seattle (WA); 1993.

Nutrition Management of Urea Cycle Disorders

16

Erin MacLeod

Contents

E. MacLeod (✉)
Rare Disease Institute – Genetics and Metabolism,
Children's National Hospital, Washington, DC, USA
e-mail: EMacLeod@childrensnational.org

L. E. Bernstein et al. (eds.), *Nutrition Management of Inherited Metabolic Diseases*,
https://doi.org/10.1007/978-3-030-94510-7_16

Core Messages

- Urea cycle disorders (UCD) differ widely in their presentation and severity.
- Correcting hyperammonemia is the priority in treating UCD.
- Dietary protein is restricted in UCD. The amount of protein provided as intact protein versus medical food protein (essential amino acid) varies.
- Preventing catabolism by providing sufficient energy is a critical part of nutrition management.
- Medications that remove nitrogen by alternative pathways help to prevent hyperammonemia and increase protein tolerance.
- Outcomes are guarded and depend on severity of the disease.
- Liver transplantation is recommended for infants with severe forms of the disorder.

16.1 Background

Urea cycle disorders (UCD) are caused by a deficiency in any one of six enzymes or two transporters in the urea cycle [1] (Fig. 16.1). In addition, a new disorder has recently been described which causes hyperammonemia (and hyperlactatemia), carbonic anhydrase VA (CA-VA [2]. Management of CA-VA will not be reviewed here. Collectively, UCD are relatively common, with an incidence of 1:35,000 births [3]. Apart from ornithine transcarbamylase deficiency (OTCD), which is x-linked, all UCD are inherited in an autosomal recessive pattern [1]. While a secondary role of the hepatic urea cycle is to produce arginine, the primary function is to remove nitrogen that is produced from amino acid metabolism to prevent accumulation of ammonia. Waste nitrogen is produced when protein intake exceeds the amount needed for protein synthesis or when endogenous protein stores are broken down to produce energy (catabolism). Nitrogen is cleaved from an amino acid and the remaining molecule is used as a source of energy (if needed) or stored as fat. Excess nitrogen is normally converted to ammonia, which enters the urea cycle and through a series of enzymatic reactions, is converted to urea and excreted (Box 16.1).

Box 16.1: Principles of Nutrition Management in UCD

Restrict:	Protein
Supplement:	Essential amino acids, arginine in ASS and ASL, citrulline in OTC and CPS.
Toxic:	Ammonia in all UCD Argininosuccinic acid (ASA) in ASL deficiency Arginine in arginase deficiency

Ammonia is neurotoxic [4, 5]. The pathophysiology of UCD and the cause of neurotoxicity is complex. It involves not only ammonia, but also the effect of ammonia and excess production of glutamine on astrocytes, causing brain edema [6]. The acute effects of hyperammonemia include poor feeding, vomiting, seizures, and lethargy that can rapidly progress to coma and death. Chronic effects of mild elevations of ammonia are less well understood but may be a cause of impaired neurocognition seen in children with UCD [7]. The potential consequences of increased ammonia concentrations are presented in Table 16.1. Note that ammonia concentrations may be expressed as μmol/L or mcg/dL.

UCD can be differentiated based on the pattern of citrulline, arginine, and ornithine on plasma amino acid analysis.

UCD can present at any age [1, 9, 10]. Typically, a neonate with a severe form of UCD will present with rapidly progressive symptoms of hyperammonemia within the first few days of life. In infants and children, presenting symptoms may include failure to thrive, cyclic vomiting, liver dysfunction, seizures, and developmental delay [1, 11, 12]. Children and adults may present after the newborn period and have a milder clinical course [10]. In some cases, adults are diagnosed with UCD after encephalopathic crises

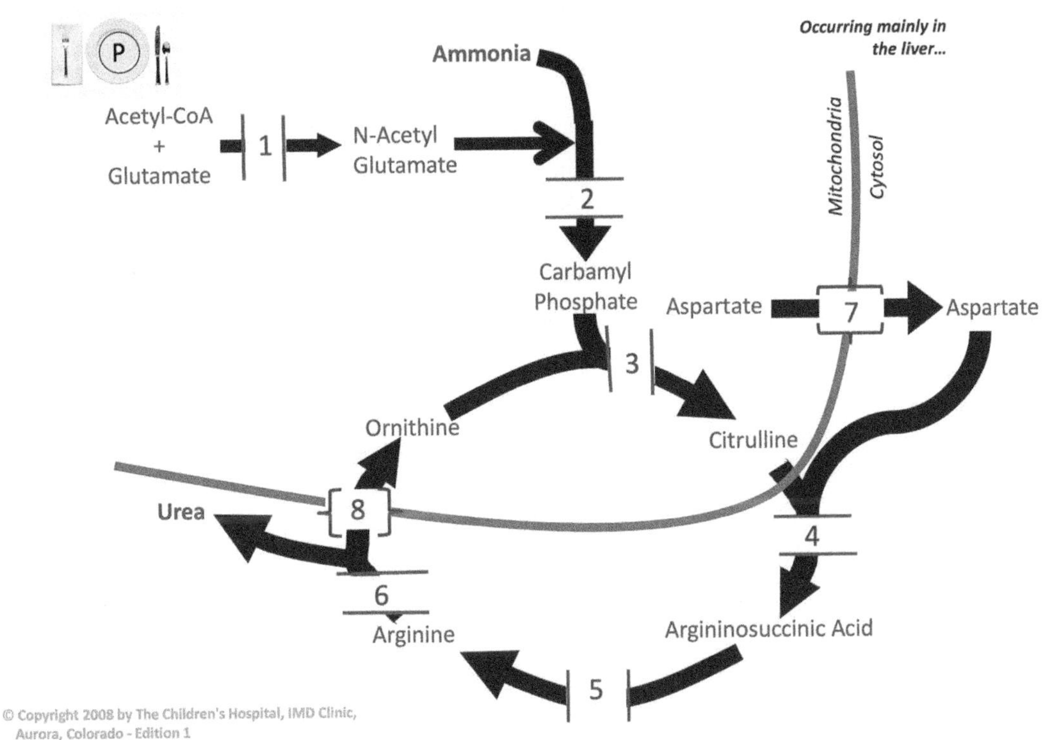

Fig. 16.1 Metabolic pathway of urea cycle disorders. The urea cycle contains six enzymes: 1. *NAGS* N-acetylglutamate synthase – activates CPS. 2. *CPS* Carbamoyl phoshate synthetase – adds bicarbonate to ammonia to form, along with a phosphate group, carbamoyl phosphate, starts the urea cycle. 3. *OTC* Ornithine transcarbamylase combines carbamoyl phosphate with ornithine to produce citrulline. 4. *ASS* Arginiosuccinate synthetase – combines citrulline and aspartate to form arginosuccinic acid. 5. *ASL* Argininosuccinate lyase – breaks down argininosuccinic acid into arginine and fumarate. 6. *Arginase* – cleaves arginine to form urea and ornithine which then feeds back into urea cycle. 7. *Citrin* – transports aspartate from the mitochondria to the cytosol. 8. *ORNT1 Ornithine translocase* – transports ornithine between the mitochondria and the cytosol, deficiency causes hyperornithinemia-hyperammonemia-homocitrullinuria (HHH) syndrome

Table 16.1 Ammonia concentrations and potential consequences

Ammonia concentration		Interpretation and symptoms
μmol/L	mcg/dL	
<35	<60	Normal concentration[a]
36–60	60–100	Mild elevation; not always associated with symptoms
61–200	150–350	Elevation: poor feeding, vomiting, irritability, lethargy, confusion
>250	>350	Hyperammonemic crisis; potentially leading to coma

[a]In newborns normal ammonia concentrations are 64–107 μmol/L (90–150 mcg/dL) and in infants age 0–2 weeks 56–92 μmol/L (79–129 mcg/dL).

Note: Norms for ammonia concentration may vary according to laboratory used. Individual symptoms may vary – some patients are more sensitive to elevations in ammonia than others. Therefore, treatment should not be based solely on ammonia concentration and needs to consider patient history, clinical, and laboratory assessments.

Ref. [8]

following catabolic stress, including infection, surgery, pregnancy, and the postpartum period [13, 14]. Finally, females who are carriers for OTC deficiency may be diagnosed following the diagnosis of a more severely affected child. Females who are carriers for OTC deficiency can still exhibit neurocognitive deficits in executive functioning and approximately 15% require treatment [1, 15]. Adolescents and adults who are diagnosed with UCD often have a history of chronic neurological and/or psychiatric symptoms [1] as well as a diet history indicating avoidance of high protein foods.

Not all individuals with UCD come to attention clinically. Some may be identified through newborn screening (NBS) [3, 11]. NBS detects high concentrations of metabolites in the blood; therefore, ASS and ASL can be identified because these disorders result in increased concentrations of citrulline and arginase deficiency because of high concentrations of arginine. However, OTC, the most common UCD, is not identified through most NBS programs because in OTC the metabolite citrulline is lower than normal. The Association of Public Health Laboratories NewSTEPS website (newsteps.org) can be accessed for state-specific screening profiles. For individuals who come to attention through NBS, the challenge is to determine how aggressively to treat infants who are flagged by NBS but who remain asymptomatic. For those who have been confirmed through biochemical testing (and in some cases molecular testing as well) but maintain normal plasma glutamine, treatment with medical foods and ammonia scavengers may not be needed, though patients should continue to be followed, supplemented with citrulline/arginine when needed, and treated conservatively when ill. Algorithms for guidance in diagnosing specific UCD are available [11].

Table 16.2 presents the 6 enzymes and 2 transporters of the urea cycle and the disorder associated with a deficiency of each. Proximal UCD, or those in the mitochondria, (NAGS, CPS, OTC) tend to be associated with marked elevations in ammonia, whereas UCD that are more distal

Table 16.2 Urea cycle disorders, associated enzymes, and altered laboratory values

Disorder	Enzyme	Abbreviation	Ammonia concentration	Plasma amino acid findings[1]
NAGS deficiency	N-Acetylglutamate synthetase	NAGS	Markedly elevated	Markedly low citrulline Low arginine
CPS deficiency	Carbomoyl phosphate synthetase	CPS	Markedly elevated	Markedly low citrulline Low arginine
OTC deficiency	Ornithine transcarbamylase[2]	OTC	Markedly elevated	Markedly low citrulline Low arginine
ASS deficiency; Citrullinemia I	Argininosuccinic acid synthetase	ASS	Elevated	Markedly elevated citrulline Low arginine
Citrin deficiency	Citrin	Citrin	Elevated	Elevated citrulline Elevated arginine
ASL deficiency; Argininosuccinic aciduria (ASA)	Argininosuccinic acid lyase[3]	ASL	Elevated	Mild elevation in citrulline Low arginine
Arginase deficiency; Argininemia	Arginase	ARG	Rarely elevated	Elevated arginine
Hyperornithinema-hyperammonemia- homocitrullinuria (HHH) syndrome	Ornithine translocase	ORNT1	Elevated	Elevated ornithine Low citrulline

[1] Plasma glutamine typically elevated in in all UCD, elevations are associated with higher risk of hyperammonemia
[2] Urine orotic acid is also present and is pathognomoic for OTC deficiency
[3] Urine argininosuccinic acid will be elevated in mild ASL deficiency even if blood level is normal

(ASS, ASL, ARG, HHH) are less likely to result in severe hyperammonemic episodes; however, all individuals with UCD are at risk of developing hyperammonemia, especially if stressed by infection and/or poor energy intake leading to catabolism of endogenous protein [16]. Although proximal UCD often have a more severe clinical course and higher risk of hyperammonemia events, there is debate about the severity of neurocognitive outcomes between the two groups [7, 9, 17].

Overall, outcomes in UCD are improving due to newborn screening for several disorders, advances in medications and nutrition management, and liver transplantation [18–20]. Traditionally, however, outcomes have been suboptimal and characterized by early mortality, growth failure, chronic liver disease, and poor development [9]. Survival rates are better for those with late onset (11% mortality) compared to neonatal onset (24% mortality) [20]. Because of shortcomings of traditional therapies, liver transplantation is becoming a more viable and attractive option for many patients with UCD [21, 22].

16.2 Nutrition Management

16.2.1 Chronic Nutrition Management

Treatment of UCD includes limiting dietary protein, providing sufficient energy to prevent catabolism, supplementing with specific amino acids, and using nitrogen-scavenging drugs [11, 14, 23–26] (Box 16.2). These strategies are typically used in combination depending on the severity of the disease. In an infant who presents with a severe form of UCD, for example, a male with OTC deficiency, emergency management is indicated [11, 27] (Sect. 16.2.2).

The goals of nutrition management are to prevent the accumulation of ammonia, normalize plasma amino acids and promote normal growth and development. The treatment of UCD differs from other metabolic disorders with respect to protein intake. In UCD, total protein is limited, unlike in many other metabolic disorders where total protein is not limited but is provided as medical food without the offending amino acid(s). The steps to initiating a diet in a newborn are presented (Box 16.3). Feeding from the breast and/or the use of pumped breast milk should be

Box 16.2: Components of Management of UCD

- Limit protein
- Prevent catabolism
- Use nitrogen scavenging drugs
- Supplement amino acids

Box 16.3: Initiating Nutrition Management in an Infant with UCD

(For the infant who is medically stable and ready to start feeding)

Goals:

- Prevent hyperammonemia
- Normalize plasma amino acids
- Promote normal growth and development

Step-by-Step:

1. Establish goals for total protein intake and (essential amino acids) (Table 16.3).
2. Determine amount needed to meet goal in step 1 and which medical food to use.
3. Determine amount of intact protein needed to meet the protein goal in step 1 and whether the source will be breast milk or standard infant formula
4. Determine if DRI for energy is met by the combination of medical food and standard infant formula/ breast milk. If not, add a protein-free energy source to meet needs.
5. Determine how much water to add to make a volume of formula that will meet the infant's fluid needs and have a caloric density of 20–25 kcal/oz.

See Sect. 16.7 Example Diet Calculation

Table 16.3 Recommended nutrient intakes for patients with UCD

Age (year)	Total protein[1] (g/kg/day)	Protein from medical food (essential amino acids) [2] (g/kg/day)	Intact protein (g/kg/day)
0–1	1.2–2.2	0.4–1.1	0.8–1.1
1–7	1.0–1.2	0.3–0.7	0.7–0.8
7–19	0.8–1.4	0.4–0.7	0.3–1.0
>19	0.8–1.0	0.2–0.5	0.6–0.7

Intakes for energy, vitamins, and minerals should meet the DRI [28] and fluid requirements [11, 29] and R.H. Singh Nutritional Management of UCD [30]

[1] Total protein goals should be considered the minimum protein required, some individuals may tolerate more total protein

[2] For some with mild disease supplementation with essential amino acids may not be required. If supplementation is needed, provide 30–50% total protein from medical food

Table 16.4 Energy and protein content of medical foods (essential amino acids) for the treatment of UCD (per 100 g powder)[1]

Medical food	Energy (kcal)	Protein (g)
Cyclinex®-1[2]	510	7.5
Cyclinex®-2[2]	440	15
EAA Supplement™[3]	288	40
Essential Amino Acid Mix[4]	316	79
UCD Anamix® Junior[4]	385	12
UCD Trio™[3]	393	15
WND® 1[5]	500	6.5
WND® 2[5]	410	8.2

[1] Available in the US (2022)

[2] Abbott Nutrition (Columbus, OH; abbottnutrition.com)

[3] Nutricia North America (Rockville, MD; nutricia-na.com)

[4] Vitaflo USA, (Alexandria, VA; vitaflousa.com)

[5] Mead Johnson Nutrition (Evansville, IN; meadjohnson.com)

encouraged as breast milk contains less total protein when compared to standard infant formula. Breast milk may need to be supplemented with a protein-free energy module to ensure energy needs are met in infants with poor feeding.

Sources of protein in the diet for infants with UCD include intact protein (breast milk or standard infant formula in infancy, baby food, table foods) and medical foods containing essential amino acids. Some patients with mild forms of UCD can be treated with breastmilk/standard infant formula (with or without protein-free energy supplement) and followed with a vegetarian diet, though continued follow-up and monitoring are required.

Practice varies widely with respect to the balance between intact protein and medical food protein. Current European guidelines suggest following FAO/WHO/UNU 2007 guidelines for protein requirements [31] and supplementing with essential amino acids with metabolic instability or use of ammonia scavengers [11]. A cross-sectional study of those enrolled in the European Registry and Network for Intoxication Type Metabolic Diseases [25] found that essential amino acid medical food was given in 32% of individuals with a UCD and provided 28–32% of total protein intake. This is congruent with previous recommendations that 20–30% of protein requirements be given as essential amino acids [14]. However in some centers, protein restriction alone (without the use of medical foods containing essential amino acids) is used [32, 33] while others recommend that approximately half of the total protein allowance be given as essential amino acids and half as intact protein [34]. Protein restriction without essential amino acid supplementation may lead to chronic protein insufficiency [35] and when intact protein is low, EAA supplementation may improve plasma branched-chain amino acid concentrations [25]. Once the current severity status of the individual patient is determined and diet goals are established, the amount of medical food and the amount of breast milk or standard infant formula necessary to meet these goals is calculated. Medical foods for the treatment of UCD are listed in Table 16.4. They provide essential amino acids as the protein source but differ in energy, vitamin, and mineral profiles.

Providing sufficient calories often necessitates the use of special protein-free medical foods, such as Pro-Phree® (Abbott Nutrition, Columbus, OH), PFD (Mead Johnson, Glenview, IL), Polycal™ (Nutricia North America, Gaithersburg, MD), Duocal® (Nutricia North America, Gaithersburg, MD), S.O.S™ (Vitaflo USA, Alexandria, VA) or Solcarb® (Solace Nutrition, Pawcatuck, CT). Nutrition education and counseling should be provided on low protein calorie-dense food options.

Preventing catabolism Catabolic stress is a major source of waste nitrogen. Episodes of hyperammonemia are often precipitated not by an overconsumption of protein, but rather by an acute infectious illness coupled with inadequate energy and protein consumption. Although a recent study found energy intakes of patients with UCD often meet recommended requirements [36], it can be challenging to provide sufficient calories to some patients with UCD as appetites at baseline can be poor. The reason for anorexia in UCD is multifactorial. Elevated blood glutamine concentrations often seen in patients with UCD, cause high brain glutamine concentrations. In the brain, glutamine is a carrier for tryptophan, which is a precursor for serotonin, the neurotransmitter that is associated with a feeling of satiety [37]. Also, patients with UCD have been shown to have higher than normal concentrations of the hormone peptide tyrosine tyrosine (also referred to as Peptide YY or PYY) that is associated with feelings of satiety [38]. It is also likely that patients with UCD have food aversions because they have been conditioned to associate intake of high protein foods with episodes of vomiting, headaches, and/or lethargy. In one study, half of the patients with UCD had feeding problems including poor appetite, food refusal, protein aversion or vomiting [39]. Given the tendency to self-restrict protein, patients with UCD need nutrition education on appropriate amounts and types of protein in the diet, particularly if EAA supplementation is not given. It is common for children with UCD, especially those with severe forms, to require nasogastric or gastrostomy tubes (G-tubes) in order to provide sufficient calories. G-tubes are especially helpful for providing medications and extra calories, especially during illness when appetites may be further diminished [11].

Use of nitrogen scavenging drugs Although there are several medications available, they remove nitrogen by one of two pathways (Fig. 16.2). Sodium benzoate binds with glycine and forms hippurate and is excreted in urine. This

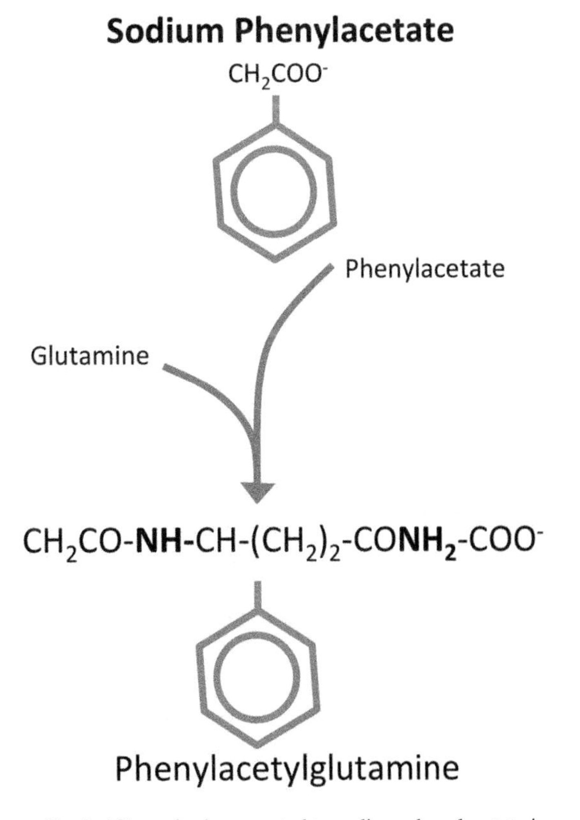

Fig. 16.2 Alternate pathways for the removal of nitrogen using sodium benzoate or sodium phenylacetate. Sodium phenylbutyrate (Buphenyl®) and glycerol phenylbutyrate (Ravicti®) are both converted to sodium phenylacetate in the liver

reaction removes one nitrogen atom. Similarly, in the second reaction, sodium phenylacetate binds with glutamine and forms phenylacetylglutamine that is excreted. In this reaction, two nitrogen atoms are bound and excreted. The pro-drug to sodium phenylacetate, sodium phenylbutyrate, is available as Buphenyl® (Hyperion Therapeutics Inc., Brisbane, CA) as well as a generic form (PAR Pharmaceuticals and Simapharm Laboratories, LLC). Glycerol phenylbutyrate (Ravicti®, Hyperion Therapeutics Inc.) works by the same mechanisms as sodium phenylbutyrate and some find it easier to administer because the dose is lower and taste is better than sodium phenylbutyrate [40]. Sodium phenylbutyrate has the secondary effect of activating branched-chain ketoacid dehydrogenase, which often results in low plasma branch chain amino acid concentrations [41]. Ammonul® (Ucyclyd Pharma, Scottsdale, AZ) is an IV form of nitrogen scavenging medication that contains a combination of sodium phenylacetate and sodium benzoate.

Carglumic acid (Carbaglu®, Recordati Rare Diseases Inc., Lebanon, NJ) is a medication for treating deficiency of the first enzyme of the urea cycle, NAGS deficiency, but it is not a nitrogen-scavenging drug. Carglumic acid is chemically analogous to N-acetylglutamine, which activates CPS. In a study of 20 patients receiving carglumic acid, 12 had NAGS deficiency and their hyperammonemia resolved [42]. Patients with NAGS deficiency receiving carglumic acid can quickly transition to a normal diet with no protein restriction. A carglumic acid trial should also be considered for all patients with CPS1 deficiency as some have been shown to have improvements in urinary nitrogen excretion and may result in increased intact protein tolerance [43].

Supplemental amino acids For all UCD except arginase deficiency, arginine becomes an essential amino acid. Arginine or citrulline supplements are given to replace the arginine that is normally produced by the urea cycle. Often, L-arginine is used in ASS and ASL deficiency whereas L-citrulline is used in CPS and OTC deficiency because it has the advantage of incorporating aspartate into the pathway and removing one additional nitrogen molecule [44]. The goal in supplementing amino acids is to keep plasma concentrations within the normal range and the doses vary for an individual as higher amounts are prescribed in acute illness [11, 27]. The typical maintenance dose of L-citrulline in OTC and CPS is 100–200 mg/kg/day [11] and should be adjusted based on plasma concentrations of citrulline. Current European guidelines recommend 100–300 mg/kg/day (2.5–6 g/m^2/d if >20 kg) L-arginine for ASS and ASL deficiency [11]. In ASL, there is evidence that lower dose arginine supplementation (100 mg/kg/day) results in lower accumulation of ASA and perhaps improved outcome since ASA may contribute to the liver and neurological disease [45]. L-arginine supplementation should be adjusted based on plasma concentrations of arginine and glutamine. The typical maintenance dose of L-citrulline in OTC and CPS is 100–200 mg/kg/day [11] and should be adjusted based on plasma concentrations of citrulline.

16.2.2 Acute Nutrition Management

16.2.2.1 Nutrition Management During Hospitalization

A hyperammonemic crisis is treated as a medical emergency whether it is in a sick neonate or an older child/adult with an acute illness. All patients should have an emergency protocol [46] to ensure they receive prompt and proper treatment. If hospitalized with hyperammonemia, protein feeds should be discontinued and IV access obtained for administration of nutrition support and medications including the nitrogen-scavenging drug, Ammonul®, and arginine. If possible, plasma amino acids should be ordered for stat analysis. In a known patient, analysis of amino acids can help to determine if hyperammonemia is due to acute illness or may be secondary to excess protein intake. If multiple essential amino acids are low on plasma amino acid analysis, essential amino acid supplementation should be given quickly to prevent further catabolism.

In severe cases of hyperammonemia, dialysis is usually required to normalize ammonia concentrations. Often patients are not able to tolerate

Box 16.4: Example of Parenteral Nutrition for a Patient with UCD in Hyperammonemic Crisis[a]

Glucose infusion rate: 10–12 mg/kg/min
Intralipid: 2–3 g/kg/d (up to 3–4 g/kg/d in neonate)
Amino acids: (after 24 h or if dialyzed):
0.25 – 0.5 g/kg/d and advanced as tolerated
Arginine HCl: 210 mg/kg/d

[a]Management in conjunction with metabolic physician

enteral feedings and parenteral nutrition (PN) is required. The PN solution focuses on providing as much energy as possible by using 20% dextrose solution and 2–3 g/kg Intralipid® and eliminating or severely restricting protein intake (Box 16.4). Goal calories should provide 120% of the DRI for age and if hyperglycemia occurs, insulin can be provided [11]. Whenever possible, enteral feeds should be utilized, even for small amounts of essential amino acids. If the patient is to be dialyzed, a limited amount of an IV amino acid solution is given, since dialysis will remove amino acids as well as ammonia, and the infant runs the risk of becoming catabolic. PN solutions that contain only essential amino acids can be ordered but may not be readily available. If enteral feeds cannot be used for EAA, standard PN solutions can be utilized to prevent further catabolism associated with inadequate protein intake. Catabolism is reversed faster when some amino acids are provided in the diet in addition to adequate energy (through glucose and/or intralipids) [47].

In a patient who is not dialyzed, protein should be eliminated for no more than 24 hours to prevent further catabolism [27]. Essential amino acids can be provided during an acute illness in order to prevent branched-chain amino acid deficiency that can occur with hyperammonemia and be further exacerbated by nitrogen scavenging medications [35, 41]. There is no consensus on how long to eliminate protein and essential amino acids in acutely ill patients with UCD and the decision is made by the medical team depending on the patient's ammonia, plasma amino acids, nutritional intake and neurological status. Enteral sources of protein can be reintroduced slowly, starting with half of the patient's intact protein needs and advancing as tolerated.

Once a neonate who presented with hyperammonemia is stabilized, he or she will usually experience a period of metabolic stability or "honeymoon period" [20]. During this time, the infant is growing rapidly and has a relatively higher protein tolerance. The diet is less complicated in the first few months since solid foods have not been introduced and protein does not yet have to be counted. The infant also has innate immunity and often limited exposure to infections. Depending on severity and desire of the family, infants with UCD can be breastfed from the breast or given pumped breast milk in combination with essential amino acids and/or a protein-free calorie supplement.

16.2.2.2 Nutrition Management During Illness at Home

Intercurrent illness is the most common cause of hyperammonemia outside of the newborn period and prompt treatment can prevent catabolism and be lifesaving [20]. Patients should have a Medic Alert® bracelet (MedicAlert, Turlock, CA). Those with mild illnesses may be managed at home if the metabolic team assesses that it is safe to do so. In such cases, ensuring adequate supplemental calories and hydration should be the focus. Given the tendency to self-restrict protein, ensuring that the patient has not been consuming less protein than recommended needs to be assessed. In some cases, the percentage of EAA to intact protein can be adjusted to ensure minimum protein needs are met during illness. Sick day plans that reduce intact protein should be given on a case-by-case basis depending on the degree of illness, how well the child has been managed at home in the past, distance to clinic, and diet history (Sect. 16.7). However, medical food containing EAA is still provided in sick day formulas as well as additional energy from fat and/or carbohydrate. If a sick day diet is prescribed, it should be used for no more than 24–48 hours [14, 23]. Its necessity beyond that requires an evaluation from the medical team.

Because fluid and energy needs are higher than normal during illness, patients need to eat more when they often feel like eating less. For patients who do not have G-tubes, getting sufficient energy and fluids by mouth may not be possible and admission for IV fluids and calories is often needed.

16.3 Monitoring

Nutrition monitoring includes assessment of anthropometrics, dietary intake, and laboratory parameters (Box 16.5). Nutrition goals should be individualized to laboratory measures and growth parameters as there may be some differences in resting energy expenditure for those with a UCD [48]. Routine laboratory measurement includes ammonia and plasma amino acids, particular attention is paid to glutamine, branched-chain amino acids, alanine, and glycine. Both ammonia and glutamine are markers for neurocognitive outcomes [20]. Collection of an accurate ammonia sample can be challenging as it must be taken from free-flowing blood and immediately placed on ice and analyzed. Ammonia measurements from send-out labs should not be considered accurate and an elevated concentration that does not coincide with the patient's clinical picture should be repeated [49].

Box 16.5: Nutrition Monitoring of Patients with UCD

- Routine assessments including anthropometrics, dietary intake, physical findings
- Laboratory Monitoring
  - Diagnosis-specific
    - Ammonia
    - Plasma amino acids, including
      - Glutamine
      - Arginine
      - Citrulline
      - Argininosuccinic acid (in ASA lyase deficiency)
      - BCAA (often low if on sodium (glycerol) phenylbutyrate therapy)
  - Nutrition laboratory monitoring of patients on protein-restricted diets may include markers of:
    - Protein sufficiency (plasma amino acids)
    - Nutritional anemia (hemoglobin, hematocrit, MCV, serum vitamin B_{12} and/or MMA, total homocysteine, ferritin, iron, folate, total iron binding capacity)
    - Vitamin and mineral status (25-hydroxy vitamin D, zinc, trace minerals)
    - Others as clinically indicated

16.3.1 Plasma Amino Acids Related to Dietary Intake

Glutamine is often a harbinger of high ammonia because it is a reservoir for ammonia, as glutamine is synthesized in the liver from glutamate and ammonia. A recent report found 20–30% of patients with UCD had low branched-chain amino acids [25] though, anecdotally, this rate could be higher. Regardless of the cause (either as a consequence of dietary restriction or sodium phenylbutyrate therapy) [50], low branched-chain amino acids indicate the need for more protein. This can be given as intact protein if the patient can tolerate it, essential amino acid medical food, or specific branched-chain amino acid supplements [11]. Low plasma branched-chain amino acids in those with a UCD have been associated with lower linear growth velocity [18, 36]. Linear growth may be related to the ratio of intact protein to energy [36, 51], and those with early-onset UCD, in particular, are at risk for poor linear growth [52]. Plasma amino acids can further be used to assess caloric intake as elevated alanine may occur if energy intake is insufficient and elevated glycine is often seen in catabolism [1].

16.3.2 Additional Plasma Amino Acids to Evaluate Based on Diagnosis

Depending on the diagnosis, analysis of an amino acid profile can help to guide management.

Arginine and citrulline should be monitored for those on L-arginine or L-citrulline supplementation as an indication of compliance or necessity of dose adjustment. Plasma citrulline will always be elevated in those with citrullinemia; however, citrulline alone is not toxic and elevations in the presence of normal glutamine is not concerning. Some labs report argininosuccinic acid (ASA) on plasma amino acid profile. For diagnosis, patients with mild ASL may only have argininosuccinic acid elevated in urine amino acids. Beyond diagnosis, ASA concentrations have not been associated with changes in dietary protein or disease outcome. Plasma arginine should be monitored in arginase deficiency with a goal to achieve concentrations as close to normal as possible [53]. Although hyperammonemia is less common in arginase deficiency, a greater restriction of intact protein may be required to achieve ideal plasma arginine concentrations [11].

Periodic laboratory monitoring to ensure that the patient is receiving adequate protein, vitamins, and minerals is recommended. Evaluation of vitamins and mineral status is of particular importance in those on a protein-restricted diet without a complete medical food supplement. Finally, compliance with nitrogen scavenger medications can be assessed using ratios of phenylacetate to phenylacetylglutamine [54]. A ratio less than 0.6 is associated with elevated plasma glutamine and may be related to suboptimal intake of nitrogen scavenger rather than excessive intake of dietary protein.

16.4 Transplantation

In patients with severe UCD outcomes are poor despite treatment and liver transplantation is often the treatment of choice [21]. The Urea Cycle Disorders Consortium and the recent European guidelines recommend that patients with UCD, other than those with NAGS, who have absent or very low enzyme activity be stabilized, aggressively managed, and placed on the liver transplant list as early as is practical [11, 20]. Even in arginase deficiency, liver transplantation has been shown to halt the progression of neurological damage [55].

Earlier United Network for Organ Sharing (UNOS) data found higher mortality when patients with UCD were transplanted before age 2 years [22]. This may be explained by the fact that, historically, only the most severely affected patients were referred for transplantation; however, current recommendations state that transplants should occur at the earliest possible time [11, 20]. Transplantation outcomes in patients with UCD have been good. In a study of 23 patients (none of whom had arginase deficiency), there was 100% patient survival and 96% graft survival [56]. Developmental outcomes were stable or improved following transplant.

Prior to liver transplantation, the goal is to maintain good metabolic control and nutritional status. Better surgical outcomes are correlated to pretransplant weight and protein status both of which can be difficult to attain on a protein-restricted diet. A minimum weight of 5 kg is usually recommended before transplantation can be performed [11]. Maintaining metabolic control is of paramount importance in order to preserve neurocognition because transplantation does not reverse neurocognitive damage [20, 57].

Pre- and postoperative nutrition protocols vary. At one center [56], patients with UCD continued to receive their usual protein-restricted diet up to approximately 6 hours prior to surgery. During surgery, patients are typically given 10% dextrose with electrolytes and Intralipid® (2 g/kg/d). After surgery, intravenous amino acids (1.5–2 g/kg/d) are added to the parenteral nutrition. After transplantation, patients with UCD no longer require a protein-restricted diet, medical food or nitrogen-scavenging drugs [56]. While a normal diet can be followed, it may be difficult for patients who have not had high protein foods in the past to readily accept unfamiliar foods. Nutrition education and guidance should be provided to expand patients' palates and introduce new foods in a healthful way.

Most patients still require L-arginine or L-citrulline supplementation, with decreased dose based on plasma amino acid concentrations. Follow-up of liver transplant patients by the metabolic dietitian in collaboration with the transplant dietitian is best. The transplant dietitian can best address issues common to all transplant patients, including possible nutrition-related side effects of anti-rejection medication, food safety concerns, and prevention of obesity, which is common in pediatric patients who have undergone liver transplantation [58].

16.5 New Treatment Options

Currently, multiple new therapies are in clinical trials for the treatment of UCD. These include targets to reduce ammonia production in the gut, supplementation of nitric oxide for ASL, enzyme replacement therapy for ARG1, and gene therapy for OTC deficiency [59]. These new treatment modalities have the potential to improve overall management and outcomes of patients with UCD as well as potentially allow for safe diet liberalization. The role of the metabolic dietitian is essential for patients who embark on these new treatment options to ensure nutrition requirements are met in a healthful way.

16.6 Summary

The primary function of the urea cycle is the removal of waste nitrogen produced during protein metabolism. Deficiency in the activity of any of the 6 enzymes or 2 transporters in the urea cycle may result in the accumulation of ammonia, often to toxic concentrations. Treatment includes restricting dietary protein, preventing catabolism, supplementing amino acids that are normally produced by the urea cycle, and promoting the excretion of nitrogen via alternative pathways. Outcomes are guarded and appear to be better for patients identified by NBS compared to patients identified clinically. Liver transplantation is a treatment option, especially for patients with a severe form of the disorder.

16.7 Diet Calculation Example

Example 1 Infant male with OTC deficiency weighing 2.9 kg who presented acutely and is ready to transition from parenteral nutrition to enteral feedings.

Patient Information	Nutrient Intake Goals
Age: 3-week-old male with OTC deficiency Weight: 2.9 kg Presented acutely with hyperammonemia Treated with dialysis Ammonul and parental nutrition Currently tolerating 1 g protein PN and ready to transition to enteral feeding	Energy: 120 kcal/kg Protein: 1.5 g/kg (half as whole protein and half as essential amino acids) Diet prescription summary for sample calculation of UCD diet

Diet prescription summary for sample calculation of UCD diet

Diet	Amount	Protein, total (g)	Protein, intact (g)	Protein, medical food (g)	Energy[1] (kcal)	Fluid[2] (mL)
Goals		4.4	2.2	2.2	348	290
Cyclinex-1 powder[3]	29 g	2.2	0	2.2	148	
Similac powder[3]	20 g	2.2	2.2		108	
Pro-Phree powder[3]	18 g		0	0	92	
Totals		4.4	2.2	2.2	348	
Total per kg		1.5	0.76	0.76	120	
Add water to make:	14–17 ounces					420–510 mL

[1] Dietary Reference Intake [28]
[2] Fluid requirement [29]
[3] Abbott Nutrition (Columbus, OH; abbottnutrition.com)
Note: Check manufacturer's website for the most up-to-date nutrient composition

Example 2 Modification of usual well-day diet during a mild illness treated at home for a 6-year-old female with ASA deficiency, weighing 24 kg (Table 16.5).

Table 16.5 Usual full protein diet prescription (when well) and sick-day modifications to diet prescription for half intact protein or no intact protein

Diet	Amount	Protein, intact[1]	Protein, medical food[1]	Energy (kcal)
Diet prescription: Usual full protein		0.7 g/kg (17 g)	0.5 g/kg (12 g)	1600[2]
Anamix Junior[3]	100 g	0	12	385
Duocal®[3]	80 g	0	0	394
Add water to make	28 oz			
Food/beverages		17 g	0	807
Diet prescription: Half intact protein, 20% more energy		0.35 g/kg (8 g)	0.7 g/kg (17 g)[5]	1900
Anamix Junior[3]	140 g	0	17	539
Duocal®[3]	140 g	0	0	689
Add water to make	44 oz[4]			
Food/beverages		8 g	0	672[6]
Diet prescription: No intact protein, 20% more energy[7]		0	0.5 g/kg (12 g)	1900
Anamix Junior[3]	100 g	0	12	385
Duocal®[3]	200 g	0	0	984
Add water to make	48 oz[4]			
Food/beverages		0 g		531[5]

[1] Singh 2007 [11, 23]
[2] Dietary Reference Intake [28]
[3] Nutricia North America (Rockville, MD; nutricia-na.com)
[4] Total amount of fluid provided in the formula is greater than usual diet in order to maintain caloric density similar to usual diet and because additional fluid is required during illness
[5] If intact protein is decreased, consider increasing EAA supplement to meet DRI for protein
[6] If patient is not able to consume sufficient amounts of food or fluids to reach energy goal, additional Pro-Phree®/Duocal and water may be added to the formula instead
[7] A sick day plan which provides less than the DRI for protein should only be given for 24–48 hours and followed up closely to ensure further decompensation does not occur at home due to catabolism

Acknowledgment Thank you to Fran Rohr, MS RD formerly of Boston Children's Hospital, for her contributions to this chapter's content in the 1st Edition of Nutrition Management of Inherited Metabolic Diseases.

References

1. Ah Mew N, Simpson KL, Gropman AL, Lanpher BC, Chapman KA, Summar ML. Urea cycle disorders overview. In: Adam MP, Ardinger HH, Pagon RA, Wallace SE, Bean LJH, Mirzaa G, et al., editors. Seattle (WA): University of Washington, Seattle 1993–2022. GeneReviews (R) [Internet].
2. van Karnebeek C, Haberle J. Carbonic anhydrase VA deficiency. In: Adam MP, Ardinger HH, Pagon RA, Wallace SE, Bean LJH, Mirzaa G, et al., editors. Seattle (WA): University of Washington, Seattle 1993–2022. GeneReviews (R) [Internet].
3. Summar ML, Koelker S, Freedenberg D, Le Mons C, Haberle J, Lee HS, et al. The incidence of urea cycle disorders. Mol Genet Metab. 2013;110(1–2):179–80.
4. Kleppe S, Mian A, Lee B. Urea cycle disorders. Curr Treat Options Neurol. 2003;5(4):309–19.
5. Albrecht J, Zielinska M, Norenberg MD. Glutamine as a mediator of ammonia neurotoxicity: a critical appraisal. Biochem Pharmacol. 2010;80(9):1303–8.
6. Dabrowska K, Skowronska K, Popek M, Obara-Michlewska M, Albrecht J, Zielinska M. Roles of glutamate and glutamine transport in ammonia neurotoxicity: state of the art and question marks. Endocr Metab Immune Disord Drug Targets. 2018;18(4):306–15.
7. Gropman AL, Batshaw ML. Cognitive outcome in urea cycle disorders. Mol Genet Metab. 2004;81 Suppl 1:S58–62.
8. Service HL, Hospital JH. The Harriet Lane handbook : a manual for pediatric house officers. 20th ed. Philadelphia: Saunders/Elsevier; 2015.

9. Ah Mew N, Krivitzky L, McCarter R, Batshaw M, Tuchman M, Urea Cycle Disorders Consortium of the Rare Diseases Clinical Research N. Clinical outcomes of neonatal onset proximal versus distal urea cycle disorders do not differ. J Pediatr. 2013;162(2):324–9 e1.
10. Ruegger CM, Lindner M, Ballhausen D, Baumgartner MR, Beblo S, Das A, et al. Cross-sectional observational study of 208 patients with non-classical urea cycle disorders. J Inherit Metab Dis. 2014;37(1):21–30.
11. Haberle J, Burlina A, Chakrapani A, Dixon M, Karall D, Lindner M, et al. Suggested guidelines for the diagnosis and management of urea cycle disorders: first revision. J Inherit Metab Dis. 2019;42(6):1192–230.
12. Gallagher RC, Lam C, Wong D, Cederbaum S, Sokol RJ. Significant hepatic involvement in patients with ornithine transcarbamylase deficiency. J Pediatr. 2014;164(4):720–5 e6.
13. Lefrere B, Ulmann G, Chartier M, Patkai J, Cynober L, Neveux N. Malnutrition with hypoaminoacidemia in a 22-year-old pregnant patient masking a likely ornithine transcarbamylase deficiency. Clin Nutr ESPEN. 2019;30:89–93.
14. Summar M, Tuchman M. Proceedings of a consensus conference for the management of patients with urea cycle disorders. J Pediatr. 2001;138(1 Suppl):S6–10.
15. Conway A. Ankyloglossia--to snip or not to snip: is that the question? J Hum Lact. 1990;6(3):101–2.
16. Summar ML, Dobbelaere D, Brusilow S, Lee B. Diagnosis, symptoms, frequency and mortality of 260 patients with urea cycle disorders from a 21-year, multicentre study of acute hyperammonaemic episodes. Acta Paediatr. 2008;97(10):1420–5.
17. Waisbren SE, Stefanatos AK, Kok TMY, Ozturk-Hismi B. Neuropsychological attributes of urea cycle disorders: a systematic review of the literature. J Inherit Metab Dis. 2019;42(6):1176–91.
18. Posset R, Garbade SF, Gleich F, Gropman AL, de Lonlay P, Hoffmann GF, et al. Long-term effects of medical management on growth and weight in individuals with urea cycle disorders. Sci Rep. 2020;10(1):11948.
19. Kido J, Nakamura K, Mitsubuchi H, Ohura T, Takayanagi M, Matsuo M, et al. Long-term outcome and intervention of urea cycle disorders in Japan. J Inherit Metab Dis. 2012;35(5):777–85.
20. Batshaw ML, Tuchman M, Summar M, Seminara J, Members of the Urea Cycle Disorders C. A longitudinal study of urea cycle disorders. Mol Genet Metab. 2014;113(1–2):127–30.
21. Gerstein MT, Markus AR, Gianattasio KZ, Le Mons C, Bartos J, Stevens DM, et al. Choosing between medical management and liver transplant in urea cycle disorders: a conceptual framework for parental treatment decision-making in rare disease. J Inherit Metab Dis. 2020;43(3):438–58.
22. Perito ER, Rhee S, Roberts JP, Rosenthal P. Pediatric liver transplantation for urea cycle disorders and organic acidemias: United Network for Organ Sharing data for 2002–2012. Liver Transpl. 2014;20(1):89–99.
23. Singh RH. Nutritional management of patients with urea cycle disorders. J Inherit Metab Dis. 2007;30(6):880–7.
24. Batshaw ML, MacArthur RB, Tuchman M. Alternative pathway therapy for urea cycle disorders: twenty years later. J Pediatr. 2001;138(1 Suppl):S46–54; discussion S-5.
25. Molema F, Gleich F, Burgard P, van der Ploeg AT, Summar ML, Chapman KA, et al. Evaluation of dietary treatment and amino acid supplementation in organic acidurias and urea-cycle disorders: on the basis of information from a European multicenter registry. J Inherit Metab Dis. 2019;42(6):1162–75.
26. Kenneson A, Singh RH. Presentation and management of N-acetylglutamate synthase deficiency: a review of the literature. Orphanet J Rare Dis. 2020;15(1):279.
27. Summar M. Current strategies for the management of neonatal urea cycle disorders. J Pediatr. 2001;138(1 Suppl):S30–9.
28. Macronutrients IoMUPo, Intakes IoMUSCotSEoDR. Dietary reference intakes for energy, carbohydrate, fiber, fat, fatty acids, cholesterol, protein, and amino acids. Washington, DC: National Academies Press; 2005. p. 1331.
29. Holliday MA, Segar WE. The maintenance need for water in parenteral fluid therapy. Pediatrics. 1957;19(5):823–32.
30. RH Singh. Nutritional management of urea cycle disorders- a practical reference for clinicians. 2014.
31. Joint WHOFAOUNUEC. Protein and amino acid requirements in human nutrition. World Health Organ Tech Rep Ser. 2007;935:1–265, back cover.
32. Adam S, Almeida MF, Assoun M, Baruteau J, Bernabei SM, Bigot S, et al. Dietary management of urea cycle disorders: European practice. Mol Genet Metab. 2013;110(4):439–45.
33. Adam S, Champion H, Daly A, Dawson S, Dixon M, Dunlop C, et al. Dietary management of urea cycle disorders: UK practice. J Hum Nutr Diet. 2012;25(4):398–404.
34. Singh RH, Rhead WJ, Smith W, Lee B, Sniderman King L, Summar M. Nutritional management of urea cycle disorders. Crit Care Clin. 2005;21(4 Suppl):S27–35.
35. Boneh A. Dietary protein in urea cycle defects: how much? Which? How? Mol Genet Metab. 2014;113(1–2):109–12.
36. Molema F, Gleich F, Burgard P, van der Ploeg AT, Summar ML, Chapman KA, et al. Decreased plasma l-arginine levels in organic acidurias (MMA and PA) and decreased plasma branched-chain amino acid levels in urea cycle disorders as a potential cause of growth retardation: options for treatment. Mol Genet Metab. 2019;126(4):397–405.
37. Delgado TC. Glutamate and GABA in appetite regulation. Front Endocrinol (Lausanne). 2013;4:103.
38. Mitchell S, Welch-Burke T, Dumitrescu L, Lomenick JP, Murdock DG, Crawford DC, et al. Peptide tyrosine tyrosine levels are increased in

patients with urea cycle disorders. Mol Genet Metab. 2012;106(1):39–42.
39. Gardeitchik T, Humphrey M, Nation J, Boneh A. Early clinical manifestations and eating patterns in patients with urea cycle disorders. J Pediatr. 2012;161(2):328–32.
40. Diaz GA, Krivitzky LS, Mokhtarani M, Rhead W, Bartley J, Feigenbaum A, et al. Ammonia control and neurocognitive outcome among urea cycle disorder patients treated with glycerol phenylbutyrate. Hepatology. 2013;57(6):2171–9.
41. Holecek M. Branched-chain amino acids and branched-chain keto acids in hyperammonemic states: metabolism and as supplements. Metabolites. 2020;10(8):324.
42. Haberle J. Role of carglumic acid in the treatment of acute hyperammonemia due to N-acetylglutamate synthase deficiency. Ther Clin Risk Manag. 2011;7:327–32.
43. Ah Mew N, Cnaan A, McCarter R, Choi H, Glass P, Rice K, et al. Conducting an investigator-initiated randomized double-blinded intervention trial in acute decompensation of inborn errors of metabolism: lessons from the N-Carbamylglutamate Consortium. Transl Sci Rare Dis. 2018;3(3–4):157–70.
44. Lichter-Konecki U, Caldovic L, Morizono H, Simpson K. Ornithine transcarbamylase deficiency. In: Adam MP, Ardinger HH, Pagon RA, Wallace SE, Bean LJH, Mirzaa G, et al., editors. Seattle (WA): University of Washington, Seattle 1993–2022. GeneReviews(R) [Internet].
45. Nagamani SC, Shchelochkov OA, Mullins MA, Carter S, Lanpher BC, Sun Q, et al. A randomized controlled trial to evaluate the effects of high-dose versus low-dose of arginine therapy on hepatic function tests in argininosuccinic aciduria. Mol Genet Metab. 2012;107(3):315–21.
46. Programs NECoM. Acute illness materials. Available from: https://www.newenglandconsortium.org/acute-illness.
47. MacLeod EL, Hall KD, McGuire PJ. Computational modeling to predict nitrogen balance during acute metabolic decompensation in patients with urea cycle disorders. J Inherit Metab Dis. 2016;39(1):17–24.
48. Brambilla A, Bianchi ML, Cancello R, Galimberti C, Gasperini S, Pretese R, et al. Resting energy expenditure in argininosuccinic aciduria and in other urea cycle disorders. J Inherit Metab Dis. 2019;42(6):1105–17.
49. Maranda B, Cousineau J, Allard P, Lambert M. False positives in plasma ammonia measurement and their clinical impact in a pediatric population. Clin Biochem. 2007;40(8):531–5.
50. Burrage LC, Jain M, Gandolfo L, Lee BH, Members of the Urea Cycle Disorders C, Nagamani SC. Sodium phenylbutyrate decreases plasma branched-chain amino acids in patients with urea cycle disorders. Mol Genet Metab. 2014;113(1–2):131–5.
51. Evans M, Truby H, Boneh A. The relationship between dietary intake, growth, and body composition in inborn errors of intermediary protein metabolism. J Pediatr. 2017;188:163–72.
52. Scaglia F. New insights in nutritional management and amino acid supplementation in urea cycle disorders. Mol Genet Metab. 2010;100 Suppl 1:S72–6.
53. Sun A, Crombez EA, Wong D. Arginase deficiency. In: Adam MP, Ardinger HH, Pagon RA, Wallace SE, Bean LJH, Mirzaa G, et al., editors. Seattle (WA): University of Washington, Seattle 1993-2022. GeneReviews (R) [Internet].
54. Jiang Y, Almannai M, Sutton VR, Sun Q, Elsea SH. Quantitation of phenylbutyrate metabolites by UPLC-MS/MS demonstrates inverse correlation of phenylacetate:phenylacetylglutamine ratio with plasma glutamine levels. Mol Genet Metab. 2017;122(3):39–45.
55. Silva ES, Cardoso ML, Vilarinho L, Medina M, Barbot C, Martins E. Liver transplantation prevents progressive neurological impairment in argininemia. JIMD Rep. 2013;11:25–30.
56. Kim IK, Niemi AK, Krueger C, Bonham CA, Concepcion W, Cowan TM, et al. Liver transplantation for urea cycle disorders in pediatric patients: a single-center experience. Pediatr Transplant. 2013;17(2):158–67.
57. Posset R, Gropman AL, Nagamani SCS, Burrage LC, Bedoyan JK, Wong D, et al. Impact of diagnosis and therapy on cognitive function in urea cycle disorders. Ann Neurol. 2019;86(1):116–28.
58. Ng VL, Alonso EM, Bucuvalas JC, Cohen G, Limbers CA, Varni JW, et al. Health status of children alive 10 years after pediatric liver transplantation performed in the US and Canada: report of the studies of pediatric liver transplantation experience. J Pediatr. 2012;160(5):820–6 e3.
59. Medicine USNLo. 2020. Available from: clinicaltrials.gov.

Nutrition Management of Maple Syrup Urine Disease

17

Sandy van Calcar

Contents

S. van Calcar (✉)
Oregon Health & Science University, Molecular and Medical Genetics, Portland, OR, USA
e-mail: vancalca@ohsu.edu

L. E. Bernstein et al. (eds.), *Nutrition Management of Inherited Metabolic Diseases*,
https://doi.org/10.1007/978-3-030-94510-7_17

Core Messages

- Maple Syrup Urine Disease (MSUD) is caused by a deficiency in the branched-chain ketoacid dehydrogenase enzyme complex that metabolizes the ketoacids of leucine, isoleucine and valine.
- Infants with classical MSUD can present with intoxication syndrome and require aggressive nutrition support to prevent or reverse catabolism.
- Nutrition management includes use of medical foods devoid of branched-chain amino acids, dietary leucine restriction, supplemental valine and isoleucine, and provision of adequate energy, protein, vitamins and minerals.
- The goal of therapy is to maintain plasma leucine concentrations of 100–200 μmol/L for infants and children <5 years and 100–300 μmol/L for those over 5 years of age.

17.1 Background

Maple Syrup Urine Disease (MSUD) is an inborn error of the branched-chain α-ketoacid dehydrogenase (BCKADH) enzyme complex required for the catabolism of the branched-chain amino acids (BCAA) leucine, valine, and isoleucine [1] (Fig. 17.1). MSUD is rare in the general population with an incidence of 1 in 200,000 live births, but in the Old Order Mennonite population, the incidence is approximately 1 in 350 live births due to a founder variant (c. 1312T > A) in the BCKADHA gene [2]. MSUD is so-named because patients with this disorder have a characteristic sweet odor detectable in the urine and cerumen.

Of the BCAA, leucine and its corresponding ketoacid, alpha-ketoisocaproic acid are the primary toxic compounds in this disorder. The pathophysiology of MSUD is not completely understood; however, all three BCAA share common transporters at the blood-brain barrier that have a higher affinity for leucine compared to other amino acids [3, 4]. In cerebral tissue, increased leucine leads to an underlying depletion of glutamate and increased

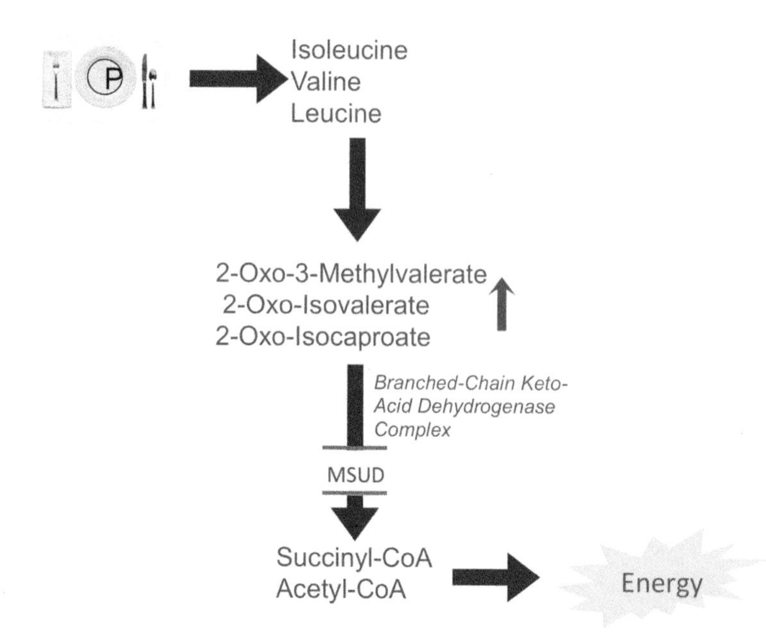

Fig. 17.1 Metabolic pathway in the metabolism of the branched-chain amino acids leucine, isoleucine, and valine

lactate concentrations. Glutamate is an excitatory neurotransmitter and depletion has been associated with learning and memory deficits, depression, and anxiety [5]. Additionally, elevated leucine in the brain alters water homeostasis, increases oxidative stress, and competes with entry of other amino acids into the central nervous system affecting protein signaling and production of other neurotransmitters [3, 6]. Elevated leucine increases renal sodium losses that can lead to hyponatremia and contribute to the development of cerebral edema [3]. Additionally, abnormal biomarkers of inflammation have been measured and may have a role in the pathophysiology [7].

Neonates with classical (severe) MSUD come to attention shortly after birth with poor feeding, weak suck, and weight loss, progressing to a metabolic intoxication crisis (Chap. 4). This is characterized by lethargy, irritability, vomiting, and fluctuating muscle tone. If the infant is not treated immediately, seizures, cerebral edema, and coma can be fatal [3, 4]. There are several classifications of disease severity, including classical (<2% enzyme activity) and intermediate, intermittent, and thiamin-responsive variants [1]. BCKADH is a thiamin-dependent enzyme and individuals with residual enzyme activity may benefit from thiamin supplementation, but those with classical MSUD do not. Nevertheless, a trial of thiamin is often completed (doses 50–200 mg/d for four weeks) to assess response [8]. Patients with variant forms of MSUD may present later in infancy or childhood with poor growth and developmental delay, or with nonspecific symptoms such as confusion, ataxia, or acute psychosis in older individuals [9]. Newborn screening identifies infants with high blood leucine, although those with classical MSUD can be symptomatic before newborn screening results are available, while those with variant forms may not be detected [9]. The diagnosis is based on clinical symptoms and a plasma amino acid profile with elevated concentrations of leucine, valine, and isoleucine and the presence of allo-isoleucine, a derivative of isoleucine that is a specific marker of MSUD [1]. Genetic testing can further confirm the diagnosis with predictive phenotype-genotype correlation [1, 10].

Nutrition management for MSUD has improved greatly (Box 17.1) and, with vigilant care, can result in good cognitive and developmental outcomes, especially if illnesses or other catabolic events are aggressively managed [11, 12]. Liver transplantation is an option for the treatment of this disorder [13].

Box 17.1: Principles of Nutrition Management for MSUD

Restrict:	Leucine
Supplement:	Valine and isoleucine, if plasma concentrations are low Thiamin[a]
Toxic metabolite:	Leucine and its keto-acid, alpha-ketoisocaproic acid

[a]A trial of 50–200 mg thiamin is given in some centers for patients with variant forms of MSUD

17.2 Nutrition Management

17.2.1 Chronic Nutrition Management

Patients who present with symptoms in the newborn period and have been medically stabilized, as well as those who are asymptomatic at diagnosis, are started on a leucine-restricted diet. Table 17.1 provides suggested goals for nutrient intakes for both symptomatic and asymptomatic infants with MSUD [4, 8, 14]. The source of intact protein to meet leucine needs can be provided by a standard infant formula; however,

Table 17.1 Suggested daily nutrient intakes for infants with classic MSUD during metabolic decompensation (initial presentation or when acutely ill) and when asymptomatic [8, 14]

	Acute [14]	Asymptomatic [8, 14]
Energy (kcal/kg)	120–140	100–120
Lipid (% of energy)	40–50%	DRI
Protein (g/kg)	3–4	2–3.5
Leucine (mg/kg)	0	40–100 mg/kg
Isoleucine (mg/kg)	80–120	30–95
Valine (mg/kg)	80–120	30–95

breast milk (mean leucine concentration of 1 mg/mL) can be considered if growth and monitoring parameters remain within goal and the mother's milk production remains adequate [8, 15].

The steps for initiating a diet in an infant with MSUD are outlined in Box 17.2.

Box 17.2: Initiating Nutrition Management of an Asymptomatic Infant with MSUD

Goal: Reduce or normalize plasma leucine.

Step-by-step:

1. Establish intake goals based on the infant's diagnostic plasma leucine level, clinical status and laboratory values.
2. Determine amount of standard infant formula or breast milk required to provide the infant's leucine needs. Determine the amount of protein and energy that will be provided by this amount of formula or breast milk.
3. Subtract the protein provided by the standard infant formula or breast milk from the infant's total protein needs.
4. Calculate the amount of BCAA-free medical food required to meet the remaining protein needs.
5. Calculate the amount of valine and isoleucine provided by the infant formula or breast milk. Determine the amount of supplemental valine and isoleucine to add to meet recommended intakes (Table 17.2). Provide valine and isoleucine in solutions of 10 mg/mL (1 g amino acid in 100 mL water).
6. Determine the number of calories provided by both the infant formula or breast milk and BCAA-free medical food. If more energy is required, provide the remaining calories from additional BCAA-free medical food. A protein-free energy module can be used if there is a concern about excessive protein intake.
7. Determine the amount of fluid required to provide a caloric density of 20–25 kcal/ounce.
8. Divide total volume into appropriate number of feedings over a 24-hour period.

Box 17.3: Recommendations for Adjusting the MSUD Diet Prescription

1. Estimate the increase or decrease in the intake of leucine, isoleucine and/or valine that will be needed to improve the plasma amino acid concentrations. Adjustments in 10% increments are typical but can be higher or lower based on BCAA concentrations.
2. Adjust the amount of infant formula or breast milk to increase or decrease leucine in the diet.
3. Recalculate the valine and isoleucine content provided by the revised amount of infant formula or breast milk.
4. Recalculate the amount of supplemental isoleucine and valine needed to meet your revised intake goals.
5. Recalculate the amount of MSUD medical food required to meet the energy goal.
6. Re-check plasma amino acid concentrations.

Once the diet has been established, adjustments in leucine, valine and isoleucine intakes should be based on blood BCAA concentrations rather than maintaining a specific mg/kg intake goal (Box 17.3). The amount of the BCAA required per kilogram of body weight decreases as the patient matures [8] (Table 17.2). Complementary feedings can be introduced to infants with MSUD at the typical age recommended for all infants, unless motor delays are present. To allow for solid food introduction, the volume of standard infant formula or breast milk is decreased and leucine from these sources is replaced with leucine from solid foods. High protein foods contain too much leucine to be incorporated into the diet in all but the mildest forms of MSUD. Foods with a moderate protein content such as starchy vegetables and regular grain products will provide the majority of leucine in the diet. Modified low protein foods made from wheat or other starch can be introduced to allow for a greater volume of food with a very low leucine content.

Table 17.2 Recommended daily nutrient intakes of BCAA, protein, and energy for individuals with MSUD when well [8, 15]

	Nutrient				
Age	LEU mg/kg	ILE mg/kg	VAL mg/kg	Protein g/kg	Energy kcal/kg
0–6 months	40–100	30–90	40–95	2.5–3.5	95–145
7–12 months	40–75	30–70	30–80	2.5–3.0	80–135
1–3 years	40–70	20–70	30–70	1.5–2.5	80–130
4–8 years	35–65	20–30	30–50	1.3–2.0	50–120
9–13 years	30–60	20–30	25–40	1.2–1.8	40–90
14–18 years	15–50	10–30	15–30	1.2–1.8	35–70
19 years +[a]	15–50	10–30	15–30	1.1–1.7	35–45

[a]Males and non-pregnant, non-lactating females

Box 17.4: Counting Leucine Intake in the MSUD Diet

Only dietary leucine must be counted

- The valine and isoleucine content of food is about half that of the leucine content.
- Patients will not consume too much valine and isoleucine if they meet their prescribed leucine intake.
- Each gram of protein contains approximately 60 mg leucine (Box 17.5).
- References listing the leucine content of foods and beverages are available.

Box 17.5: Estimated Leucine from the Protein Content of Foods

- Use serving size and grams of protein listed on "How Much Phe" or other resource.
- To estimate the leucine content:
  - Breads and cereals: 70 mg leucine/g protein
  - Vegetables: 50 mg leucine/g protein
  - Fruit: 40 mg leucine/g protein
  - Mixed foods: 60 mg leucine/g protein

In MSUD, only the leucine content of foods and beverages need to be counted (Box 17.4). There is no need for caregivers to calculate the valine and isoleucine content of foods. Unless there is a concern about low energy intake, caregivers do not need to count calories from foods or beverages since the medical food provides the majority of energy, especially for infants.

Resources are available to provide the leucine content of foods and beverages [16, 17] or the leucine content can be estimated from resources listing the protein content of foods, such as "How Much Phe" (howmuchphe.org). Low protein recipes from cookbooks/websites are available for MSUD; or resources for PKU can be adapted for MSUD by estimating the leucine content from the provided protein content (Box 17.5). For older individuals with MSUD, counting protein rather than leucine may be appropriate and easier for the patient, if metabolic control can be maintained with this less accurate method. Some clinics have adapted the "simplified diet" for PKU and successfully managed patients with MSUD using similar guidance (Chap. 10).

Medical Food For the great majority of individuals with MSUD, a medical food is required for life (Table 17.3). In patients with classical MSUD, medical foods provide up to 80–90% of protein needs and a majority of energy needs, especially in infancy.

Infants with MSUD are prescribed a complete medical food containing all amino acids except BCAA with a fat, carbohydrate, and micronutrient content similar to standard infant formulas. Toddlers and young children are transitioned to

Table 17.3 Selected medical foods for the treatment of MSUD

Infant/Toddler (complete[a])	Older Child/Adult (complete[a])	Older Child/Adult (incomplete[b])
Complex Essential MSD Mix[c] MSUD Anamix Early Years[c] Ketonex-1[d] Ketonex-2[d] BCAD-1[e] BCAD-2[e]	Complex Junior MSD Drink Mix[c] Ketonex-2[d] MSUD Lophlex LQ[c] BCAD-2[e] Vilactin AA Plus[f]	Complex MSD Amino Acid Blend[c] Camino Pro MSUD Drink[f] MSUD Maxamum[c] MSUD Gel[g] MSUD Cooler 15[g] MSUD Express[g]

Examples of medical foods available in the US (as of March 2021)
[a]Contains L-amino acids (without BCAA), as well as fat, carbohydrate, vitamins, and minerals
[b]Contains L-amino acids (without BCAA), but low in or devoid of fat, carbohydrate, vitamins, and/or minerals. See company websites for specific nutrient composition
[c]Nutricia North America (Rockville MD; nutricia-na.com)
[d]Abbott Nutrition (Columbus, OH; abbottnutrition.com)
[e]Mead Johnson Nutrition (Evansville, IN; meadjohnson.com)
[f]Cambrooke Therapeutics (Ayer, MA; cambrookefoods.com)
[g]Vitaflo USA (Alexandria, VA; vitaflousa.com)

complete medical foods designed for those over age 2 years that contain all amino acids except BCAA with age-appropriate fat, carbohydrate, and micronutrient profiles [18]. There are several other medical foods on the market, as well, including those more concentrated in amino acids with little or no fat and some with reduced carbohydrate content. These can decrease the amount of medical food required to meet an individual's protein needs and, thus, can be helpful if excess energy intake is a concern. However, decreasing energy from medical food may lead to excessive intake of leucine-containing foods or may decrease energy intake to a point that the individual is losing weight. Both of these situations can cause elevations in blood leucine. The vitamin and mineral content of medical foods vary. Intake needs to be assessed and supplemental vitamins and minerals provided, if necessary [8].

Isoleucine and valine supplements When leucine intake is reduced sufficiently to maintain leucine concentrations in the goal range, the plasma concentrations of isoleucine and valine may be lower than recommended and supplementation with either or both of these amino acids is often necessary, especially for those with classical MSUD [4, 8, 14, 15]. Without supplementation, deficiency of isoleucine can lead to skin lesions similar to that seen in acrodermatitis enteropathica [19, 20]. A 10% oral solution (10 mg/mL) of these amino acids can be made by dissolving 1 g of valine or isoleucine in 100 mL water. Maintaining plasma concentrations of 200–400 μmol/L for valine and 100–400 isoleucine is suggested to prevent deficiency [4, 8, 14]. Alternatively, some clinics prescribe medical foods designed for treatment of isovaleric acidemia that are devoid of leucine but contain valine and isoleucine (i.e., I-Valex®, Abbott Nutrition) for their patients with MSUD to avoid the need for valine or isoleucine supplements [21] although this may make it more difficult to individualize intake of these two amino acids.

17.2.2 Acute Nutrition Management

Symptomatic MSUD in a neonate is a medical emergency and requires the immediate initiation of medical and nutrition support to reverse catabolism [3, 4, 6, 8, 14, 15]. Additionally, individuals of any age are at risk for metabolic decompensation with any intercurrent illness or other stress leading to catabolism. During these episodes, altered mental status, ataxia, acute dystonia, and seizures can develop; progression to cerebral edema can be fatal [3, 4]. Families and individuals with MSUD should know the signs of metabolic decompensation and be provided with an emergency protocol that includes directions for both the family and for emergency personnel who may become involved in their care. Information for contacting the on-call metabolic physician must be included in any protocol.

There are many factors to consider during an illness and the entire metabolic team must be aware of the potential of an impending emergency. Often, a "sick-day" diet prescription is provided for use at the first sign of an illness [4, 8]. For minor illnesses, use of the sick-day diet may allow for management of the disorder on an outpatient basis, but many factors go into this decision, including age of the child, severity of MSUD (i.e., classical vs. variant MSUD), severity and length of illness, and ability of the family to manage a complicated protocol at home. Home monitoring with dinitrophenylhydrazine (DNPH) solution can be used as an immediate marker to assess diet modifications. DNPH specifically reacts with the α-ketoacids produced in MSUD and can be detected in urine [4]. If DNPH is not available, measuring urine ketones with Ketostix® can be a substitute. Although measuring urine ketones is not as specific as utilizing DNPH, ketones can be used as a marker of impending crisis [3]. Many clinics use ketone measurements to adjust at-home diet composition since the availability of DNPH is limited. Sick-day diets must be individualized for each patient and general guidelines for designing these diets are outlined (Box 17.6).

Box 17.6: Guidelines for Designing a "Sick-Day" Diet for Patients with MSUD

- The "sick-day" diet must provide enough energy to meet the individual's estimated requirement, which may be higher than their usual caloric intake.
- Increase protein equivalents by increasing medical food to approximately 120% of usual intake. This also supplies more energy from carbohydrate and/or fat.
- Decrease the leucine prescription. Remove 50–100% of usual leucine intake, depending on the degree of illness, for 24 hours and reassess with the medical team.
- Prevent low blood concentrations of isoleucine and valine. Provide the same amount of isoleucine and valine as in the patient's usual diet by supplementing with isoleucine and/or valine. Additional isoleucine and valine may be required to prevent low concentrations.
- Provide small, frequent feedings throughout a 24-hour period.
- Monitor plasma concentrations of the BCAA to guide appropriate diet adjustments.

There should be a low threshold when deciding if a patient's clinical condition warrants an emergency department visit or admission. Admissions require a medical team specialized in treating inborn errors of metabolism, access to frequent and rapid turnaround time for plasma amino acids, electrolytes, and other critical laboratory values [4, 8], as well as all components for providing the diet, including medical foods and specialized parenteral solutions, if necessary. General guidelines for nutrition management during hospital admissions are provided (Box 17.7). Promoting protein anabolism is key to reducing BCAA concentrations and requires an energy intake above maintenance requirements, removal or significant reduction in leucine intake, and prevention of valine and isoleucine deficiency. Non-protein calories are often provided by peripheral or central line access. An energy intake of 1.25–1.5 times the patient's estimated energy requirement (EER) is necessary from both dextrose (50–70% of calories) and lipids (30–50% of calories); however, energy needs may be as high as three times the EER, especially in older children and adults [4]. A continuous insulin infusion is often required to prevent hyperglycemia. Administration of excess fluid and use of hypotonic solutions needs to be avoided given the high risk of cerebral edema [3, 4].

To reduce the leucine concentration, a sufficient supply of all other amino acids, including valine and isoleucine, must be provided. A source of BCAA-free amino acids is needed as soon as possible to provide total protein equivalents of 2–3.5 g/kg in infants and greater than DRI needs for all ages [3, 4, 8]. Protein equivalent needs can be met with continuous nasogastric feedings of an MSUD medical food (0.7–1.2 kcal/mL at a rate of 30–60 mL/hour) with peripheral administration of dextrose and lipid solutions for addi-

Box 17.7: Management During Admission for Illness in MSUD

The initial treatment of intoxication syndrome is a medical emergency and is managed by the metabolic physician[a].

- Provide appropriate energy and leucine-free amino acid sources for acute illness from parenteral and/or enteral sources (Table 17.1).
- Maintain blood isoleucine and valine concentrations >200 µmol/L as leucine decreases. When anabolic, leucine can decrease very rapidly, and isoleucine and valine needs exceed the patient's usual isoleucine and valine tolerance.
- Reassess plasma amino acids every 12–24 hours, or as clinically indicated.
- Monitor electrolytes and fluid volume.
- Restart a source of leucine when plasma concentrations are <200 µmol/L in infants and children <5 years, and <300 µmol/L in those >5 years of age.
- Do not discharge patient until plasma leucine has decreased sufficiently, and patient is tolerating enteral feedings.

[a]Chapter 4 provides additional information for managing metabolic decompensation

tional energy [4]. However, if sufficient gastrointestinal administration of medical food is not possible, BCAA-free parenteral solutions can be obtained from specialty compounding pharmacies. During metabolic decompensation, blood concentrations of isoleucine and valine are typically lower than leucine. If the patient is only provided a BCAA-free medical food, concentrations of these two amino acids can become deficient before the leucine concentration normalizes. Supplementation of enteral or parenteral isoleucine and valine at 20–120 mg/kg/d is needed to maintain sufficiently elevated blood concentrations of 400–800 µmol/L for both amino acids to promote a rapid reduction in blood leucine [4, 8]. Sources of leucine are not added back into the diet until the leucine concentration decreases to at least the upper limit of the target range (200 µmol/L for infants and young children and 300 µmol/L for older individuals) [8, 22].

With aggressive management during a metabolic crisis, the leucine concentration can be expected to decrease by 50% after 24 hours [6, 8, 22], or at a rate of 500–1000 µmol/L per day [4]. A slower rate of decrease in leucine concentration is noted during admissions with infection or illness compared to the decrease in leucine when the patient is admitted because of inadequate dietary adherence [22].

Finally, caregivers and individuals with MSUD need to be aware that metabolic decompensation can be precipitated by events other than illness – significant injury and surgery are also catabolic events that need attention from the metabolic team. For surgical procedures, reducing the fasting time by providing an energy source (i.e., IV dextrose) during and after the procedure until oral intake can be restarted is often necessary [3, 6].

17.3 Monitoring

In addition to frequent monitoring of BCAA concentrations, a complete amino acid profile should be periodically evaluated. It is best to collect blood samples at a consistent time during the day, either after an overnight fast or approximately 2–3 hours after a meal [4, 8]. Table 17.4 provides recommended blood BCAA concentrations for healthy individuals with MSUD [4, 8]. Home collection of dried blood spots for monitoring BCAA and other amino acids allows for an increased frequency of monitoring that positively correlates with improved metabolic control [23].

Table 17.4 Recommended blood BCAA concentrations in MSUD [4, 8]

	µmol/L	mg/dL	Normal (µmol/L)
Leucine: < 5 years	100–200[a]	1.3-2.6	50–215
Leucine: > 5 years	100–300	1.3–3.9	
Valine	200–400	2.3–4.6	85–200
Isoleucine	100–300	1.3–3.9	25–90

[a]Recommended maximum blood concentration is 200 µmol/L for infants and children <5 years of age and 300 µmol/L for those >5 years of age

If leucine concentrations are elevated with routine monitoring, but the patient is not exhibiting signs of illness or other stress, there are several parameters to consider:

Evaluate energy intake Significant weight loss may increase BCAA concentrations due to catabolism. Increasing energy intake from medical food promotes weight gain (or maintenance in older patients) and also helps to reduce hunger so the individual may be less tempted to consume more leucine than prescribed. If a low fat or protein-concentrated medical food is prescribed, consider addition of a product with a greater calorie to protein ratio.

Evaluate the distribution of medical food throughout the day As in PKU, medical food distributed in 3 or 4 servings per day and given with a source of leucine at the same time will result in better utilization of BCAA and, thus, lower and more consistent leucine concentrations (Chap. 6).

Consider recommending additional protein equivalents from medical food Given the rapid oxidation of amino acids compared to intact protein sources, protein requirements for patients with metabolic disorders are often higher than recommended for the general population (Chap. 6). If excess energy intake is a concern, adding a low/no fat medical food concentrated in protein equivalents can increase total protein without significantly increasing energy intake from the medical food.

With your metabolic team, consider the possibility of a hidden illness, infection, or other catabolic stressors Urinary tract infections, sinus infections, or dental problems often increase leucine concentrations but may not be clinically obvious to the patient. Because of hormonal effects on protein metabolism, some women with MSUD have higher leucine concentrations just before menstruation [11]. Reduction in the leucine prescription and additional energy sources may be needed during these times.

Evaluate the amount of isoleucine and valine supplements added to the diet In the plasma amino acid profile, aim to maintain a 1 to 1 ratio of isoleucine to leucine concentrations, and at least a 2 to 1 ratio of valine to leucine concentrations [4]. If low concentrations of valine and/or isoleucine are found, increase the amount of supplements (10 mg/mL) to improve blood concentrations and normalize the ratios between the BCAA.

Box 17.8: Considerations if Plasma Leucine Concentrations Are Elevated (Without Signs of Illness or Stress)

1. Is the patient consuming sufficient energy?
2. Is all the medical food being consumed and distributed throughout the day?
3. Is protein intake from the medical food too low?
4. Are there hidden illnesses or infections?
5. Are blood concentrations of valine and/or isoleucine too low?
6. Is the patient taking the prescribed amount of leucine?
7. Is a decrease in the leucine prescription required?

Consider decreasing the patient's leucine prescription First, determine if the patient is taking the prescribed amount of leucine. Inadequate adherence to the diet regimen, especially "guessing" portion sizes, can lead to chronically elevated leucine concentrations. Typically, decreasing the leucine prescription is the last diet component to adjust since leucine tolerance is relatively constant throughout the lifespan. However, during periods of slowed growth, such as late infancy or late adolescence, a decrease in the prescribed amount of leucine may be needed. Assuring adequate energy intake is crucial when decreasing leucine in the diet prescription (Box 17.8).

Other laboratory parameters also need to be considered for diet monitoring (Box 17.9).

17.4 Transplantation

Liver transplantation is a treatment option for patients with MSUD to significantly decrease their risk of developing cerebral edema and other complications associated with high leucine con-

Box 17.9: Nutrition Monitoring of a Patient with MSUD[a]

- Routine assessments including anthropometrics, dietary intake, physical findings
- Laboratory Monitoring
  - Diagnosis-specific
    - Plasma amino acids
      - Leucine
      - Valine
      - Isoleucine
  - Nutrition-related laboratory monitoring of patients on BCAA-restricted diets may include markers of:
    - Protein sufficiency (plasma amino acids, prealbumin)
    - Nutritional anemia (hemoglobin, hematocrit, MCV, serum vitamin B12 and/or methylmalonic acid, total homocysteine, ferritin, iron, folate, total iron binding capacity)
    - Vitamin and mineral status (total 25-hydroxyvitamin D, zinc, trace minerals)
    - Others, as clinically indicated

[a]Suggested frequency of monitoring can be found in the GMDI/SERN MSUD Guidelines [15] (southeastgenetics.org/ngp)

centrations during illness or other catabolic stress [13, 24]. Liver transplantation restores 9–13% of whole-body BCKADH activity in the patient with MSUD, which is sufficient to allow for a diet without protein restriction or medical food. After transplantation, episodes of metabolic decompensation rarely occur, although there are two reports of decompensation in transplanted patients [25, 26]. Plasma BCAA concentrations range from 1.5 to 2 times normal during intercurrent catabolic stress. Long-term cognitive and adaptive functioning remains steady, or improves in some, following transplant [27, 28]. Since BCKADH activity is not found solely in the liver but is also active in muscle, heart, kidney, brain, and other tissues, a liver that is removed from a patient with MSUD can be donated to a recipient without MSUD in a domino liver transplant [25].

The goal of nutrition management for liver transplantation is to maintain good metabolic control prior to the surgery and prevent decompensation with administration of IV dextrose during pre-surgical fasting and the surgical procedure. The diet can be advanced to an unrestricted diet following the transplant [8]. Outcomes in liver transplantation for MSUD have been good. In 54 patients with MSUD who received a liver transplant, the overall survival rate was 98–100% [24]. After transplantation, patients tolerate unrestricted diets and have stable plasma BCAA concentrations [13]. However, studies have found that patients do not gain significant improvement in cognitive scores after transplant compared to their pre-transplant intelligence scores (mean IQ 78+/-24), although many of these patients had cognitive impairment prior to transplantation. Thus, for young patients with severe MSUD, undergoing a transplant early in life before brain damage is sustained is a viable treatment option [13, 24].

17.5 Summary

Early identification, aggressive treatment during catabolic events, and diligent nutrition management with frequent monitoring can result in positive outcomes for patients with MSUD. Treatment includes restricting BCAA with the use of medical foods, intact protein restriction, and isoleucine and valine supplementation, as needed, to maintain plasma BCAA concentrations in the target ranges. Regardless of the patient's age, acute metabolic decompensation in MSUD remains life-threatening and should be treated as a medical emergency with rapid, aggressive management to reverse catabolism. Liver transplantation is a viable option to prevent episodes of decomposition and allows for a diet without medical food and protein restriction.

17.6 Diet Calculation Example

17.6.1 MSUD Diet Calculation Example Using Standard Infant Formula as the Source of Leucine and Intact Protein

Patient Information	Nutrient intake goals (per day) (Table 17.5)
Weight: 4 kg Age: 8 days This patient presents asymptomatically. Plasma leucine concentration is 600 μmol/L, isoleucine is 80 μmol/L and valine is 180 μmol/L. Since this patient is asymptomatic with a relatively low leucine concentration, recommend leucine at the higher end of range	Leucine (LEU): 90 mg/kg (Range 40–100 mg/kg) Isoleucine (ILE): 50 mg/kg (Range 30–95 mg/kg) Valine (VAL): 50 mg/kg (Range 30–95 mg/kg) Protein: 3.0 g/kg (Range 2–3.5 g/kg) Energy: 100–120 kcal/kg Fluid: 150 mL/kg

Table 17.5 Selected Nutrient Composition of Formulas for MSUD Diet Calculation Using a Standard Infant Formula as the Source of Intact Protein

Medical Food	Amount	LEU (mg)	VAL (mg)	ILE (mg)	Protein (g)	Energy (kcal)
Anamix MSUD Early Years[a]	100 g	0	0	0	13.5	473
Enfamil Premium Newborn powder[b]	100 g	1250	640	640	10.8	510

[a] Nutricia North America (Rockville, MD)
[b] Mead Johnson Nutrition (Evansville, IN)
Note: Check manufacturer's website for the most up-to-date nutrient composition

Step-by-Step Calculation

Step 1 Calculate the infant's nutrient needs

Nutrient goal/kg × Infant weight
LEU: 90 mg LEU/kg × 4 kg = 360 mg/day
ILE: 50 mg/kg × 4 kg = 200 mg
VAL: 50 mg/kg × 4 kg = 200 mg
Protein: 3.0 g/kg protein × 4 kg = 12 g total protein
Energy: 110–120 kcal/kg × 4 kg = 440–480 kcal
Fluid: 150 mL × 4 kg = 600 mL (20 fluid ounces)

Step 2 Calculate the amount of standard infant formula needed to meet daily LEU requirement.

Amount of LEU required per day ÷ amount of LEU in 100 g of standard formula

$$360\,\text{mg}\,LEU \div 1250\,\text{mg}\,LEU = 0.29$$

$$0.29 \times 100 = 29\,\text{g Enfamil Premium needed to meet daily}\ LEU\ \text{requirement.}$$

Step 3 Calculate protein provided from the standard infant formula.

Amount of standard formula × amount of protein provided in 100 g of standard formula

$$0.29 \times 10.8\,\text{g protein in}\,100\,\text{g Enfamil} = 3.1\,\text{g protein from Enfamil}$$

Step 4 Determine the remaining amount of protein to be provided from BCAA-free medical food to meet the total protein prescription.

$$\text{Total protein needs} - \text{protein from standard formula} = \text{protein needed from medical food}$$

$$12\,\text{g} - 3.1\,\text{g}\,(\text{from Enfamil}) = 8.9\,\text{g protein needed from medical food}$$

Step 5 Calculate the amount of BCAA-free medical food needed to provide 8.9 g protein.

Protein needed to fill diet prescription ÷ protein provided in 100 g of medical food

$$8.9\ \text{g protein needed} \div 13\ \text{g protein in}100\ \text{g Anamix MSUD Early Years} = 0.68$$

$$0.68 \times 100 = 68\ \text{g Anamix MSUD Early Years required in the diet prescription}$$

Step 6 Calculate the amount of isoleucine and valine provided from standard infant formula (note no ILE or VAL in BCAA-free medical food)

Amount of standard formula × ILE in 100 g of standard formula

$$0.29(\text{Enfamil}) \times 640\,\text{mg}\,ILE = 186\,\text{mg}\,ILE$$

Amount of standard formula × VAL in 100 g of standard formula

$$0.29(\text{Enfamil}) \times 640\,\text{mg}\,VAL = 186\,\text{mg}\,VAL$$

Step 7 Calculate the remaining amount of ILE and VAL to be provided by supplements to meet requirements determined in step 1 (Goal minus amount in Enfamil)

$$ILE : 200\,\text{mg} - 186\,\text{mg} = 14\,\text{mg}\,ILE\ \text{to be provided}\ by\ ILE\ \text{supplement}$$

$$VAL : 200\,\text{mg} - 186\,\text{mg} = 14\,\text{mg}\,VAL\ \text{to be provided}\ by\ VAL\ \text{supplement}$$

Step 8 Determine how much amino acid solution is needed to provide remaining ILE and VAL.

Use amino acid solutions containing 10 mg/mL. This is made by adding 1 gram of amino acid (ILE or VAL) powder and adding water to make total volume of 100 mL

(This is equivalent to 1000 mg VAL or 1000 mg ILE in 100 mL = 10 mg/mL)

14 mg ILE divided by 10 mg/mL = 1.4 mL ILE solution (containing 10 mg/mL)

14 mg VAL divided by 10 mg/mL = 1.4 mL VAL solution (containing 10 mg/mL)

Round up to 2 ml of each solution.

Step 9 Calculate total energy provided from standard infant formula and BCAA-free medical food.

Amount of standard infant formula × kcal in 100 g of standard formula.

$$0.29(\text{Enfamil}) \times 510\,\text{kcal} = 148\,\text{kcal}$$

Amount of BCAA-free medical food × kcal of 100 g of BCAA-free medical food.

$$0.68\,(\text{Anamix MSUD Early Years}) \times 473\ \text{kcal} = 322\ \text{kcal}$$

Add standard formula + BCAA-free medical food for total kcal provided in diet prescription.

$$148\ \text{kcal} + 322\ \text{kcal} = 470\ \text{kcal}$$

Step 10 Calculate the final volume of the formula to make a formula concentration of 20–25 kcal per ounce (Table 17.6).

470 kcal ÷ 20 kcal/ounce = 23.5 ounces of formula (round to 24 ounces)

470 kcal ÷ 25 kcal/ounce = 18.8 ounces of formula (round to 19 ounces)

19–24 ounces meets the initial fluid goal of 600 mL (20 ounces)

(The volume prescribed will depend on infant's usual intake and growth)

Table 17.6 Diet Prescription Summary for Sample Calculation of MSUD Diet Using Standard Infant Formula as the Source of Intact Protein[a]

Medical Food	Amount	LEU (mg)	VAL (mg)	ILE (mg)	Protein (g)	Energy (kcal)
Anamix MSUD Early Years[b]	68 g	0	0	0	9.0	322
Enfamil Premium powder[c]	29 g	362	186	186	3.1	148
ILE Supplement	2 mL[d]			20		
VAL Supplement	2 mL[d]		20		–	
Total per day		362	206	206	12.1	470
Total per kg		90 mg/kg	52 mg/kg	52 mg/kg	3.0 g/kg	118 kcal/kg

[a]Rounded to nearest whole number for amount of formula powders, leucine, isoleucine, valine, and energy and to the nearest 0.1 g for protein

[b] Nutricia North America (Rockville, MD)

[c] Mead Johnson Nutrition (Evansville IN)

[d]Amino acid solution containing 10 mg/mL

References

1. Strauss KA, Puffenberger EG, Carson VJ. Maple syrup urine disease. In: Adam MP, Ardinger HH, Pagon RA, Wallace SE, Bean LJH, Mirzaa G, et al., editors. GeneReviews. Seattle: University of Washington; 1993–2021. Updated 2020, Apr 23.
2. Chapman KA, Gramer G, Vial S, Summar ML. Incidence of maple syrup urine disease, propionic acidemia, and methylmalonic aciduria from newborn screening data. Mol Genet Metab Rep. 2018;15:106–9.
3. Rodan LH, Aldubayan SH, Berry GT, Levy HL. Acute illness protocol for maple syrup urine disease. Pediatr Emerg Care. 2018;34(1):64–7.
4. Strauss KA, Carson VJ, Soltys K, Young ME, Bowser LE, Puffenberger EG, et al. Branched-chain alphaketoacid dehydrogenase deficiency (maple syrup urine disease): treatment, biomarkers, and outcomes. Mol Genet Metab. 2020;129(3):193–206.
5. Xu J, Jakher Y, Ahrens-Nicklas RC. Brain branched-chain amino acids in maple syrup urine disease: implications for neurological disorders. Int J Mol Sci. 2020;21(20):7490.
6. Blackburn PR, Gass JM, Vairo FPE, Farnham KM, Atwal HK, Macklin S, et al. Maple syrup urine disease: mechanisms and management. Appl Clin Genet. 2017;10:57–66.
7. Scaini G, Tonon T, Moura de Souza CF, Schuck PF, Ferreira GC, Quevedo J, et al. Evaluation of plasma biomarkers of inflammation in patients with maple syrup urine disease. J Inherit Metab Dis. 2018;41(4):631–40.
8. Frazier DM, Allgeier C, Homer C, Marriage BJ, Ogata B, Rohr F, et al. Nutrition management guideline for maple syrup urine disease: an evidence- and consensus-based approach. Mol Genet Metab. 2014;112(3):210–7.
9. Pode-Shakked N, Korman SH, Pode-Shakked B, Landau Y, Kneller K, Abraham S, et al. Clues and challenges in the diagnosis of intermittent maple syrup urine disease. Eur J Med Genet. 2020;63(6):103901.
10. Khalifa OA, Imtiaz F, Ramzan K, Zaki O, Gamal R, Elbaik L, et al. Genotype-phenotype correlation of 33 patients with maple syrup urine disease. Am J Med Genet A. 2020;182(11):2486–500.
11. Abi-Warde MT, Roda C, Arnoux JB, Servais A, Habarou F, Brassier A, et al. Long-term metabolic follow-up and clinical outcome of 35 patients with maple syrup urine disease. J Inherit Metab Dis. 2017;40(6):783–92.
12. Kenneson A, Osara Y, Pringle T, Youngborg L, Singh RH. Natural history of children and adults with maple syrup urine disease in the NBS-MSUD connect registry. Mol Genet Metab Rep. 2018;15:22–7.
13. Diaz VM, Camarena C, de la Vega A, Martinez-Pardo M, Diaz C, Lopez M, et al. Liver transplantation for classical maple syrup urine disease: long-term follow-up. J Pediatr Gastroenterol Nutr. 2014;59(5):636–9.
14. Morton DH, Strauss KA, Robinson DL, Puffenberger EG, Kelley RI. Diagnosis and treatment of maple syrup disease: a study of 36 patients. Pediatrics. 2002;109(6):999–1008.
15. GMDI-SERN. Nutrition Management Guideline for MSUD, 2014. Available from: https://southeastgenetics.org/ngp/guidelines-msud/php.
16. Singh R. MSUD food list. Atlanta: Emory University, Department of Human Genetics; 2008.
17. Genetic Metabolic Dietitians International. Leucine and protein content of foods appropriate for individuals on a leucine-restricted diet. 2013. Available from: https://www.gmdi.org/resources/leucine-and-protein-content-of-foods.
18. Strauss KA, Wardley B, Robinson D, Hendrickson C, Rider NL, Puffenberger EG, et al. Classical maple syrup urine disease and brain development: principles of management and formula design. Mol Genet Metab. 2010;99(4):333–45.
19. Flores K, Chikowski R, Morrell DS. Acrodermatitis dysmetabolica in an infant with maple syrup urine disease. Clin Exp Dermatol. 2016;41(6):651–4.
20. Dominguez-Cruz JJ, Bueno-Delgado M, Pereyra J, Bernabeu-Wittel J, Conejo-Mir J. Acrodermatitis enteropathica-like skin lesions secondary to isoleucine deficiency. Eur J Dermatol. 2011;21(1):115–6.
21. Sowa M. Personal communication. Orange CA: Children's Hospital of Orange County; 2020.
22. Scott AI, Cusmano-Ozog K, Enns GM, Cowan TM. Correction of hyperleucinemia in MSUD patients on leucine-free dietary therapy. Mol Genet Metab. 2017;122(4):156–9.
23. Kaur J, Nagy L, Wan B, Saleh H, Schulze A, Raiman J, et al. The utility of dried blood spot monitoring of branched-chain amino acids for maple syrup urine disease: a retrospective chart review study. Clin Chim Acta. 2020;500:195–201.
24. Mazariegos GV, Morton DH, Sindhi R, Soltys K, Nayyar N, Bond G, et al. Liver transplantation for classical maple syrup urine disease: long-term follow-up in 37 patients and comparative united network for organ sharing experience. J Pediatr. 2012;160(1):116–21 e1.
25. Feier F, Schwartz IV, Benkert AR, Seda Neto J, Miura I, Chapchap P, et al. Living related versus deceased donor liver transplantation for maple syrup urine disease. Mol Genet Metab. 2016;117(3):336–43.
26. Al-Shamsi A, Baker A, Dhawan A, Hertecant J. Acute metabolic crises in maple syrup urine disease after liver transplantation from a related heterozygous living donor. JIMD Rep. 2016;30:59–62.
27. Muelly ER, Moore GJ, Bunce SC, Mack J, Bigler DC, Morton DH, et al. Biochemical correlates of neuropsychiatric illness in maple syrup urine disease. J Clin Invest. 2013;123(4):1809–20.
28. Shellmer DA, DeVito Dabbs A, Dew MA, Noll RB, Feldman H, Strauss KA, et al. Cognitive and adaptive functioning after liver transplantation for maple syrup urine disease: a case series. Pediatr Transplant. 2011;15(1):58–64.

Part III

Organic Acidemias

Organic Acidemias

18

Janet A. Thomas

Contents

J. A. Thomas (✉)
Department of Pediatrics, Section of Clinical Genetics and Metabolism, University of Colorado School of Medicine, Aurora, CO, USA
e-mail: janet.thomas@childrenscolorado.org

L. E. Bernstein et al. (eds.), *Nutrition Management of Inherited Metabolic Diseases*,
https://doi.org/10.1007/978-3-030-94510-7_18

Core Messages

- Organic acidemias (OA) are defects in the degradation of leucine, isoleucine, and valine.
- OA can present as either a severe neonatal onset form (poor feeding, vomiting, lethargy, tachypnea, progressing to acidosis, respiratory distress, coma, death) or late-onset (usually recurrent ketoacidosis or lethargy with catabolic stress).
- Nutrition treatment involves use of propiogenic amino acid free medical foods and restriction of natural protein in PROP and MMA and protein restriction with or without leucine-free medical food and supplemental glycine in IVA.
- Outcomes in PROP and MMA have been guarded with frequent neurological complications, renal dysfunction, cardiomyopathy and optic atrophy but are improving with earlier identification and treatment, as well as with liver or liver-kidney transplantation; outcomes in IVA are often normal.

18.1 Background

Organic acidemias are disorders of branched chain amino metabolism in which non-amino organic acids accumulate in serum and urine. They are defects in the degradation pathways of leucine, isoleucine, and valine. These conditions are usually diagnosed by examining organic acids in urine with abnormal metabolites also notable on acylcarnitine profile. Organic acidemias comprise a variety of disorders and include methylmalonic acidemia (MMA), propionic acidemia (PROP), isovaleric acidemia (IVA), glutaric acidemia, type 1 (GA-1), 3- methylcrotonyl carboxylase deficiency (3-MCC), 3-methylglutaconic acidemia (3-MGA), methylmalonyl-CoA epimerase deficiency (MCEE), and vitamin B_{12} uptake, transport, and synthesis defects [1–3].

All are autosomal recessive with the exception of the rare, x-linked disorder, 2-methyl-3-hydroxybutyryl-CoA dehydrogenase deficiency (MHBD). The two primary disorders of isoleucine and valine catabolism are propionic acidemia (PROP) and methylmalonic acidemia (MMA) and the primary organic acidemia of leucine catabolism is isovaleric acidemia (IVA). These three disorders will be discussed in detail in this chapter. GA-1 is addressed in Chaps. 19 and 20. The incidence of MMA ranges from 1:83,000 in Quebec to 1:115,000 in Italy to 1:169,000 in Germany and that of PROP from 1:17,400 in Japan to 1:165,000 in Italy to 1:277,000 in Germany [4–7]. On the basis of newborn screening data, the incidence of IVA has a range of 1:62,500 live births in Germany to ~1:250,000 in the United States [7, 8]. Newborn screening via tandem mass spectrometry has allowed earlier diagnosis and has revealed a higher incidence of these disorders than previously noted based on clinical presentation suggesting a broader phenotype with milder and/or asymptomatic individuals [4, 5, 7, 9–13]. Techniques for newborn screening continue to be refined to aid in increased sensitivity and specificity of screening [14, 15].

The oxidation of threonine, valine, methionine, and isoleucine results in propionyl-CoA, which propionyl-CoA carboxylase converts into L-methylmalonyl-CoA, which is metabolized through methylmalonyl-CoA mutase to succinyl-CoA. Whereas the breakdown of the above amino acids is felt to contribute to ~50% of the propionyl-CoA production, gut bacteria and the breakdown of odd-chain-length fatty acids also substantially contribute to propionyl-CoA production (~ 25% each) with a minimal contribution by cholesterol metabolism [16–19] (Fig. 18.1).

PROP is caused by a deficiency of the mitochondrial enzyme, propionyl-CoA carboxylase (PCC) [9, 19]. The enzyme is composed of two subunits, an alpha and beta subunit, each encoded by a different gene, *PCCA* and *PCCB*, respectively [9]. The enzyme is biotin-dependent with biotin binding to the alpha subunit [19, 20]. Deficiency of the enzyme results in the accumulation of propionyl-CoA and increased concentrations of free propionate in blood and urine. Identification of methylcitrate and 3-hydroxypropionate are the major diagnostic metabolites seen on organic acid analysis [19,

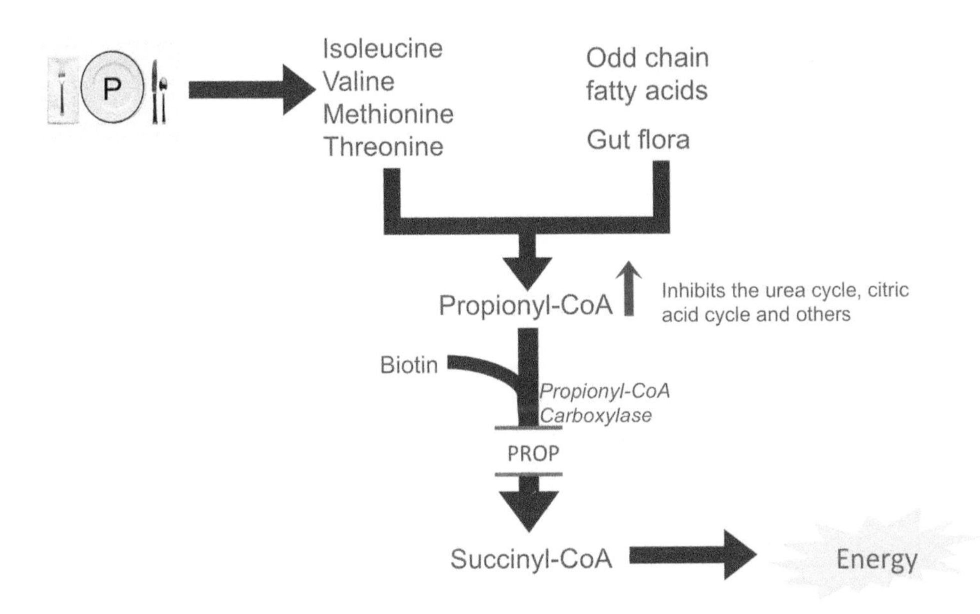

Fig. 18.1 Metabolic pathway of propionic acidemia (PROP)

21]. Elevation of propionylcarnitine (C3) can be seen on acylcarnitine profile [9, 21].

Classic MMA is caused by a deficiency of the enzyme, methylmalonyl-CoA mutase, an adenosylcobalamin (AdoCbl)-dependent enzyme consisting of two identical subunits (2α) [9, 19, 21] (Fig. 18.2). About 50% of cases of MMA are due to a defect in the mutase apoenzyme; in others, it is due to a defect in the uptake, transport, or synthesis of its adenosyl-B_{12} coenzyme causing variant forms of MMA that may or may not be associated with homocystinuria. Individuals who are deficient in mutase activity may be further designated as mut^- or mut^0 pending residual enzyme activity [19]. There is good correlation between residual enzyme activity and severity of the clinical phenotype [21]. Acquired methylmalonic aciduria can also be seen with acquired deficiency of vitamin B_{12} in pernicious anemia and in transcobalamin II deficiency [9]. Hence, vitamin B_{12} deficiency must be excluded in all individuals with elevated methylmalonic acid concentrations [9, 19]. Deficiency of the mutase enzyme results in the accumulation of methylmalonyl-CoA and propionyl-CoA and is reflected in elevations of methylmalonic acid and propionic acid in blood and urine [19, 21]. Methylmalonic acid, methylcitrate, 3-hydroxypropionate, and 3-hydroxyisovalerate are found on urine organic acid analysis [9, 19, 21]. Propionylcarnitine (C3) is also found on acylcarnitine profile in MMA [9, 21].

IVA was initially described in 1966 and was the first organic acidemia described. IVA is caused by a deficiency of the enzyme, isovaleryl-CoA dehydrogenase, an enzyme important in leucine catabolism and also important in the transfer of electrons to the respiratory chain [9, 19]. The consequent accumulating metabolites include isovaleric acid, isovalerylglycine, 3-hydroxyisovaleric acid, and isovalerylcarnitine (C5) [9, 19] (Fig. 18.3). These are easily identified on urine organic acid analysis and the

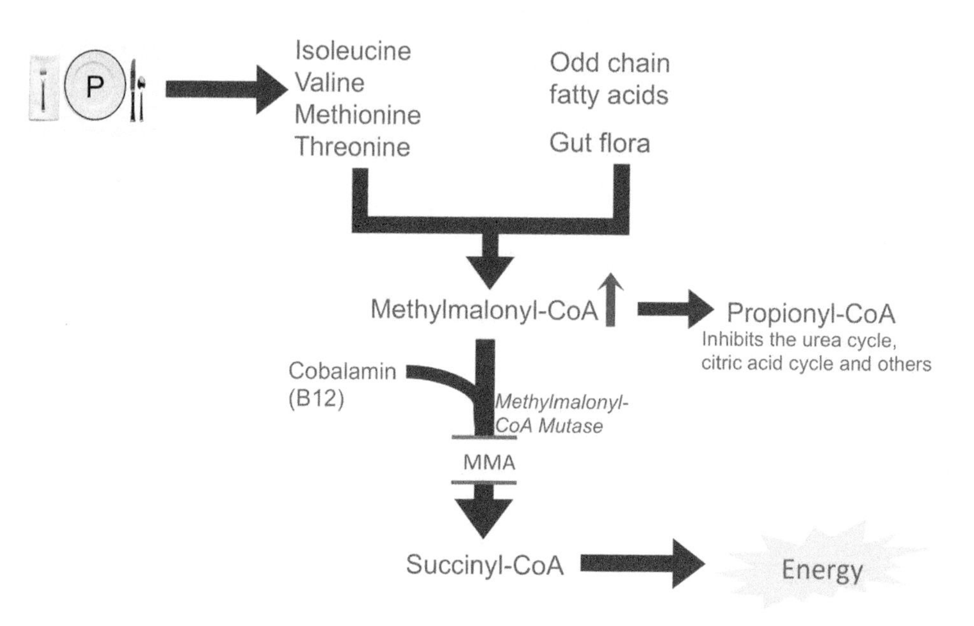

Fig. 18.2 Metabolic pathway of methylmalonic scidemia (MMA)

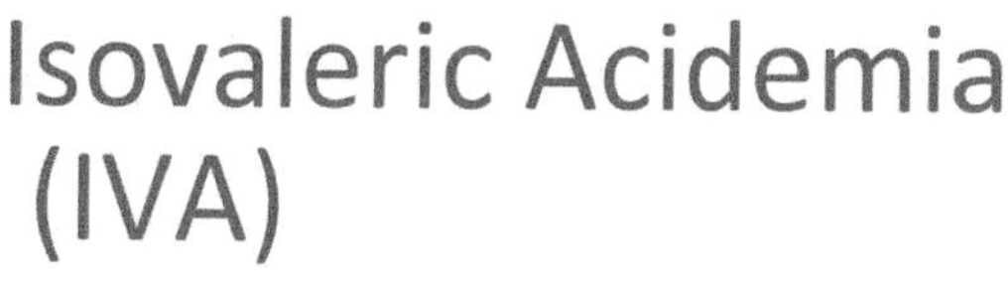

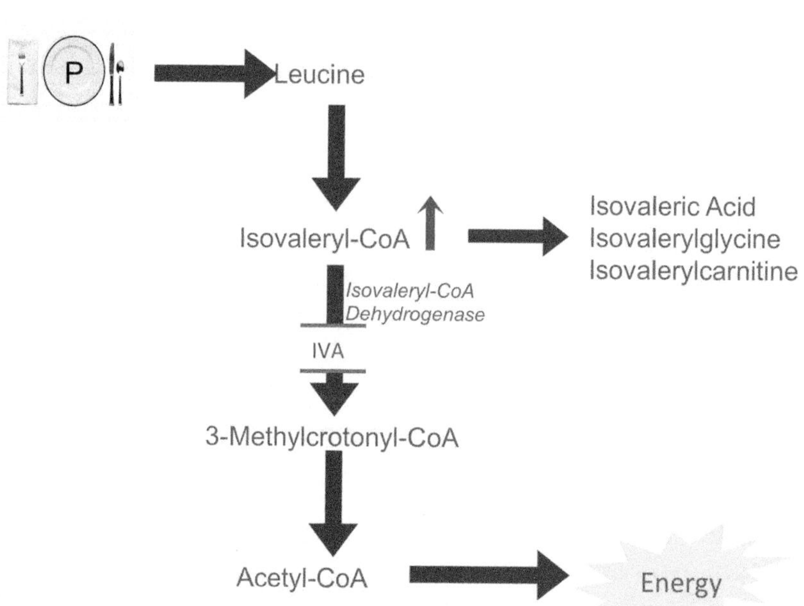

Fig. 18.3 Metabolic pathway of isovaleric acidemia (IVA)

latter on acylcarnitine profile. The excretion of isovalerylglycine and 3-hydroxyisovaleric acid are diagnostic.

18.2 Clinical Presentation

Organic acidemias may present at any age. In general, they can be divided into two broad groups—a severe, neonatal presentation and a chronic late-onset presentation.

18.2.1 Severe Neonatal Onset Form

The clinical presentation of the severe, neonatal onset form of these disorders can be quite similar for all three disorders. As is typical with inborn errors of metabolism, the pregnancy and birth history for the child is often unremarkable. Following an initial symptom-free period which may last from hours to weeks, the infant then develops nonspecific symptoms, such as poor feeding, vomiting, dehydration, lethargy, tachypnea, and hypothermia and if unrecognized, quickly progresses to respiratory distress, apnea, bradycardia, coma, cerebral edema, and death [9, 13, 16, 19, 21]. Despite newborn screening, many children are critically ill at the time of initial presentation [13]. At the time of presentation, the physical examination is primarily one of altered mental status and encephalopathy, but dehydration, hepatomegaly, abnormal tone, and seizure-like activity may also be seen [9, 13, 16, 19]. A sweaty feet or dirty sock smell is classically described for IVA secondary to excretion of 3-hydroxyisovaleric acid [9–11]. An antenatal presentation of PROP with nephromegaly and acute neonatal kidney injury has also been reported [22].

18.2.2 Chronic Late Onset Form

The late onset form typically presents after 30 days of age and maybe much later including into adolescence or adulthood [19]. McCrory et al. noted one-third of patients with PROP were ascertained by clinical presentation after one year of age [13]. Individuals may present with recurrent attacks of ketoacidosis with coma or lethargy and ataxia during times of catabolic stress such as during an illness or following a high protein meal [9, 19]. The presentation may mimic diabetic ketoacidosis [23–26]. Childhood and adolescent onset patients have presented with chronic renal failure [27]. Other individuals may present with acute hemiplegia, hemianopsia, or cerebral edema, or symptoms that mimic a cerebral vascular accident, cerebral tumor, or acute encephalitis [13, 19]. In addition, symptoms may simulate a neurologic disorder presenting with hypotonia, weakness, ataxia, seizures, progressive spasticity, movement disorder, vision loss, or developmental delay. Symptoms may also be misdiagnosed as a gastrointestinal disorder secondary to presenting with failure to thrive, anorexia, chronic vomiting, or a Reye-like presentation [9, 13, 19, 21, 27]. Some individuals may present with hematologic manifestations or present with recurrent infections [9, 19]. Adult presentations have included acute metabolic acidosis with renal and respiratory failure [28] and isolated dilated cardiomyopathy [29].

18.2.3 Laboratory Studies and Diagnosis

Laboratory studies typically reveal a severe metabolic acidosis with an elevated anion gap, ketosis, and hyperammonemia [9, 16, 19, 21]. Hyperuricemia, hyperlacticacidemia, and hypocalcemia may also be seen. Blood glucose can be reduced, normal, or elevated [16, 19]. Bone marrow involvement as reflected by neutropenia, anemia, thrombocytopenia, or pancytopenia can also be observed and is a rather unique finding of organic acidemias [9, 16, 19]. Diagnostic metabolites, as noted above, are seen on urine organic acid analysis and acylcarnitine profile. Quantitative plasma amino acids and urine amino acids are useful to investigate the possibility of combined MMA and homocystinuria due to vitamin B_{12} synthesis defects. Striking elevations of glycine and alanine can be seen in blood and urine and may be an early clue to diagnosis and explains the historical descriptive term of "ketotic hyperglycinemias" [9, 21]. The diagnosis may be confirmed by enzyme assay or molecular studies. Organic acidemias are increasingly identified via newborn screening with elevations in propionylcarnitine (C3) for PROP and MMA and elevated isovalerylcarnitine (C5) for IVA.

18.2.4 Complications

Organic acidemias are multisystem disorders with individuals at risk for a variety of complications. Complications arise despite apparent good metabolic control [30–32]. Neurologic complications include metabolic stroke with edema evolving into necrosis of the basal ganglia, especially the globus pallidus, and leading to a disabling movement disorder, motor dysfunction, and hypotonia [19, 21, 33–35]. Cortical volume loss, basal ganglia lesions, cerebral and vermian atrophy, and delayed myelination may be seen on neuroimaging [9, 19, 21, 34, 36, 37]. Restricted diffusion may be noted during acute events [36]. Clinically, seizures, deafness, optic nerve atrophy, neuropathy, myopathy, developmental delay, attention deficit-hyperactivity disorder (ADHD), and autistic features are seen [33, 35, 38–41] (Box 18.1). One study reported approximately 50% of affected individuals have an IQ < 80 [33], while another study suggested >70% of individuals with PROP have cognitive deficits [42]. The etiology of this neurologic damage is unclear. Theories include direct toxic effects of methylmalonic acid, propionic acid, and methylcitrate, impairment of energy metabolism as mediated by synergistic inhibition of the Krebs cycle and mitochondrial respiratory chain by the three metabolites, accumulation of decarboxylates in the central nervous system, neuroinflammation, interference of cytoskeleton assembly in neuronal and glial cells, and disruption of signaling pathways that promote apoptosis of neuronal cells [30, 42–50]. Elevations in lactate and ammonia in plasma and lactate, glutamine, glycine, and alanine in cerebrospinal fluid have also been detected in a patient with neurologic symptoms but no signs of catabolism suggesting that neurologic abnormalities may be related to localized metabolic derangements [31, 51]. Data suggests a synergistic effect of methylmalonic acid and ammonia disturbing the redox homeostasis and causing morphological brain abnormalities, including vacuolization, ischemic neurons, and pericellular edema in a rat model [52]. Propionate accumulation also results in morphological alterations in cerebral cortex astrocytes [35].

Another complication of organic acidemias is renal tubular acidosis with hyperuricemia leading to chronic renal impairment and eventually to renal failure [9, 19, 40] (Box 18.2). This is espe-

Box 18.1: Neurological Complications of Organic Acidemias

- Metabolic stroke with edema evolving into necrosis of the basal ganglia and globus pallidus which leads to disabling movement disorder, motor dysfunction and hypotonia
- Cerebral atrophy and delayed myelination
- Seizures
- Optic nerve atrophy, deafness
- Neuropathy or skeletal myopathy
- Developmental delay, autistic features

Box 18.2: Complications of Organic Acidemias

- Renal tubular acidosis (RTA) with hyperuricemia; chronic renal impairment leading to renal failure
- Superficial desquamation and alopecia due to nutrient or essential amino acid deficiency
- Cardiomyopathy, long QT syndrome
- Pancreatitis – acute, chronic and/or recurrent
- Carnitine deficiency
- Osteopenia or osteoporosis
- Ovarian failure
- Liver disease including nonalcoholic steatohepatitis, fibrosis, and cirrhosis
- Possible increased risk of infections

cially prominent in individuals with MMA; however, renal disease and failure have also been reported in individuals with propionic acidemia with an age-dependent decline [53–56]. Renal histology reveals tubulointerstitial nephritis with fibrosis, tubular atrophy, and mononuclear inflammatory infiltrate [55, 57–59]. Renal disease is found in the majority of individuals with MMA who are over 6 years of age and may be due to chronic glomerular hyperfiltration secondary to excessive methylmalonic acid excretion [10, 19, 34, 46]. The risk of developing renal failure seems to correlate with methylmalonic acid exposure over time and depends on the disease type with mutase-deficient patients at greater risk than patients with cobalamin defects [58]. Thus, minimizing renal injury may require strict metabolic control to maintain methylmalonic acid concentrations as low as possible [19].

Furthermore, cardiomyopathy, more common in PROP than MMA and more commonly dilated than hypertrophic, may occur during acute decompensations or be the presenting feature and may be rapidly fatal [19, 60–64]. The pathogenesis of the cardiomyopathy is unclear—carnitine or micronutrient deficiency, infection, or acute energy deprivation have all been postulated [21, 32, 51]. Cardiomyopathy appears to develop independent of any specific metabolic profile and appears to occur at any age [32, 51, 62]. The mean age of presentation in one series was 7 years [62]. Long QT syndrome (delayed repolarization of the heart) is also reported and may occur in as high as 70% of patients with PROP [32, 65–68].

A secondary carnitine deficiency due to accumulation of propionyl-CoA and increased concentration of acylcarnitines is also common [19]. Superficial desquamation, alopecia, and corneal ulcerations similar to staphylococcal scalded skin syndrome or acrodermatitis enteropathica-like syndrome, typically associated with diarrhea, may be seen secondary to acute protein malnutrition or essential amino acid deficiency, especially isoleucine deficiency [51, 69–71]. Immune dysfunction has also been suggested with an increased risk for viral or bacterial infections, but good studies are lacking [51]. Chronic moniliasis has been described and reflects the effect of propionyl-CoA and methylmalonate on T-cell number and function [9]. Finally, acute, chronic, and recurrent pancreatitis, osteopenia or osteoporosis, ovarian failure, and liver abnormalities including nonalcoholic steatohepatitis, fibrosis, and cirrhosis may also occur; the etiologies of which remain unclear [9, 21, 32, 40, 51, 54, 72–79].

18.3 Pathophysiology

The pathogenesis of the clinical features of organic acidemias remains complex and incompletely understood. The metabolic blocks cause metabolite accumulation triggering an endogenous intoxication. Propionyl-CoA and its metabolites inhibit the Krebs cycle resulting in reduced GTP and ATP synthesis, inhibit potassium channel flow, and are known to have inhibitory effects on pyruvate dehydrogenase complex, succinyl-CoA synthetase, ATP-citrate lyase, and N-acetylglutamate synthetase activities, and on the glycine cleavage system [9, 17, 18, 42, 80, 81]. Furthermore, methylmalonyl-CoA is known to inhibit pyruvate carboxylase [17, 82, 83]. Similarly, isovaleric acid causes marked inhibition of Na(+), K(+) ATPase activity [84]. Methylcitrate, itself, inhibits citrate synthase, aconitase, isocitrate dehydrogenase, and glutamate dehydrogenase activities, disturbs mitochondrial energy homeostasis, decreases ATP generation [42, 81, 85] and has been shown to cause morphologic changes and apoptosis of brain cells [43]. Thus, there is an energy deficit secondary to substrate insufficiency and toxin accumulation [86], as well as a direct impact on Krebs cycle intermediates resulting in secondary effects on other pathways [42, 44]. These inhibitory effects appear to explain some of the clinical signs seen in MMA and PROP, such as the hypoglycemia, lactic acidemia, hyperglycinemia, and hyperammonemia [17].

In addition, it has become increasingly evident that there is significant mitochondrial dysfunction, impairment of the oxidative phosphorylation system, increased production of reactive oxygen species (ROS), and increased autophagy [30, 35, 42, 46, 59, 87–95]. The chronic effect of inhibition of mitochondrial energy production leads to oxidative stress, mitochondrial DNA damage, and altered mitochondrial morphology [44, 96]. The oxidative stress is mediated by increased levels of reactive oxygen species (ROS) and reduced ROS-protective levels of glutathione [44]. In addition, there are extensive mitochondrial ultrastructural changes in liver and kidney samples from MMA patients providing more evidence of mitochondrial dysfunction and respiratory chain impairment [59, 87, 89, 92, 97]. Mutase deficiency has been linked to mechanisms that cause mitophagy dysfunction and accumulation of damaged mitochondria that generate epithelial stress and tissue damage [87, 97]. Proteomic studies also suggest disturbances in proteins involved in energy metabolism, cellular detoxification, oxidative stress, cytoskeleton assembly, gluconeogenesis, and Kreb cycle anaplerosis [98, 99]. Finally, Storgaard et al. also suggested involvement of impaired lipolysis, blunted fatty acid oxidation, compensatory increase in carbohydrate utilization, and low work capacity as contributors to the pathophysiology of organic acidemias [100].

The etiology of the hyperammonemia seen in organic acidemias is different than that seen in urea cycle disorders. Recall that in the urea cycle, carbamoyl-phosphate synthesis is activated by N-acetylglutamate (NAG) [101]. Propionyl-CoA, which is accumulating in PROP, and isovaleryl-CoA, accumulating in IVA, are potent inhibitors of N-acetylglutamate synthase (NAGS) [11, 102]. Thus, NAG production is reduced and lack of NAG results in carbamoyl-phosphate synthetase inhibition and elevated ammonia concentrations [102]. It has also been suggested that hyperammonemia may be related to the inability to maintain adequate concentrations of glutamate precursors through a dysfunctional Krebs cycle secondary to accumulating methylcitrate and the decline in citric acid excretion [101].

18.4 Management

The goal of treatment of an individual with an organic acidemia is to reduce the accumulation of toxic metabolites, maintain normal growth, development, and nutritional status, prevent catabolism, and minimize complications [19, 44]. Therapy is multifaceted and typically involves a diet based on restriction of propiogenic amino acids, medication supplementation, and life-long monitoring [44]. Individualized dietary prescriptions, as prescribed by a metabolic nutritionist, balance the necessary intake of the restricted amino acids, other protein, and energy to provide the recommended daily allowances of nutrients and allow for adequate growth [103]. This is frequently accomplished by the use of special propiogenic amino acid-restricted medical foods combined with a prescribed amount of intact protein provided by breast milk or regular infant formula in infancy and regular solid foods in older children [19]. Provision of total protein intake modestly above the dietary reference intake (DRI) is well-tolerated and can provide a buffer against catabolism [32]. The target plasma range for restricted amino acids in PROP and MMA (isoleucine, valine, methionine, threonine) is low normal to normal [104]. In IVA, it is often sufficient to restrict natural protein to the recommended minimum daily requirements without the use of a leucine-free medical food [19, 104]. The target plasma range for leucine is 50–180 μM or normal range for the laboratory and 200–400 μM for glycine [104].

For all patients, particular attention must be paid to adequate energy intake. Energy requirements have been reported to be lower than predicted for age and sex during the well-fed state secondary to lower energy expenditure [105–107]. During illness, however, resting energy expenditure increases, requiring increased caloric intake to prevent catabolism and decompensation [19, 103]. These needs may require the use of additional fat and carbohydrate sources or protein-free modules. Catabolism is the major reason for acute decompensation [32]. If individual amino acids are found to be low, supplementation may be required, but no studies prove the efficiency of consistent supplementation of isoleucine and valine [107]. Nutrition management guidelines have been published by Yannicelli, Knerr et al., and Jurecki et al. [103, 104, 108] and are described in Chap. 21.

Therapy of IVA varies slightly from that of PROP and MMA. Isovaleryl-CoA conjugates with glycine via the enzyme, glycine-N-acylase, forming isovalerylglycine, and also binds with carnitine, via carnitine N-acylase, to form isovalerylcarnitine [109, 110]. Both products, isovalerylglycine and isovalerylcarnitine, are easily excreted in the urine. This feature is exploited for both acute and chronic management. Thus, glycine (150–300 mg/kg/d) and carnitine (50–100 mg/kg/d) are both supplemented in individuals with IVA resulting in excretion of isovaleric acid [9, 11, 16, 19, 82, 83, 104, 109–114]. Subsequently, a strict metabolic diet may not be needed.

Supplementation of L-carnitine (100–400 mg/kg/d divided 2–3 times per day) is also an important aspect of the treatment of PROP and MMA [9, 19, 21, 32, 33, 103]. Provision of oral carnitine is effective in preventing carnitine depletion, regenerating the intracellular pool of free coenzyme A (CoA), and allows urinary excretion of propionylcarnitine, thereby reducing propionate toxicity [19, 104]. High doses of carnitine may cause a fishy odor due to overproduction of methylamines and may cause diarrhea [9, 103] but may be particularly helpful in PROP [32].

All patients with MMA should be tested for responsiveness to vitamin B_{12} [9, 19]. Testing regimes vary, but responsiveness can be determined by monitoring quantitative plasma or urine methylmalonic acid concentrations or by measuring metabolites via urine organic acid analysis. Vitamin B_{12} responsiveness leads to prompt and sustained decrease of propionyl-CoA byproducts [19]. Results should be confirmed by additional studies. Many vitamin B_{12}-responsive patients may need minimal to no protein or amino acid restriction [19]. In responsive patients, vitamin B_{12} is supplemented orally once per day or intramuscularly or subcutaneously daily or weekly with a beginning dose of 1 mg [19, 104]. A biotin responsive form of PROP has not been seen, but biotin dosed at 5–20 mg/d is sometimes supplemented in PROP [9, 32, 33, 103, 104].

As propionate production may result from gut bacteria, an intermittent antibiotic regime to reduce gut propionate production is sometimes implemented. The antibiotic, metronidazole, has been reported to be effective in reducing urinary excretion of propionate metabolites when used at a dose of 10–20 mg/kg once per day [16, 19, 103, 104]. The regime of therapy varies, but 7–10 consecutive days each month is a common practice [19, 33, 37, 104]. Some care providers prefer neomycin (50 mg/kg) because it is not absorbed [9]. Care must be taken to avoid complications associated with chronic antibiotic use including leukopenia, peripheral neuropathy, and pseudomembranous colitis. Metronidazole may also cause anorexia and dystonia [32, 103]. There are no studies that evaluate the clinical efficacy of metronidazole in improving clinical outcome, reducing ammonia concentrations, or reducing episodes of acute decompensation [32]. Overall, results of intermittent antibiotic use have been variable as measured by change in metabolite excretion, likely reflecting a variable colonization of gut bacteria by organisms which may or may not produce propionate [9].

Administration of N-carbamylglutamate (100–250 mg/kg/d) with or without ammonia scavengers has been suggested to help restore ureagenesis and improve acute hyperammonemia [18, 32, 44, 115, 116]. Increasing data is beginning to also suggest benefit of chronic use of N-carbamylglutamate (50 mg/kg/d) including a decrease in mean ammonia concentrations and a decrease in acute episodes of decompensation [44, 117]. Similarly, chronic therapy with sodium benzoate (150–250 mg/kg/d) has been proposed to help correct chronic hyperammonemia and hyperglycinemia [33]; however, there is no evidence that supports a role of sodium benzoate in chronic treatment especially given the evidence that higher glycine concentrations may be indicative of good metabolic control [32, 118]. Multivitamins may be given to reduce the risk of micronutrient deficiency. Citric acid and ornithine alpha-ketoglutarate have also been proposed to help sustain Krebs cycle flux and promote anaplerosis during illness and chronic management [96, 101, 119] with citric acid being most efficacious in one study of three agents [120]. In addition, coenzyme Q10 and vitamin E have been suggested as possible therapies for MMA-related optic neuropathy or secondary respiratory chain deficiency [46, 121, 122] and angiotension II inhibition has been suggested to help delay renal disease [123]. The role of growth hormone and supplemental alanine to promote anabolism has been suggested, but experience is limited [9, 32, 124–126]. Glutathione deficiency treated with high doses of ascorbate has also been reported [127].

In addition, prompt treatment of intercurrent illnesses, particularly those placing the individual at risk for catabolism (e.g., vomiting, diarrhea, fever), and avoidance of fasting is paramount to reduce the risk of acute decompensations. Many children develop anorexia and feeding difficulties necessitating the placement of a gastrostomy tube to prevent fasting and ensure adequate dietary intake [33, 75, 128]. Patients and families should be provided an emergency medical letter as well as a sick day protocol [32]. A medical alert bracelet or necklace is also recommended [32].

Management of an acute decompensation involves reduction or discontinuation of protein and provision of energy to stop catabolism and promote anabolism by infusion of glucose and intralipid [21]. Fluid recommendations are standard for age. Using a 10% dextrose solution at 120–150 mL/kg/day (or 1.5 times maintenance) often can provide the necessary level of glucose delivery [37, 104]. Rehydration should occur over a 48-hour period to prevent cerebral edema [104]. Additional calories are added by using intralipid at 1–3 gm/kg/day [37, 104]. If hyperglycemia develops, an insulin drip (0.01–0.1 units/kg/h) may be necessary, but the dextrose delivery rate or amount should not be decreased [9, 37, 104]. Bicarbonate supplementation (1–2 mEq/kg) may be necessary to help correct acidosis [104]. If severe hyperammonemia is present, hemodialysis, hemofiltration, continuous chronic renal replacement (CCRT), extracorporeal membrane oxygenation (ECMO), and/or ammonia scavenging medications may be necessary [33, 37, 104, 129, 130]. Sodium benzoate and sodium phenylacetate, however, should be used with caution in patients with organic acidemias because glutamine concentrations can already be low and they may potentiate ammonia toxicity by blocking the urea cycle through sequestration of CoA [44, 115]. Carbamylglutamute (100–250 mg/kg/d) has been demonstrated to be beneficial in controlling the hyperammonemia associated with an acute decompensation [33, 44, 102, 115, 131–135]. Administration of intravenous L-carnitine in relatively high doses (100–400 mg/kg/d) is used in acute illness [37, 104]. Metabolic decompensation in PROP may be complicated by hyperlacticacidemia due to thiamin deficiency, requiring supplementation (10 mg/kg/d) [104, 136, 137]. If the illness is prolonged, total parenteral nutrition may be necessary. Otherwise, reintroduction of protein occurs as tolerated, but should be reintroduced within 24–36 hours of therapy initiation [37, 104]. Frequent monitoring of laboratory studies and for possible complications is required.

For a fragile, medically intractable individual, liver, kidney, or combined liver kidney transplantation may be considered [138–148]. Transplantation is not a cure as it only partially corrects the enzymatic defect, but may result in improved survival, metabolic stability, neurologic function, and quality of life [32, 33, 86, 138–141, 149–155]. Perioperative complications, especially vascular complications, however, are common [138]. Liver transplantation has also been shown to improve cardiomyopathy [62, 156, 157], but cardiomyopathy has also recurred following transplantation [158]. Dietary therapy, perhaps liberalized, and L-carnitine supplementation are continued following transplantation [142, 145, 147, 149, 159]. Neurologic dysfunction, including metabolic stroke, and renal disease are not always prevented with transplantation [9, 17, 19, 32, 33, 160, 161]. One-year survival rate following transplantation was 72.2% in a multi-site, retrospective study of 12 individuals with PROP [32, 150] and may be up to 100% at experienced centers [138, 141, 162]. Therapies under investigation include import of transactivation of transcription (TAT) conjugated enzymes, viral vector-mediated gene transfer, systemic messenger RNA therapy, and genome editing [163–166].

18.5 Monitoring

Monitoring of patients with organic acidemias will vary according to each clinics' practice but should occur with some degree of regularity.

Patients should be seen routinely in clinic with routine monitoring of laboratory studies. Quantitative plasma amino acids should be obtained at least monthly in all patients managed with a restricted diet, although this practice varies between clinics. Quantitative methylmalonic acid is available in selected laboratories and may be used to follow individuals with MMA [9]. There is no established biomarker for monitoring therapeutic control in IVA [11]. Propionate concentrations may be difficult to obtain for individuals with PROP; some advocate following the methylcitrate to ctirate ratio via quantitative urine organic acid analysis or dried blood spots, if available [167, 168]. Propionylcarnitine has not been demonstrated to correlate with severity or level of control [32]. Ammonia, acid-base balance, and anion gap have been demonstrated to be important biochemical parameters in identifying an impending metabolic decompensation and to assess severity of PROP and MMA patients [169, 170]. The frequency of monitoring laboratory studies varies pending the patient's age and clinical stability. Laboratory studies to obtain every 6–12 months include complete blood count, complete metabolic panel (to include electrolytes, renal and liver function studies), carnitine, urinalysis, β-type natriuretic peptide, cystatin C, and calculated glomerular filtration rate, as well as annual nutrition monitoring studies to include prealbumin, 25-hydroxyvitamin D, vitamin B_{12}, iron, ferritin, and other micronutrients (thiamin, selenium) [32]. Additional laboratory studies to consider during acute illness include complete blood count, complete metabolic panel (to include electrolytes, renal and liver function studies), amylase, lipase, ammonia, osmolality, lactate, coagulation studies, creatine kinase, and urine ketones. Families can also be taught to test for urine ketones using ketone reagent strips at home as an early warning sign for pending decompensation [9] (Box 18.3).

Box 18.3: Laboratory Monitoring in Organic Acidemias[a]

- Routine:
  - Plasma amino acids
  - Prealbumin
  - Serum methylmalonic acid concentrations (MMA)
  - Urine Organic Acids
    Urinary methylcitrate to citrate ratio (MC ≤ 2 times citrate in PROP)
- Annual
  - Complete blood count
  - Electrolytes, renal and liver function tests
  - Calculated creatinine clearance and glomerular filtration rate (GFR)
  - Carnitine (total, free and esterified)
  - Nutrient adequacy: vitamin D, B12, thiamin, iron studies, minerals (zinc, selenium)
  - β-type naturiuretic peptide
  - Urinalysis
  - Cystatin C
- Acute illness (additional)
  - Amylase, lipase, ammonia, ketones, lactate, coagulation studies, osmolality, CK

[a]Frequency depends on age of patient and clinical status, recommended monthly routine laboratory evaluations.

Recent evidence suggests fibroblast growth factor 21 (FGF21) may be a predictive biomarker for metabolic stress in patients with MMA and PROP [171, 172]. The plasma concentrations of FGF21 appear to correlate with disease subtype and markers of mitochondrial dysfunction and are not affected by nutritional status or renal disease [171, 172]. Molema et al. suggested FGF21 levels >1500 during stable metabolic periods predicted an increase in long-term complications in patients with MMA and PROP [171]. This laboratory study, however, is not yet readily available for clinical use.

In addition to laboratory studies, management of an individual with an organic acidemia often requires the involvement of additional subspecialty services including neurology, nephrology, cardiology, neuropsychology, endocrinology, and ophthalmology. The utilization of these subspecialties is individualized to the clinical presentation of the patient. The patient may be seen yearly if monitoring is only required to assess increased risk or may be seen more frequently if organ system involvement is already noted [32]. Cardiology evaluation, however, with echocardiogram, ECG, and 24-hour Holter monitoring is recommended yearly in individuals with PROP [32] and MMA and during acute illnesses [27]. Schreiber et al. also recommended a baseline electroencephalogram and repeat studies as clinically indicated in all patients with PROP [35]. Long-term and repeated neuropsychological assessment is an excellent tool for tracking developmental progress or decline over time. Early evaluation and, if necessary, intervention are recommended beginning at a young age. Routine bone densitometry (DEXA scan) is also recommended for all patients typically beginning at age 5 years [27, 173]. Baseline endocrinology evaluation should be considered for female patients in late adolescence or thereafter. Nephrotoxic medications and medications that prolong the QT interval should be used with caution [27].

18.6 Summary

The outcome of individuals with organic acidemias is quite variable. In general for PROP and MMA, late onset forms appear to have a better prognosis as compared with early onset forms, mut^- MMA patients appear to do better than mut^0 patients, and individuals with vitamin B_{12} responsive MMA appear to have improved outcome over patients with vitamin B_{12} unresponsive forms [10, 21, 34, 40, 58, 128, 174, 175]. In MMA, an earlier age of onset, the presence of hyperammonemia at diagnosis, and a history of seizures also predict more severe impairment [176]. The duration of hyperammonemia, abnormal acid–base balance with metabolic acidosis, and coma correlate with poor neurologic outcome [44]. Also, in general, individuals with IVA appear to have a better outcome than those with MMA or PROP; however, in contrast to MMA and PROP, the neurocognitive outcome in patients with a neonatal presentation is more favorable than in patients with a late diagnosis [177, 178]. Mortality has been reported to be >80% in the neonatal onset form of these disorders and as high as 40% before 16 years of age in the late onset forms [33, 179]. Survival has improved [33]. The survival at one year of age in patients with mut^0 was 65% in the 1970s but has increased up to 90% in the 1990s [17]. Death may be due to cerebral edema, cerebral or cerebellar hemorrhage, infection, renal failure, heart failure, arrhythmias, cardiomyopathy, pancreatitis, or irreversible metabolic decompensation [9, 51, 63, 68, 179–181].

Morbidity is also high with frequent complications, poor growth and nutritional status, poor neurodevelopmental progress with frequent progressive neurocognitive deterioration, abnormal neurologic signs such as chorea and dystonia, and frequent and severe relapses of metabolic decompensation [6, 10, 21, 33, 68]. Overall, developmental outcome is poor in PROP and MMA with the majority of patients demonstrating developmental delay [6, 33, 51, 68, 75, 86, 178]. Martin-Hernandez et al. reported on the long-term needs of adult patients with organic acidemias [40]. In this series of 15 patients, largely with late onset disease, two-thirds of the patients had neurologic or visceral complications, and three-quarters of them required some kind of social support [40]. In contrast, developmental outcome in IVA is normal in 60% or more of the patients [86, 178]. In addition, long-term complications and the risk of metabolic decompensations associated with catabolic stress in individuals with IVA are also much less frequent than compared to PROP and MMA [40, 178]. Evaluation of older patients is beginning to suggest a risk of psychiatric disorders [86].

Outcome and prognosis, however, may be changing and improving with early identification via newborn screening. A benign MMA phenotype has been described and some patients with MMA have remained symptom-free [4, 182, 183]. In addition, infants diagnosed with IVA by newborn screen have also remained asymptomatic with carnitine supplementation and mild or no dietary restriction and retrospectively identified siblings ranging in age from 3 to 11 years were also asymptomatic [7, 11]. Dionisi-Vici et al. compared the outcome of 29 patients with MMA, PROP, or IVA diagnosed clinically to 18 similar patients diagnosed by newborn screening. The newborn screened population demonstrated an earlier diagnosis, significantly reduced mortality (11% compared to 51%) and an increased number of patients with normal development at <1 year of age [10]. A more stable clinical course with less frequent relapses of decompensation was also demonstrated [10]. Similar findings were also found by Grünert et al. in a population of patients with PROP, however, they did not demonstrate a reduction of complications in patients diagnosed by newborn screening [184]. Overall, newborn screening and early diagnosis may result in decreased early mortality, decrease severity of initial symptoms, and improved neurodevelopmental outcome [10]. Outcome data, however, is early and limited and more long-term follow-up studies are needed.

References

1. Abily-Donval L, Torre S, Samson A, Sudrie-Arnaud B, Acquaviva C, Guerrot AM, et al. Methylmalonyl-CoA epimerase deficiency mimicking propionic aciduria. Int J Mol Sci. 2017;18(11):2294.
2. Heuberger K, Bailey HJ, Burda P, Chaikuad A, Krysztofinska E, Suormala T, et al. Genetic, structural, and functional analysis of pathogenic variations causing methylmalonyl-CoA epimerase deficiency. Biochim Biophys Acta Mol basis Dis. 2019;1865(6):1265–72.
3. Waters PJ, Thuriot F, Clarke JT, Gravel S, Watkins D, Rosenblatt DS, et al. Methylmalonyl-coA epimerase deficiency: a new case, with an acute metabolic presentation and an intronic splicing mutation in the MCEE gene. Mol Genet Metab Rep. 2016;9:19–24.
4. Sniderman LC, Lambert M, Giguere R, Auray-Blais C, Lemieux B, Laframboise R, et al. Outcome of individuals with low-moderate methylmalonic aciduria detected through a neonatal screening program. J Pediatr. 1999;134(6):675–80.
5. Yorifuji T, Kawai M, Muroi J, Mamada M, Kurokawa K, Shigematsu Y, et al. Unexpectedly high prevalence of the mild form of propionic acidemia in Japan: presence of a common mutation and possible clinical implications. Hum Genet. 2002;111(2):161–5.
6. Rafique M. Propionic acidaemia: demographic characteristics and complications. J Pediatr Endocrinol Metab. 2013;26(5–6):497–501.
7. Ensenauer R, Vockley J, Willard JM, Huey JC, Sass JO, Edland SD, et al. A common mutation is associated with a mild, potentially asymptomatic phenotype in patients with isovaleric acidemia diagnosed by newborn screening. Am J Hum Genet. 2004;75(6):1136–42.
8. Ensenauer R, Fingerhut R, Maier EM, Polanetz R, Olgemoller B, Roschinger W, et al. Newborn screening for isovaleric acidemia using tandem mass spectrometry: data from 1.6 million newborns. Clin Chem. 2011;57(4):623–6.
9. Nyhan WL, Barshop BA, Ozand PT. Propionic acidemia, methylmalonic acidemia, isovaleric acidemia. In: Atlas of metabolic disease, 2nd ed. London: Hodder Arnold; 2005.
10. Dionisi-Vici C, Deodato F, Roschinger W, Rhead W, Wilcken B. 'Classical' organic acidurias, propionic aciduria, methylmalonic aciduria and isovaleric aciduria: long-term outcome and effects of expanded newborn screening using tandem mass spectrometry. J Inherit Metab Dis. 2006;29(2–3):383–9.
11. Vockley J, Ensenauer R. Isovaleric acidemia: new aspects of genetic and phenotypic heterogeneity. Am J Med Genet C Semin Med Genet. 2006;142C(2):95–103.
12. Cappuccio G, Atwal PS, Donti TR, Ugarte K, Merchant N, Craigen WJ, et al. Expansion of the phenotypic spectrum of propionic acidemia with isolated elevated propionylcarnitine. JIMD Rep. 2017;35:33–7.
13. McCrory NM, Edick MJ, Ahmad A, Lipinski S, Scott Schwoerer JA, Zhai S, et al. Comparison of methods of initial ascertainment in 58 cases of propionic acidemia enrolled in the inborn errors of metabolism information system reveals significant differences in time to evaluation and symptoms at presentation. J Pediatr. 2017;180:200–5 e8.
14. Monostori P, Klinke G, Richter S, Barath A, Fingerhut R, Baumgartner MR, et al. Simultaneous determination of 3-hydroxypropionic acid, methylmalonic acid and methylcitric acid in dried blood spots: second-tier LC-MS/MS assay for newborn screening of propionic acidemia, methylmalonic acidemias and combined remethylation disorders. PLoS One. 2017;12(9):e0184897.
15. Peng G, Shen P, Gandotra N, Le A, Fung E, Jelliffe-Pawlowski L, et al. Combining newborn metabolic and DNA analysis for second-tier testing of methylmalonic acidemia. Genet Med. 2019;21(4):896–903.
16. Ogier de Baulny H, Saudubray JM. Branched-chain organic acidurias. Semin Neonatol. 2002;7(1):65–74.
17. Tanpaiboon P. Methylmalonic acidemia (MMA). Mol Genet Metab. 2005;85(1):2–6.
18. Soyucen E, Demirci E, Aydin A. Outpatient treatment of propionic acidemia-associated hyperammonemia with N-carbamoyl-L-glutamate in an infant. Clin Ther. 2010;32(4):710–3.
19. Ogier de Baulny H, Dionisi-Vici C, Wendel U. Branched-chain organic acidurias/acidemias. In:

Saudubray JM, editor. Inborn metabolic diseases. 5th ed. Heidelberg: Springer-Verlag; 2012.
20. Dionisi-Vici C, Ogier de Baulny H. Emergency treatment. In: Saudubray J-M, van den Berghe G, Walter JH, editors. Inborn metabolic diseases diagnosis and treatment. Berlin: Springer-Verlag; 2012. p. 104–11.
21. Deodato F, Boenzi S, Santorelli FM, Dionisi-Vici C. Methylmalonic and propionic aciduria. Am J Med Genet C Semin Med Genet. 2006;142C(2):104–12.
22. Bernheim S, Deschenes G, Schiff M, Cussenot I, Niel O. Antenatal nephromegaly and propionic acidemia: a case report. BMC Nephrol. 2017;18(1):110.
23. Erdem E, Cayonu N, Uysalol E, Yildirmak ZY. Chronic intermittent form of isovaleric acidemia mimicking diabetic ketoacidosis. J Pediatr Endocrinol Metab. 2010;23(5):503–5.
24. Dweikat IM, Naser EN, Abu Libdeh AI, Naser OJ, Abu Gharbieh NN, Maraqa NF, et al. Propionic acidemia mimicking diabetic ketoacidosis. Brain Dev. 2011;33(5):428–31.
25. Joshi R, Phatarpekar A. Propionic acidemia presenting as diabetic ketoacidosis. Indian Pediatr. 2011;48(2):164–5.
26. Guven A, Cebeci N, Dursun A, Aktekin E, Baumgartner M, Fowler B. Methylmalonic acidemia mimicking diabetic ketoacidosis in an infant. Pediatr Diabetes. 2012;13(6):e22–5.
27. Fraser JL, Venditti CP. Methylmalonic and propionic acidemias: clinical management update. Curr Opin Pediatr. 2016;28(6):682–93.
28. Zhao Z, Chu CC, Chang MY, Chang HT, Hsu YL. Management of adult-onset methylmalonic acidemia with hypotonia and acute respiratory failure: a case report. Medicine (Baltimore). 2018;97(25):e11162.
29. Riemersma M, Hazebroek MR, Helderman-van den Enden A, Salomons GS, Ferdinandusse S, Brouwers M, et al. Propionic acidemia as a cause of adult-onset dilated cardiomyopathy. Eur J Hum Genet. 2017;25(11):1195–201.
30. de Keyzer Y, Valayannopoulos V, Benoist JF, Batteux F, Lacaille F, Hubert L, et al. Multiple OXPHOS deficiency in the liver, kidney, heart, and skeletal muscle of patients with methylmalonic aciduria and propionic aciduria. Pediatr Res. 2009;66(1):91–5.
31. Scholl-Burgi S, Haberlandt E, Gotwald T, Albrecht U, Baumgartner Sigl S, Rauchenzauner M, et al. Stroke-like episodes in propionic acidemia caused by central focal metabolic decompensation. Neuropediatrics. 2009;40(2):76–81.
32. Sutton VR, Chapman KA, Gropman AL, MacLeod E, Stagni K, Summar ML, et al. Chronic management and health supervision of individuals with propionic acidemia. Mol Genet Metab. 2012;105(1):26–33.
33. de Baulny HO, Benoist JF, Rigal O, Touati G, Rabier D, Saudubray JM. Methylmalonic and propionic acidaemias: management and outcome. J Inherit Metab Dis. 2005;28(3):415–23.
34. Cosson MA, Benoist JF, Touati G, Dechaux M, Royer N, Grandin L, et al. Long-term outcome in methylmalonic aciduria: a series of 30 French patients. Mol Genet Metab. 2009;97(3):172–8.
35. Schreiber J, Chapman KA, Summar ML, Ah Mew N, Sutton VR, MacLeod E, et al. Neurologic considerations in propionic acidemia. Mol Genet Metab. 2012;105(1):10–5.
36. Pfeifer CM, Van Tassel DC, Miller JH. Unique neuroradiological findings in propionic acidemia. Radiol Case Rep. 2018;13(6):1207–11.
37. Chapman KA, Gropman A, MacLeod E, Stagni K, Summar ML, Ueda K, et al. Acute management of propionic acidemia. Mol Genet Metab. 2012;105(1):16–25.
38. Sindgikar SP, Shenoy KD, Kamath N, Shenoy R. Audit of organic acidurias from a single centre: clinical and metabolic profile at presentation with long term outcome. J Clin Diagn Res. 2017;11(9):SC11–SC4.
39. Ianchulev T, Kolin T, Moseley K, Sadun A. Optic nerve atrophy in propionic acidemia. Ophthalmology. 2003;110(9):1850–4.
40. Martin-Hernandez E, Lee PJ, Micciche A, Grunewald S, Lachmann RH. Long-term needs of adult patients with organic acidaemias: outcome and prognostic factors. J Inherit Metab Dis. 2009;32(4):523–33.
41. Williams ZR, Hurley PE, Altiparmak UE, Feldon SE, Arnold GL, Eggenberger E, et al. Late onset optic neuropathy in methylmalonic and propionic acidemia. Am J Ophthalmol. 2009;147(5):929–33.
42. Wongkittichote P, Ah Mew N, Chapman KA. Propionyl-CoA carboxylase - a review. Mol Genet Metab. 2017;122(4):145–52.
43. Cudre-Cung HP, Zavadakova P, do Vale-Pereira S, Remacle N, Henry H, Ivanisevic J, et al. Ammonium accumulation is a primary effect of 2-methylcitrate exposure in an in vitro model for brain damage in methylmalonic aciduria. Mol Genet Metab. 2016;119(1–2):57–67.
44. Haberle J, Chakrapani A, Ah Mew N, Longo N. Hyperammonaemia in classic organic acidaemias: a review of the literature and two case histories. Orphanet J Rare Dis. 2018;13(1):219.
45. Kolker S, Schwab M, Horster F, Sauer S, Hinz A, Wolf NI, et al. Methylmalonic acid, a biochemical hallmark of methylmalonic acidurias but no inhibitor of mitochondrial respiratory chain. J Biol Chem. 2003;278(48):47388–93.
46. Morath MA, Okun JG, Muller IB, Sauer SW, Horster F, Hoffmann GF, et al. Neurodegeneration and chronic renal failure in methylmalonic aciduria--a pathophysiological approach. J Inherit Metab Dis. 2008;31(1):35–43.
47. Ballhausen D, Mittaz L, Boulat O, Bonafe L, Braissant O. Evidence for catabolic pathway of propionate metabolism in CNS: expression pattern of methylmalonyl-CoA mutase and propionyl-CoA carboxylase alpha-subunit in developing and adult rat brain. Neuroscience. 2009;164(2):578–87.
48. Broomfield A, Gunny R, Prabhakar P, Grunewald S. Spontaneous rapid resolution of acute basal gan-

glia changes in an untreated infant with propionic acidemia: a clue to pathogenesis? Neuropediatrics. 2010;41(6):256–60.
49. Ribeiro LR, Della-Pace ID, de Oliveira Ferreira AP, Funck VR, Pinton S, Bobinski F, et al. Chronic administration of methylmalonate on young rats alters neuroinflammatory markers and spatial memory. Immunobiology. 2013;218(9):1175–83.
50. Schuck PF, Alves L, Pettenuzzo LF, Felisberto F, Rodrigues LB, Freitas BW, et al. Acute renal failure potentiates methylmalonate-induced oxidative stress in brain and kidney of rats. Free Radic Res. 2013;47(3):233–40.
51. Pena L, Burton BK. Survey of health status and complications among propionic acidemia patients. Am J Med Genet A. 2012;158A(7):1641–6.
52. Viegas CM, Zanatta A, Grings M, Hickmann FH, Monteiro WO, Soares LE, et al. Disruption of redox homeostasis and brain damage caused in vivo by methylmalonic acid and ammonia in cerebral cortex and striatum of developing rats. Free Radic Res. 2014;48(6):659–69.
53. Shchelochkov OA, Manoli I, Sloan JL, Ferry S, Pass A, Van Ryzin C, et al. Chronic kidney disease in propionic acidemia. Genet Med. 2019;21(12):2830–5.
54. Lam C, Desviat LR, Perez-Cerda C, Ugarte M, Barshop BA, Cederbaum S. 45-year-old female with propionic acidemia, renal failure, and premature ovarian failure; late complications of propionic acidemia? Mol Genet Metab. 2011;103(4):338–40.
55. Vernon HJ, Bagnasco S, Hamosh A, Sperati CJ. Chronic kidney disease in an adult with propionic acidemia. JIMD Rep. 2014;12:5–10.
56. Kasapkara CS, Akar M, Yuruk Yildirim ZN, Tuzun H, Kanar B, Ozbek MN. Severe renal failure and hyperammonemia in a newborn with propionic acidemia: effects of treatment on the clinical course. Ren Fail. 2014;36(3):451–2.
57. Rutledge SL, Geraghty M, Mroczek E, Rosenblatt D, Kohout E. Tubulointerstitial nephritis in methylmalonic acidemia. Pediatr Nephrol. 1993;7(1):81–2.
58. Horster F, Baumgartner MR, Viardot C, Suormala T, Burgard P, Fowler B, et al. Long-term outcome in methylmalonic acidurias is influenced by the underlying defect (mut0, mut-, cblA, cblB). Pediatr Res. 2007;62(2):225–30.
59. Zsengeller ZK, Aljinovic N, Teot LA, Korson M, Rodig N, Sloan JL, et al. Methylmalonic acidemia: a megamitochondrial disorder affecting the kidney. Pediatr Nephrol. 2014;29(11):2139–46.
60. Massoud AF, Leonard JV. Cardiomyopathy in propionic acidaemia. Eur J Pediatr. 1993;152(5):441–5.
61. Lee TM, Addonizio LJ, Barshop BA, Chung WK. Unusual presentation of propionic acidaemia as isolated cardiomyopathy. J Inherit Metab Dis. 2009;32 Suppl 1:S97–101.
62. Romano S, Valayannopoulos V, Touati G, Jais JP, Rabier D, de Keyzer Y, et al. Cardiomyopathies in propionic aciduria are reversible after liver transplantation. J Pediatr. 2010;156(1):128–34.
63. Prada CE, Al Jasmi F, Kirk EP, Hopp M, Jones O, Leslie ND, et al. Cardiac disease in methylmalonic acidemia. J Pediatr. 2011;159(5):862–4.
64. Laemmle A, Balmer C, Doell C, Sass JO, Haberle J, Baumgartner MR. Propionic acidemia in a previously healthy adolescent with acute onset of dilated cardiomyopathy. Eur J Pediatr. 2014;173(7):971–4.
65. Kakavand B, Schroeder VA, Di Sessa TG. Coincidence of long QT syndrome and propionic acidemia. Pediatr Cardiol. 2006;27(1):160–1.
66. Baumgartner D, Scholl-Burgi S, Sass JO, Sperl W, Schweigmann U, Stein JI, et al. Prolonged QTc intervals and decreased left ventricular contractility in patients with propionic acidemia. J Pediatr. 2007;150(2):192–7, 7 e1.
67. Jameson E, Walter J. Cardiac arrest secondary to long QT(C)in a child with propionic acidemia. Pediatr Cardiol. 2008;29(5):969–70.
68. Grunert SC, Mullerleile S, De Silva L, Barth M, Walter M, Walter K, et al. Propionic acidemia: clinical course and outcome in 55 pediatric and adolescent patients. Orphanet J Rare Dis. 2013;8:6.
69. De Raeve L, De Meirleir L, Ramet J, Vandenplas Y, Gerlo E. Acrodermatitis enteropathica-like cutaneous lesions in organic aciduria. J Pediatr. 1994;124(3):416–20.
70. Ozturk Y. Acrodermatitis enteropathica-like syndrome secondary to branched-chain amino acid deficiency in inborn errors of metabolism. Pediatr Dermatol. 2008;25(3):415.
71. Dominguez-Cruz JJ, Bueno-Delgado M, Pereyra J, Bernabeu-Wittel J, Conejo-Mir J. Acrodermatitis enerophatica-like skin lesions secondary to isoleucine deficiency. Eur J Dermatol. 2011;21(1):115–6.
72. Choe JY, Jang KM, Min SY, Hwang SK, Kang B, Choe BH. Propionic acidemia with novel mutation presenting as recurrent pancreatitis in a child. J Korean Med Sci. 2019;34(47):e303.
73. Imbard A, Garcia Segarra N, Tardieu M, Broue P, Bouchereau J, Pichard S, et al. Long-term liver disease in methylmalonic and propionic acidemias. Mol Genet Metab. 2018;123(4):433–40.
74. Sag E, Cebi AH, Kaya G, Karaguzel G, Cakir M. A rare cause of recurrent acute pancreatitis in a child: isovaleric acidemia with novel mutation. Pediatr Gastroenterol Hepatol Nutr. 2017;20(1):61–4.
75. North KN, Korson MS, Gopal YR, Rohr FJ, Brazelton TB, Waisbren SE, et al. Neonatal-onset propionic acidemia: neurologic and developmental profiles, and implications for management. J Pediatr. 1995;126(6):916–22.
76. Kahler SG, Sherwood WG, Woolf D, Lawless ST, Zaritsky A, Bonham J, et al. Pancreatitis in patients with organic acidemias. J Pediatr. 1994;124(2):239–43.
77. Burlina AB, Dionisi-Vici C, Piovan S, Saponara I, Bartuli A, Sabetta G, et al. Acute pancreatitis in propionic acidaemia. J Inherit Metab Dis. 1995;18(2):169–72.

78. Bultron G, Seashore MR, Pashankar DS, Husain SZ. Recurrent acute pancreatitis associated with propionic acidemia. J Pediatr Gastroenterol Nutr. 2008;47(3):370–1.
79. Mantadakis E, Chrysafis I, Tsouvala E, Evangeliou A, Chatzimichael A. Acute pancreatitis with rapid clinical improvement in a child with isovaleric acidemia. Case Rep Pediatr. 2013;2013:721871.
80. Grunert SC, Bodi I, Odening KE. Possible mechanisms for sensorineural hearing loss and deafness in patients with propionic acidemia. Orphanet J Rare Dis. 2017;12(1):30.
81. Brusque AM, Borba Rosa R, Schuck PF, Dalcin KB, Ribeiro CA, Silva CG, et al. Inhibition of the mitochondrial respiratory chain complex activities in rat cerebral cortex by methylmalonic acid. Neurochem Int. 2002;40(7):593–601.
82. Ozand PT, Gascon GG. Organic acidurias: a review. Part 2. J Child Neurol. 1991;6(4):288–303.
83. Ozand PT, Gascon GG. Organic acidurias: a review. Part 1. J Child Neurol. 1991;6(3):196–219.
84. Ribeiro CA, Balestro F, Grando V, Wajner M. Isovaleric acid reduces Na+, K+-ATPase activity in synaptic membranes from cerebral cortex of young rats. Cell Mol Neurobiol. 2007;27(4):529–40.
85. Amaral AU, et al. 2-methylcitric acid impairs glutamate metabolism and induces permeability transition in brain mitochondria. J Neurochem. 2016;137(1):62–75.
86. Nizon M, Ottolenghi C, Valayannopoulos V, Arnoux JB, Barbier V, Habarou F, et al. Long-term neurological outcome of a cohort of 80 patients with classical organic acidurias. Orphanet J Rare Dis. 2013;8:148.
87. Luciani A, Schumann A, Berquez M, Chen Z, Nieri D, Failli M, et al. Impaired mitophagy links mitochondrial disease to epithelial stress in methylmalonyl-CoA mutase deficiency. Nat Commun. 2020;11(1):970.
88. Ruppert T, Schumann A, Grone HJ, Okun JG, Kolker S, Morath MA, et al. Molecular and biochemical alterations in tubular epithelial cells of patients with isolated methylmalonic aciduria. Hum Mol Genet. 2015;24(24):7049–59.
89. Chandler RJ, Zerfas PM, Shanske S, Sloan J, Hoffmann V, DiMauro S, et al. Mitochondrial dysfunction in mut methylmalonic acidemia. FASEB J. 2009;23(4):1252–61.
90. Wajner M, Goodman SI. Disruption of mitochondrial homeostasis in organic acidurias: insights from human and animal studies. J Bioenerg Biomembr. 2011;43(1):31–8.
91. Melo DR, Kowaltowski AJ, Wajner M, Castilho RF. Mitochondrial energy metabolism in neurodegeneration associated with methylmalonic acidemia. J Bioenerg Biomembr. 2011;43(1):39–46.
92. Wilnai Y, Enns GM, Niemi AK, Higgins J, Vogel H. Abnormal hepatocellular mitochondria in methylmalonic acidemia. Ultrastruct Pathol. 2014;38(5):309–14.
93. Richard E, Alvarez-Barrientos A, Perez B, Desviat LR, Ugarte M. Methylmalonic acidaemia leads to increased production of reactive oxygen species and induction of apoptosis through the mitochondrial/caspase pathway. J Pathol. 2007;213(4):453–61.
94. Solano AF, Leipnitz G, De Bortoli GM, Seminotti B, Amaral AU, Fernandes CG, et al. Induction of oxidative stress by the metabolites accumulating in isovaleric acidemia in brain cortex of young rats. Free Radic Res. 2008;42(8):707–15.
95. Fernandes CG, Borges CG, Seminotti B, Amaral AU, Knebel LA, Eichler P, et al. Experimental evidence that methylmalonic acid provokes oxidative damage and compromises antioxidant defenses in nerve terminal and striatum of young rats. Cell Mol Neurobiol. 2011;31(5):775–85.
96. Collado MS, Armstrong AJ, Olson M, Hoang SA, Day N, Summar M, et al. Biochemical and anaplerotic applications of in vitro models of propionic acidemia and methylmalonic acidemia using patient-derived primary hepatocytes. Mol Genet Metab. 2020;130(3):183–96.
97. Luciani A, Devuyst O. Methylmalonyl acidemia: from mitochondrial metabolism to defective mitophagy and disease. Autophagy. 2020;16(6):1159–61.
98. Caterino M, Chandler RJ, Sloan JL, Dorko K, Cusmano-Ozog K, Ingenito L, et al. The proteome of methylmalonic acidemia (MMA): the elucidation of altered pathways in patient livers. Mol Biosyst. 2016;12(2):566–74.
99. Imperlini E, Santorelli L, Orru S, Scolamiero E, Ruoppolo M, Caterino M. Mass spectrometry-based metabolomic and proteomic strategies in organic acidemias. Biomed Res Int. 2016;2016:9210408.
100. Storgaard JH, Madsen KL, Lokken N, Vissing J, van Hall G, Lund AM, et al. Impaired lipolysis in propionic acidemia: a new metabolic myopathy? JIMD Rep. 2020;53(1):16–21.
101. Filipowicz HR, Ernst SL, Ashurst CL, Pasquali M, Longo N. Metabolic changes associated with hyperammonemia in patients with propionic acidemia. Mol Genet Metab. 2006;88(2):123–30.
102. Gebhardt B, Dittrich S, Parbel S, Vlaho S, Matsika O, Bohles H. N-carbamylglutamate protects patients with decompensated propionic aciduria from hyperammonaemia. J Inherit Metab Dis. 2005;28(2):241–4.
103. Yannicelli S. Nutrition therapy of organic acidaemias with amino acid-based formulas: emphasis on methylmalonic and propionic acidaemia. J Inherit Metab Dis. 2006;29(2–3):281–7.
104. Knerr I, Gibson KM. Disorders of leucine, isoleucine and valine metabolism. In: Blau N, editor. Physician's guide to the diagnosis, treatment and follow-up of inherited metabolic diseases. Berlin: Springer-Verlag; 2014.
105. Feillet F, Bodamer OA, Dixon MA, Sequeira S, Leonard JV. Resting energy expenditure in disorders of propionate metabolism. J Pediatr. 2000;136(5):659–63.

106. Thomas JA, Bernstein LE, Greene CL, Koeller DM. Apparent decreased energy requirements in children with organic acidemias: preliminary observations. J Am Diet Assoc. 2000;100(9):1074–6.
107. Hauser NS, Manoli I, Graf JC, Sloan J, Venditti CP. Variable dietary management of methylmalonic acidemia: metabolic and energetic correlations. Am J Clin Nutr. 2011;93(1):47–56.
108. Jurecki E, Ueda K, Frazier D, Rohr F, Thompson A, Hussa C, et al. Nutrition management guideline for propionic acidemia: an evidence- and consensus-based approach. Mol Genet Metab. 2019;126(4):341–54.
109. Roe CR, Millington DS, Maltby DA, Kahler SG, Bohan TP. L-carnitine therapy in isovaleric acidemia. J Clin Invest. 1984;74(6):2290–5.
110. de Sousa C, Chalmers RA, Stacey TE, Tracey BM, Weaver CM, Bradley D. The response to L-carnitine and glycine therapy in isovaleric acidaemia. Eur J Pediatr. 1986;144(5):451–6.
111. Chinen Y, Nakamura S, Tamashiro K, Sakamoto O, Tashiro K, Inokuchi T, et al. Isovaleric acidemia: therapeutic response to supplementation with glycine, l-carnitine, or both in combination and a 10-year follow-up case study. Mol Genet Metab Rep. 2017;11:2–5.
112. Berry GT, Yudkoff M, Segal S. Isovaleric acidemia: medical and neurodevelopmental effects of long-term therapy. J Pediatr. 1988;113(1 Pt 1):58–64.
113. Naglak M, Salvo R, Madsen K, Dembure P, Elsas L. The treatment of isovaleric acidemia with glycine supplement. Pediatr Res. 1988;24(1):9–13.
114. Fries MH, Rinaldo P, Schmidt-Sommerfeld E, Jurecki E, Packman S. Isovaleric acidemia: response to a leucine load after three weeks of supplementation with glycine, L-carnitine, and combined glycine-carnitine therapy. J Pediatr. 1996;129(3):449–52.
115. Valayannopoulos V, Baruteau J, Delgado MB, Cano A, Couce ML, Del Toro M, et al. Carglumic acid enhances rapid ammonia detoxification in classical organic acidurias with a favourable risk-benefit profile: a retrospective observational study. Orphanet J Rare Dis. 2016;11:32.
116. Ah Mew N, McCarter R, Daikhin Y, Nissim I, Yudkoff M, Tuchman M. N-carbamylglutamate augments ureagenesis and reduces ammonia and glutamine in propionic acidemia. Pediatrics. 2010;126(1):e208–14.
117. Tummolo A, Melpignano L, Carella A, Di Mauro AM, Piccinno E, Vendemiale M, et al. Long-term continuous N-carbamylglutamate treatment in frequently decompensated propionic acidemia: a case report. J Med Case Reports. 2018;12(1):103.
118. Al-Hassnan ZN, Boyadjiev SA, Praphanphoj V, Hamosh A, Braverman NE, Thomas GH, et al. The relationship of plasma glutamine to ammonium and of glycine to acid-base balance in propionic acidaemia. J Inherit Metab Dis. 2003;26(1):89–91.
119. Siekmeyer M, Petzold-Quinque S, Terpe F, Beblo S, Gebhardt R, Schlensog-Schuster F, et al. Citric acid as the last therapeutic approach in an acute life-threatening metabolic decompensation of propionic acidemia. J Pediatr Endocrinol Metab. 2013;26(5–6):569–74.
120. Longo N, et al. Anaplerotic therapy in propionic acidemia. Mol Genet Metab. 2018;122(1–2):51–9.
121. Pinar-Sueiro S, Martinez-Fernandez R, Lage-Medina S, Aldamiz-Echevarria L, Vecino E. Optic neuropathy in methylmalonic acidemia: the role of neuroprotection. J Inherit Metab Dis. 2010;33 Suppl 3:S199–203.
122. Fragaki K, Cano A, Benoist JF, Rigal O, Chaussenot A, Rouzier C, et al. Fatal heart failure associated with CoQ10 and multiple OXPHOS deficiency in a child with propionic acidemia. Mitochondrion. 2011;11(3):533–6.
123. Ha TS, Lee JS, Hong EJ. Delay of renal progression in methylmalonic acidemia using angiotensin II inhibition: a case report. J Nephrol. 2008;21(5):793–6.
124. Kelts DG, Ney D, Bay C, Saudubray JM, Nyhan WL. Studies on requirements for amino acids in infants with disorders of amino acid metabolism. I. Effect of alanine. Pediatr Res. 1985;19(1):86–91.
125. Wolff JA, Kelts DG, Algert S, Prodanos C, Nyhan WL. Alanine decreases the protein requirements of infants with inborn errors of amino acid metabolism. J Neurogenet. 1985;2(1):41–9.
126. Marsden D, Barshop BA, Capistrano-Estrada S, Rice M, Prodanos C, Sartoris D, et al. Anabolic effect of human growth hormone: management of inherited disorders of catabolic pathways. Biochem Med Metab Biol. 1994;52(2):145–54.
127. Treacy E, Arbour L, Chessex P, Graham G, Kasprzak L, Casey K, et al. Glutathione deficiency as a complication of methylmalonic acidemia: response to high doses of ascorbate. J Pediatr. 1996;129(3):445–8.
128. Touati G, Valayannopoulos V, Mention K, de Lonlay P, Jouvet P, Depondt E, et al. Methylmalonic and propionic acidurias: management without or with a few supplements of specific amino acid mixture. J Inherit Metab Dis. 2006;29(2–3):288–98.
129. Gander JW, Rhone ET, Wilson WG, Barcia JP, Sacco MJ. Veno-venous extracorporeal membrane oxygenation for continuous renal replacement in a neonate with propionic acidemia. J Extra Corpor Technol. 2017;49(1):64–6.
130. Aygun F, Varol F, Aktuglu-Zeybek C, Kiykim E, Cam H. Continuous renal replacement therapy with high flow rate can effectively, safely, and quickly reduce plasma ammonia and leucine levels in children. Children (Basel). 2019;6(4):53.
131. Jones S, Reed CA, Vijay S, Walter JH, Morris AA. N-carbamylglutamate for neonatal hyperammonaemia in propionic acidaemia. J Inherit Metab Dis. 2008;31 Suppl 2:S219–22.
132. Filippi L, Gozzini E, Fiorini P, Malvagia S, la Marca G, Donati MA. N-carbamylglutamate in emergency management of hyperammonemia in neonatal acute onset propionic and methylmalonic aciduria. Neonatology. 2010;97(3):286–90.

133. Schwahn BC, Pieterse L, Bisset WM, Galloway PG, Robinson PH. Biochemical efficacy of N-carbamylglutamate in neonatal severe hyperammonaemia due to propionic acidaemia. Eur J Pediatr. 2010;169(1):133–4.
134. Kasapkara CS, Ezgu FS, Okur I, Tumer L, Biberoglu G, Hasanoglu A. N-carbamylglutamate treatment for acute neonatal hyperammonemia in isovaleric acidemia. Eur J Pediatr. 2011;170(6):799–801.
135. Abacan M, Boneh A. Use of carglumic acid in the treatment of hyperammonaemia during metabolic decompensation of patients with propionic acidaemia. Mol Genet Metab. 2013;109(4):397–401.
136. Matern D, Seydewitz HH, Lehnert W, Niederhoff H, Leititis JU, Brandis M. Primary treatment of propionic acidemia complicated by acute thiamine deficiency. J Pediatr. 1996;129(5):758–60.
137. Mayatepek E, Schulze A. Metabolic decompensation and lactic acidosis in propionic acidaemia complicated by thiamine deficiency. J Inherit Metab Dis. 1999;22(2):189–90.
138. Critelli K, McKiernan P, Vockley J, Mazariegos G, Squires RH, Soltys K, et al. Liver transplantation for propionic acidemia and methylmalonic acidemia: perioperative management and clinical outcomes. Liver Transpl. 2018;24(9):1260–70.
139. Chu TH, Chien YH, Lin HY, Liao HC, Ho HJ, Lai CJ, et al. Methylmalonic acidemia/propionic acidemia - the biochemical presentation and comparing the outcome between liver transplantation versus non-liver transplantation groups. Orphanet J Rare Dis. 2019;14(1):73.
140. Jain-Ghai S, Joffe AR, Bond GY, Siriwardena K, Chan A, Yap JYK, et al. Pre-school neurocognitive and functional outcomes after liver transplant in children with early onset urea cycle disorders, maple syrup urine disease, and propionic acidemia: an inception cohort matched-comparison study. JIMD Rep. 2020;52(1):43–54.
141. Quintero J, Molera C, Juamperez J, Redecillas S, Meavilla S, Nunez R, et al. The role of liver transplantation in propionic acidemia. Liver Transpl. 2018;24(12):1736–45.
142. Van Calcar SC, Harding CO, Lyne P, Hogan K, Banerjee R, Sollinger H, et al. Renal transplantation in a patient with methylmalonic acidaemia. J Inherit Metab Dis. 1998;21(7):729–37.
143. van't Hoff WG, Dixon M, Taylor J, Mistry P, Rolles K, Rees L, et al. Combined liver-kidney transplantation in methylmalonic acidemia. J Pediatr. 1998;132(6):1043–4.
144. Lubrano R, Scoppi P, Barsotti P, Travasso E, Scateni S, Cristaldi S, et al. Kidney transplantation in a girl with methylmalonic acidemia and end stage renal failure. Pediatr Nephrol. 2001;16(11):848–51.
145. Nagarajan S, Enns GM, Millan MT, Winter S, Sarwal MM. Management of methylmalonic acidaemia by combined liver-kidney transplantation. J Inherit Metab Dis. 2005;28(4):517–24.
146. Lubrano R, Elli M, Rossi M, Travasso E, Raggi C, Barsotti P, et al. Renal transplant in methylmalonic acidemia: could it be the best option? Report on a case at 10 years and review of the literature. Pediatr Nephrol. 2007;22(8):1209–14.
147. Mc Guire PJ, Lim-Melia E, Diaz GA, Raymond K, Larkin A, Wasserstein MP, et al. Combined liver-kidney transplant for the management of methylmalonic aciduria: a case report and review of the literature. Mol Genet Metab. 2008;93(1):22–9.
148. Clothier JC, Chakrapani A, Preece MA, McKiernan P, Gupta R, Macdonald A, et al. Renal transplantation in a boy with methylmalonic acidaemia. J Inherit Metab Dis. 2011;34(3):695–700.
149. Yorifuji T, Muroi J, Uematsu A, Nakahata T, Egawa H, Tanaka K. Living-related liver transplantation for neonatal-onset propionic acidemia. J Pediatr. 2000;137(4):572–4.
150. Barshes NR, Vanatta JM, Patel AJ, Carter BA, O'Mahony CA, Karpen SJ, et al. Evaluation and management of patients with propionic acidemia undergoing liver transplantation: a comprehensive review. Pediatr Transplant. 2006;10(7):773–81.
151. Kasahara M, Horikawa R, Tagawa M, Uemoto S, Yokoyama S, Shibata Y, et al. Current role of liver transplantation for methylmalonic acidemia: a review of the literature. Pediatr Transplant. 2006;10(8):943–7.
152. Chen PW, Hwu WL, Ho MC, Lee NC, Chien YH, Ni YH, et al. Stabilization of blood methylmalonic acid level in methylmalonic acidemia after liver transplantation. Pediatr Transplant. 2010;14(3):337–41.
153. Vara R, Turner C, Mundy H, Heaton ND, Rela M, Mieli-Vergani G, et al. Liver transplantation for propionic acidemia in children. Liver Transpl. 2011;17(6):661–7.
154. Brassier A, Boyer O, Valayannopoulos V, Ottolenghi C, Krug P, Cosson MA, et al. Renal transplantation in 4 patients with methylmalonic aciduria: a cell therapy for metabolic disease. Mol Genet Metab. 2013;110(1–2):106–10.
155. Nagao M, Tanaka T, Morii M, Wakai S, Horikawa R, Kasahara M. Improved neurologic prognosis for a patient with propionic acidemia who received early living donor liver transplantation. Mol Genet Metab. 2013;108(1):25–9.
156. Arrizza C, De Gottardi A, Foglia E, Baumgartner M, Gautschi M, Nuoffer JM. Reversal of cardiomyopathy in propionic acidemia after liver transplantation: a 10-year follow-up. Transpl Int. 2015;28(12):1447–50.
157. Ou P, Touati G, Fraisse A, Sidi D, Kachaner J, Saudubray JM, et al. A rare cause of cardiomyopathy in childhood: propionic acidosis. Three case reports. Arch Mal Coeur Vaiss. 2001;94(5):531–3.
158. Berry GT, Blume ED, Wessel A, Singh T, Hecht L, Marsden D, et al. The re-occurrence of cardiomyopathy in propionic acidemia after liver transplantation. JIMD Rep. 2020;54(1):3–8.

159. Kasahara M, Sakamoto S, Kanazawa H, Karaki C, Kakiuchi T, Shigeta T, et al. Living-donor liver transplantation for propionic acidemia. Pediatr Transplant. 2012;16(3):230–4.
160. Chakrapani A, Sivakumar P, McKiernan PJ, Leonard JV. Metabolic stroke in methylmalonic acidemia five years after liver transplantation. J Pediatr. 2002;140(2):261–3.
161. Nyhan WL, Gargus JJ, Boyle K, Selby R, Koch R. Progressive neurologic disability in methylmalonic acidemia despite transplantation of the liver. Eur J Pediatr. 2002;161(7):377–9.
162. Collard R, Majtan T, Park I, Kraus JP. Import of TAT-conjugated propionyl coenzyme a carboxylase using models of propionic acidemia. Mol Cell Biol. 2018;38(6):e00491–17.
163. An D, Schneller JL, Frassetto A, Liang S, Zhu X, Park JS, et al. Systemic messenger RNA therapy as a treatment for methylmalonic acidemia. Cell Rep. 2017;21(12):3548–58.
164. Erlich-Hadad T, Hadad R, Feldman A, Greif H, Lictenstein M, Lorberboum-Galski H. TAT-MTS-MCM fusion proteins reduce MMA levels and improve mitochondrial activity and liver function in MCM-deficient cells. J Cell Mol Med. 2018;22(3):1601–13.
165. An D, Frassetto A, Jacquinet E, Eybye M, Milano J, DeAntonis C, et al. Long-term efficacy and safety of mRNA therapy in two murine models of methylmalonic acidemia. EBioMedicine. 2019;45:519–28.
166. Chandler RJ, Venditti CP. Gene therapy for methylmalonic acidemia: past, present, and future. Hum Gene Ther. 2019;30(10):1236–44.
167. Al-Dirbashi OY, Alfadhel M, Al-Thihli K, Al Dhahouri N, Langhans CD, Al Hammadi Z, et al. Assessment of methylcitrate and methylcitrate to citrate ratio in dried blood spots as biomarkers for inborn errors of propionate metabolism. Sci Rep. 2019;9(1):12366.
168. Arnold GL, et al. Methylcitrate/citrate ratio as a predictor of clinical control in propionic acidemia. J Inherit Metab Dis. 2003:37.
169. Zwickler T, Haege G, Riderer A, Horster F, Hoffmann GF, Burgard P, et al. Metabolic decompensation in methylmalonic aciduria: which biochemical parameters are discriminative? J Inherit Metab Dis. 2012;35(5):797–806.
170. Zwickler T, Riderer A, Haege G, Hoffmann GF, Kolker S, Burgard P. Usefulness of biochemical parameters in decision-making on the start of emergency treatment in patients with propionic acidemia. J Inherit Metab Dis. 2014;37(1):31–7.
171. Molema F, Jacobs EH, Onkenhout W, Schoonderwoerd GC, Langendonk JG, Williams M. Fibroblast growth factor 21 as a biomarker for long-term complications in organic acidemias. J Inherit Metab Dis. 2018;41(6):1179–87.
172. Manoli I, Sysol JR, Epping MW, Li L, Wang C, Sloan JL, et al. FGF21 underlies a hormetic response to metabolic stress in methylmalonic acidemia. JCI Insight. 2018;3(23):e124351.
173. Propionic acidemia: care plan & shared dataset. Mountain States Genetics Regional Collaborative; 2013.
174. Surtees RA, Matthews EE, Leonard JV. Neurologic outcome of propionic acidemia. Pediatr Neurol. 1992;8(5):333–7.
175. Nicolaides P, Leonard J, Surtees R. Neurological outcome of methylmalonic acidaemia. Arch Dis Child. 1998;78(6):508–12.
176. O'Shea CJ, Sloan JL, Wiggs EA, Pao M, Gropman A, Baker EH, et al. Neurocognitive phenotype of isolated methylmalonic acidemia. Pediatrics. 2012;129(6):e1541–51.
177. Szymanska E, Jezela-Stanek A, Bogdanska A, Rokicki D, Ehmke Vel Emczynska-Seliga E, Pajdowska M, et al. Long term follow-up of polish patients with isovaleric aciduria. Clinical and molecular delineation of isovaleric aciduria. Diagnostics (Basel). 2020;10(10):738.
178. Grunert SC, Wendel U, Lindner M, Leichsenring M, Schwab KO, Vockley J, et al. Clinical and neurocognitive outcome in symptomatic isovaleric acidemia. Orphanet J Rare Dis. 2012;7:9.
179. van der Meer SB, Poggi F, Spada M, Bonnefont JP, Ogier H, Hubert P, et al. Clinical outcome of long-term management of patients with vitamin B12-unresponsive methylmalonic acidemia. J Pediatr. 1994;125(6 Pt 1):903–8.
180. Fischer AQ, Challa VR, Burton BK, McLean WT. Cerebellar hemorrhage complicating isovaleric acidemia: a case report. Neurology. 1981;31(6):746–8.
181. van der Meer SB, Poggi F, Spada M, Bonnefont JP, Ogier H, Hubert P, et al. Clinical outcome and long-term management of 17 patients with propionic acidaemia. Eur J Pediatr. 1996;155(3):205–10.
182. Ledley FD, Levy HL, Shih VE, Benjamin R, Mahoney MJ. Benign methylmalonic aciduria. N Engl J Med. 1984;311(16):1015–8.
183. Treacy E, Clow C, Mamer OA, Scriver CR. Methylmalonic acidemia with a severe chemical but benign clinical phenotype. J Pediatr. 1993;122(3):428–9.
184. Grunert SC, Mullerleile S, de Silva L, Barth M, Walter M, Walter K, et al. Propionic acidemia: neonatal versus selective metabolic screening. J Inherit Metab Dis. 2012;35(1):41–9.

Glutaric Acidemia Type I: Diagnosis and Management

19

Curtis R. Coughlin II

Contents

C. R. Coughlin II (✉)
Clinical Genetics and Metabolism, Children's Hospital Colorado, University of Colorado Denver - Anschutz Medical Campus, Aurora, CO, USA
e-mail: curtis.coughlin@childrenscolorado.org

L. E. Bernstein et al. (eds.), *Nutrition Management of Inherited Metabolic Diseases*,
https://doi.org/10.1007/978-3-030-94510-7_19

Core Messages

- Glutaric acidemia type 1 (GA-1) is an autosomal recessive disorder of lysine, hydroxylysine, and tryptophan metabolism caused by a deficiency of glutaryl-CoA dehydrogenase. It results in the accumulation of 3-hydroxyglutaric and glutaric acid.
- Patients can present with brain atrophy and macrocephaly, often with concurrent acute dystonia triggered by an intercurrent childhood infection and often with fever. This can occur anytime during the first 6 years of life with a vulnerable period between 8 and 18 months of age.
- GA-1 is identified by elevated glutaryl carnitine (C5DC) on the newborn screening panel.

19.1 Background

Glutaric acidemia type 1 (also referred to as glutaric aciduria type 1) is an organic aciduria characterized by a striatal injury and a progressive movement disorder that occurs in early childhood [1]. Neurologic symptoms are often precipitated by an intercurrent illness [2], and aggressive treatment of illness or other catabolic stress is central to the management of glutaric acidemia type 1 (GA-1) [3]. Approximately 10–20% of patients develop a striatal injury without a clear illness or encephalopathic crisis emphasizing the importance of early diagnosis [4, 5]. Newborn screening and neonatal treatment have dramatically improved the natural history of this disease [6]. Due to early diagnosis facilitated by newborn screening programs and appropriate medical management, most patients remain healthy into adulthood.

This chapter will focus on the underlying enzymatic defect that results in GA-1 and subsequent rationale for medical management. The reader should use the information in this chapter and the reference material within, to gain an understanding of laboratory studies integral to the diagnosis of GA-1. Other laboratories may also be used for monitoring nutrition management in general, although there is no treatment metabolite specific to GA-1 that correlates with either the risk of striatal injury or overall clinical outcome. The best predictor of clinical outcome is adherence to medical management recommendations [6].

19.2 Clinical, Genetic, and Biochemical Findings

Phenotype The initial patients reported with GA-1 were siblings who, after a period of normal development, experienced significant neurological deterioration in the first year of life [1]. As more patients with GA-1 were identified, a distinctive neurologic phenotype began to emerge including a complex movement disorder [2] and acute bilateral striatal injury identified on brain imaging [7]. The highest risk for encephalopathic crisis occurs during a critical period of brain development (age 3–36 months), and 95% of affected individuals have an encephalopathic crisis prior to 24 months of age [2, 3, 8]. The vulnerable period for neurologic injury is often reported as the first 6 years of life as the oldest reported patient with an encephalopathic crisis experienced a repeat crisis at 70 months of age [2]. As a result, the benefit of treatment regimens after the age of 6 years is unclear [3].

Dystonia and axial hypotonia are reported to be the predominant neurologic findings following an encephalopathic crisis, although dyskinesia and slight spastic signs have also been reported [9, 10]. The phenotype of GA-1 evolves with time and a fixed dystonia and akinetic-rigid parkinsonism has been reported in older patients [11].

Brain imaging (typically through magnetic resonance imaging or computerized tomography) is often performed following an encephalopathic crisis, and certain imaging findings have been suggested as pathognomonic for GA-1. Patients are often noted to have widening of sylvian fissures and frontotemporal atrophy, and these findings may be evident in the newborn period. A subset of patients have developed an acute subdural hemorrhage, which is an important clinical entity as parents have even been investigated for non-accidental trauma prior to the diagnosis of GA-1 [12–14]. Following an acute crisis, the basal ganglia is affected, and this injury typically affects the putamen and caudate as well as the pallidum [7, 15]. White matter changes are also noted on magnetic resonance imaging (MRI) of patients as they age, including those patients who remain asymptomatic.

It is important to note that the phenotype of GA-1 has dramatically improved by early diagnosis and medical management. Prior to newborn screening, approximately 80–90% of untreated patients developed a striatal injury [16]. Following institution of newborn screening for GA-1, approximately 70% of patients remain asymptomatic through adolescence [6]. Of course, not all diagnosed patients remain asymptomatic and it is currently unclear whether the residual risk for patients is due to poor compliance with treatment guidelines or some other unknown risk factor [17]. There is growing recognition of a late onset phenotype marked by headaches, transient ataxic gaits, and peripheral polyneuropathy with noted white matter findings on brain MRI [18, 19]. There are also limited reports of older patients with GA-1 who had brain tumors [2, 19–22], although it is unclear if these case reports suggest an increased risk for brain tumors or coincidental diagnosis.

Biochemistry and Genetics GA-1 results from the deficiency of the enzyme glutaryl-CoA dehydrogenase (GCDH), which catalyzes the decarboxylation of glutaryl-CoA to crotonyl-CoA [23]. GCDH is involved in the degradation of the amino acids lysine, hydroxylysine, and tryptophan and the deficiency of GCDH results in the accumulation of glutaryl-CoA, glutaconic acid, glutaric acid (GA), and 3-hydroxyglutaric acid (3OHGA) (Fig. 19.1). These metabolites are pathognomonic for GA-1 and, therefore, are important for diagnosis. The role of these metabolites in disease pathology is less clear.

As noted above, GCDH is involved in the degradation and decarboxylation of lysine, and to a lesser effect, hydroxylysine and tryptophan. Patients may also be treated with L-arginine although the use of arginine supplementation in the

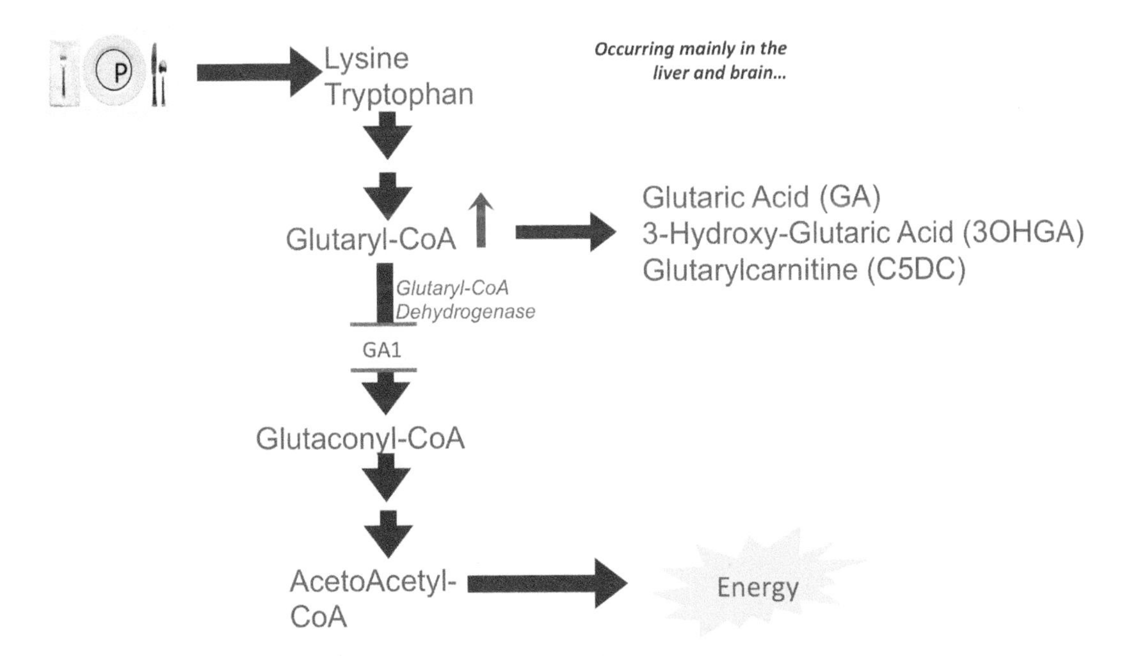

Fig. 19.1 Metabolism of lysine and tryptophan in GA-1 – defects in GCDH results in the accumulation of glutaryl-CoA and subsequently GA, 3OHGA, and C5DC

treatment of this disease is controversial [3]. Lysine crosses the blood–brain barrier through a specific sodium-independent, facilitative amino acid transporter known as γ+. Lysine competes with arginine, ornithine, and homoarginine for cellular uptake through the transporter. As a result, arginine supplementation has been suggested as a possible adjunct therapy as arginine would theoretically reduce the cerebral uptake of lysine by overwhelming the γ + transporter with arginine [24, 25].

GCDH is encoded by the gene *GCDH* located at chromosome 19p13.3 (chr19: 12,891,128-12,915,344, GRCh38) [26]. Although a few recurrent variants have been identified, especially in isolated genetic populations, the majority of individuals have private or familial variants [27, 28]. There is a limited genotype–phenotype correlation among patients except for the low-excretor biochemical phenotype. There are multiple criteria for the low-excretor phenotype although a common criterion is a urine GA level of <100 mmol/mol creatinine [5] or a urine 3OHGA > urine GA level. The low-excretor variants have been hypothesized to act as biochemical-dominant mutations [29], and patients with at least one low-excretor variant are more likely to have a false negative newborn screen [30]. It is important to emphasize that patients with a low-excretor phenotype have the same risk of developing a striatal injury as any other patient with GA-1 [31].

GA-1 is a rare autosomal recessive disorder and estimated to have a worldwide incidence of 1:100,000 live births. The incidence of GA-1 is significantly higher in genetically isolated communities including the Amish community, Canadian Oji-Cree natives, and the Irish Travellers [16, 32, 33]. A few ancestries also have higher incidences of GA-1 including 1:65,000 newborns in Victoria, Australia [34], 1:70,0000 births in Taiwan [35], and 1:112,000 births in Germany [17]. Initially, dedicated screening programs focused on these high-risk populations and have allowed for prospective treatment of patients prior to neurologic injury and have significantly reduced the risk of striatal injury. In those communities with a high prevalence of low-excretor genotypes, a DNA-based screening approach was also utilized [32].

19.3 Diagnosis and Management

Diagnosis Prior to the initiation of screening programs, the diagnosis of GA-1 was suspected either as a result of characteristic brain imaging or the presence of a movement disorder. Abnormal biochemical findings would then support the already suspected diagnosis of GA-1. As previously discussed, the defect in GCDH subsequently results in the accumulation of GA, 3OHGA, and glutarylcarnitine (C5DC). The latter metabolite can be identified on newborn screening platforms that utilize mass spectrometry platforms [36]. As a result of newborn screening, the majority of individuals with GA-1 are now diagnosed shortly after birth and prior to striatal injury, but individuals with a low-excretor phenotype may be "missed" on newborn screening as previously described [30]. Other congenital or acquired disorders can also result in false suspicion for GA-1. Individuals with renal insufficiency have decreased excretion of C5DC, which results in increased retention of C5DC in blood [37]. Also, other inborn errors of metabolism may have elevations of C5DC or elevations of C10-OH (C10-OH cannot easily be differentiated from C5DC) requiring further testing to differentiate GA-1 from other inborn errors of metabolism [38].

To correctly diagnosis true positives for GA-1 following a positive screen, further metabolite testing is often recommended. This can include an acylcarnitine profile for repeat measurement of C5DC, urine organic acids, and quantification of GA and 3OHGA. In a retrospective review of serum GA and 3OHGA, there was significant overlap between the metabolite values of those individuals with confirmed GA-1 (true positives) and those who were false positive (Fig. 19.2). Due to this significant overlap, the value of GA and 3OHGA alone is not always suitable to identify affected individuals. Of note, elevations of GA are also common in other inborn errors of metabolism as well as acquired disorders, and patients should be evaluated for other conditions when appropriate (Table 19.1). The diagnosis of GA-1 can be confirmed by deficient GCDH enzyme activity or the presence of two known disease-causing variants in *GCDH* [3]. This is

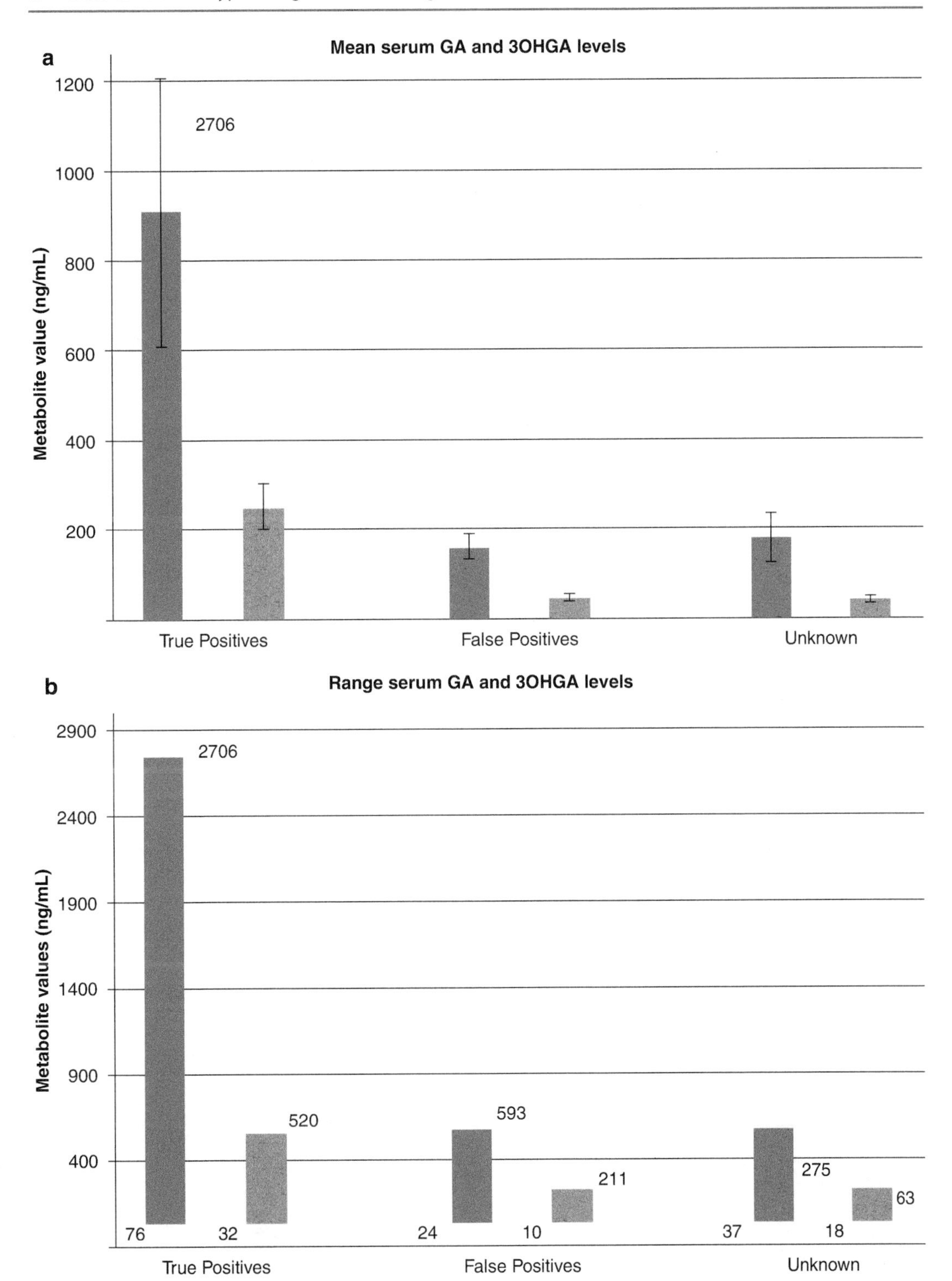

Fig. 19.2 Glutaric acid and 3-hydroxy glutaric acid concentrations in affected and unaffected subjects (**a**) Mean serum GA (blue) and 3OHGA (orange) levels are significantly different between affected and unaffected patients. (**b**) There is overlap in the range of GA and 3OHGA levels between affected and unaffected patients often making a single metabolite uninformative. Subjects affected status was classified as true positive, false positive or unknown by the referring physician through a retrospective survey. All serum samples were analyzed in the Goodman Biochemical Laboratory, University of Colorado

especially important in cases of non-accidental trauma and in those asymptomatic individuals identified through screening programs.

Despite its significant benefits, treatment does place a burden on the family. As a result, it is desirable to only treat those individuals who are deemed "at-risk" for neurologic injury. Unfortunately, there is no discernable biochemical marker associated with neurologic outcome in GA-1. As reported by Christensen et al., the clinical outcome in those patients with a low excretor phenotype is identical to those individuals with a high excretor phenotype (Fig. 19.3) [31]. Similarly, Kölker et al. reported that the age at encephalopathic crisis between high and low-excretors are similar (Fig. 19.4) [2]. This suggests that the degree of metabolite excretion does not correlate with the risk for neurologic damage. Even patients with significant residual enzyme activity (up to 30% of enzyme activity) have had severe neurologic damage following an encephalopathic crisis [39].

Table 19.1 Known causes of glutaric acid elevations in plasma or urine

Inborn errors of metabolism
Glutaric aciduria type I
Glutaric aciduria type II (multiple acyl-CoA dehydrogenase deficiency)
Glutaric aciduria type III (glutaryl-CoA oxidase deficiency)
Glycerol kinase deficiency
HMG-CoA lyase deficiency
Methylmalonic aciduria
Mitochondrial disorders
2-Oxoadipic aciduria
Propionic aciduria
Additional causes
Bacterial production
MCT containing formulas
Riboflavin deficiency (acquired)
Valproic acid

In the absence of a genetic, enzymatic, or biochemical correlation with phenotype, it is important that every patient with GA-1 be treated similarly and that no patient be labeled as having a mild clinical phenotype [3]. Inadequate treatment can lead to irreversible neurologic damage, and as a result, a marker of disease control would be ideal.

The use of accumulating metabolites for disease control is a common paradigm in the treatment of most inborn errors of metabolism such as the use of phenylalanine to evaluate the treatment of an individual with phenylketonuria. As already discussed, the degrees to which metabolites accumulate differ significantly between affected individuals with GA-1, as exemplified by the low excretor phenotype. But just as these metabolites are not indicative of overall outcome, there is no evidence that GA, 3OHGA, or C5DC are reliable biochemical markers for the monitoring of nutrition treatment [2].

19.4 Treatment

Emergency Management In the majority of cases, striatal necrosis occurs during an encephalopathic crisis usually precipitated by an infectious illness, although in 10–20% of patients, neurologic symptoms are present without a precipitating event [4]. As a result, emergency treatment of infectious illness is paramount to

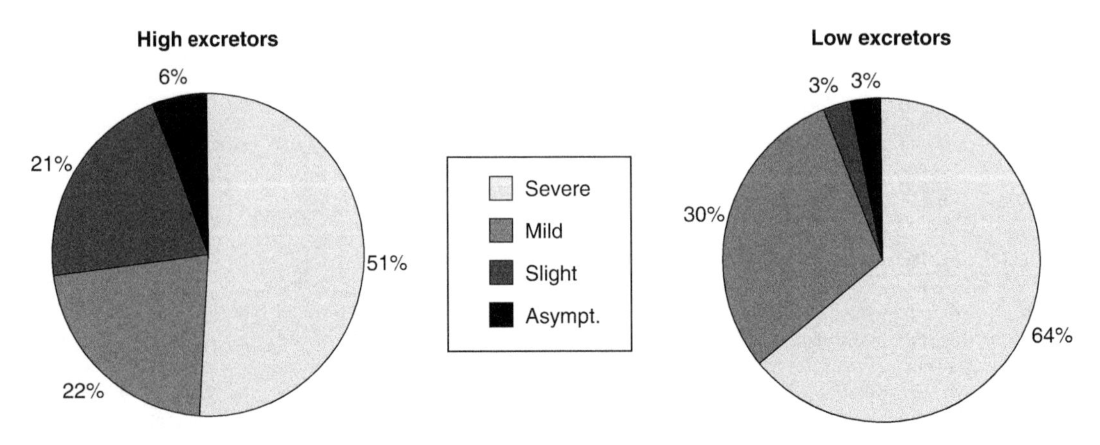

Fig. 19.3 Phenotype of 76 GA-1 patients classified as previously published [5, 31]

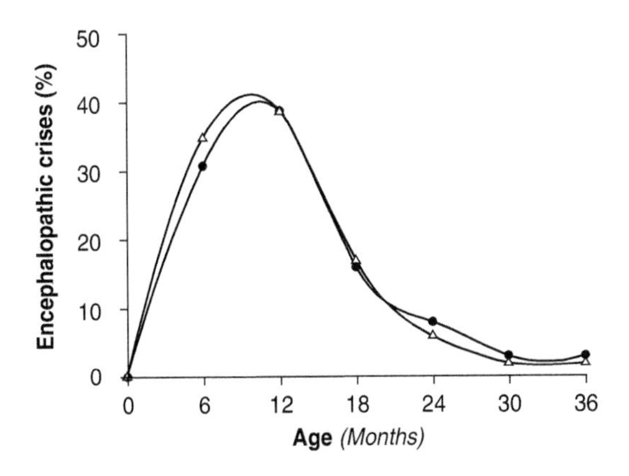

Fig. 19.4 Acute encephalopathic crises. Age at first encephalopathic crisis in high (●) and low excretors (△) [2]

avoiding an encephalopathic crisis and striatal injury. Since it is impossible to determine when an acute crisis may occur, patients should receive emergency management during every illness and surgical intervention. Emergency treatment in GA-1 is similar to that of other IEM and includes avoidance or reversal of the catabolic state by providing a source of energy, reduction of lysine or intact protein, L-carnitine supplementation for detoxification, and treatment of the present illness [40]. Consensus recommendations have developed to implement emergency treatment at the first sign of an intercurrent illness [3].

19.5 Summary

Individuals with GA-1 are at risk for irreversible neurologic damage resulting in a debilitating, complex movement disorder. Without a reliable biomarker to stratify those at risk, treatment should be initiated in all affected patients, and emergency management should be implemented at the first sign of illness.

Acknowledgements We are grateful to the late Distinguished Professor Stephen Goodman of the University of Colorado for his dedication to the diagnosis and treatment of GA-1 and his mentorship to many in the field of metabolism. We are also grateful to Daryl Goodman and Susana San Roman, as well as the members of the Goodman Biochemical Laboratory, for their previous retrospective analysis of metabolites in individuals with GA-1.

References

1. Goodman SI, Markey SP, Moe PG, Miles BS, Teng CC. Glutaric aciduria; a "new" disorder of amino acid metabolism. Biochem Med. 1975;12(1):12–21.
2. Kolker S, Garbade SF, Greenberg CR, Leonard JV, Saudubray JM, Ribes A, et al. Natural history, outcome, and treatment efficacy in children and adults with glutaryl-CoA dehydrogenase deficiency. Pediatr Res. 2006;59(6):840–7.
3. Boy N, Muhlhausen C, Maier EM, Heringer J, Assmann B, Burgard P, et al. Proposed recommendations for diagnosing and managing individuals with glutaric aciduria type I: second revision. J Inherit Metab Dis. 2017;40(1):75–101.
4. Hoffmann GF, Athanassopoulos S, Burlina AB, Duran M, de Klerk JB, Lehnert W, et al. Clinical course, early diagnosis, treatment, and prevention of disease in glutaryl-CoA dehydrogenase deficiency. Neuropediatrics. 1996;27(3):115–23.
5. Busquets C, Merinero B, Christensen E, Gelpi JL, Campistol J, Pineda M, et al. Glutaryl-CoA dehydrogenase deficiency in Spain: evidence of two groups of patients, genetically, and biochemically distinct. Pediatr Res. 2000;48(3):315–22.
6. Boy N, Mengler K, Thimm E, Schiergens KA, Marquardt T, Weinhold N, et al. Newborn screening: a disease-changing intervention for glutaric aciduria type 1. Ann Neurol. 2018;83(5):970–9.
7. Boy N, Garbade SF, Heringer J, Seitz A, Kolker S, Harting I. Patterns, evolution, and severity of striatal injury in insidious- versus acute-onset glutaric aciduria type 1. J Inherit Metab Dis. 2018. https://doi.org/10.1007/s10545-018-0187-y.
8. Bjugstad KB, Goodman SI, Freed CR. Age at symptom onset predicts severity of motor impairment and clinical outcome of glutaric acidemia type 1. J Pediatr. 2000;137(5):681–6.
9. Kyllerman M, Skjeldal O, Christensen E, Hagberg G, Holme E, Lonnquist T, et al. Long-term follow-up, neurological outcome and survival rate in 28 Nordic patients with glutaric aciduria type 1. Eur J Paediatr Neurol. 2004;8(3):121–9.
10. Cerisola A, Campistol J, Perez-Duenas B, Poo P, Pineda M, Garcia-Cazorla A, et al. Seizures versus dystonia in encephalopathic crisis of glutaric aciduria type I. Pediatr Neurol. 2009;40(6):426–31.
11. Gitiaux C, Roze E, Kinugawa K, Flamand-Rouviere C, Boddaert N, Apartis E, et al. Spectrum of movement disorders associated with glutaric aciduria type 1: a study of 16 patients. Mov Disord. 2008;23(16):2392–7.
12. Morris AA, Hoffmann GF, Naughten ER, Monavari AA, Collins JE, Leonard JV. Glutaric aciduria and suspected child abuse. Arch Dis Child. 1999;80(5):404–5.
13. Bodamer O. Subdural hematomas and glutaric aciduria type I. Pediatrics. 2001;107(2):451.
14. Vester ME, Bilo RA, Karst WA, Daams JG, Duijst WL, van Rijn RR. Subdural hematomas: glutaric

aciduria type 1 or abusive head trauma? A systematic review. Forensic Sci Med Pathol. 2015;11(3):405–15.
15. Harting I, Neumaier-Probst E, Seitz A, Maier EM, Assmann B, Baric I, et al. Dynamic changes of striatal and extrastriatal abnormalities in glutaric aciduria type I. Brain. 2009;132(Pt 7):1764–82.
16. Strauss KA, Puffenberger EG, Robinson DL, Morton DH. Type I glutaric aciduria, part 1: natural history of 77 patients. Am J Med Genet C Semin Med Genet. 2003;121C(1):38–52.
17. Heringer J, Boy SP, Ensenauer R, Assmann B, Zschocke J, Harting I, et al. Use of guidelines improves the neurological outcome in glutaric aciduria type I. Ann Neurol. 2010;68(5):743–52.
18. Bahr O, Mader I, Zschocke J, Dichgans J, Schulz JB. Adult onset glutaric aciduria type I presenting with a leukoencephalopathy. Neurology. 2002;59(11):1802–4.
19. Pierson TM, Nezhad M, Tremblay MA, Lewis R, Wong D, Salamon N, et al. Adult-onset glutaric aciduria type I presenting with white matter abnormalities and subependymal nodules. Neurogenetics. 2015;16(4):325–8.
20. Herskovitz M, Goldsher D, Sela BA, Mandel H. Subependymal mass lesions and peripheral polyneuropathy in adult-onset glutaric aciduria type I. Neurology. 2013;81(9):849–50.
21. Korman SH, Jakobs C, Darmin PS, Gutman A, van der Knaap MS, Ben-Neriah Z, et al. Glutaric aciduria type 1: clinical, biochemical and molecular findings in patients from Israel. Eur J Paediatr Neurol. 2007;11(2):81–9.
22. Serrano Russi A, Donoghue S, Boneh A, Manara R, Burlina AB, Burlina AP. Malignant brain tumors in patients with glutaric aciduria type I. Mol Genet Metab. 2018;125(3):276–80.
23. Lenich AC, Goodman SI. The purification and characterization of glutaryl-coenzyme a dehydrogenase from porcine and human liver. J Biol Chem. 1986;261(9):4090–6.
24. Strauss KA, Brumbaugh J, Duffy A, Wardley B, Robinson D, Hendrickson C, et al. Safety, efficacy and physiological actions of a lysine-free, arginine-rich formula to treat glutaryl-CoA dehydrogenase deficiency: focus on cerebral amino acid influx. Mol Genet Metab. 2011;104(1–2):93–106.
25. Kolker S, Boy SP, Heringer J, Muller E, Maier EM, Ensenauer R, et al. Complementary dietary treatment using lysine-free, arginine-fortified amino acid supplements in glutaric aciduria type I - a decade of experience. Mol Genet Metab. 2012;107(1–2):72–80.
26. Goodman SI, Kratz LE, DiGiulio KA, Biery BJ, Goodman KE, Isaya G, et al. Cloning of glutaryl-CoA dehydrogenase cDNA, and expression of wild type and mutant enzymes in Escherichia coli. Hum Mol Genet. 1995;4(9):1493–8.
27. Goodman SI, Stein DE, Schlesinger S, Christensen E, Schwartz M, Greenberg CR, et al. Glutaryl-CoA dehydrogenase mutations in glutaric acidemia (type I): review and report of thirty novel mutations. Hum Mutat. 1998;12(3):141–4.
28. Zschocke J, Quak E, Guldberg P, Hoffmann GF. Mutation analysis in glutaric aciduria type I. J Med Genet. 2000;37(3):177–81.
29. Goodman SI, Woontner M. An explanation for metabolite excretion in high- and low-excretor patients with glutaric acidemia type 1. Mol Genet Metab. 2019;127(4):325–6.
30. Schillaci LA, Greene CL, Strovel E, Rispoli-Joines J, Spector E, Woontner M, et al. The M405V allele of the glutaryl-CoA dehydrogenase gene is an important marker for glutaric aciduria type I (GA-I) low excretors. Mol Genet Metab. 2016;119(1–2):50–6.
31. Christensen E, Ribes A, Merinero B, Zschocke J. Correlation of genotype and phenotype in glutaryl-CoA dehydrogenase deficiency. J Inherit Metab Dis. 2004;27(6):861–8.
32. Greenberg CR, Prasad AN, Dilling LA, Thompson JR, Haworth JC, Martin B, et al. Outcome of the first 3-years of a DNA-based neonatal screening program for glutaric acidemia type 1 in Manitoba and northwestern Ontario, Canada. Mol Genet Metab. 2002;75(1):70–8.
33. Naughten ER, Mayne PD, Monavari AA, Goodman SI, Sulaiman G, Croke DT. Glutaric aciduria type I: outcome in the Republic of Ireland. J Inherit Metab Dis. 2004;27(6):917–20.
34. Boneh A, Beauchamp M, Humphrey M, Watkins J, Peters H, Yaplito-Lee J. Newborn screening for glutaric aciduria type I in Victoria: treatment and outcome. Mol Genet Metab. 2008;94(3):287–91.
35. Hsieh CT, Hwu WL, Huang YT, Huang AC, Wang SF, Hu MH, et al. Early detection of glutaric aciduria type I by newborn screening in Taiwan. J Formos Med Assoc. 2008;107(2):139–44.
36. Lindner M, Kolker S, Schulze A, Christensen E, Greenberg CR, Hoffmann GF. Neonatal screening for glutaryl-CoA dehydrogenase deficiency. J Inherit Metab Dis. 2004;27(6):851–9.
37. Hennermann JB, Roloff S, Gellermann J, Gruters A, Klein J. False-positive newborn screening mimicking glutaric aciduria type I in infants with renal insufficiency. J Inherit Metab Dis. 2009;32(Suppl 1):S355–9.
38. Moore T, Le A, Cowan TM. An improved LC-MS/MS method for the detection of classic and low excretor glutaric acidemia type 1. J Inherit Metab Dis. 2012;35(3):431–5.
39. Muhlhausen C, Christensen E, Schwartz M, Muschol N, Ullrich K, Lukacs Z. Severe phenotype despite high residual glutaryl-CoA dehydrogenase activity: a novel mutation in a Turkish patient with glutaric aciduria type I. J Inherit Metab Dis. 2003;26(7):713–4.
40. Kolker S, Greenberg CR, Lindner M, Muller E, Naughten ER, Hoffmann GF. Emergency treatment in glutaryl-CoA dehydrogenase deficiency. J Inherit Metab Dis. 2004;27(6):893–902.

Nutrition Management of Glutaric Acidemia Type 1

20

Laurie E. Bernstein

Contents

L. E. Bernstein (✉)
University of Colorado Hospital, Children's Hospital
Colorado, Aurora, CO, USA
e-mail: laurie.bernstein@met-ed.net

L. E. Bernstein et al. (eds.), *Nutrition Management of Inherited Metabolic Diseases*,
https://doi.org/10.1007/978-3-030-94510-7_20

Core Messages

- Glutaric acidemia type-1 (GA-1) is an autosomal recessive disorder of lysine, hydroxylysine, and tryptophan metabolism.
- A defect of glutaryl-CoA dehydrogenase results in the accumulation of 3-hydroxyglutaric acid and glutaric acid.
- Nutrition management of GA-1 consists of restricting lysine and tryptophan, supplementing L-carnitine and providing sufficient energy to prevent catabolism.
- Patients with GA-1 have a particularly high risk of permanent cerebral damage from a metabolic crisis.

20.1 Background

Glutaric acidemia type-1 (GA-1) is an autosomal recessive disorder of lysine, hydroxylysine, and tryptophan metabolism caused by a deficiency of glutaryl-CoA dehydrogenase (Fig. 20.1). GA-1 results in the accumulation of 3-hydroxyglutaric acid and glutaric acid in the urine [1, 2], the metabolites most likely associated with the risk of neurological damage (Box 20.1). However, concentrations of these metabolites have not been shown to correlate to patient outcomes [3].

Box 20.1: Principles of Nutrition Management in GA-1

- *Restrict*: Lysine and tryptophan
- *Supplement*: L-carnitine, riboflavin[a], pantothenic acid[a]
- *Toxic metabolites*: 3-hydroxyglutaric acid and glutaric acid[b]

[a]Practice varies - supplemented in some clinics.

[b]These metabolites accumulate but concentrations are not related to patient outcomes.

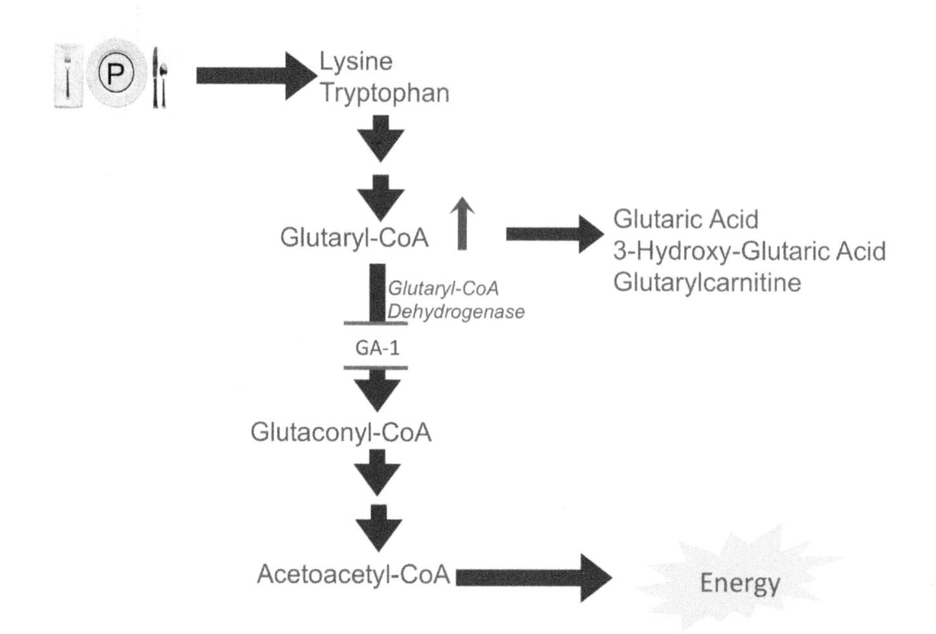

Fig. 20.1 Metabolic pathway of glutaric acidemia type-1 (GA-1)

The management of GA-1 poses several challenges: (1) metabolic decompensations are associated with a very high risk of permanent neurological insult, (2) good biomarkers to guide therapy have not been identified, and (3) there is a lack of agreement about how long strict dietary treatment is necessary. The risk for neurological damage appears to be greatest in newborns and early childhood when cerebral lysine uptake is the highest [1, 2]. There are no published reports of acute encephalopathic crises in children over age 6 years, but there are documented cases of chronic neurological deterioration in patients with late onset disease who did not experience metabolic crises [4–12]. Diet management using a lysine-free, tryptophan-reduced medical food and intact protein restriction rather than treatment with protein restriction alone may be advisable. The dietary treatment after age 6 years is discussed in Sect. 20.4 of this chapter. A further description of the diagnosis and management of GA-1 is described in Chap. 19. [4, 13]

20.2 Nutrition Management

20.2.1 Chronic Nutrition Management

Expanded newborn screening allows for early diagnosis of GA-1 that leads to timely, preventive management thereby reducing the risk of acute neurological damage associated with untreated GA-1 [3]. Minimizing the risk of cerebral damage while maintaining normal development and growth are the overarching goals of the nutrition management of GA-1 [14, 15]. The most critical component of management in patients with GA-1 is the prompt emergency treatment of intercurrent illnesses. L-carnitine supplementation is also an integral component of management.

The diet for a patient with GA-1 is restricted in the amino acids lysine and tryptophan. The goals for nutrient intake are provided in Table 20.1. When well, the patient with GA-1 has normal requirements for most other nutrients, including energy, vitamins, and minerals (Box 20.2) Medical foods free of lysine and low in tryptophan are used to meet protein goals (Table 20.2). These medical foods provide varying amounts of essential amino acids, fat, carbohydrate, vitamins, and minerals, as well as L-arginine. In the dietary management of GA-1, it is important to note that there is less tryptophan in whole protein than lysine (on a molar basis); therefore, restricting lysine may cause an over-restriction of tryptophan. Blood concentrations of both amino acids require close monitoring (Table 20.3) [1].

Table 20.1 Recommended intake for a patient with GA-1 [1, 4, 16]

Age	Protein (g/kg)	Lysine (mg/kg)	Tryptophan (mg/kg)
Birth–6 months	2.75–3.0	65–100	10–20
6 months to 1 year	2.5–3.0	55–90	10–12
1 year to 4 years	1.8–2.6	50–80	8–12
4 years to 7 years	1.6–2.0	40–70	7–11

Energy, vitamin[a] and mineral intakes should meet the DRI and normal fluid requirements met

Adjustments should be made based on growth, laboratory findings, and health status

aSome clinics recommend supplemental riboflavin (100 mg/d) and pantothenic acid (400–600ug/kg/d). These are average ranges

Arginine competes with lysine for uptake across the blood–brain barrier and should be provided at 1.5– 2 times that of dietary lysine. Strauss et al. 2011 recommend providing measured amounts of both arginine and lysine at the same time as the key to efficacy [16]. Reports of improved outcomes in patients consuming a diet providing the recommended lysine to arginine ratio have been published, although brain concentrations of these amino acids have not been quantified [16]. Boy et al. (2017) reported that there is no evidence for an oral high dose supplement of L-arginine for maintenance or for IV arginine for emergency treatment [18]. Adequate arginine should be provided by a lysine-free, tryptophan-reduced, arginine-containing medical food. It may also be provided by intact protein within a low lysine diet, but the amount of arginine consumed from protein-containing foods is more difficult to quantify.

Standard infant formula or breast milk provides the recommended amount of lysine and tryptophan during infancy. Due to the risk of neurological consequences associated with energy-deprivation and catabolism, close monitoring of intake and appropriate weight gain is crucial in all infants. In breast-fed infants, weight gain is the primary measure of

Box 20.2: Initiating Nutrition Management in an Asymptomatic Infant with GA-1

Goal: Prevent neurological insult associated with metabolic crises.

Step-by-Step:

1. Establish intake goals based on clinical status and laboratory values.

Intake Goals

Age (days)	Protein [1] (g/kg)	Lys [1, 16] (mg/kg)	Lysine/arginine ratio [16]	Carnitine [16] (mg/kg)	Riboflavin[a] [17] (mg)	Pantothenate[b] [16] (µg/kg)
5	2.75–3.5	65–100	1:1.5–1:2	75–100	100	400–600

2. Calculate the amount of infant formula/breast milk[c] needed to meet lysine needs. Determine the amount of protein provided by the whole protein source.
3. Calculate amount of medical food required to meet remaining total protein needs (Table 20.3).
4. Calculate arginine provided by GA-1 medical food to ensure lysine to arginine ratio is correct.
5. Determine the calories provided by both the whole protein source and GA-1 medical food. Provide the remaining calories from a protein-free medical food.
6. Determine the amount of fluid required to make a formula that provides 20–25 kcal/ounce (depending on energy needs and volume tolerated).

[a]Some clinics supplement riboflavin. Administer 15–25 mg mixed into 3–4 feedings per day for maximum absorption [17]

[b]May not be supplemented by all clinics. Check individual clinical protocols for guidance

[c]In severe forms, expressed breast milk is recommended

Table 20.2 GA-1 formula comparison

Formulas available in the United States				
	Arginine (mg)/100 g	Tryptophan (mg)/100 g	Carnitine (mg)/100 g	Calories (kcal)/100 g
GA-1 Anamix Early Years[a]	1180	90	10	473
Glutarade essential GA-1[a]	2700	150	40	385
Glutarade GA-1 amino acid Blend	8690	480	200	324
Glutarade GA-1 Junior[a]	1080	60	30	410
GA gel[b]	4190	310	46	339
GA express[b]	6030	450	64	297
Glutarex-1[c]	1550	0	900	480
Glutarex-2[c]	3100	0	370	410
GA Infant[d]	1040	0	0	500
Formulas not available in the United States				
GA explore5[b]	4110	310	44	342
GA Amino5[b]	8390	630	0	332

[a]Nutricia North America (Rockville MD; medicalfood.com)

[b]Vitaflo USA (Alexandria VA; vitaflousa.com)

[c]Abbott Nutrition (Columbus OH; abbottnutrition.com)

[d]Mead Johnson Nutrition (Evansville IN; meadjohnson.com)

Table 20.3 Plasma concentration reference ranges for arginine, lysine, and tryptophan for patients with GA-1

Amino acid	0–1 month	1–24 months	2–18 years	Adult
Arginine (µmol/mL)	6–140	12–133	10–140	15–128
Lysine (µmol/mL)	92–325	52–196	48–284	100–250
Tryptophan (µmol/mL)	–	5–60	34–47	42–106

Reference ranges for Children's Hospital Colorado; check your laboratory for reference ranges

caloric adequacy. Solid foods that are naturally low in protein (lysine) may be introduced when the infant is developmentally ready, and specialty low protein foods may be used to provide sufficient energy and variety to the diet. Providing sufficient energy can be challenging in patients with GA-1. Those who have sustained cerebral damage usually present with severe dystonia and choreoathetosis, interfering with the patient's ability to eat normally. If severe enough, the patient may require a gastrostomy tube [15]. Energy needs may be increased in patients with dystonia [19] or decreased in patients who are non-ambulatory [15].

L-carnitine supplementation is routinely provided to patients with GA-1 as a way to reduce intramitochondrial glutaryl-CoA and provide extracellular release without the synthesis of glutaric acid and 3-hydroxyglutaric acid. L-carnitine conjugates with coenzyme A esters to form acylcarnitines. The typical L-carnitine dose is 100 mg/kg/day or sufficient quantities to maintain free L-carnitine concentrations within the normal range [4]. Large doses of enteral L-carnitine may cause loose stools or diarrhea [20]. In the hospitalized patient with acute illness, a continuous infusion of intravenous L-carnitine is preferably provided.

Glutaryl-CoA dehydrogenase is a riboflavin-dependent enzyme that converts glutaryl-CoA to glutaconyl-CoA. Once the diagnosis of GA-1 is confirmed, a trial of pharmacological doses of riboflavin (100–200 mg/day) may be successful in reducing glutaric acid or 3-hydroxyglutaric acid concentrations in some patients with specific responsive mutations [21]. Some centers recommend routine riboflavin supplementation regardless of response. Many preparations of riboflavin are distasteful and cause staining due to the bright orange color of the vitamin [16, 22]. High doses of riboflavin have been reported to cause gastric distress. Kolker et al. 2006 reported that there is no evidence that riboflavin improves the clinical outcome, and there are no established standards to evaluate riboflavin responsiveness [23].

20.2.2 Acute Nutrition Management

Sick day protocols for home use are used extensively for many inherited metabolic diseases, including organic acidemias, but the practice is different with GA-1. The risk for neurological injury is greatest during illnesses with reduced energy intake, fever, and associated catabolism. Very aggressive treatment and a zero tolerance with regard to hospital admission during any of these presentations can help prevent permanent neurological damage. Thus, if a patient has an illness in which he or she is not consuming adequate energy due to vomiting, poor intake, or diarrhea, and/or if the patient has a fever (>38.5 °C), it is considered a medical emergency, and the patient must be seen in the emergency department immediately. The consequences of an acute metabolic crisis are dire and include irreversible neurologic squeal involving damage to the basal ganglia (striatal necrosis), which can cause a normally developing infant or child to have a lifetime of severe physical and developmental disabilities. During an illness that is associated with catabolism, maintaining usual therapy ("well-day" diet) and supplementing L-carnitine, is NOT sufficient to prevent an acute crisis; additional non-protein energy sources must be provided. Management of a sick day diet at home requires the guidance of the metabolic physician and the threshold for seeking emergency treatment is very low, even for relatively minor illnesses, particularly during the first 6 years of vulnerability. Sick day management includes reducing intact protein intake, continuing consumption of a lysine- and tryptophan-free medical food and providing extra sources of protein-free energy (e.g., Prophree,® Duocal,® Solcarb,® Polycal®) (Box 20.3). Additionally, the dose of L-carnitine dose is often increased.

Sick day management is difficult to achieve at home; the key is to reduce intact protein intake, provide sufficient L-carnitine, and consume enough energy to prevent catabolism. All patients

Box 20.3: "Sick-Day" Nutrition Management of a Patient with GA-1

The diet may be used at home for minor illnesses. If the patient does not improve or energy intake is inadequate it is considered a medical emergency in GA-1.

	Children's Hospital Colorado[a]	Strauss [16]
Energy	110–120% of usual intake	95–115 kcal/kg
Whole (natural) protein (g/kg/day)	0.6–0.7	0.5
Lysine-free medical food (g/kg/day)	Maintain current	1.5–2.0
L-carnitine[b] (mg/kg/day)	50	100

[a]Children's Hospital Colorado, GA-1 IMD Clinic protocol; please check your clinic's protocol
[b]Use caution in diarrheal illnesses [16]

Box 20.4: Transitioning a Hospitalized Patient with GA-1 from a "Sick Day" to a "Well Day" Diet

1. Introduce the sick-day diet (Box 20.3) as soon as the child can tolerate feedings, initially given in combination with IV dextrose to meet energy goals.
2. Wean IV dextrose[a] as formula intake approaches maintenance well-day diet volume.
3. Transition gradually to well-day formula to provide at least half of the protein/lysine intake, starting within 24–36 h after admission.
4. Gradually transition to full intake of the well-day formula prescription before discharge.

[a]See Appendix I

with GA-1 should have a written emergency department protocol that can be referenced if the patient is seen at a hospital unfamiliar with the management of GA-1. In such cases, the patient's metabolic physician should be contacted and consulted regarding management. Acute medical management must commence quickly to avoid catabolism and includes reducing intact protein by 50% and increasing lysine-free medical food by 50%, providing sufficient energy intake, and managing the underlying illness. When admitted to the emergency room, intravenous dextrose of 10% concentration is provided at a rate of 1.5 times maintenance fluid needs and Intralipid® (Baxter Healthcare, Deerfield, IL) at 2 g/kg/day are often rapidly added, particularly for children with compromised oral intake due to illness. Usually within 24–36 h of administering the inpatient emergency diet, the patient can begin to transition back to his or her usual diet (Box 20.4).

20.3 Monitoring

Laboratory markers that are good indicators of the clinical status of patients with GA-1 are lacking. Frequent outpatient visits with plasma amino acid analysis at each visit along with phone follow-up is the protocol for most centers.

Nutrition monitoring includes ensuring adequate growth and nutrient intake, especially markers of protein status (Chap. 6). Monitoring plasma amino acids is necessary to ensure that concentrations of the essential amino acids lysine and tryptophan are maintained within the normal range for age (based on the metabolic laboratory's reference ranges) (Table 20.4).

Table 20.4 Estimation of lysine intake

Food[a]	Lysine content (% of total protein)
Fish	9
Meat and meat products	8
Breast milk	8
Cow's milk, milk products	7
Eggs (whole)	6
Potatoes	6
Soy and soy products	6
Nuts	2–8.5
Vegetables	4–6.5
Fruit	2–6.5
Cereal and cereal products	2–4

[a]BGVV-Computer Program Berlin

Box 20.5: Nutrition Monitoring of a Patient with GA-1

- Routine assessments including anthropometrics, dietary intake, physical findings
- Laboratory monitoring
  - Diagnosis-specific
    - Carnitine (total, free, esterified)
    - Plasma amino acids, including
      - Lysine
      - Arginine
      - Tryptophan
- Nutrition laboratory monitoring of patients on lysine and/or protein-restricted diets may include markers of:
  - Protein sufficiency
  - Nutritional anemia (hemoglobin, hematocrit, MCV, serum vitamin B_{12} and/or methylmalonic acid (MMA), total homocysteine, ferritin, iron, folate, total iron binding capacity)
  - Vitamin and mineral status (25-hydroxyvitamin D, zinc, trace minerals)
  - Others as clinically indicated

Care must be taken to avoid essential amino acid deficiencies, particularly tryptophan. Tryptophan is difficult to quantify using certain methodologies [24]. Albumin binds tryptophan in circulation, with one binding site per albumin molecule. Variable albumin binding may make free tryptophan concentrations variable [24]. The frequency of monitoring depends on the patient's age and health status. During early infancy, many clinics measure plasma amino acids along with anthropometrics each week, but at least monthly (Box 20.5).

20.4 Diet After the Age of 6

After 6 years of age, the recommendation is to transition to an individualized age-appropriate "protein-controlled" diet [18]. A recent survey [13] found that, despite this recommendation, fewer than half of survey respondents (45%) recommend diet liberalization after age 6 years in patients who were identified via newborn screening and have not experienced a striatal injury. Twenty percent of respondents "never" liberalize diet. The time of liberalization is variable and individualized. Some respondents from the survey approach liberalization slowly after 6 years of age and may continue the use of a medical food.

Eighty-five percent of survey respondents defined a "protein-controlled diet" to mean providing only the amount of protein recommended by the US DRI (or similar standard recommendation for protein intake if outside the United States). For 44% of respondents, "protein-controlled diet" also meant that the clinician prescribes a certain number of grams of protein that the patient counts and 27% consider "protein-controlled diet" to mean not allowing meat or other high biological value protein sources. For patients who are instructed to count intact protein, 76% count grams of protein from food, whereas only 20% count milligrams of lysine and 6% use an exchange system. There was overall consensus that the dietitian needs to approach each patient as an individual and may initiate counting lysine during infancy and then transition to counting protein as the child ages.

Further study and consensus of diet recommendations, along with development of educational materials, are needed that include sources of intact protein with a low lysine content (Table 20.4) and sources of lysine-rich foods. Counseling from a metabolic dietitian to support growth and optimal nutrition is imperative for treatment success.

20.5 Summary

The nutrition management of GA-1 presents a clinical challenge because the benefit of a life-long lysine and tryptophan-restricted diet is not established, there are not good biomarkers to guide treatment decisions, and an acute metabolic crisis can result in striatal damage causing irreversible neurological sequelae. Preventing acute metabolic crises is the primary goal of treatment. Lysine-restricted, arginine-supplemented diets are believed to confer some benefit, perhaps by altering the flux of lysine and arginine across the blood–brain barrier. L-carnitine conjugates and removes glutaric acid and 3-hydroxyglutaric acid from circulation and is a key part of therapy. The revised guidelines recommend a low lysine diet with amino acid based medical foods up to age 6 years [18]. After 6 years, the recommendation is to transition to an individualized age-appropriate "protein-controlled" diet; however, the treatment approach among dietitians varies. A clearer definition of both a "liberalized" and "protein-controlled" diets needed.

20.6 Diet Calculation Example

Patient information and nutrient intake goals	Laboratory results
Age: 4 days	Newborn Screen C5DC: 0.37 (reference range 0.35 μmol/L)
Weight: 3.2 kg	Plasma 3-OH glutaric acid on day of life 5: 104 (reference range < 65 μmol/L)
Currently drinking 14 ounces formula	Plasma lysine (Lys) on day of life 6: 59 μmol/L (reference range: 55–196 μmol/L)
Lysine goal: 70 mg/kg (range: 70–100 mg/kg)	
Tryptophan goal: 20–25 mg/kg	
Protein goal: 2.6 g/kg	
Energy goal: 127 kcal/kg (range: 95–145 kcal/kg)	

Table 20.5 Select nutrient composition of formulas for GA-1 diet calculation example (using standard infant formula as a source of whole protein)

Medical food	Amount (g)	LYS (mg)	ARG (mg)	TRP (mg)	Protein (g)	Energy (kcal)
GA-1 Anamix Early Years[a]	100	–	1180	–	13.5	473
Enfamil Premium Infant Powder[b]	100	750	240	163	10.1	510

[a]Nutricia North America (Rockville, MD)
[b]Mead Johnson Nutrition (Evansville, IN)
Note: Check manufacturer's website for the most up-to-date nutrient composition

Step-by-Step Calculation (using formulas found in Table 20.5)

Step 1. Calculate the amount of Lys required each day.

Lys goal × infant weight = mg Lys per day

70 mg/kg Lys × 3.2 kg = 224 mg Lys per day

Step 2. Calculate the amount of standard infant formula needed to meet the daily Lys requirement.

Amount of Lys required per day 224 mg/day ÷ 910 mg Lys = 0.25

0.25 × 100 = 25 g Enfamil Infant needed to meet daily Lys requirement

Step 3. Calculate protein and energy provided from standard infant formula

Amount of standard formula × protein provided in 100 g of standard formula.

0.25 × 10.1 g protein = 2.5 g protein in standard infant formula

0.25 × 510 kcals = 128 kcals provided in standard infant formula

Step 4. Calculate the amount of protein needed to fill the diet prescription.

Protein goal × infant weight

2.6 g protein × 3.2 kg = 8.3 g daily protein requirement

8.3 g – 2.5 g = 5.8 g protein needed to fill in the diet prescription.

Step 5. Calculate the amount of protein required from Lys/Trp-free medical food.

Protein needed to fill diet prescription ÷ protein provided in 100 g of medical food.

5.8 g protein needed ÷ 13.5 g protein in GA-1 Anamix Early Years = 0.43

0.43 × 100 = 43 g GA-1 Anamix Early Years required to fill the diet prescription

Step 6. Calculate the total energy provided from standard infant formula and Lys/Trp-free medial food.

Amount of standard infant formula × kcal in 100 g of standard formula.

0.25 (Enfamil Infant) × 510 kcal = 128 kcal

Amount of Lys/Trp-free medical food x kcal of 100 g of Lys/Trp-free medical food.

0.43 (GA-1 Anamix Early Years) × 473 kcal = 203 kcals

Add standard formula + Lys/Trp-free medical food for total kcal provided in diet prescription.

$$128\ \text{kcal} + 203\ \text{kcal} = 331\ \text{kcal}$$

$$331\ \text{kcal} \div 3.2\ \text{kg} = 103\ \text{kcal/kg}$$

Step 7. Calculate the final volume of the formula to make a concentration of approximately 20–22 kcal per ounce

Divide total calories by desired concentration to find final volume.

331 kcals ÷ 22 = 15 oz (Table 20.6)

Table 20.6 Diet prescription summary for diet calculation example of GA-1. (Using standard infant formula as a source of whole protein[a])

Medical food	Amount (g)	LYS (mg)	ARG (mg)	TRP (mg)	Protein (g)	Energy (kcal)
GA-1 Anamix Early Years	51	–	561	–	6.6	242
Enfamil Premium Infant Powder	30	225	72	49	3	153
Total per day		225	633	49	9.6	395
Total per kg		70 mg/kg	198 mg/kg	15 mg/kg	3.3 g/kg (1.2 g/kg of natural protein)	123 kcal/kg

[a]Values rounded to nearest whole number for amount of formula powders, phenylalanine, protein, and energy and rounded to the nearest 0.1 g for protein

Note: Check manufacturer's website for the most up-to-date nutrient composition

References

1. Acosta PB. Nutrition management of patients with inherited metabolic disorders. 1st ed. Sudbury: Jones & Bartlett Learning; 2009.
2. Pusti S, Das N, Nayek K, Biswas S. A treatable neurometabolic disorder: glutaric aciduria type 1. Case Rep Pediatr. 2014;2014:256356.
3. Hedlund GL, Longo N, Pasquali M. Glutaric acidemia type 1. Am J Med Genet C Semin Med Genet. 2006;142C(2):86–94.
4. Kolker S, Christensen E, Leonard JV, Greenberg CR, Boneh A, Burlina AB, et al. Diagnosis and management of glutaric aciduria type I—revised recommendations. J Inherit Metab Dis. 2011;34(3):677–94.
5. Harting I, Neumaier-Probst E, Seitz A, Maier EM, Assmann B, Baric I, et al. Dynamic changes of striatal and extrastriatal abnormalities in glutaric aciduria type I. Brain. 2009;132(Pt 7):1764–82.
6. Bahr O, Mader I, Zschocke J, Dichgans J, Schulz JB. Adult onset glutaric aciduria type I presenting with a leukoencephalopathy. Neurology. 2002;59(11):1802–4.
7. Busquets C, Coll MJ, Merinero B, Ugarte M, Ruiz MA, Martinez Bermejo A, et al. Prenatal molecular diagnosis of glutaric aciduria type I by direct mutation analysis. Prenat Diagn. 2000;20(9):761–4.
8. Fernandez-Alvarez E, Garcia-Cazorla A, Sans A, Boix C, Vilaseca MA, Busquets C, et al. Hand tremor and orofacial dyskinesia: clinical manifestations of glutaric aciduria type I in a young girl. Mov Disord. 2003;18:1076–9.
9. Hoffmann GF, Athanassopoulos S, Burlina AB, Duran M, de Klerk JB, Lehnert W, et al. Clinical course, early diagnosis, treatment, and prevention of disease in glutaryl-CoA dehydrogenase deficiency. Neuropediatrics. 1996;27(3):115–23.
10. Kulkens S, Harting I, Sauer S, Zschocke J, Hoffmann GF, Gruber S, et al. Late-onset neurologic disease in glutaryl-CoA dehydrogenase deficiency. Neurology. 2005;64(12):2142–4.
11. Pierson TM, Nezhad M, Tremblay MA, Lewis R, Wong D, Salamon N, et al. Adult-onset glutaric aciduria type I presenting with white matter abnormalities and subependymal nodules. Neurogenetics. 2015;16(4):325–8.
12. Strauss KA, Lazovic J, Wintermark M, Morton DH. Multimodal imaging of striatal degeneration in Amish patients with glutaryl-CoA dehydrogenase deficiency. Brain. 2007;130(Pt 7):1905–20.
13. Bernstein L, Coughlin CR, Drumm M, Yannicelli S, Rohr F. Inconsistencies in the nutrition management of glutaric aciduria type 1: an international survey. Nutrients. 2020;12(10):3162.
14. Strauss KA, Puffenberger EG, Robinson DL, Morton DH. Type I glutaric aciduria, part 1: natural history of 77 patients. Am J Med Genet C Semin Med Genet. 2003;121C(1):38–52.
15. Thomas JA, Bernstein LE, Greene CL, Koeller DM. Apparent decreased energy requirements in children with organic acidemias: preliminary observations. J Am Diet Assoc. 2000;100(9):1074–6.
16. Strauss KA, Brumbaugh J, Duffy A, Wardley B, Robinson D, Hendrickson C, et al. Safety, efficacy and physiological actions of a lysine-free, arginine-rich formula to treat glutaryl-CoA dehydrogenase deficiency: focus on cerebral amino acid influx. Mol Genet Metab. 2011;104(1–2):93–106.
17. Zempleni J, Galloway JR, McCormick DB. Pharmacokinetics of orally and intravenously administered riboflavin in healthy humans. Am J Clin Nutr. 1996;63(1):54–66.
18. Boy N, Muhlhausen C, Maier EM, Heringer J, Assmann B, Burgard P, et al. Proposed recommendations for diagnosing and managing individuals with glutaric aciduria type I: second revision. J Inherit Metab Dis. 2017;40(1):75–101.
19. Boy N, Haege G, Heringer J, Assmann B, Muhlhausen C, Ensenauer R, et al. Low lysine diet in glutaric aciduria type I--effect on anthropometric and biochemical follow-up parameters. J Inherit Metab Dis. 2013;36(3):525–33.
20. Winter SC, Szabo-Aczel S, Curry CJ, Hutchinson HT, Hogue R, Shug A. Plasma carnitine deficiency. Clinical observations in 51 pediatric patients. Am J Dis Child. 1987;141(6):660–5.
21. Brandt NJ, Gregersen N, Christensen E, Gron IH, Rasmussen K. Treatment of glutaryl-CoA dehydrogenase deficiency (glutaric aciduria). Experience with diet, riboflavin, and GABA analogue. J Pediatr. 1979;94(4):669–73.
22. Chalmers RA, Bain MD, Zschocke J. Riboflavin-responsive glutaryl CoA dehydrogenase deficiency. Mol Genet Metab. 2006;88(1):29–37.
23. Kolker S, Sauer SW, Okun JG, Hoffmann GF, Koeller DM. Lysine intake and neurotoxicity in glutaric aciduria type I: towards a rationale for therapy? Brain. 2006;129(Pt 8):e54.
24. Mc MR, Oncley JL. The specific binding of L-tryptophan to serum albumin. J Biol Chem. 1958;233(6):1436–47.

Nutrition Management of Propionic Acidemia and Methylmalonic Acidemia

21

Mary Sowa

Contents

M. Sowa (✉)
Division of Medical Genetics, CHOC Children's,
Orange, CA, USA
e-mail: MSowa@choc.org

L. E. Bernstein et al. (eds.), *Nutrition Management of Inherited Metabolic Diseases*,
https://doi.org/10.1007/978-3-030-94510-7_21

Core Messages

- Infants with propionic acidemia (PROP) or methylmalonic acidemia (MMA) can be identified by newborn screening, although those with severe phenotypes may suffer a metabolic crisis before screening results are available.
- Nutrition management of PROP or MMA involves limiting intact protein and providing a medical food free of the propiogenic amino acids valine, methionine, isoleucine and threonine to meet the DRI for protein.
- Providing adequate energy to prevent catabolism, especially during periods of illness, is a key component of therapy.
- Individualized therapy is based on the severity of disease as well as monitoring of metabolic and nutrition parameters.
- Treatment often includes L-carnitine supplementation for both disorders.

21.1 Background

Propionic acidemia (PROP) and methylmalonic acidemia (MMA) are inherited disorders of the metabolism of the propiogenic amino acids (AA) valine, methionine, isoleucine, and threonine, and odd-chain fatty acids (Figs. 21.1 and 21.2, respectively). Either disorder can be identified by newborn screening (NBS) with elevated propionylcarnitine (C3) on the acylcarnitine profile and some NBS programs use secondary markers, such as the ratio of C3 to acetylcarnitine (C2) [1, 2]. Distinction between these two disorders requires additional confirmatory laboratory testing including urine organic acids [1, 2]. Serum methylmalonic acid will be elevated in methylmalonic acidemia but not propionic acidemia. Molecular testing confirms the disorder [1, 2]. Patients with MMA can either have an absence (mut^0) or deficiency (mut^-) of the methylmalonyl CoA mutase enzyme or a defect in cobalamin

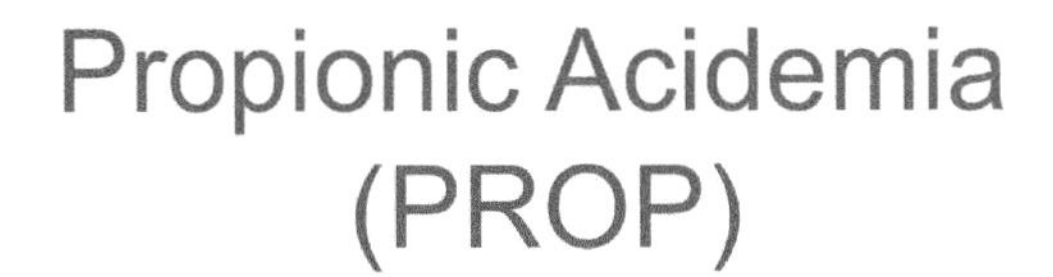

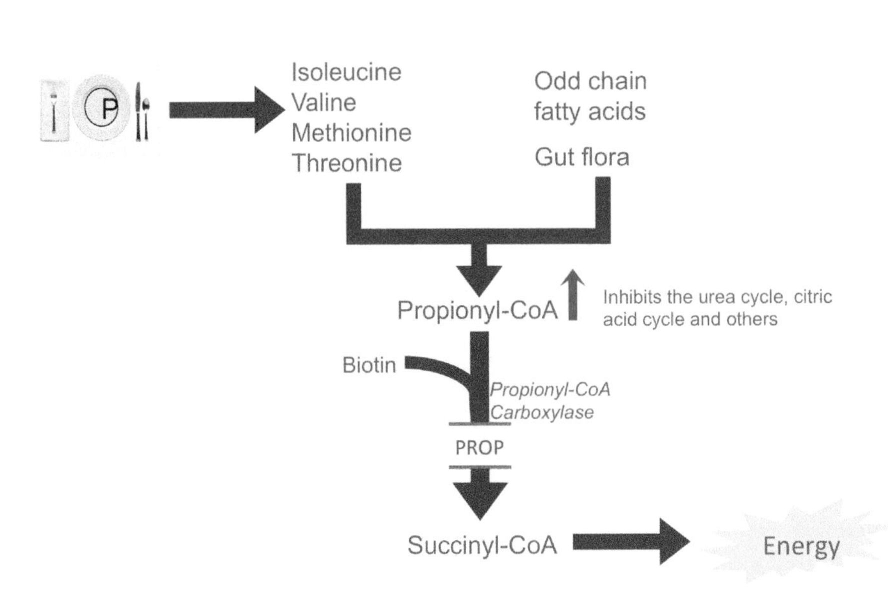

Fig. 21.1 Metabolic pathway of propionic acidemia

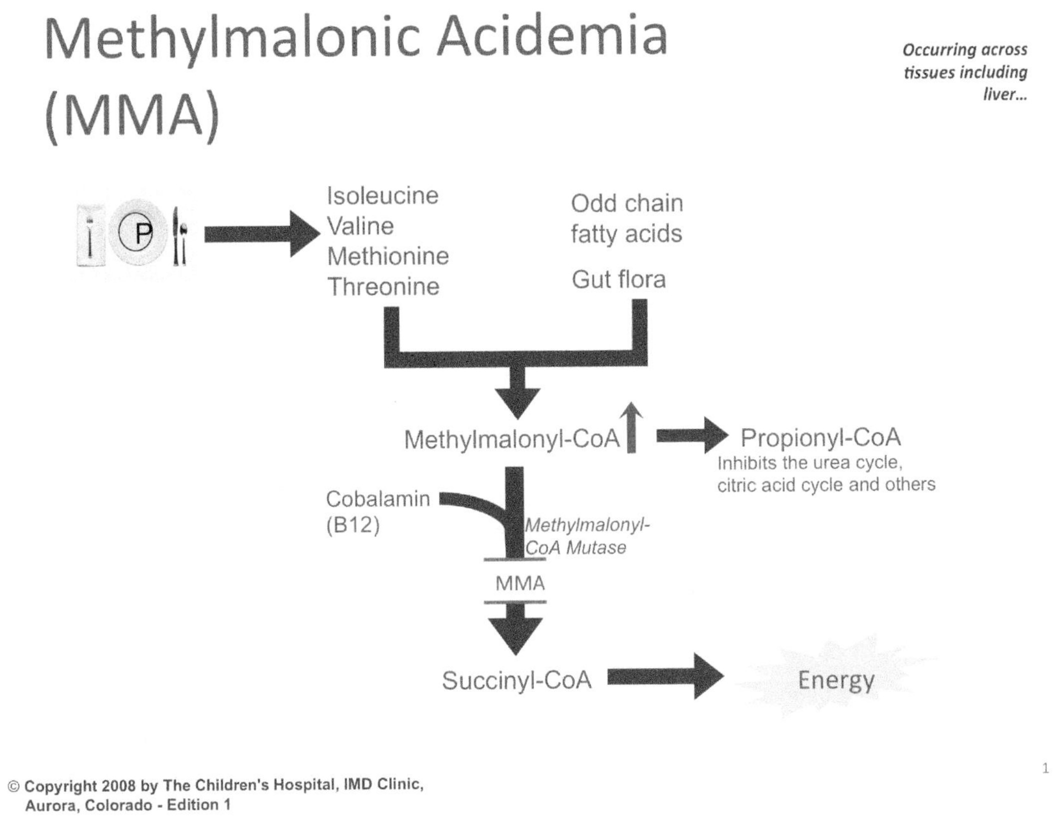

Methylmalonic Acidemia (MMA)

Occurring across tissues including liver...

Isoleucine
Valine
Methionine
Threonine

Odd chain fatty acids

Gut flora

Methylmalonyl-CoA ↑

Propionyl-CoA
Inhibits the urea cycle, citric acid cycle and others

Cobalamin (B12)

Methylmalonyl-CoA Mutase

MMA

Succinyl-CoA

Energy

1

Fig. 21.2 Metabolic pathway of methylmalonic acidemia

synthesis or utilization (e.g., cobalamin A or cobalamin B deficiency). Cobalamin defects are covered in detail in Chap. 15. Those with the mut^0 or mut$^-$ form of MMA have absent or minimal mutase activity and often develop a more severe phenotype than those who have some residual enzyme activity [1]. There is a wide range of clinical severity in both PROP and MMA and nutrition management needs to be individualized. Further discussion of organic acidemias, including PROP and MMA, is found in Chap. 18.

Long-term clinical complications include poor growth, cognitive delay, pancreatitis, seizures, and optic nerve atrophy. In addition, cardiomyopathy is more common in PROP, whereas chronic renal disease can develop in MMA caused by mutase deficiency [1–3]. These complications will be discussed later in the chapter (Box 21.1).

Box 21.1: Principles of Nutrition Management for PROP and MMA

Restrict: Intact protein, while maintaining normal plasma levels of propiogenic amino acids (Val, Met, Ile and Thr).

Provide: Medical food (without propiogenic amino acids) to meet total protein needs (100–120% of the DRI for age).

Ensure: Adequate calories to meet energy needs for growth.

Supplement: L-carnitine

21.2 Nutrition Management

21.2.1 Initial Nutrition Management of the Acutely Ill Newborn

Infants with severe forms of either PROP or MMA may present with metabolic ketoacidosis, hyperammonemia with vomiting, lethargy, and coma before newborn screening results are available. In these cases, elimination of all protein and the provision of adequate energy from intravenous (IV) glucose starting with 10% dextrose (D10) with appropriate electrolytes at 1–1.5 times maintenance fluid needs (8–10 mg/kg/min) and lipid (2 g/kg/d) by peripheral or central access to slow protein catabolism [4–6]. This initial non-protein calorie support can supply ~70 kcal/kg/d and the calories can be increased further with placement of a central line to allow for a higher volume or concentration of dextrose and a further increase in the IV lipid source. Once hyperammonemia improves, the addition of a standard parenteral source of essential amino acids can be initiated at 0.5 gm/kg/d and advanced 0.25 gm/kg/d as tolerated in infants where enteral nutrition is delayed. Frequent monitoring of clinical status and both metabolic and critical labs is required [7].

Once the newly diagnosed infant is stable, enteral nutrition (usually nasogastric) can be initiated. The use of a medical food with propiogenic amino acid-free protein equivalents can be used to meet the total protein requirement. The metabolic formula "recipe" will likely consist of three components to meet the infant's energy, intact protein, and total protein needs (Appendix K-4). The intact protein source can be either expressed breast milk or a term infant formula. A propiogenic amino acid-free medical food is selected to meet the remainder of the total protein requirement and a protein-free modular is added to meet total energy needs. The concept of the "24-hour batch recipe" is useful to ensure the patient is receiving the complete nutrition prescription (Box 21.2).

Box 21.2: The "24-Hour Batch Recipe"

- Parents should make the formula the same time each day.
- The recipe provides the prescribed amount of protein (both intact and medical food).
- Making another batch before the end of the 24-hour period would provide the infant with more protein than recommended.
- Not finishing the batch before the end of the 24-hour period would provide the infant with less protein than recommended.
- Use a protein-free carbohydrate/fat module (i.e., Pro-Phree®) to bridge the gap after 24-hour batch is completed.
- Parents should call the metabolic dietitian for a recipe change if they are taking more than 4 oz of Pro-Phree® per day.

Over-restriction of intact protein sources needs to be avoided as poor growth, weight gain, and wound healing have been reported [7]. A skin rash due to isoleucine deficiency has been reported in propionic acidemia [6]. Increasing intact protein is preferred versus the use of supplementary single amino acids to correct any low concentrations of propiogeninc amino acids [6]. Avoiding excessive intake of medical food improves plasma ratios of the branched chain amino acids (BCAA) [9]. In addition, this reduces the reliance of isoleucine and/or valine supplements to achieve desired plasma amino acid profiles [8].

Prior to discharge following the initial metabolic crisis, an infant will often require feeding assessments and therapy to improve oral intake and may benefit from a gastrostomy tube (g-tube) placement [7]. A g-tube can be very helpful to assure adequate intake while an infant continues to work on oral feeding skills at home. Availability of a g-tube can be critical to provide sufficient energy intake during any subsequent illnesses. The patient that has suffered a metabolic crisis during the newborn period will need to be monitored very closely in the clinic setting once discharged. Dietitians should work with the family on a home feeding schedule that not only meets the nutritional needs of the patient but meets the family's needs as well [10] (Box 21.3).

Box 21.3: Initiating Nutrition Management for a Symptomatic Infant with PROP/MMA

Goals:

- Provide adequate energy to prevent catabolism
- Normalize plasma concentrations of propiogenic AA (valine, methionine, isoleucine, threonine)
- Reduce production of abnormal metabolites (see Monitoring).

Step by Step:

1. Establish energy needs.
2. Determine the amount of intact protein needed from either a standard infant formula or breast milk.
3. Determine the amount of PROP/MMA medical food to provide the remainder of the infant's total protein needs.
4. Determine the calories provided by both the intact protein source and PROP/MMA medical food. Provide the remaining calories from a protein-free medical food. These formulas contain only carbohydrate, fat, and micronutrients.
5. Determine the amount of fluid necessary to make a final formula concentration of 20–24 kcal/oz, depending on energy needs and volume tolerated.
6. Initially the infant may be unable to consume adequate volumes to meet his needs and may require enteral feedings.

21.2.2 Chronic Nutrition Management

For typically developing infants with PROP or MMA, solids can be started at the same age as their unaffected peers, usually at 4–6 months age [11]. Feeding therapy should be recommended for those patients who are unable to meet their feeding milestones. As solid foods are introduced, counting grams of protein rather than milligrams of valine is appropriate as intact protein tolerance is typically higher in this population compared to PKU and some other inherited metabolic diseases and availability of lists of valine content of foods is limited. Applications such as "How Much Phe" (https://howmuchphe.org/) can be more accurate for protein counting than using food labels. As a patient's solid food intake advances, the volume of the formula can be reduced to allow greater intake of intact protein from foods. Careful monitoring of amino acids is important in this transition.

Other concepts to review with families during the first year of life include general nutrition principles, selection of lower protein foods, label reading, advancement of feeding textures, use of protein-free and low protein specialty foods in a meal plan, and dental care.

Caregivers should be given guidelines to avoid prolonged fasting which can lead to catabolism. Suggested maximum time between feedings for individuals <12 months is 4–6 hours and 8 hours for those >12 months of age [6].

For infants and young children needing a medical food, a "complete" medical food that contains propiogenic-free amino acids, as well as carbohydrates, fat, and micronutrients is recommended. For older individuals, medical foods that are concentrated in protein equivalents and low-fat or fat-free may allow the patient to meet their total protein requirement with a lower volume of medical food. Low-volume medical foods are also appropriate for overweight patients or those who can consume the majority of their energy from foods and thus require fewer calories from medical food.

21.3 Adjunct Treatments for Propionic Acidemia and Methylmalonic Acidemia

Since carnitine conjugates with the toxic acyl-CoA metabolites produced in PROP and MMA, patients often develop a secondary carnitine deficiency. To prevent this, L-carnitine in doses of 100–300 mg/kg/day, divided in 2–4 doses throughout the day, is routinely prescribed to maintain plasma-free carnitine concentrations in the normal range [3, 6, 7]. Some medical foods designed for PROP and MMA contain L-carnitine, and this should be considered when determining the amount of supplement to prescribe. The IV form of L-carnitine is often used during hospitalization for acute illness [4].

Some forms of MMA may be responsive to vitamin B_{12}. Responsiveness can be determined by administration of 1.0 mg hydroxocobalamin (IM or IV) for 5 days. A reduction in serum methylmalonic acid concentrations of 50% or greater indicates responsiveness [12]. For those with cobalamin-responsive forms of MMA, intramuscular (IM) hydroxocobalamin injections of 1.0–2.0 mg are often administered daily. A decreased frequency of IM injections or use of oral supplements may be appropriate for older individuals. Injections of hydroxocobalamin rather than cyanocobalamin are necessary in these disorders [13]. See Chap. 15.

A biotin supplement may be given during the initial diagnostic work-up for propionic acidemia, while multiple carboxylase deficiency is ruled out. Once PROP is confirmed, biotin should be discontinued [6].

Metronidazole has been used by some clinics to help reduce the production of propionic and methylmalonic acid by gut bacteria in the large intestine, in the hope of improving overall metabolic stability [6, 14].

Carbamylglutamate is a synthetic form of N-acetylglutamate, the co-factor required for carbamoyl phosphate synthase-1 (CPS), the initial step in the urea cycle. Stimulation of the first step of the urea cycle by prescribing this co-factor can reduce the secondary production of ammonia in patients with PROP and MMA [6, 15]. The efficacy and safety profile of these medications need to be evaluated by the medical team.

21.4 Monitoring

21.4.1 Nutritional Evaluation

A comprehensive evaluation of a patient's nutritional status should be completed at routine clinic visits. This includes a review of dietary intake using food records, food frequency or 24-hour recalls, physical activity, and nutrition-focused physical exam. Nutrient analysis should be conducted to ensure that a patient's macronutrient, essential fatty acid, vitamin, and mineral needs are met. MetabolicPro©, a software program designed specifically for nutrient analysis of metabolic disorders, is available (https://www.metabolicpro.org).

21.4.2 Anthropometrics

Monitoring a patient's weight, length or height, weight-for-length, and/or body mass index (BMI) is essential in PROP and MMA. Failure to thrive is a common finding in patients with these disorders due to oral motor delays and anorexia secondary to elevated metabolite concentrations. When adjusting energy and protein content, use the patient's ideal weight rather than actual weight to prevent underestimation of needs. See Chap. 6. However, because of lower lean body mass and decreased physical activity in patients with PROP and MMA, the resting energy expenditure in patients with these disorders may be lower than predicted by standard equations [6, 16, 17].

21.4.3 Laboratory Monitoring

The GMDI and SERN Nutrition Guidelines for PROP (https://southeastgenetics.org/ngp) provide recommendations for routine and conditional biochemical markers. Routine tests include

Box 21.4: Amino Acid Profiles in PROP and MMA

- *Goal:* Maintain the concentration of the propiogenic amino acids, Val, Met, Ile, and Thr in the low normal range.
- Glycine is often elevated in PROP, but not MMA. This is caused by propionic acid inhibition of the glycine cleavage system. How to interpret abnormal glycine concentrations is not well established. Glycine concentrations may be associated with energy intake, but not protein intake [18, 19].
- Low concentrations of BCAA (Val, Ile and Leu) have been associated with over-restriction of intact protein [6]. If low, incrementally increase the intact protein.

plasma amino acids, carnitine profile, total protein, albumin, prealbumin, complete blood count, 25-hydroxyvitamin D, and urine ketones. Plasma amino acid profiles are essential to help identify over-restriction of intact protein which results in low concentrations of the propiogenic and branched chain amino acids. Glycine is often elevated in PROP but not in MMA. This is caused by propionic acid inhibition of the glycine cleavage system. High glycine concentrations may be associated with low energy intake but are not related to protein intake (Box 21.4) [18–20].

In addition to plasma amino acids, concentrations of albumin and prealbumin (also called transthyretin) can be used to assess protein status. Albumin, with a half-life of 18–20 days, reflects a longer period of protein intake. Prealbumin is a more acute marker with a 2–3-day half-life. Albumin may be unreliable in liver disease and prealbumin can be altered with inflammation and renal disease (Chap. 6). A carnitine profile includes total carnitine, free carnitine, and carnitine esters (esterified) concentrations. Low concentrations of free carnitine suggest a need to increase the dose of supplemental L-carnitine. With supplementation, the total and ester fractions are often elevated.

Other biochemical markers should be considered during acute illness and for monitoring of chronic complications [6]. Some of these conditional biochemical markers include ammonia, chemistry panel, acylcarnitine profiles, urine organic acids, and other nutritional markers including serum vitamin B12, vitamin B6, erythrocyte folate, ferritin, zinc, selenium, and essential fatty acids (Box 21.5) [6].

Box 21.5: Nutrition Monitoring of a Patient with PROP or MMA

- Routine assessments include anthropometrics, dietary intake, physical findings
- Laboratory Monitoring
  - Diagnosis-specific
    - Plasma amino acids
      - Propiogenic (VAL, ILE, MET, THR)
      - Glycine
    - Serum methylmalonic acid (MMA)
    - Carnitine profile (total, free, esterified)
  - Nutrition-related laboratory monitoring of patients on BCAA-restricted diets may include markers of:
    - Protein sufficiency (plasma amino acids, prealbumin)
    - Nutritional anemia (hemoglobin, hematocrit, MCV, serum vitamin B12 and/or methylmalonic acid, total homocysteine, ferritin, iron, folate, total iron binding capacity)
    - Vitamin and mineral status (Total 25-hydroxyvitamin D, zinc, trace minerals)
    - Others as clinically indicated

21.5 Acute Nutrition Management During Illness

Patients with PROP and MMA are at risk for metabolic decompensation with any intercurrent illness, serious injury, or surgery [7]. The goal of treatment is to reduce or prevent catabolism by providing adequate energy. Patients should be provided with a plan for illness and the contact information to reach the on-call metabolic team. Common signs of metabolic decompensation include vomiting, decreased oral intake, lethargy, and/or decreased consciousness. Based on the severity of symptoms, a caregiver may be instructed to test for urine ketones, which can be used as an indicator of the degree of illness. Moderate to large ketones indicate compromised metabolic control, and the child will likely need medical attention.

A "sick day" protocol can be provided for at-home treatment of minor illnesses. The age of the child, severity of illness, and comfort level of caregivers dictate the length of time that home treatment can be continued. Caretakers need to be instructed to contact the metabolic team for further instructions if the child is unable to tolerate the sick day plan. A gastrostomy tube can help a child tolerate a sick day recipe when oral intake is reduced due to nausea and vomiting (Box 21.6).

Box 21.6: "Sick-Day" Diet for PROP/MMA

- Develop an individualized sick day plan for each patient.
- Emphasis should be placed on increasing energy and fluid needs rather than prolonged protein restriction that can exacerbate catabolism [3, 4].
- Reduce protein no longer than 24–48 hours, depending on degree of illness.
- Provide protein-free, carbohydrate-based fluids [5, 21].
- Caregivers need to follow-up with the metabolic team and be provided with an emergency protocol if emergency attention is required.

Box 21.7: Management of Acute Illness for a Patient with PROP or MMA [6, 7]

- Remove all protein sources and provide sufficient energy.
- After 24–48 hours of initiating treatment, restart a source of intact protein.
- Once intact protein needs have been optimized, add medical food to meet total. protein needs. Start with 0.5 g/kg/d, and increase 0.25 g/kg/d, as tolerated to goal
- If oral intake is inadequate or not possible, NG feedings are initiated.
- Provide L-carnitine. If oral L-carnitine is not tolerated, IV L-carnitine (100–300 mg/kg) may be prescribed.

Refer to Chap. 4 for acute medical management.

If hospitalization is necessary, and enteral nutrition is poorly tolerated, increased energy needs can be met with intravenous administration, often including 10% dextrose with appropriate electrolytes at 1.5–2 times maintenance fluid needs [6]. Protein sources are often reduced or discontinued for 24–48 hours; however, prolonged reduction of protein intake should be avoided to prevent catabolism [6]. When the patient is clinically stable, protein can be reintroduced at 0.5 g protein/kg/d and advanced by 0.25 g/kg/d, as tolerated, to a patient's usual prescription of intact and medical food sources. If enteral feeds are not tolerated and parenteral support is required for >48 hours, a combination of standard AA solutions and specialty AA solutions are available (Box 21.7) [6, 7].

21.6 Long-Term Complications

There are a number of long-term complications that can develop in these disorders that require close monitoring. Patients with either PROP or MMA are at risk for inadequate nutritional intake due to feeding difficulties caused by vomiting and anorexia. Repeated admissions may lead to poor growth and/or failure-to-thrive [1, 6]. Gastrostomy tube feedings, adaptive feeding devices, and feeding therapy can help ameliorate under-nutrition.

Those with PROP or MMA are susceptible to pancreatitis [14]. If a patient presents to the emergency room with vomiting, pancreatic enzymes should be monitored. Reduced physical activity and poor nutrition status can lead to inadequate bone mineralization. Vitamin D status along with bone density assessments should be monitored in patients at risk. Optic atrophy is a known concern in both conditions and should be monitored by an eye specialist. Cardiomyopathy is a known complication in PROP. Routine cardiology assessments may include the laboratory markers brain natriuretic peptide (BNP) and troponin, along with ECHO and EKG evaluations. Renal impairment is a known complication of MMA but can also develop in PROP. Biochemical markers to assess renal function include creatinine, cystatin-C, and glomerular filtration rate [1]. See Chap. 18 for more details.

21.7 Transplantation

Severe forms of MMA and PROP are associated with significant complications including frequent metabolic crises, cardiomyopathy, renal disease, and developmental delay. Liver transplantation becomes an option, especially for those patients with recurrent metabolic episodes that are not adequately controlled using conventional strategies [3]. Liver transplantation improves the quality of life and metabolic stability in patients with MMA and PROP and reduces the likelihood of a metabolic crisis and progressive cardiac and neurologic disability [22, 23]. In patients with MMA who received either a liver or combined liver-kidney transplant, neurological development was stabilized [24]. However, in PROP and MMA, transplantation is less curative than in some metabolic disorders and chronic complications in other organ systems can persist [6]. Metabolic stroke has been reported after liver transplantation [22, 25]. Patients with PROP or MMA who have undergone liver transplantation show improved measures of metabolic status including glycine in PROP, methylmalonic acid in MMA, and ammonia in both [23]. However, some metabolites such as urine methylcitrate and propionylcarnitine do not normalize [22, 25].

Patients with MMA can still develop renal disease and optic atrophy despite transplantation. Combined liver-kidney transplantation (LKT) may be performed in MMA, especially if renal disease is already present [26]. Plasma MMA decreases but does not normalize after LKT [23]. These patients remain at risk for neurological complications and optical atrophy [27]. After liver transplantation, protein restriction may be liberalized in both MMA and PROP, but the optimal intake of protein has not been determined. Protein tolerance ranges from mild protein restriction to an unrestricted diet [6, 23]. As an increase in intact protein is tolerated, the use of medical foods can be decreased but often not eliminated. L-carnitine will need to be continued to treat the secondary carnitine depletion [23].

21.8 Summary

The clinical outcome and lifespan of patients with PROP and MMA have improved through nutrition management, adjunct therapies, and aggressive treatment during metabolic crises. The Nutrition Guideline and Toolkit for Propionic Acidemia (https://southeastgenetics.org/ngp/) answers many questions about optimal treatment in both acute and chronic settings for the individual with this disorder. Future research will help improve these recommendations and allow for development of similar guidelines for MMA. For patients undergoing transplantation, continued support from a metabolic team is needed to assure optimal long-term outcomes.

21.9 Diet Case Examples

The GMDI/SERN Nutrition Guideline for Propionic Acidemia contains five cases with diet calculations (available at https://southeastgenetics.org/ngp/toolkit.php).

1. Infancy (or at diagnosis)
2. Toddlers (introduction of solids)
3. Liver transplantation in school-aged child
4. Adolescence and adults
5. Before and during pregnancy and in the post-partum period

Acknowledgments Thank you to Sandy van Calcar of Oregon Health & Science University for her contributions to this chapter's content in the first Edition of Nutrition Management of Inherited Metabolic Diseases.

References

1. Manoli I, Sloan JL, Venditti CP. Isolated Methylmalonic Acidemia. 2005 Aug 16 [Updated 2016 Dec 1]. In: Adam MP, Ardinger HH, Pagon RA, et al., editors. GeneReviews® [Internet]. Seattle (WA): University of Washington, Seattle; 1993–2022.
2. Shchelochkov OA, Carrillo N, Venditti C. Propionic acidemia. In: Adam MP, Ardinger HH, Pagon RA, Wallace SE, Bean LJH, Stephens K, et al., editors. GeneReviews((R)). Seattle: University of Washington, Seattle; 2016.
3. Sutton VR, Chapman KA, Gropman AL, MacLeod E, Stagni K, Summar ML, et al. Chronic management and health supervision of individuals with propionic acidemia. Mol Genet Metab. 2012;105(1):26–33.
4. Chapman KA, Gropman A, MacLeod E, Stagni K, Summar ML, Ueda K, et al. Acute management of propionic acidemia. Mol Genet Metab. 2012;105(1):16–25.
5. Yannicelli S. Nutrition management of patients with inherited disorders of organic acid metabolism. In: Nutrition management of patients with inherited metabolic disorders. 1st ed. Sudbury: Jones and Bartlett; 2010.
6. Jurecki E, Ueda K, Frazier D, Rohr F, Thompson A, Hussa C, et al. Nutrition management guideline for propionic acidemia: an evidence- and consensus-based approach. Mol Genet Metab. 2019;126(4):341–54.
7. Baumgartner MR, Horster F, Dionisi-Vici C, Haliloglu G, Karall D, Chapman KA, et al. Proposed guidelines for the diagnosis and management of methylmalonic and propionic acidemia. Orphanet J Rare Dis. 2014;9:130.
8. Bernstein L, Burns C, Drumm M, Gaughan S, Sailer-Hammons M, Baker P. Impact on isoleucine and valine supplementation when decreasing use of medical food in the nutritional management of methylmalonic acidemia. Nutrients. 2020;12(2):473.
9. Myles JG, Manoli I, Venditti CP. Effects of medical food leucine content in the management of methylmalonic and propionic acidemias. Curr Opin Clin Nutr Metab Care. 2018;21(1):42–8.
10. Lea D, Shchelochkov O, Cleary J, Koehly LM. Dietary management of propionic acidemia: parent caregiver perspectives and practices. JPEN J Parenter Enteral Nutr. 2019;43(3):434–7.
11. Breastfeeding and the use of human milk. Pediatrics. 2012;129(3):e827–41.
12. Fowler B, Leonard JV, Baumgartner MR. Causes of and diagnostic approach to methylmalonic acidurias. J Inherit Metab Dis. 2008;31(3):350–60.
13. Andersson HC, Shapira E. Biochemical and clinical response to hydroxocobalamin versus cyanocobalamin treatment in patients with methylmalonic acidemia and homocystinuria (cblC). J Pediatr. 1998;132(1):121–4.
14. Saudubray J-M. Inborn metabolic diseases: diagnosis and treatment. 6th ed. New York: Springer; 2016. pages cm p. 281, 287.
15. Haberle J, Chakrapani A, Ah Mew N, Longo N. Hyperammonaemia in classic organic acidaemias: a review of the literature and two case histories. Orphanet J Rare Dis. 2018;13(1):219.
16. Feillet F, Bodamer OA, Dixon MA, Sequeira S, Leonard JV. Resting energy expenditure in disorders of propionate metabolism. J Pediatr. 2000;136(5):659–63.
17. Hauser NS, Manoli I, Graf JC, Sloan J, Venditti CP. Variable dietary management of methylmalonic acidemia: metabolic and energetic correlations. Am J Clin Nutr. 2011;93(1):47–56.
18. Yannicelli S, Acosta PB, Velazquez A, Bock HG, Marriage B, Kurczynski TW, et al. Improved growth and nutrition status in children with methylmalonic or propionic acidemia fed an elemental medical food. Mol Genet Metab. 2003;80(1–2):181–8.
19. Al-Hassnan ZN, Boyadjiev SA, Praphanphoj V, Hamosh A, Braverman NE, Thomas GH, et al. The relationship of plasma glutamine to ammonium and of glycine to acid-base balance in propionic acidaemia. J Inherit Metab Dis. 2003;26(1):89–91.
20. Yannicelli S. Nutrition therapy of organic acidaemias with amino acid-based formulas: emphasis on methylmalonic and propionic acidaemia. J Inherit Metab Dis. 2006;29(2–3):281–7.
21. Van Hove JL, Myers S, Kerckhove KV, Freehauf C, Bernstein L. Acute nutrition management in the prevention of metabolic illness: a practical approach with glucose polymers. Mol Genet Metab. 2009;97(1):1–3.
22. Vara R, Turner C, Mundy H, Heaton ND, Rela M, Mieli-Vergani G, et al. Liver transplantation for propionic acidemia in children. Liver Transpl. 2011;17(6):661–7.
23. Critelli K, McKiernan P, Vockley J, Mazariegos G, Squires RH, Soltys K, et al. Liver transplantation for propionic acidemia and methylmalonic acidemia: perioperative management and clinical outcomes. Liver Transpl. 2018;24(9):1260–70.
24. Niemi AK, Kim IK, Krueger CE, Cowan TM, Baugh N, Farrell R, et al. Treatment of methylmalonic acidemia by liver or combined liver-kidney transplantation. J Pediatr. 2015;166(6):1455–61 e1.

25. Kasahara M, Sakamoto S, Kanazawa H, Karaki C, Kakiuchi T, Shigeta T, et al. Living-donor liver transplantation for propionic acidemia. Pediatr Transplant. 2012;16(3):230–4.
26. Mazariegos G, Shneider B, Burton B, Fox IJ, Hadzic N, Kishnani P, et al. Liver transplantation for pediatric metabolic disease. Mol Genet Metab. 2014;111(4):418–27.
27. Vernon HJ, Bagnasco S, Hamosh A, Sperati CJ. Chronic kidney disease in an adult with propionic acidemia. JIMD Rep. 2014;12:5–10.

Part IV

Fatty Acid Oxidation Disorders

22 Fatty Acid Oxidation Disorders

Curtis R. Coughlin II

Contents

C. R. Coughlin II (✉)
Clinical Genetics and Metabolism, Children's Hospital Colorado, University of Colorado Denver - Anschutz Medical Campus, Aurora, CO, USA
e-mail: curtis.coughlin@childrenscolorado.org

L. E. Bernstein et al. (eds.), *Nutrition Management of Inherited Metabolic Diseases*,
https://doi.org/10.1007/978-3-030-94510-7_22

Core Messages

- Fatty acid oxidation disorders often present with intermittent symptoms triggered by prolonged fasting.
- Avoidance of fasting is a key component of treatment.
- Cardiac or skeletal muscle dysfunction are more difficult to treat that the hypoglycemia that defines many of these disorders. Early and consistent treatment with alternate energy sources is helpful although not always effective.

22.1 Background

Fatty acids are the primary energy source for the heart, skeletal muscle, and liver [1]. As one would expect, patients with fatty acid oxidation disorders (FAOD) can present with cardiac symptoms (cardiomyopathy and arrhythmias), muscular symptoms, such as rhabdomyolysis, and liver disorders (hypoglycemia, hepatomegaly, and rarely liver failure) [2]. It is important to recognize that glucose metabolism transitions from gluconeogenesis to lipolysis and ketogenesis starting at 12–14 hours of fasting. Therefore, limitation of extended fasting is a primary management strategy for all FAODs, regardless of the specific enzyme defect. Historically, a number of undiagnosed patients died as a result of an early intercurrent illness resulting in poor feeding and extended fasting [3, 4]. Newborn screening has dramatically improved the natural history for most FAODs [5], although universal newborn screening for long-chain defects is not available in all countries and false negative newborn screening results have been reported [6]. Therefore, it is paramount for clinicians to recognize the early symptoms of these fatal yet highly treatable disorders.

22.2 Biochemistry

Fatty acids are long alkanes with a single carboxylic acid. The most common saturated fatty acids in our body are palmitic acid with 16 carbons and stearic acid with 18 carbons [7]. Unsaturated fatty acids have a single unsaturated bond as in oleic acid with 18 carbons and a single cis-unsaturated bond at position 9 designated as C18:1 (the number after the colon denotes the number of unsaturated bonds). Fatty acids are derived from dietary sources and stored in fat tissue as triglycerides. Fatty acids are released by lipolysis to free fatty acids and glycerol and transported in the blood to the tissues that use them. Fatty acids contain an even number of carbons and are catabolized in sequential cycles to acetyl-coenzyme A. This process is called β-oxidation and occurs inside the mitochondria [8]. First, fatty acids need to enter the mitochondria, a process which occurs via the carnitine cycle.

22.2.1 Carnitine Cycle

In a first step after entering the cell, fatty acids move to the outer mitochondrial membrane bound to fatty acid binding proteins. At the outer mitochondrial membrane, the fatty acids are converted into their respective acyl-CoA (a coenzyme A ester of a fatty acid) by acyl-CoA synthases with the use of ATP. Acyl-CoA esters are then converted into acylcarnitines by transferring the acyl-moiety from coenzyme A to carnitine through the action of carnitine palmitoyltransferase I (CPT-I). This first step is the regulatory step of fatty acid oxidation. The acylcarnitine then enters the mitochondria in exchange for carnitine by the action of the carnitine:acylcarnitine translocase (CACT). Once inside the mitochondria, the acylcarnitine is exchanged for coenzyme A to an acyl-CoA ester through the action of carnitine palmitoyltransferase II (CPT-II). This process is reversible, and acyl-CoA that accumulates in the mitochondria can exit the mitochondria as acylcarnitine esters (Fig. 22.1). This process is taken advantage of in acylcarnitine analysis.

22.2.2 Fatty Acid Beta-Oxidation

Fatty acid β-oxidation is depicted in Fig. 22.2. In the first step, the acyl-CoA is oxidized by acyl-

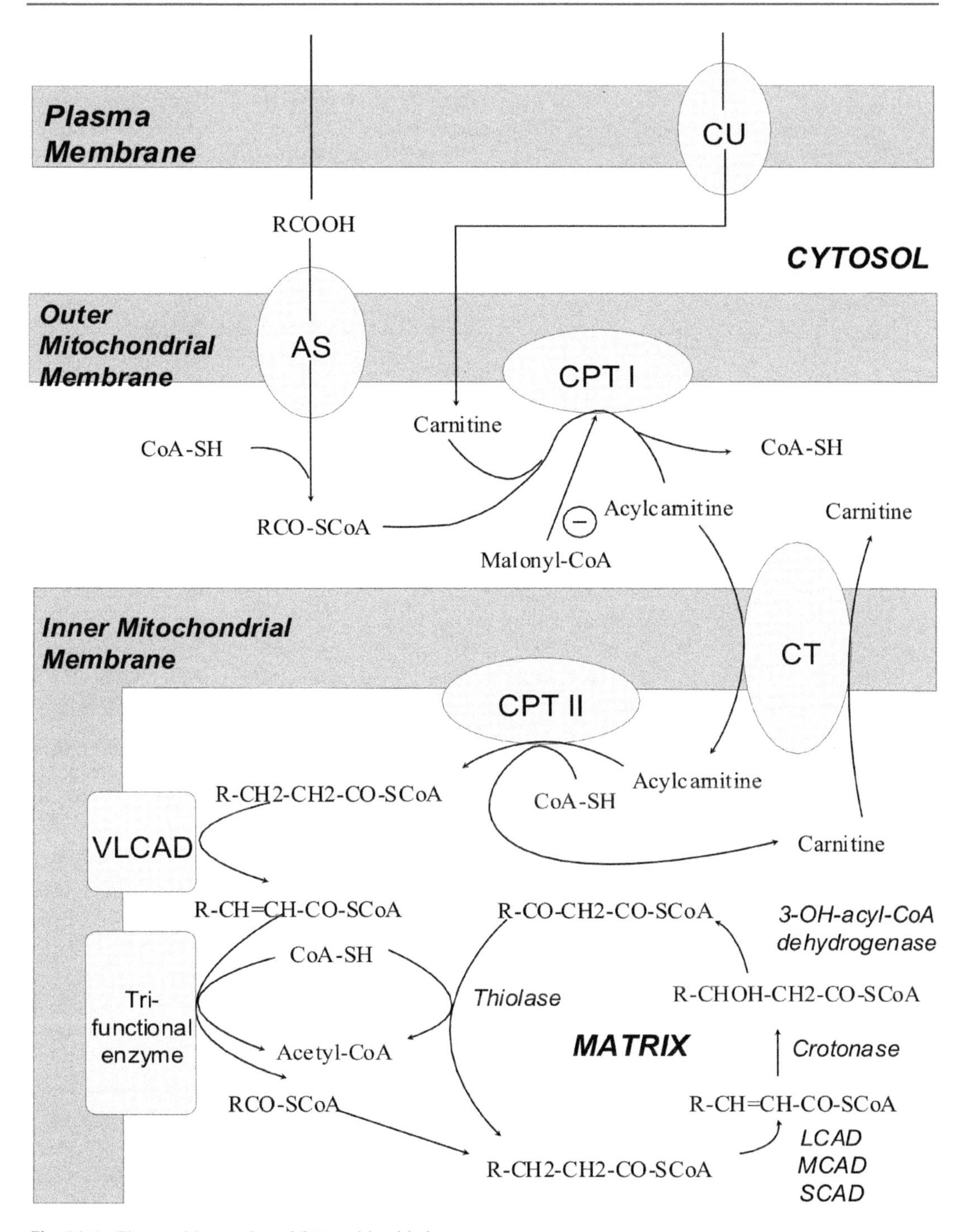

Fig. 22.1 The carnitine cycle and fatty acid oxidation

CoA dehydrogenase removing two hydrogens and transferring them to FAD (flavin adenine dinucleotide) resulting in 2,3-enoyl-CoA. The unsaturated bond is between atoms 2 and 3 on the beta-carbon. There are several different acyl-CoA dehydrogenases, which differ in the chain length specificity of their substrates. Short chain acyl-CoA dehydrogenase (SCAD) acts on fatty acids with 4–6 carbons [9]. Medium-chain acyl-CoA dehydrogenase (MCAD) acts on fatty acids with 6–10 carbons [10]. Long-chain acyl-CoA dehydrogenase (LCAD) acts on fatty acids with

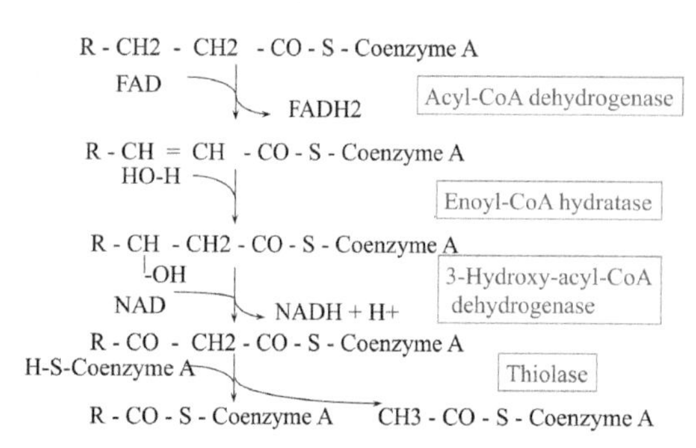

Fig. 22.2 Beta-oxidation of fatty acids

10–18 carbons but has limited activity in fatty acid oxidation [11]. These three enzymes (LCAD, MCAD, and SCAD) occur in the mitochondrial matrix. Very long chain acyl-CoA dehydrogenase (VLCAD) acts on fatty acids of 10–20 carbons and acts in the inner mitochondrial membrane. VLCAD is the enzyme that first starts β-oxidation for dietary fatty acids of 16 and 18 carbons [12].

The second step then uses water and places one hydrogen on carbon 2 and a hydroxyl-group on carbon 3. This hydratase enzyme thus makes a 3-hydroxy-acyl-CoA. There are two hydratases: long chain enoyl-CoA hydratase, present in the inner mitochondrial membrane, and short chain enoyl-CoA hydratase, present in the matrix. The next step removes two hydrogens from the hydroxyl group on carbon 3 and transfers them to NAD making NADH and H+ by the enzyme 3-hydroxy-acyl-CoA dehydrogenase. There are two enzymes, a long-chain 3-hydroxyacyl-CoA dehydrogenase (LCHAD) present in the inner mitochondrial membrane and a short-chain 3-hydroxyacyl-CoA dehydrogenase (SCHAD) present in the mitochondrial matrix. In the last step, the enolase enzyme cleaves the carbon chain between carbon 2 and 3 and transfers the shortened carbon chain onto coenzyme A making a new acyl-CoA that is 2 carbons shorter and releasing acetyl-CoA. There is a long chain enolase in the inner mitochondrial membrane and a short chain enolase in the mitochondrial matrix. The three long chain enzymes, long chain hydratase, long chain 3-hydroxyacyl-CoA dehydrogenase, and long chain enolase are part of the same single trifunctional enzyme, which consists of an α and a β chain and resides in the inner mitochondrial membrane close to the VLCAD enzyme. The VLCAD and the trifunctional enzyme are responsible for β-oxidation of acyl-CoAs from 12–20 carbons, before releasing them to the enzymes in the mitochondrial matrix.

22.2.3 Ketogenesis and Ketone Utilization

When fatty acid oxidation occurs at a high rate, the liver will generate excess acetyl-CoA molecules that are used in ketogenesis. Ketones are generated by first making 3-hydroxy-3-methylglutaryl-CoA (HMG-CoA) by HMG-CoA synthase, which is then converted to acetoacetate by HMG-CoA lyase. The free acetoacetate is in equilibrium with 3-hydroxybutyrate with a usual ratio of 3:1 (3-hydroxybutyrate:acetoacetate). Other tissues can use ketones by three steps: in a first step, acetoacetate enters the mitochondria by the monocarboxylate transporter MCT1, it is then activated by coenzyme A transfer from succinyl-CoA by succinyl-CoA:3-oxoacid transferase (SCOT), and then acetoacetyl-CoA is cleaved by acetoacetyl-CoA thiolase, of which there are two, α- and β-ketothiolase. Lack of one of the enzymes in ketone generation will result in insufficient ketogenesis, whereas a lack of an enzyme in ketone utilization will result in excessive ketosis.

The rate at which fatty acid β-oxidation occurs is related to the availability of its substrates, the free fatty acids. Free fatty acids are released from fat tissue when glucose and insulin concentrations are low. The production of ketones is dependent on the availability of free fatty acids and a ratio of ketones:free fatty acids is the best measure of the efficacy of this process. Therefore, free fatty acids, 3-hydroxybutyrate, and acetoacetate should be measured in a patient with hypoglycemia. An insufficient concentration of ketones for the concentration of free fatty acids indicates a defect in β-oxidation or in ketogenesis. Excessive ketones for the concentration of free fatty acids indicate a defect in ketone utilization. There is a relationship between low glucose concentrations and the release of free fatty acids and hence of ketone generation, which can also be used as an indicator of a ketone disorder but is more indirect.

After a meal, the preferred substrate is carbohydrate with very limited fatty acid oxidation, less than 10% of total capacity. Hence, only patients with severe disorders of fatty acid oxidation will be symptomatic at this stage. During short-term fasting, glucose from glycogen breakdown is primarily used. In children over 1 year of age, lipolysis occurs after a prolonged fast of at least 12–15 hours before fatty acid oxidation commences at a maximum rate. The highest rates of ketogenesis occur in children ages 1 and 3 years, decreasing thereafter. After 12–15 hours of fasting, even patients with mild fatty acid oxidation defects will be unable to handle the high rate of fatty acid β-oxidation and can become symptomatic.

The fasting associated with illness is a common trigger for fatty acid oxidation defects. The cytokines and hormones released with the stress of infection further promote lipolysis and hence shorten the duration of fasting before high rates of β-oxidation occur, and symptoms can be expected in fatty acid oxidation defects. Most fatty acid oxidation defects thus typically occur with intermittent symptoms. These patients tend to be asymptomatic between episodes but have intermittent problems usually elicited by fasting and infections or other illnesses. Typically, only patients with severe fatty acid oxidation defects will present in the neonatal period.

Finally, muscle cells use fatty acid β-oxidation during prolonged exercise. During short exercise, muscle will use blood glucose and endogenous glycogen stores. During prolonged exercise, muscle will switch to the use of fat as an energy substrate. At that time, patients with fatty acid oxidation defects can exhibit muscle symptoms, including weakness, cramps, and lysis of muscle cells called rhabdomyolysis.

22.3 Phenotypic Overview of Fatty Acid Oxidation Disorders

Fatty acids are a primary source of energy for the heart, skeletal muscle, and during hepatic glycogen depletion [1]; therefore, symptoms of FAODs include elements of cardiac, skeletal muscle, and/or liver dysfunction. Severe hypoglycemia is common to all FAODs [2] and typically occurs during periods of fasting for more than 12–24 hours. Historically, patients presented in early childhood after an intercurrent illness resulting in poor intake [13] although case reports emphasize the risk of severe hypoglycemia in adulthood following significant illness or alcohol-related intoxications [14–16]. These symptoms constitute a Reye-like syndrome of hypoglycemia, elevated transaminases, mild hyperammonemia, and brain edema with lethargy and coma. Uric acid is usually elevated due to energy failure [17, 18]. All fatty acid oxidation defects can present with Reye-like syndrome. In fact, most cases of idiopathic Reye-like syndrome diagnosed before 1990 were patients with an unrecognized fatty acid oxidation defect. Long chain 3-hydroxyacyl-CoA dehydrogenase (LCHAD) deficiency is exceptional, in that it causes chronic cholestasis. In addition, carrier women during pregnancy with a fetus affected with LCHAD deficiency have a high rate of acute fatty liver of pregnancy [19, 20].

Fatty acid oxidation is the preferred energy source for the heart, and patients with FAODs can exhibit several cardiac abnormalities. Defects in long chain fatty acid oxidation enzymes are associated with early onset cardiomyopathy [21]. Early and aggressive therapy has been associated with the reversal of severe cardiomyopathy, which emphasizes the importance to recognize this phenotype [22, 23]. Cardiomyopathy may also present as a late-onset symptom due to both acute decompensation and chronic disease pathology [24]. Conduction abnormalities and ventricular arrhythmias (ventricular tachycardia, ventricular fibrillation, torsades de pointes) occur in FAODs. They are frequent in severe fatty acid oxidation defects of long chain fatty acids and particularly prominent in carnitine acylcarnitine translocase (CACT) deficiency [25] but can also occur in all FAODs during a severe decompensation [26]. Atrioventricular block can occur but is rare.

In skeletal muscle, symptoms are usually triggered by prolonged exercise. They most often consist of acute cramping followed by rhabdomyolysis, and muscle weakness can be a feature but is not common [27]. Rhabdomyolysis results in the large release of muscle cell proteins in blood and can result in precipitation of small proteins such as myoglobin in the renal tubules resulting in acute renal blockade and renal insufficiency. Prevention of acute renal failure thus requires hyperhydration, often needing large amounts of intravenous fluids. Some patients exhibit recurrent rhabdomyolysis, whereby any excessive exercise will immediately result in symptomatic rhabdomyolysis. Finally, even fatty acid oxidation defects such as MCAD can have elevated creatine kinase concentrations with metabolic decompensations without muscle symptoms.

22.4 Diagnostic Testing

The diagnosis of a FAOD is often established by biochemical testing, such as a characteristic acylcarnitine profile, although a FAOD may be suggested by routine clinical tests. In patients presenting with hypoglycemia, it is prudent to measure free fatty acids and quantitative ketones (3-hydroxybutyrate and acetoacetate). It is important to note that patients with FAODs are hypoketotic, but still may generate some degree of ketones [28]. As noted above, other clinical testing such as hyperuricemia may also indicate a generalized energy failure seen in FAOD [17, 18]. These laboratory findings in the setting of classic phenotypic findings may suggest the presence of a FAOD, although further testing is warranted.

Most patients with FAODs are diagnosed based on a characteristic carnitine or acylcarnitine profile. Acylcarnitine analysis can be performed through a number of methodologies although most laboratories will utilize liquid chromatography with tandem mass spectrometry (LC-MS/MS) and are used for both diagnostic testing of symptomatic patients and for newborn screening [29, 30]. An increase in a specific acylcarnitine species is often indicative of a specific enzymatic block. It is important to note several other physiologic conditions can cause elevated acylcarnitines such as fasting itself [31, 32]. Most FAOD can be diagnosed by an acyclarnitine profile measured in blood except for carnitine palmitoyltransferase I (CPT-I) where a decrease in palmitoylcarnitine is more readily identified in blood spots [33]. Urine organic acids can show increased dicarboxylic acids, but these have very limited specificity. Medium chain fatty acid oxidation defects (MCAD) and multiple acyl-CoA dehydrogenase deficiency (MADD) have increased acylglycine esters (hexanoylglycine and suberylglycine) that can be recognized on urine organic acid analysis or can be quantified in specific acylglycine analysis. SCAD deficiency and MADD can have increased ethylmalonic acid concentrations. A profile of free fatty acids in serum can be diagnostic, for instance, by showing increased cis-4-decenoic acid in MCAD deficiency but is nowadays rarely used.

Occasionally, an acylcarnitine profile may not be diagnostic. This is often due to a combination of a mild enzyme deficiency and a patient who is in the fed (non-catabolic) state [34]. Several strategies can be used to confirm the diagnosis. The sensitivity of the acylcarnitine analysis can be increased by first loading a biological sample with fatty acids and is often referred to as fatty acid oxidation flux studies or fatty acid oxidation probe studies. This testing is often performed in vitro by incubating fibroblasts with both fatty acids and carnitine before measuring acylcarnitines in the medium and the cell pellet. Enzyme assays exist for most fatty acid oxidation defects in either fibroblasts or in leukocytes [35]. These functional tests are valuable to establishing the diagnosis of patients with biochemical testing results that are unclear [36]. There are limitations of functional testing such as there is overlap between results from mildly affected patients and those patients who are heterozygote (i.e., carriers of a disease) with no clinical risk.

Genetic testing can further clarify those patients with indeterminate biochemical and functional test results. As with all testing, genetic results may be inconclusive in isolation although should be interpreted in the context of clinical symptoms, biochemical results, and functional testing when possible. There is also some genotype–phenotype correlation, which may help guide the clinical team and family [37, 38].

22.5 Overview of Selected Fatty Acid Oxidation Disorders

22.5.1 Medium Chain Acyl-Coenzyme A Dehydrogenase (MCAD) Deficiency

MCAD deficiency is the most common fatty acid oxidation defect in North America and Northern Europe [39, 40]. The medium-chain acyl-CoA dehydrogenase has substrate specificity for fatty acyl-CoAs with chain lengths of 6, 8, and 10 carbons, including the unsaturated C10:1 acyl-CoA derived from unsaturated fatty acids [41]. There are overlapping substrate specificities at each chain length with other acyl-CoA dehydrogenases such as SCAD for shorter chain lengths and LCAD for longer chain lengths. As a result, even in patients with two severe mutations with no residual activity of the MCAD enzyme, there is still about 20% of residual enzyme activity due to the overlapping substrate specificities [42]. Thus, during the normal fed state, there is sufficient capacity of fatty acid oxidation that a normal flux of fatty acid metabolism is measured. As a result, outside of acute episodes, patients with MCAD deficiency are asymptomatic. Only when the demand for fatty acid oxidation is increased, such as during prolonged fasting, will the reduction in fatty acid oxidation capacity become evident and symptoms develop.

Clinical symptoms usually present during the first 2 years of life but can occur at any age (Box 22.1). Up to 5% of patients present in the first 3 days of life, often with fatal consequences [13, 43]. These patients were exclusively breast fed, and breast milk production was somewhat delayed resulting in inadvertent fasting. Triggering factors are always prolonged fasting and often infections. Typical symptoms involve a Reye-like syndrome with hypoglycemia, elevated transaminases with mild hepatomegaly, elevated uric acid, and mild hyperammonemia (with values usually in the hundreds). There is brain edema resulting in lethargy and coma. Cardiac arrhythmias have been recognized as a terminal event in many children. Elevated creatine kinase is seen in half the children, but frank rhabdomyolysis is very rare [44]. There is hypoketosis for the duration of fasting, as production of ketones from free fatty acids is reduced and the degree of hypoglycemia presents as hypoketotic hypoglycemia. The unrecognized condition has a mortality of 20% and a high morbidity with resulting learning problems. Children who become ill in the evening and do not receive typical treatment can be found dead in their crib as sudden unexplained death syndrome (SUDS). At autopsy, fatty infiltration of liver and heart is found as well as brain edema, distinguishing it on pathology from SUDS [45]. Postmortem analysis of acylcarnitine in a blood spot or in bile can be diagnostic, or molecular analysis can be pursued.

Box 22.1: Clinical Presentation of MCAD Deficiency

- Age:
  - Most common: Infancy up to 2 years
  - Neonatal period: 5% of MCAD patients present in first 3 days of life; usually breast fed
  - Can occur at any age under stress.
- Triggering factors: fasting and infections
- Symptoms
  - Reye-like syndrome
  - Hypoglycemia
  - Heart: arrhythmia, sudden death
  - SIDS-like
  - Autopsy: fatty liver, heart, brain edema

MCAD is an autosomal recessive disorder and is caused by mutations in the *ACADM* gene. The most common mutation is c.985A > G resulting in p.K329E [46]. The mutation is present in 90% of symptomatic cases and in about 50% of cases identified on newborn screening [47]. The mutation is most prevalent in Northern European populations. The incidence of MCAD deficiency ranges from 1:24,000 to 1:17,000 births. Diagnosis is usually made by acylcarnitine analysis showing elevated C6, C8, C10, and C10:1 acylcarnitines with an increase in C8 greater than the increase in C10 [30]. Other diagnostic metabolites include increased concentrations of the acylglycines, suberylglycine, and hexanoylglycine in urine. Total carnitine concentrations are often decreased. Sequencing the *ACADM* gene is used as a confirmatory test. Given the high frequency of MCAD deficiency, and its intermittent symptomatology, it is necessary to screen family members including not only siblings but also parents, as asymptomatic affected status of parents has been observed (pseudodominant inheritance). This condition requires not only a conducive genotype but also a strong environmental stress factor, most importantly long duration fasting before becoming symptomatic, which makes it also well amenable to treatment. Thus, this condition satisfies all criteria for newborn screening and has been added in most countries to the universal newborn screening programs.

Foremost in the treatment of MCAD deficiency is the avoidance of long fasting at all times (Box 22.2). In one retrospective study, the shortest fasting time at which children with MCAD deficiency were observed to exhibit hypoglycemia was 12 hours [48]. Families are often instructed in counting fasting time, and it is important to consider the last meal that provided good caloric intake. Children over 1 year of age should be able to fast for 15–18 hours. Practically, families are instructed to limit fasting to 12 hours, which provides a few hours in which to try different strategies to provide calories to the child before requiring intravenous support.

Box 22.2: Treatment of MCAD Deficiency

- AVOID prolonged fasting under any circumstances
  - Infections, medical procedures, alcohol consumption
  - Provide caloric support in illness
- Provide L-carnitine in acute episodes - consider utility in chronic management
- Avoid Medium Chain Triglycerides (MCT)
- Rarely supplement uncooked cornstarch at night

During clinic visits, scenarios where long fasting can occur are reviewed such as illness in the morning after an overnight physiologic fast of sleep. With an illness in the evening and reduced oral intake or vomiting, long fasting will occur overnight. Parents are then instructed to wake up their child and to try to feed them; and if unsuccessful, to bring them to the emergency room and not to wait until the morning. All caregivers in the family must be educated, and families that do not attend clinic visits and show poor compliance must be particularly paid attention to as this is a risk factor for metabolic decompensation and a risk of fatality during illness [49]. Furthermore, instructions must be given to other medical professionals to avoid long fasting associated with medical or dental procedures and to institute prophylactic intravenous glucose support in cases of long procedure-associated fasting. Enteral intake of sufficient calories must be ensured before patients can be released to home after an anesthesia or dental extraction without complications of nausea, vomiting, or trismus. Dietary fat restriction is not needed except to avoid very high fat diets such as Atkins diet or ketogenic diet. Valproate interferes with fatty acid oxidation and should be avoided. Low concentrations of carnitine are common in patients with MCAD deficiency. The degree of carnitine deficiency outside of acute episodes is, for most children, mild and does not interfere with fatty acid oxidation. However, during acute episodes, carnitine concentrations can fall precipitously worsening the fatty acid oxidation flux and carnitine supplementation is then indicated. Some children, particularly young infants, have limited capacity to produce carnitine and can have very low concentrations, in which case, chronic carnitine supplementation can be indicated. Additional risk factors for low carnitine include heterozygosity for carnitine transporter defect, vegetarian diet, renal disease, or pregnancy. Adults have a longer fasting tolerance but can still develop a fatal Reye-like syndrome. Care should be taken with alcohol consumption, since excessive amounts of alcohol interferes with fatty acid oxidation and liver function, as well as creates a risk for hypoglycemia with prolonged fasting (e.g., vomiting during hangover) and decreased consciousness.

Outcome of treatment is excellent. Patients with MCAD have become Olympic athletes or attained professions of the highest education. With careful management, particularly of fasting avoidance and prophylactic admissions during illness, episodes of metabolic decompensation can be avoided. Both mortality and morbidity can be significantly reduced.

22.5.2 Long Chain 3-Hydroxyacyl-Coenzyme A Dehydrogenase (LCHAD) Deficiency

The trifunctional protein is a mitochondrial inner membrane enzyme that consists of an α-chain with the 3-hydroxyacyl-CoA dehydrogenase enzyme activity and a β-chain with the hydratase and thiolase activity. A common mutation c.1528C>G, comprising 60% of the alleles, specifically impairs the 3-hydroxyacyl-CoA dehydrogenase enzyme activity while leaving the other two enzyme activities intact [50]. Other mutations impair all three enzyme activities and are called trifunctional protein deficient [51, 52]. Patients with the c.1528G>C mutation tend to have higher concentrations of 3-hydroxyacylcarnitines and, thus, have a greater incidence of symptoms such as retinal dysfunction [53]. Genotypes with two severe variants without residual enzyme activity or overlapping activity of other TFP enzymes can result in patient phenotypes at higher risk to develop severe symptoms such as cardiomyopathy [19].

Patients with LCHAD deficiency can have Reye-like syndrome, cardiomyopathy, and myopathic symptoms of recurrent rhabdomyolysis [54]. Patients with LCHAD deficiency have additional symptoms that are specific to this fatty acid oxidation disorder. Infants can present with prolonged cholestasis with fibrosis leading to liver insufficiency. They tend to have chronic lactic acidosis that can be confused with respiratory chain enzyme deficiency and can have decreased activities of respiratory chain enzymes on biopsy. In childhood, patients can develop a retinal dystrophy with retinitis pigmentosa leading to loss of vision. The incidence and progression of retinitis pigmentosa is related to the elevation of 3-hydroxyacylcarnitines and is more common in isolated LCHAD deficiency with c.1528G>C variants [55]. Patients can develop disabling and painful peripheral neuropathies [56]. Finally, during pregnancy of a fetus affected with LCHAD deficiency, the mother who is an obligate heterozygote can develop acute fatty liver of pregnancy or hemolysis, elevated liver enzymes, and low platelets (HELLP) syndrome. This complication is particularly prevalent in fetuses affected with the c.1528G>C variant compared to fetuses with trifunctional protein deficiency [19, 20]. However, the incidence of the common c.1528G>C mutation in prospective mothers who develop HELLP syndrome is low (<1%) [57].

The diagnosis of LCHAD deficiency is often based on an acylcarnitine profile with elevated long chain acylcarnitines C12, C14, C18, and C18:1 but also show elevations of 3-hydroxyacylcarnitines, including hydroxyl-C14, hydroxyl-C16, and hydroxyl-C18:1 [58]. Urine organic analysis shows dicarboxylic acids and 3-hydroxydicarboxylic acids. These latter metabolites can rarely also be observed in certain patients with respiratory chain enzyme deficiencies. Lactate and the lactate:pyruvate ratio are often elevated. The incidence of LCHAD deficiency on newborn screening is estimated at 1:60,000 births. The diagnosis is usually confirmed by mutation analysis of the genes for the α-chain *HADHA* and the β-chain *HADHB*.

The treatment of LCHAD deficiency is similar to other long-chain FAOD such as VLCAD deficiency. Strict treatment is necessary in order to reduce the development of long-term complications such as retinal dystrophy [55]. Treatment consists of avoidance of fasting, severe reduction of dietary fat, provision of medium chain triglycerides, while providing sufficient amounts of polyunsaturated fatty acids, in particular docosahexaenoic acid (DHA). Fat restriction and particularly providing sufficient quantities of MCT is associated with reduced concentrations of 3-hydroxyacylcarnitines.

22.5.3 Very Long Chain Acyl-Coenzyme A Dehydrogenase (VLCAD) Deficiency

The very long chain acyl-coenzyme A dehydrogenase (VLCAD) enzyme has substrate specificity for long chain acyl-CoAs of 10–20 carbons [12]. VLCAD is the main enzyme for oxidation of acyl-CoAs of this chain length, and there is very little other enzyme activity. Therefore, variants that completely abolish residual activity will result in a near complete block of fatty acid oxidation flux and can cause symptoms outside of fasting, often in the neonatal period. The majority of variants of patients identified with VLCAD on newborn screening are mild and have remaining residual activity. These patients are still at risk for intermittent symptoms at times of increased fatty acid oxidation flux such as during fasting or in the muscle with prolonged exercise.

There are three clinical presentations for VLCAD deficiency (Box 22.3) [37]. All patients, regardless of genotype, are at risk of developing a Reye-like syndrome identical to that of MCAD deficiency. The triggers are similarly prolonged fasting and infection. All patients are also at risk of myopathic symptoms with intermittent episodes of rhabdomyolysis, sometimes with painful cramping but rarely with muscle weakness [59]. Some patients have frequent recurrent episodes of severe rhabdomyolysis. These can be triggered by prolonged exercise, fasting, stress, or exposure to cold [35]. Even patients with mild variants can experience recurrent rhabdomyolysis. Only the patients with severe VLCAD deficiency can develop cardiomyopathy, although cardiac symptoms are not always present in the neonatal period. The cardiomyopathy is usually hypertrophic. It can range from mild hypertrophy without involvement of cardiac contractility to severe dysfunction. Cardiac ventricular arrhythmias is also possible with prolonged QT, ventricular tachycardia, torsades de pointes, and ventricular fibrillation [21].

Box 22.3: Clinical Presentation of VLCAD Deficiency

- Cardiac (severe form): Acute cardiomyopathy with severe ventricular arrhythmia risk
- Liver: Reye-like syndrome (hypoglycemia, elevated transaminases, mild hyperammonemia, and brain edema with lethargy and coma)
- Muscle: Myopathy, rhabdomyolysis
  - Often associated with prolong exercise, fasting, stress, or exposure to cold

VLCAD deficiency is often identified on acylcarnitine profile by elevations of long chain acylcarnitines C12, C12:1, C14, C14:1, C14:2, C16, and C18:1. Characteristic of VLCAD is a pronounced elevation of C14:1 that is higher than C14 and C14:2. Care must be taken to use fasting-appropriate normal values, as fasting causes a mild elevation of C14:1 and C14 in unaffected individuals reflecting the greater fatty acid oxidation flux [32]. In neonates with mild VLCAD, the acylcarnitine profile can be abnormal on the first newborn screen at 24 hours of life but can then normalize in the next days, while the patient can still be vulnerable to life threatening Reye-like syndrome in the context of illness or other stress [60, 61]. There are case reports of patients who had false negative newborn screening results emphasizing the importance of exploring this diagnosis in symptomatic patients regardless of screening results [61–63]. Following an abnormal newborn screen, confirmation of the diagnosis can be accomplished through either genetic or enzymatic testing [64, 65].

The primary treatment for VLCAD is the avoidance of long duration fasting, similar to that of MCAD deficiency [64, 66]. For patients with severe VLCAD deficiency (with the cardiac phenotype), the allowed fasting duration is shorter than for MCAD and must be strictly adhered to. Extra energy can be provided as medium chain triglycerides. For patients with the severe form, long-chain fat intake must be severely restricted to about 10% of total energy, and up to 30% of calories as medium chain triglycerides. During such severe fat restriction, care must be taken to provide sufficient sources of essential fatty acids. Diet modification improves cardiomyopathy [22], reduces long chain acylcarnitine concentrations, and reduces the frequency of episodes of rhabdomyloysis but does not prevent them. Odd-carbon medium-chain length triglycerides, such as triheptanoin oil, also provide an alternate energy source and has been shown to have added benefit over medium chain triglycerides [67]. Chapter 23 further addresses nutrition management of long-chain FAOD.

For the prevention of rhabdomyolysis, prolonged exercise must be avoided with breaks of 15–30 minutes instituted after 30–45 minutes of activity. Carbohydrates and medium chain triglyceride supplements can be consumed prior to exercise and reduce the incidence of rhabdomyolysis and muscle cramps, as well as improve exercise capacity of medium intensity. These interventions are also effective to improve cardiac symptoms, prevent symptoms of Reye-like syndrome, and reduce but do not prevent episodes of rhabdomyolysis. The cardiomyopathy responds to dietary intervention but can be so severe as to require cardiac transplantation.

22.6 Overview of Ketogenesis and Ketolysis Defects

22.6.1 Ketogenesis

3-hydroxy-3-methylglutarylcoenzyme A synthase is the first step in the synthesis of ketones [68]. Patients with deficiency present with hypoketotic hypoglycemia and hepatomegaly, but respond promptly to treatment with glucose. The primary treatment for disorders of ketone metabolism is avoidance of long-term fasting [69]. No metabolites accumulate, and urine organic acids and plasma acylcarnitines are normal. The primary diagnostic sign is a low ratio of ketones:free fatty acids, in the presence of hypoglycemia. If not identified on acute presentation, then a careful fasting test can help establish the diagnosis. Confirmatory testing is best completed by molecular analysis by sequencing the *HMGCS2* gene [70].

22.6.2 Ketolysis Defects

After the activation to its coenzyme A ester of acetoacetate by succinyl-coenzyme A oxoacid transferase, the acetoacetyl-coenzyme A must be cleaved into acetyl-CoA by thiolase [71]. There are cytosolic and mitochondrial thiolase enzymes, although the main enzyme only cleaves acetoacetyl-CoA and provides a baseline thiolase activity. The other enzyme cleaves both acetoacetyl-CoA and 2-methylacetoacetyl-CoA derived from isoleucine metabolism. The added capacity of this latter enzyme is required to metabolize the high flux of ketones generated during fasting and full ketogenesis. The accumulation of ketoacids causes an anion gap metabolic ketoacidosis. Clinical symptoms usually reflect the metabolic acidosis with Kussmaul breathing and vomiting [72]. Unresolved, the accumulation of ketoacids can result in brain damage including basal ganglia stroke and developmental delays. Treatment consists of reducing ketosis by providing glucose and preventive treatment consists of avoidance of long duration fasting. β-ketothiolase also metabolizes branched methylketones such as methylacetoacetate derived from isoleucine [71]. Rarely, metabolic decompensation can be triggered by excessive protein intake and a modest reduction in protein intake to a maximum of 2 g/kg/day for infants is usually indicated. Diagnosis requires the recognition of hyperketosis (>6 mM ketones in blood) and the presence of methylketones in urine organic acids (2-methylacetoacetate, 2-methyl-3-hydroxybutyrate). During the fed state, these metabolites can be very low, and it can be difficult to establish a diagnosis without confirmatory testing. Confirmatory testing includes measuring β-ketothiolase activity in fibroblasts or by sequencing the *ACAT1* gene [73].

Patients with succinyl-coenzyme A oxoacid transferase (SCOT) deficiency have genetic variants that completely abolish the function of the enzyme [74]. They cannot metabolize even the low flux of normal ketone body generation and metabolism, resulting in metabolic ketoacidosis in the neonatal period. Patients with SCOT deficiency have excessive ketones even in the fed state, resulting in neonatal acidosis, tachypnea, hypotonia, vomiting, obtundation, and coma [75]. A few rare patients have been reported to have variants with some residual activity. These patients present with hyperketosis upon fasting similar to β-ketothiolase deficiency. Treatment is difficult. Diagnosis requires enzyme assay in fibroblasts or variant analysis of the *OXCT1* gene [76].

Patients with variants in the monocarboxylate carrier exhibit intermittent hyperketotic metabolic acidosis. Patients with biallelic variants have more profound acidosis than patients with a variant on a single allele. The primary diagnostic method is sequencing of the *SLC16A1* gene encoding the MCT1 protein [77].

22.7 Summary

Fatty acid oxidation disorders and ketone metabolism disorders often present with intermittent symptoms triggered by prolonged fasting. Avoidance of fasting is a key component of treatment, and its practical application requires continued education of caregivers to maintain vigilance. Symptoms of cardiac and skeletal muscle pose significant problems particularly in patients with long chain fatty acid oxidation disorders, for which current treatment is only partially effective.

Acknowledgments We are grateful to Professor Johan Van Hove from the University of Colorado who authored the initial version of this chapter on fatty acid oxidation disorders and for his mentorship on fatty acid oxidation disorders and the importance of anabolism in general.

References

1. Longo N, Amat di San Filippo C, Pasquali M. Disorders of carnitine transport and the carnitine cycle. Am J Med Genet C Semin Med Genet. 2006;142C(2):77–85.
2. Baruteau J, Sachs P, Broue P, Brivet M, Abdoul H, Vianey-Saban C, et al. Clinical and biological features at diagnosis in mitochondrial fatty acid beta-oxidation defects: a French pediatric study of 187 patients. J Inherit Metab Dis. 2013;36(5):795–803.
3. Boles RG, Buck EA, Blitzer MG, Platt MS, Cowan TM, Martin SK, et al. Retrospective biochemical screening of fatty acid oxidation disorders in postmortem livers of 418 cases of sudden death in the first year of life. J Pediatr. 1998;132(6):924–33.
4. Chace DH, DiPerna JC, Mitchell BL, Sgroi B, Hofman LF, Naylor EW. Electrospray tandem mass spectrometry for analysis of acylcarnitines in dried postmortem blood specimens collected at autopsy from infants with unexplained cause of death. Clin Chem. 2001;47(7):1166–82.
5. Nennstiel-Ratzel U, Arenz S, Maier EM, Knerr I, Baumkotter J, Roschinger W, et al. Reduced incidence of severe metabolic crisis or death in children with medium chain acyl-CoA dehydrogenase deficiency homozygous for c.985A>G identified by neonatal screening. Mol Genet Metab. 2005;85(2):157–9.
6. Ficicioglu C, Coughlin CR 2nd, Bennett MJ, Yudkoff M. Very long-chain acyl-CoA dehydrogenase deficiency in a patient with normal newborn screening by tandem mass spectrometry. J Pediatr. 2010;156(3):492–4.
7. Emken EA, Adlof RO, Rohwedder WK, Gulley RM. Influence of linoleic acid on desaturation and uptake of deuterium-labeled palmitic and stearic acids in humans. Biochim Biophys Acta. 1993;1170(2):173–81.
8. Rinaldo P, Matern D, Bennett MJ. Fatty acid oxidation disorders. Annu Rev Physiol. 2002;64:477–502.
9. Turnbull DM, Bartlett K, Stevens DL, Alberti KG, Gibson GJ, Johnson MA, et al. Short-chain acyl-CoA dehydrogenase deficiency associated with a lipid-storage myopathy and secondary carnitine deficiency. N Engl J Med. 1984;311(19):1232–6.

10. Stanley CA, Hale DE, Coates PM, Hall CL, Corkey BE, Yang W, et al. Medium-chain acyl-CoA dehydrogenase deficiency in children with non-ketotic hypoglycemia and low carnitine levels. Pediatr Res. 1983;17(11):877–84.
11. Eder M, Krautle F, Dong Y, Vock P, Kieweg V, Kim JJ, et al. Characterization of human and pig kidney long-chain-acyl-CoA dehydrogenases and their role in beta-oxidation. Eur J Biochem. 1997;245(3):600–7.
12. Aoyama T, Ueno I, Kamijo T, Hashimoto T. Rat very-long-chain acyl-CoA dehydrogenase, a novel mitochondrial acyl-CoA dehydrogenase gene product, is a rate-limiting enzyme in long-chain fatty acid beta-oxidation system. cDNA and deduced amino acid sequence and distinct specificities of the cDNA-expressed protein. J Biol Chem. 1994;269(29):19088–94.
13. Derks TG, Reijngoud DJ, Waterham HR, Gerver WJ, van den Berg MP, Sauer PJ, et al. The natural history of medium-chain acyl CoA dehydrogenase deficiency in the Netherlands: clinical presentation and outcome. J Pediatr. 2006;148(5):665–70.
14. Mayell SJ, Edwards L, Reynolds FE, Chakrapani AB. Late presentation of medium-chain acyl-CoA dehydrogenase deficiency. J Inherit Metab Dis. 2007;30(1):104.
15. Wilhelm GW. Sudden death in a young woman from medium chain acyl-coenzyme A dehydrogenase (MCAD) deficiency. J Emerg Med. 2006;30(3):291–4.
16. Raymond K, Bale AE, Barnes CA, Rinaldo P. Medium-chain acyl-CoA dehydrogenase deficiency: sudden and unexpected death of a 45 year old woman. Genet Med. 1999;1(6):293–4.
17. Mayatepek E, Koch HG, Hoffmann GF. Hyperuricaemia and medium-chain acyl-CoA dehydrogenase deficiency. J Inherit Metab Dis. 1997;20(6):842–3.
18. Davidson-Mundt A, Luder AS, Greene CL. Hyperuricemia in medium-chain acyl-coenzyme A dehydrogenase deficiency. J Pediatr. 1992;120(3):444–6.
19. Ibdah JA, Dasouki MJ, Strauss AW. Long-chain 3-hydroxyacyl-CoA dehydrogenase deficiency: variable expressivity of maternal illness during pregnancy and unusual presentation with infantile cholestasis and hypocalcaemia. J Inherit Metab Dis. 1999;22(7):811–4.
20. Strauss AW, Bennett MJ, Rinaldo P, Sims HF, O'Brien LK, Zhao Y, et al. Inherited long-chain 3-hydroxyacyl-CoA dehydrogenase deficiency and a fetal-maternal interaction cause maternal liver disease and other pregnancy complications. Semin Perinatol. 1999;23(2):100–12.
21. Mathur A, Sims HF, Gopalakrishnan D, Gibson B, Rinaldo P, Vockley J, et al. Molecular heterogeneity in very-long-chain acyl-CoA dehydrogenase deficiency causing pediatric cardiomyopathy and sudden death. Circulation. 1999;99(10):1337–43.
22. Cox GF, Souri M, Aoyama T, Rockenmacher S, Varvogli L, Rohr F, et al. Reversal of severe hypertrophic cardiomyopathy and excellent neuropsychologic outcome in very-long-chain acyl-coenzyme A dehydrogenase deficiency. J Pediatr. 1998;133(2):247–53.
23. Brown-Harrison MC, Nada MA, Sprecher H, Vianey-Saban C, Farquhar J Jr, Gilladoga AC, et al. Very long chain acyl-CoA dehydrogenase deficiency: successful treatment of acute cardiomyopathy. Biochem Mol Med. 1996;58(1):59–65.
24. Cavicchi C, Donati M, Parini R, Rigoldi M, Bernardi M, Orfei F, et al. Sudden unexpected fatal encephalopathy in adults with OTC gene mutations-clues for early diagnosis and timely treatment. Orphanet J Rare Dis. 2014;9:105.
25. Choong K, Clarke JT, Cutz E, Pollit RJ, Olpin SE. Lethal cardiac tachyarrhythmia in a patient with neonatal carnitine-acylcarnitine translocase deficiency. Pediatr Dev Pathol. 2001;4(6):573–9.
26. Bonnet D, Martin D, Pascale De L, Villain E, Jouvet P, Rabier D, et al. Arrhythmias and conduction defects as presenting symptoms of fatty acid oxidation disorders in children. Circulation. 1999;100(22):2248–53.
27. El-Gharbawy A, Vockley J. Inborn errors of metabolism with myopathy: defects of fatty acid oxidation and the carnitine shuttle system. Pediatr Clin N Am. 2018;65(2):317–35.
28. Fletcher JM, Pitt JJ. Fasting medium chain acyl-coenzyme a dehydrogenase--deficient children can make ketones. Metabolism. 2001;50(2):161–5.
29. Millington DS, Kodo N, Norwood DL, Roe CR. Tandem mass spectrometry: a new method for acylcarnitine profiling with potential for neonatal screening for inborn errors of metabolism. J Inherit Metab Dis. 1990;13(3):321–4.
30. Van Hove JL, Zhang W, Kahler SG, Roe CR, Chen YT, Terada N, et al. Medium-chain acyl-CoA dehydrogenase (MCAD) deficiency: diagnosis by acylcarnitine analysis in blood. Am J Hum Genet. 1993;52(5):958–66.
31. Bonnefont JP, Specola NB, Vassault A, Lombes A, Ogier H, de Klerk JB, et al. The fasting test in paediatrics: application to the diagnosis of pathological hypo- and hyperketotic states. Eur J Pediatr. 1990;150(2):80–5.
32. Costa CC, de Almeida IT, Jakobs C, Poll-The BT, Duran M. Dynamic changes of plasma acylcarnitine levels induced by fasting and sunflower oil challenge test in children. Pediatr Res. 1999;46(4):440–4.
33. Fingerhut R, Roschinger W, Muntau AC, Dame T, Kreischer J, Arnecke R, et al. Hepatic carnitine palmitoyltransferase I deficiency: acylcarnitine profiles in blood spots are highly specific. Clin Chem. 2001;47(10):1763–8.
34. Hesse J, Braun C, Behringer S, Matysiak U, Spiekerkoetter U, Tucci S. The diagnostic challenge in very-long chain acyl-CoA dehydrogenase deficiency (VLCADD). J Inherit Metab Dis. 2018;41(6):1169–78.
35. Hoffmann L, Haussmann U, Mueller M, Spiekerkoetter U. VLCAD enzyme activity determinations in newborns identified by screening: a valuable tool for risk assessment. J Inherit Metab Dis. 2012;35(2):269–77.

36. Wanders RJ, Ruiter JP, IJLst L, Waterham HR, Houten SM. The enzymology of mitochondrial fatty acid beta-oxidation and its application to follow-up analysis of positive neonatal screening results. J Inherit Metab Dis. 2010;33(5):479–94.
37. Andresen BS, Olpin S, Poorthuis BJ, Scholte HR, Vianey-Saban C, Wanders R, et al. Clear correlation of genotype with disease phenotype in very-long-chain acyl-CoA dehydrogenase deficiency. Am J Hum Genet. 1999;64(2):479–94.
38. Coughlin CR 2nd, Ficicioglu C. Genotype-phenotype correlations: sudden death in an infant with very-long-chain acyl-CoA dehydrogenase deficiency. J Inherit Metab Dis. 2010;33 Suppl 3:S129–31.
39. Sander S, Janzen N, Janetzky B, Scholl S, Steuerwald U, Schafer J, et al. Neonatal screening for medium chain acyl-CoA deficiency: high incidence in Lower Saxony (northern Germany). Eur J Pediatr. 2001;160(5):318–9.
40. Chace DH, Kalas TA, Naylor EW. The application of tandem mass spectrometry to neonatal screening for inherited disorders of intermediary metabolism. Annu Rev Genomics Hum Genet. 2002;3:17–45.
41. Rinaldo P, Raymond K, al-Odaib A, Bennett MJ. Clinical and biochemical features of fatty acid oxidation disorders. Curr Opin Pediatr. 1998;10(6):615–21.
42. Heales SJ, Thompson GN, Massoud AF, Rahman S, Halliday D, Leonard JV. Production and disposal of medium-chain fatty acids in children with medium-chain acyl-CoA dehydrogenase deficiency. J Inherit Metab Dis. 1994;17(1):74–80.
43. Anderson DR, Viau K, Botto LD, Pasquali M, Longo N. Clinical and biochemical outcomes of patients with medium-chain acyl-CoA dehydrogenase deficiency. Mol Genet Metab. 2020;129(1):13–9.
44. Ruitenbeek W, Poels PJ, Turnbull DM, Garavaglia B, Chalmers RA, Taylor RW, et al. Rhabdomyolysis and acute encephalopathy in late onset medium chain acyl-CoA dehydrogenase deficiency. J Neurol Neurosurg Psychiatry. 1995;58(2):209–14.
45. Arens R, Gozal D, Jain K, Muscati S, Heuser ET, Williams JC, et al. Prevalence of medium-chain acyl-coenzyme A dehydrogenase deficiency in the sudden infant death syndrome. J Pediatr. 1993;122(5 Pt 1):715–8.
46. Gregersen N, Winter V, Curtis D, Deufel T, Mack M, Hendrickx J, et al. Medium-chain acyl-CoA dehydrogenase (MCAD) deficiency: the prevalent mutation G985 (K304E) is subject to a strong founder effect from northwestern Europe. Hum Hered. 1993;43(6):342–50.
47. Andresen BS, Dobrowolski SF, O'Reilly L, Muenzer J, McCandless SE, Frazier DM, et al. Medium-chain acyl-CoA dehydrogenase (MCAD) mutations identified by MS/MS-based prospective screening of newborns differ from those observed in patients with clinical symptoms: identification and characterization of a new, prevalent mutation that results in mild MCAD deficiency. Am J Hum Genet. 2001;68(6):1408–18.
48. Derks TG, van Spronsen FJ, Rake JP, van der Hilst CS, Span MM, Smit GP. Safe and unsafe duration of fasting for children with MCAD deficiency. Eur J Pediatr. 2007;166(1):5–11.
49. Yusupov R, Finegold DN, Naylor EW, Sahai I, Waisbren S, Levy HL. Sudden death in medium chain acyl-coenzyme a dehydrogenase deficiency (MCADD) despite newborn screening. Mol Genet Metab. 2010;101(1):33–9.
50. IJlst L, Ruiter JP, Hoovers JM, Jakobs ME, Wanders RJ. Common missense mutation G1528C in long-chain 3-hydroxyacyl-CoA dehydrogenase deficiency. Characterization and expression of the mutant protein, mutation analysis on genomic DNA and chromosomal localization of the mitochondrial trifunctional protein alpha subunit gene. J Clin Invest. 1996;98(4):1028–33.
51. Brackett JC, Sims HF, Rinaldo P, Shapiro S, Powell CK, Bennett MJ, et al. Two alpha subunit donor splice site mutations cause human trifunctional protein deficiency. J Clin Invest. 1995;95(5):2076–82.
52. Ushikubo S, Aoyama T, Kamijo T, Wanders RJ, Rinaldo P, Vockley J, et al. Molecular characterization of mitochondrial trifunctional protein deficiency: formation of the enzyme complex is important for stabilization of both alpha- and beta-subunits. Am J Hum Genet. 1996;58(5):979–88.
53. Fletcher AL, Pennesi ME, Harding CO, Weleber RG, Gillingham MB. Observations regarding retinopathy in mitochondrial trifunctional protein deficiencies. Mol Genet Metab. 2012;106(1):18–24.
54. den Boer ME, Wanders RJ, Morris AA, IJlst L, Heymans HS, Wijburg FA. Long-chain 3-hydroxyacyl-CoA dehydrogenase deficiency: clinical presentation and follow-up of 50 patients. Pediatrics. 2002;109(1):99–104.
55. Gillingham MB, Weleber RG, Neuringer M, Connor WE, Mills M, van Calcar S, et al. Effect of optimal dietary therapy upon visual function in children with long-chain 3-hydroxyacyl CoA dehydrogenase and trifunctional protein deficiency. Mol Genet Metab. 2005;86(1–2):124–33.
56. Ibdah JA, Tein I, Dionisi-Vici C, Bennett MJ, IJlst L, Gibson B, et al. Mild trifunctional protein deficiency is associated with progressive neuropathy and myopathy and suggests a novel genotype-phenotype correlation. J Clin Invest. 1998;102(6):1193–9.
57. Yang Z, Yamada J, Zhao Y, Strauss AW, Ibdah JA. Prospective screening for pediatric mitochondrial trifunctional protein defects in pregnancies complicated by liver disease. JAMA. 2002;288(17):2163–6.
58. Van Hove JL, Kahler SG, Feezor MD, Ramakrishna JP, Hart P, Treem WR, et al. Acylcarnitines in plasma and blood spots of patients with long-chain 3-hydroxyacyl-coenzyme A dehydrogenase defiency. J Inherit Metab Dis. 2000;23(6):571–82.
59. Ogilvie I, Pourfarzam M, Jackson S, Stockdale C, Bartlett K, Turnbull DM. Very long-chain acyl coenzyme A dehydrogenase deficiency presenting

with exercise-induced myoglobinuria. Neurology. 1994;44(3 Pt 1):467–73.
60. Schymik I, Liebig M, Mueller M, Wendel U, Mayatepek E, Strauss AW, et al. Pitfalls of neonatal screening for very-long-chain acyl-CoA dehydrogenase deficiency using tandem mass spectrometry. J Pediatr. 2006;149(1):128–30.
61. Boneh A, Andresen BS, Gregersen N, Ibrahim M, Tzanakos N, Peters H, et al. VLCAD deficiency: pitfalls in newborn screening and confirmation of diagnosis by mutation analysis. Mol Genet Metab. 2006;88(2):166–70.
62. Sahai I, Bailey JC, Eaton RB, Zytkovicz T, Harris DJ. A near-miss: very long chain acyl-CoA dehydrogenase deficiency with normal primary markers in the initial well-timed newborn screening specimen. J Pediatr. 2011;158(1):172; author reply -3.
63. Spiekerkoetter U, Mueller M, Sturm M, Hofmann M, Schneider DT. Lethal undiagnosed very long-chain acyl-CoA dehydrogenase deficiency with mild C14-Acylcarnitine abnormalities on Newborn screening. JIMD Rep. 2012;6:113–5.
64. Arnold GL, Van Hove J, Freedenberg D, Strauss A, Longo N, Burton B, et al. A Delphi clinical practice protocol for the management of very long chain acyl-CoA dehydrogenase deficiency. Mol Genet Metab. 2009;96(3):85–90.
65. Spiekerkoetter U, Sun B, Zytkovicz T, Wanders R, Strauss AW, Wendel U. MS/MS-based newborn and family screening detects asymptomatic patients with very-long-chain acyl-CoA dehydrogenase deficiency. J Pediatr. 2003;143(3):335–42.
66. Spiekerkoetter U, Lindner M, Santer R, Grotzke M, Baumgartner MR, Boehles H, et al. Treatment recommendations in long-chain fatty acid oxidation defects: consensus from a workshop. J Inherit Metab Dis. 2009;32(4):498–505.
67. Gillingham MB, Heitner SB, Martin J, Rose S, Goldstein A, El-Gharbawy AH, et al. Triheptanoin versus trioctanoin for long-chain fatty acid oxidation disorders: a double blinded, randomized controlled trial. J Inherit Metab Dis. 2017;40(6):831–43.
68. Robinson AM, Williamson DH. Physiological roles of ketone bodies as substrates and signals in mammalian tissues. Physiol Rev. 1980;60(1):143–87.
69. Thompson GN, Hsu BY, Pitt JJ, Treacy E, Stanley CA. Fasting hypoketotic coma in a child with deficiency of mitochondrial 3-hydroxy-3-methylglutaryl-CoA synthase. N Engl J Med. 1997;337(17):1203–7.
70. Aledo R, Zschocke J, Pie J, Mir C, Fiesel S, Mayatepek E, et al. Genetic basis of mitochondrial HMG-CoA synthase deficiency. Hum Genet. 2001;109(1):19–23.
71. Korman SH. Inborn errors of isoleucine degradation: a review. Mol Genet Metab. 2006;89(4):289–99.
72. Sovik O. Mitochondrial 2-methylacetoacetyl-CoA thiolase deficiency: an inborn error of isoleucine and ketone body metabolism. J Inherit Metab Dis. 1993;16(1):46–54.
73. Abdelkreem E, Harijan RK, Yamaguchi S, Wierenga RK, Fukao T. Mutation update on ACAT1 variants associated with mitochondrial acetoacetyl-CoA thiolase (T2) deficiency. Hum Mutat. 2019;40(10):1641–63.
74. Fukao T, Mitchell G, Sass JO, Hori T, Orii K, Aoyama Y. Ketone body metabolism and its defects. J Inherit Metab Dis. 2014;37(4):541–51.
75. Fukao T, Sass JO, Kursula P, Thimm E, Wendel U, Ficicioglu C, et al. Clinical and molecular characterization of five patients with succinyl-CoA:3-ketoacid CoA transferase (SCOT) deficiency. Biochim Biophys Acta. 2011;1812(5):619–24.
76. Fukao T, Mitchell GA, Song XQ, Nakamura H, Kassovska-Bratinova S, Orii KE, et al. Succinyl-CoA:3-ketoacid CoA transferase (SCOT): cloning of the human SCOT gene, tertiary structural modeling of the human SCOT monomer, and characterization of three pathogenic mutations. Genomics. 2000;68(2):144–51.
77. van Hasselt PM, Ferdinandusse S, Monroe GR, Ruiter JP, Turkenburg M, Geerlings MJ, et al. Monocarboxylate transporter 1 deficiency and ketone utilization. N Engl J Med. 2014;371(20):1900–7.

Nutrition Management of Fatty Acid Oxidation Disorders

23

Fran Rohr

Contents

F. Rohr (✉)
Met Ed Co, Boulder, CO, USA
e-mail: fran.rohr@met-ed.net

L. E. Bernstein et al. (eds.), *Nutrition Management of Inherited Metabolic Diseases*,
https://doi.org/10.1007/978-3-030-94510-7_23

Core Messages

Long-Chain Fatty Acid Oxidation Disorders

Management of acute illness and the avoidance of prolonged fasting are important treatment strategies to minimize the reliance on fat as an energy source.

- Nutrition management depends on the degree of disease severity; in the most severe forms, long-chain fat is limited to 10% of total energy intake.
- Diets restricted in long-chain fat require monitoring of essential fatty acids and fat-soluble vitamins.

Medium-Chain Acyl-CoA Dehydrogenase Deficiency (MCAD)

- Management of acute illness and the avoidance of prolonged fasting are important treatment strategies to minimize the reliance on fat as an energy source.
- MCT should be avoided in MCAD, however, the restriction of other fats is not indicated, and a normal, healthy diet is recommended.

23.1 Background

The pathophysiology of fatty acid oxidation disorders is described in detail in Chap. 22. In summary, when fat is needed as an energy source, for example during prolonged fasting, lipolysis occurs. Plasma-free fatty acids are released from triglycerides, esterified, conjugated with carnitine and transported into the mitochondria where beta-oxidation occurs. Here, a series of carbon chain-length-specific enzymes break down the fatty acids into acetyl-CoA for entry in to the Krebs cycle or for ketone formation [1]. A deficiency in any of the LC-FOAD enzymes can cause a metabolic disorder. LC-FAOD disorders include carnitine palmitoyl transferase deficiency type 1 (CPT-1), carnitine palmitoyl transferase deficiency type 2 (CPT-2), carnitine-acylcarnitine translocase (CACT), very long-chain acyl-CoA dehydrogenase deficiency (VLCAD), long-chain hydroxy acyl-CoA dehydrogenase deficiency (LCHAD) and trifunctional protein disorder (TFP). CPT-1, CACT, and CPT-2 are disorders in transporting fatty acids into the mitochondria, whereas VLCAD, LCHAD, and TFP are disorders in the mitochondrial beta oxidation process [2] (Table 23.1). All can cause symptoms associated with energy deprivation to the heart, liver, and/or muscle. Approaches to managing LC-FAOD are similar, involving avoidance of prolonged fasting, ensuring adequate energy intake and supplementation with medium-chain triglycerides or triheptanoin.

Medium-chain acyl-CoA dehydrogenase deficiency (MCAD), described in Chap. 22, is also a mitochondrial enzyme involved in the

Table 23.1 Fatty acid oxidation disorders identified by plasma acylcarnitine analysis [5]

Disorders
Disorders of carnitine metabolism
Carnitine uptake defect
Carnitine-acylcarnitine translocase deficiency (CACT)
Carnitine palmitoyl transferase I & II deficiency (CPT I & II)
Long chain fatty acid (12–20 carbons) oxidation disorders
Very long chain acyl-CoA dehydrogenase deficiency (VLCAD)
Long chain 3-hydroxyacyl-CoA dehydrogenase deficiency (LCHAD)
Trifunctional protein deficiency (TFP)
Medium-chain fatty acid (6–12 carbons) oxidation disorders
Medium-chain acyl-CoA dehydrogenase deficiency (MCAD)
Medium-chain 3-ketoacyl-CoA thiolase deficiency (MCKAT)
2,4 dienoyl-CoA reductase deficiency
Short-chain fatty acid (<6 carbons) oxidation disorders
Short-chain acyl-CoA dehydrogenase deficiency (SCAD)
Short-chain L-3-hydroxyacyl-CoA dehydrogenase deficiency (SCHAD)
Other
Multiple acyl-CoA dehydrogenase deficiency (MADD) or Glutaric aciduria II (GAII)

Adapted from Rinaldo et al. [5]

metabolism of fatty acids with 6–8 carbons [3], and its management will be addressed in this chapter. Short-chain acyl-CoA dehydrogenase deficiency (SCAD) is not treated with a special diet and presents as a benign condition (Table 23.1) [4].

23.2 Management of Long-Chain Fatty Acid Oxidation Disorders (LC-FAOD)

23.2.1 Chronic Nutrition Management

In LC-FAOD, one or more enzymes in the mitochondrial beta-oxidation of long-chain fatty acids is deficient and fat is not oxidized normally to acetyl co-A for entry into the Krebs cycle nor are ketones formed. The main principle of nutrition management is to avoid reliance upon long-chain fat as an energy substrate. This is accomplished by avoiding physiological stress and modifying the diet (Box 23.1).

Specific nutrition recommendations depend on the patient's state of health and the severity of the disease [6]. Historically, infants with LC-FAOD presented clinically with cardiomyopathy or hypoketotic hypoglycemia and most required strict diet modification. Presently in many countries, newborn screening identifies infants who may have LC-FAOD, many of whom are asymptomatic. Clinical judgment is needed to determine how aggressively to treat asymptomatic infants while evaluating the extent of their disease, and, moreover, how to properly classify the severity of disease. Current molecular and enzyme assessments are imperfect in predicting who is likely to become symptomatic [7]. While practices variation occurs [8–10] there is a trend toward less stringent management of asymptomatic patients [6]. The recommendations for LC-FAOD are based primarily on evidence for treating very long-chain acyl-CoA dehydrogenase deficiency but can be applied to the other long-chain disorders, as well.

Box 23.1: Principles of Management of Long-Chain Fatty Acid Oxidation Defects

Minimize long-chain fat as energy substrate by:

- Avoiding physiological stress:
  - Illness
  - Prolonged fasting
  - Exercise without sufficient energy intake
- Modifying the diet to:
  - Limit long-chain fat intake
  - Provide alternative energy sources such as:
    - Medium-chain triglycerides
    - Triheptanoin

23.2.2 Treating Illness

Perhaps the most important aspect of treating patients with LC-FAOD or MCAD is to counsel families about the urgency of seeking medical attention if the patient becomes ill. Especially if a patient has had poor intake or vomiting, a quick energy source (i.e., carbohydrate) is needed. Carbohydrate can be provided as regular foods and beverages, medical foods containing glucose polymers (Appendix C), or IV glucose, depending on the patient's ability to tolerate feedings. Families are provided with an emergency protocol that describes the disease, emergency management, and laboratory testing to be done when the patient is ill [11].

23.2.3 Fasting

Fat is normally oxidized for energy when glucose and glycogen stores are depleted, generally after 12 hours of fasting (Chap. 5). Although an infant with a LC-FAOD can tolerate a 12-hour fast without difficulty, clinics vary widely in their recommendations for the amount of time allowed between feedings [12] and most recommend shorter feeding intervals than 12 hours to provide a margin of safety. The infant's ability to tolerate a fast will depend on the absence or presence of illness, when the last meal was consumed, and body weight [12]. Table 23.2 shows recommendations for maximum fasting intervals in LC-FAOD [6]. Since newborns generally feed every 2–4 hours, the recommended safe intervals between feedings do not generally interfere with an infant's normal feeding schedule. In infants with severe disease, it may be necessary to wake the child at night to feed; however, in milder forms of LC-FAOD, this practice may cause overfeeding and unnecessary stress for the family.

The goal is to provide the individual with the recommended energy intake during the day and to follow fasting guidelines at night. If energy needs have not been met during the day, a nighttime snack containing complex carbohydrate is recommended [6]. Unlike in glycogen storage disease, the use of uncooked cornstarch to extend feeding intervals is not necessary. It is important to note that hypoglycemia is rarely the first symptom to present when a patient with LC-FAOD is ill [6]; therefore, monitoring blood glucose with glucometers is not recommended as it may lead to a false sense of security for families (Table 23.2).

23.2.4 Diet Modifications

Infants with LC-FAOD who are asymptomatic can continue to receive standard infant formula or breast milk, as long as the mother's breast milk supply is adequate (if the infant is breast fed), the infant is feeding according to the guidelines provided (Table 23.3), and the infant remains clinically normal [6]. Asymptomatic infants should be monitored closely and provided an emergency treatment protocol to be used in the case of illness. In moderate or severe forms of LC-FAOD, the goal of the diet is to reduce long-chain fat and provide an alternative energy source.

The total amount of fat in the diet is not restricted, only the source of the fat. Recommended long-chain fat intakes range from 10% of energy in patients with severe forms of LC-FAOD to 45% of energy for infants with mild forms of the disease (Table 23.3) [6]. All other nutrients except fat should be provided in amounts to meet the DRI (Appendix D). A high protein intake (25% of energy) is associated with preservation of lean body mass and lower lipid profiles when compared to lower protein intakes (12% of energy) [14] (Table 23.3) [13]

Medium-chain triglycerides (MCT) are frequently used as an alternative energy source. MCT use in LCFOAD has been shown to reverse cardiomyopathy [15]. MCT contain even chain fatty acids and are 6–12 carbons in length. They are readily absorbed via the portal vein, do not require L-carnitine for transport in the mitochondria, and do not depend on long-chain acyl-CoA

Table 23.2 Maximum duration between feeds in individuals with very long chain Acyl-CoA dehydrogenase deficiency when well

Age	Hours
0– 4 months	3–4
4–6 months	4–6
6–9 months	6–8
9–12 months	8–10
>12 months	10–12

Adapted from GMDI/SERN Nutrition Guidelines (www.southeastgenetics/ngp) [13]

Table 23.3 Recommended intakes of fat (total, long chain, and medium chain) for individuals with very long-chain acyl-CoA dehydrogenase deficiency

Age	Disease severity	Total fat (% of total energy)	Long-chain fat (% of total energy)	Medium-chain fat (% of total energy)
0–6 mos	Severe	40–55	10–15	30–45
	Moderate		15–30	10–30
	Mild		30–55	0–20
7–12 mos	Severe	35–45	10–15	25–30
	Moderate		15–30	10–25
	Mild		30–40	0–10
1–3 years	Severe	30–40	10–15	10–30
	Moderate		20–30	10–20
	Mild		20–40	0–10
4–18 years	Severe	25–35	10	15–25
	Moderate		15–25	10–20
	Mild		20–35	0–10
>19 years	Severe	20–35	10	10–25
	Moderate		15–20	10–20
	Mild		20–35	0–10

Adapted from GMDI/SERN Nutrition Guidelines (www.southeastgenetics/ngp) [13]

dehydrogenases for oxidation [16]. MCT supplies 10–45% of energy in the diet for LC-FAOD, depending on the severity of the disease [6, 17]. Higher amounts of MCT are impractical because high concentrations of MCT can cause gastrointestinal cramping, vomiting, and diarrhea [18]. Some prescribe MCT on a weight basis, using 2–3 g/kg in infancy and 1–1.25 g/kg after the first year [19].

Triheptanoin (C7) is an odd-chain medium fat that contains 7 carbons in each fatty acid side chain. Like MCT, it does not require carnitine to be transported into the mitochondria and uses short and medium-chain acyl-CoA dehydrogenases for beta-oxidation, resulting in 2 acetyl-CoA molecules and one propionyl-CoA molecule for each 7-carbon fatty acid. Acetyl Co A enters the Krebs cycle for energy production or is diverted to the liver to produce ketones. Propionyl CoA is metabolized to succinyl-CoA where it enters the Krebs cycle. Krebs intermediates are thought to be deficient in patients with LC-FAOD, and the resupplying of these intermediates, known as anaplerois, can help provide energy for gluconeogenesis [20].

Dojolvi® (Ultragenyx, Novato, CA) is a liquid form of triheptanoin approved in the United States as a source of calories for the treatment of pediatric and adult patients with molecularly confirmed LCFOAD [21]. Clinical studies comparing subjects with LC-FAOD who received triheptanoin vs. even-chain MCT showed improvement in the cardiac phenotype (e.g., improved ejection fraction, reduction in left ventricular wall mass, and lower resting heart rate) [22, 23], as well as a lower frequency and duration of major clinical events associated with LC-FAOD [24]. Drug side effects are similar to those encountered with MCT, primarily mild to moderate gastrointestinal disturbances [25].

The prescribing information recommends providing up to 35% of the patients' total recommended energy intake from Dojolvi®. Dojolvi® is used instead of even-chain MCT, not in addition to it. If patients who are receiving MCT as part of their treatment regimen, it should be discontinued, and Dojolvi® started at the current percent of energy that the MCT provided, then titrated up to 35% of energy intake. For patients not previously prescribed even-chain MCT, initially provide 10% of total energy intake as Dojolvi® and titrate up to 35% of energy, as tolerated. Dojolvi® is divided into at least four dose per day and administer at mealtimes or with snacks [21].

23.2.5 Diet After Infancy

The diet follows the same principles as for infants with the same balance between the amounts of long-chain fat and medium-chain fat depending on disease severity. The source of long-chain fat in the diet shifts from standard infant formula or breast milk to food sources. Patients who require severe long-chain fat restriction (10–15% of total energy) are prescribed a daily limit in the number grams of long-chain fat allowed in the diet and are counseled about how to count grams of fat in food. If the patient is receiving MCT as part of their treatment regimen, they will either continue on their usual MCT-containing medical formulas or switch to another source of MCT supplementation (Table 23.4).

Table 23.4 MCT supplements

Product	% of kcal as MCT	MCT content	Kcal[d]
MCT Procal (Vitaflo[a])	92	10 g per 16 g powder (16 g = 1 packet)	105
MCT oil (Nestle[b])	100	14 g per tablespoon	116
Liquigen (Nutricia[c])	96	45 g per bottle (250 mL)	450
Betaquik (Vitaflo[a])	89	45 g per bottle (225 mL)	420

[a]Vitaflo USA, Alexandria VA (vitaflousa.com)
[b]Nestle Nutrition, Florham Park, NJ (nestle-nutrition.com)
[c]Nutricia North America, Rockville MD (medicalfood.com)
[d]Per amount listed in column "MCT Content"

23.2.6 Supplements

Patients with LCHAD should receive supplemental docosohexaenoic acid (DHA) (60 mg/d for patients weighing <20 kg and 100 mg/d if ≥20 kg) because DHA stabilizes the retinopathy that is seen in this disorder [17]. For other LC-FAOD, DHA supplementation in infancy is not necessary if the patient is receiving a FAOD medical food, because DHA and arachadonic acid (ARA) are added to these formulas [6]. For infants on Dojolvi, and for older children who are no longer taking an FAOD formula, DHA or essential fatty acid (EFA) supplementation may be necessary depending on the dietitian's assessments of EFA intake and laboratory monitoring. Supplementing specific oils, such as walnut or flax oil, as a source of EFA may be necessary [26]. Fat-soluble vitamin intake is likely to be low for patients with severe long-chain fat restrictions, and supplementation is often necessary.

Box 23.2: Nutrition Monitoring of a Patient with a LC-FAOD

- Routine assessments including anthropometrics, dietary intake, physical findings
- Laboratory Monitoring
  - Diagnosis-specific
    - Creatine kinase
    - Plasma carnitine profile (total, esterified, free)
    - Plasma acylcarnitine profile
    - Liver function tests
    - Blood glucose
- Nutrition laboratory monitoring of patients on fat-restricted diets may include markers of:
  - Essential fatty acid sufficiency: Plasma fatty acids
  - Fat-soluble vitamin status: 25-hydroxy vitamin D, Vitamins A and E.
  - Others as clinically indicated

23.2.7 Diet for Exercise

Providing additional sources of energy for prolonged exercise may help prevent or reduce episodes of rhabdomyolysis in patients with LC-FAOD. Recommendations include providing a source of complex carbohydrate and supplemental MCT (0.3 per kg total body weight) for improved exercise tolerance [27]. Ideally, MCT supplementation should be given 20–45 minutes prior to exercise [6]. During exercise, adequate fluid intake, a source of simple carbohydrate and rest, as needed, are encouraged.

23.3 Monitoring of Patients with LC-FAOD

Nutritional monitoring of FAOD includes standard anthropometric measurements, as well as assessment of nutrition intake and physical signs and symptoms (Box 23.2). Routine laboratory monitoring includes creatine kinase and plasma carnitine profiles, and additional monitoring of individuals on fat-restricted diets is recommended. Patients are at risk for developing deficiencies of essential fatty acids, DHA, and fat-soluble vitamins. Erythrocyte or plasma fatty acid profiles and fat-soluble vitamins should be monitored at least yearly or more often if clinically indicated (Appendix H).

Creatine kinase (CK) is a biomarker that is associated with the clinical condition of patients with VLCAD and other LC-FAOD and should be routinely monitored [6]. Elevated CK is a sign of physiological stress, especially a lack of energy production in skeletal muscle. Very high CK concentrations are associated with rhabdomyolysis which, if not corrected, can lead to renal failure. Troponin and beta-natriuretic protein (BNP) are markers of cardiac muscle stress and are followed in patients with severe LFAOD-associated cardiomyopathy.

Plasma carnitine profiles (total, esterified, and free carnitine) are monitored in LC-FAOD but whether or not L-carnitine should be supplemented is an area of uncertainty. Supplementation is often recommended if plasma-free carnitine is very low (<10 μmol/L) [6], yet some clinicians feel that carnitine has not been shown to be beneficial and supplementation is not recommended [28]. (Appendix F).

Plasma acylcarnitine profiles indicate whether the patient is accumulating acylcarnitines and can be useful to monitor for patients with LC-FAOD. However, acylcarnitines are affected by several factors, such as the timing of feeding and/or exercise, as well as genotype [29]; therefore, they are helpful for assessing trends in metabolic control over time rather than being a specific indicator of the need for a diet change, unlike in patients with PKU where the diet is fine-tuned based on one marker: blood phenylalanine. In patients with LCHAD, reducing long-chain fat in the diet has been shown to reduce plasma acylcarnitine concentrations and is associated with improved retinopathy [17]; however in patients with VLCAD, the clinical benefit of lowering acylcarnitine concentrations has not been shown.

23.4 Nutrition Management of Medium-Chain Acyl Co-A Dehydrogenase Deficiency (MCAD)

23.4.1 Chronic Management

Patients with MCAD should avoid medium-chain triglycerides (MCT) but otherwise do not need dietary intervention when they are well. In infancy, breast-feeding is allowed as long as the supply of breast milk is adequate. However, some infants present with MCAD in the first days after birth when breast-feeding is being established and the infant's energy intake is insufficient. Formula-feeding with standard infant formulas is acceptable as long as the formula does not contain MCT. Recommended fasting duration is 8 hours in children between 6 months and 1 year of age, 10 hours in the second year of life, and 12 hours thereafter [30].

Carnitine supplementation in MCAD is controversial, and there is variation in practice [10]. Unlike in LC-FAOD, in MCAD acylcarnitines do not accumulate so there is less concern about toxicity. In some centers, carnitine is recommended on a daily basis but in others it is provided only during illness (Chap. 22). Many clinicians base their decision regarding supplementation by monitoring plasma-free carnitine and supplementing if the free carnitine is low.

23.5 Acute Nutrition Management in FAOD (MCAD and LC-FAOD)

Patients with FAOD who become ill may be treated at home as long as they continue to eat well and are not vomiting or having diarrhea [6, 31]. Any illness has the potential to be life threatening and must be evaluated with the guidance of a metabolic physician. Whether the patient needs to be seen urgently for medical evaluation and/or IV nutrition support is dependent on whether or not the patient is able to ingest sufficient energy to prevent relying on fat as an energy source. The amount of carbohydrate a sick patient at home should consume is described in Chap. 5 and presented in Appendix C.

Individuals with MCAD and LC-FAOD are at risk of metabolic decompensation throughout life whenever there is a circumstance that could lead to energy deprivation, including illness, prolonged fasting (for religious or other reasons), vigorous or prolonged exercise without the provision of adequate energy, skipping meals, excessive dieting, or vomiting associated with illness, eating disorders, or binge drinking. Iatrogenic causes of prolonged fasting such as sedation, anesthesia, and surgical or dental procedures may require that IV glucose be given as an energy source when the patient is not allowed to eat by mouth. The metabolic physician should be consulted prior to elective surgical procedures and the emergency protocol used in case of an unplanned surgery. Counseling early in life about cautionary measures under these circumstances and continuing to follow patients with FAOD can help prevent problems.

Note that in MCAD, those most at risk for metabolic decompensation include patients who are homozygous for the A985G mutation [32] and patients with illnesses that include vomiting [33]. Special attention needs to be paid to make certain that families understand the risks associated with FAOD and have sufficient social support to respond quickly to emergency situations.

23.6 Summary

Fatty acid oxidation defects cover a wide range of enzyme deficiencies in the metabolism of long, medium, and short-chain fats. Patients with LC-FAOD and MCAD can present with severe illness or be asymptomatic. Chronic nutrition management of LC-FAOD focuses on avoiding reliance on fat as source of energy and providing sufficient energy by other means. In severe LC-FAOD, long-chain fat is restricted to 10% of energy and supplementation with MCT or triheptanoin provides alternate energy sources. Patients with MCAD do not need day-to-day modifications in their diets but are at risk of acute metabolic crisis if fasted due to illness, stress, or other causes. Acute management of both LC-FAOD and MCAD is to provide sufficient energy to prevent catabolism.

23.7 Diet Calculations Examples

Example 23.1

Patient Information	Nutrient intake goals (per day)
Age: 8-year-old male with moderate VLCAD Weight: 25 kg	Energy: 1900 kcal (DRI) Total fat intake: approximately 30% (normal fat intake) LCF: 20% energy; 380 kcal = 42 g of LCF MCT: 10% of energy = 190 kcal = 23 g MCT (keep in mind that MCT provides 8.3 kcal/g) Linoleic acid 10 g (DRI) α-Linolenic acid 0.9 g (DRI)

How much of Liquigen® supplement would you need to meet MCT goals?

- Liquigen® contains 45.4 g MCT per 100 mL
- 23 g MCT divided by 45.4/100 mL = 50.6 mL (51 mL)
- Give 17 mL, three times daily

How much fat from food?

- 42 g
- (10 g per meal and 4 g per snack- assuming 3 meals, 3 snacks per day)

Additional Examples

The GMDI/SERN Nutrition Guideline for Very Long-Chain Acyl-CoA Dehydrogenase Deficiency Toolkit contains 6 cases with diet calculations: (available at https://southeastgenetics.org/ngp/toolkit.php)

- Infant with cardiomyopathy
- Asymptomatic infant
- Toddler transitioning off medical food
- Adolescent participating in sports
- Adult with rhabdomyolysis
- Pregnant woman

References

1. Aoyama T, Uchida Y, Kelley RI, Marble M, Hofman K, Tonsgard JH, et al. A novel disease with deficiency of mitochondrial very-long-chain acyl-CoA dehydrogenase. Biochem Biophys Res Commun. 1993;191(3):1369–72.
2. Knottnerus SJG, Bleeker JC, Wust RCI, Ferdinandusse S, IJlst L, Wijburg FA, et al. Disorders of mitochondrial long-chain fatty acid oxidation and the carnitine shuttle. Rev Endocr Metab Disord. 2018;19(1):93–106.
3. Merritt JL 2nd, Chang IJ. Medium-chain acyl-coenzyme A dehydrogenase deficiency. In: Adam MP, Ardinger HH, Pagon RA, Wallace SE, LJH B, Mirzaa G, et al., editors. GeneReviews((R)). Seattle: University of Washington, Seattle; 1993.
4. Gallant NM, Leydiker K, Tang H, Feuchtbaum L, Lorey F, Puckett R, et al. Biochemical, molecular, and clinical characteristics of children with short chain acyl-CoA dehydrogenase deficiency detected by newborn screening in California. Mol Genet Metab. 2012;106(1):55–61.
5. Rinaldo P, Cowan TM, Matern D. Acylcarnitine profile analysis. Genet Med. 2008;10(2):151–6.
6. Van Calcar SC, Sowa M, Rohr F, Beazer J, Setlock T, Weihe TU, et al. Nutrition management guideline for very-long chain acyl-CoA dehydrogenase deficiency (VLCAD): an evidence- and consensus-based approach. Mol Genet Metab. 2020;131(1–2):23–37.
7. Hesse J, Braun C, Behringer S, Matysiak U, Spiekerkoetter U, Tucci S. The diagnostic challenge in very-long chain acyl-CoA dehydrogenase deficiency (VLCADD). J Inherit Metab Dis. 2018;41(6):1169–78.
8. Arnold GL, Van Hove J, Freedenberg D, Strauss A, Longo N, Burton B, et al. A Delphi clinical practice protocol for the management of very long chain acyl-CoA dehydrogenase deficiency. Mol Genet Metab. 2009;96(3):85–90.
9. Spiekerkoetter U, Lindner M, Santer R, Grotzke M, Baumgartner MR, Boehles H, et al. Treatment recommendations in long-chain fatty acid oxidation defects: consensus from a workshop. J Inherit Metab Dis. 2009;32(4):498–505.
10. Potter BK, Little J, Chakraborty P, Kronick JB, Evans J, Frei J, et al. Variability in the clinical management of fatty acid oxidation disorders: results of a survey of Canadian metabolic physicians. J Inherit Metab Dis. 2012;35(1):115–23.
11. New England Consortium. Acute illness protocols for very long chain acyl-CoA dehydrogenase deficiency. 2020. Available from: https://www.newenglandconsortium.org/vlcadd.
12. Walter JH. Tolerance to fast: rational and practical evaluation in children with hypoketonaemia. J Inherit Metab Dis. 2009;32(2):214–7.
13. GMDI/SERN nutrition management guidelines for VLCAD. 2019. Available from: www.southeastgenetics/ngp.
14. Gillingham MB, Elizondo G, Behrend A, Matern D, Schoeller DA, Harding CO, et al. Higher dietary protein intake preserves lean body mass, lowers liver lipid deposition, and maintains metabolic control in participants with long-chain fatty acid oxidation disorders. J Inherit Metab Dis. 2019;42(5):857–69.
15. Cox GF, Souri M, Aoyama T, Rockenmacher S, Varvogli L, Rohr F, et al. Reversal of severe hypertrophic cardiomyopathy and excellent neuropsychologic outcome in very-long-chain acyl-coenzyme A dehydrogenase deficiency. J Pediatr. 1998;133(2):247–53.
16. Odle J. New insights into the utilization of medium-chain triglycerides by the neonate: observations from a piglet model. J Nutr. 1997;127(6):1061–7.
17. Gillingham MB, Connor WE, Matern D, Rinaldo P, Burlingame T, Meeuws K, et al. Optimal dietary therapy of long-chain 3-hydroxyacyl-CoA dehydrogenase deficiency. Mol Genet Metab. 2003;79(2):114–23.
18. Liu YM. Medium-chain triglyceride (MCT) ketogenic therapy. Epilepsia. 2008;49:33–6.
19. Saudubray JM, Martin D, de Lonlay P, Touati G, Poggi-Travert F, Bonnet D, et al. Recognition and management of fatty acid oxidation defects: a series of 107 patients. J Inherit Metab Dis. 1999;22(4):488–502.
20. Roe CR, Brunengraber H. Anaplerotic treatment of long-chain fat oxidation disorders with triheptanoin: review of 15 years experience. Mol Genet Metab. 2015;116(4):260–8.
21. Food and Drug Administration. Dojolvi prescribing information. Available from: https://www.accessdata.fda.gov/drugsatfda_docs/label/2020/213687s000lbl.pdf.
22. Gillingham MB, Heitner SB, Martin J, Rose S, Goldstein A, El-Gharbawy AH, et al. Triheptanoin versus trioctanoin for long-chain fatty acid oxidation disorders: a double blinded, randomized controlled trial. J Inherit Metab Dis. 2017;40(6):831–43.
23. Vockley J, Charrow J, Ganesh J, Eswara M, Diaz GA, McCracken E, et al. Triheptanoin treatment in patients with pediatric cardiomyopathy associated with long chain-fatty acid oxidation disorders. Mol Genet Metab. 2016;119(3):223–31.
24. Vockley J, Burton B, Berry G, Longo N, Phillips J, Sanchez-Valle A, et al. Effects of triheptanoin (UX007) in patients with long-chain fatty acid oxidation disorders: results from an open-label, long-term extension study. J Inherit Metab Dis. 2021;44(1):253–63.
25. Vockley J, Burton B, Berry GT, Longo N, Phillips J, Sanchez-Valle A, et al. UX007 for the treatment of long chain-fatty acid oxidation disorders: safety and efficacy in children and adults following 24weeks of treatment. Mol Genet Metab. 2017;120(4):370–7.
26. Roe CR, Roe DS, Wallace M, Garritson B. Choice of oils for essential fat supplements can enhance produc-

tion of abnormal metabolites in fat oxidation disorders. Mol Genet Metab. 2007;92(4):346–50.
27. Gillingham MB, Weleber RG, Neuringer M, Connor WE, Mills M, van Calcar S, et al. Effect of optimal dietary therapy upon visual function in children with long-chain 3-hydroxyacyl CoA dehydrogenase and trifunctional protein deficiency. Mol Genet Metab. 2005;86(1–2):124–33.
28. Spiekerkoetter U, Bastin J, Gillingham M, Morris A, Wijburg F, Wilcken B. Current issues regarding treatment of mitochondrial fatty acid oxidation disorders. J Inherit Metab Dis. 2010;33(5):555–61.
29. Gillingham MB, Matern D, Harding CO. Effect of feeding, exercise and genotype on plasma 3-hydroxyacylcarnitines in children with LCHAD deficiency. Top Clin Nutr. 2009;24(4):359–65.
30. Derks TG, van Spronsen FJ, Rake JP, van der Hilst CS, Span MM, Smit GP. Safe and unsafe duration of fasting for children with MCAD deficiency. Eur J Pediatr. 2007;166(1):5–11.
31. Van Hove JL, Myers S, Kerckhove KV, Freehauf C, Bernstein L. Acute nutrition management in the prevention of metabolic illness: a practical approach with glucose polymers. Mol Genet Metab. 2009;97(1):1–3.
32. Maier EM, Gersting SW, Kemter KF, Jank JM, Reindl M, Messing DD, et al. Protein misfolding is the molecular mechanism underlying MCADD identified in newborn screening. Hum Mol Genet. 2009;18(9):1612–23.
33. Yusupov R, Finegold DN, Naylor EW, Sahai I, Waisbren S, Levy HL. Sudden death in medium chain acyl-coenzyme a dehydrogenase deficiency (MCADD) despite newborn screening. Mol Genet Metab. 2010;101(1):33–9.

Part V

Disorders of Carbohydrate Metabolism

Nutrition Management of Galactosemia

24

Laurie E. Bernstein and Sandy van Calcar

Contents

L. E. Bernstein (✉)
University of Colorado Hospital, Children's Hospital Colorado, Aurora, CO, USA
e-mail: laurie.bernstein@met-ed.net

S. van Calcar
Oregon Health & Science University, Molecular and Medical Genetics, Portland, OR, USA
e-mail: vancalca@ohsu.edu

L. E. Bernstein et al. (eds.), *Nutrition Management of Inherited Metabolic Diseases*,
https://doi.org/10.1007/978-3-030-94510-7_24

Core Messages

- Classical galactosemia can result in life-threatening complications including failure to thrive, hepatocellular damage, and *E. coli* sepsis in untreated infants.
- Initiation of a soy-based infant formula or other lactose-free medical food within the first few days of life can mitigate these complications.
- Patients with classical galactosemia are at increased risk for developmental delay, speech problems and neurological complications, even with life-long dietary treatment.
- Dairy products are the primary source of dietary galactose.
- Galactose is produced endogenously and accounts for a greater contribution to the total galactose pool than the small amounts of galactose found in plant-based foods.

24.1 Background

Galactosemia is an autosomal recessive disorder of carbohydrate metabolism with an incidence of 1 in 10,000 to 30,000 live births in the United States [1]. Over 250 different mutations have been identified in the gene for galactose-1-phosphate uridyltransferase (GALT), located on chromosome 9p13 [2–4].

Lactose is a disaccharide that is hydrolyzed in the small intestine into the monosaccharides, glucose and galactose. Galactose must be converted to glucose via the Leloir pathway in order to be used for energy production [5]. This occurs primarily in the liver. GALT is the second enzyme in this pathway and a severe deficiency of GALT leads to classical galactosemia (Fig. 24.1; Box 24.1).

Classical galactosemia can result in life-threatening complications including failure to thrive, hepatocellular damage, and *E. coli* sepsis in untreated infants (Box 24.2). Initiation of a soy-based infant formula or a lactose-free medi-

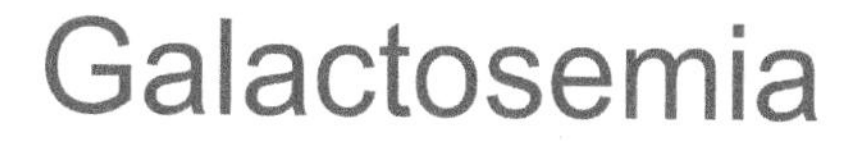

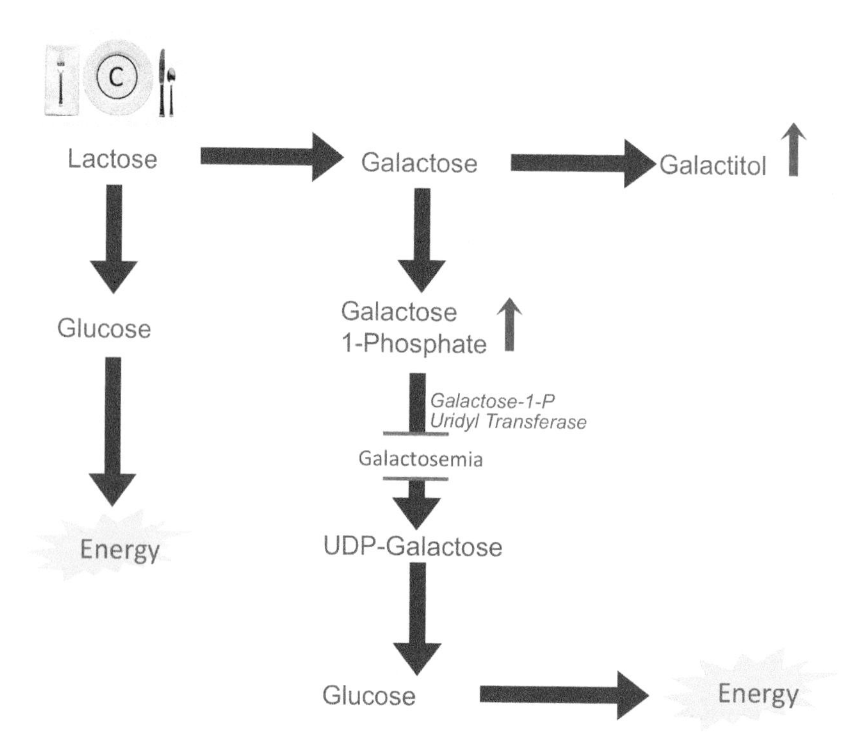

Fig. 24.1 Metabolic pathway of galactosemia

Box 24.1: Principles of Nutrition Management for Galactosemia

- *Restrict:* Lactose and galactose
- *Supplement:* Calcium and vitamin D[a]
- *Toxic metabolites:* galactose-1-phosphate and galactitol[b]

[a]Intake is often low due to lack of dairy products in diet.

[b]These metabolites accumulate but concentrations are not necessarily related to patient outcome.

Box 24.2: Clinical Manifestations of the Newborn with Untreated Classical Galactosemia

- Poor weight gain
- Feeding difficulties
- Jaundice
- Vomiting
- Diarrhea
- Lethargy/Coma
- Hypotonia
- Brain edema/bulging fontanel
- Cataracts
- Hepatomegaly
- Coagulopathy
- Sepsis

cal food within the first few days of life usually resolves these acute complications. However, despite identification by newborn screening and early initiation of a galactose-restricted diet, patients with classical galactosemia often experience long-term complications such as growth delay, impaired cognitive function, speech abnormalities, motor dysfunction, and in females, premature ovarian insufficiency, even if diet treatment is continued throughout life [6, 7].

Elevated galactose-1-phosphate and increased concentrations of galactitol and/or other metabolites, combined with reduced synthesis of UDP-galactose likely leads to the long-term complications commonly seen in patients with classical galactosemia [8–10]. However, the mechanism for galactose toxicity is not well defined [11, 12]. In an exploratory study of patients with classical galactosemia with poor neurological and intellectual outcomes, both white matter (WM) and gray matter (GM) pathology and severe brain abnormalities were found on MRI scan [13]. However, widespread WM lesions were absent in those with classical galactosemia suggesting that this is primarily a GM disease with secondary damage to the WM as a result of neuronal degeneration [13].

24.2 Nutrition Management

Newborns with galactosemia require the same macro- and micronutrients for growth and development as other typically developing infants. However, due to the high lactose content, breast milk or milk-based formulas should not be given to infants with galactosemia and infant formulas containing minimal or no galactose are required [14–18]. Soy-based formulas containing soy protein isolate or elemental formulas containing L-amino acids are recommended (Box 24.3).

Ready-to-feed and liquid concentrate soy formulas contain more galactose than powdered soy formula because liquid formulas have carrageenan added as an emulsifier. However, the galactose in carrageenan is not digested or absorbed by the human gastrointestinal tract [19]. Therefore, the amount of free galactose in liquid soy formulas is equivalent to that found in powdered formula and

Box 24.3: Infant Formulas for the Treatment of Galactosemia

Soy Formula

Protein source: soy protein isolate (extracted from soybeans)

- *Contains small amounts of galactose*
- Both powdered and liquid soy formulas are acceptable

Elemental Formula

Protein source: L-amino acids.

- *Contains no detectable galactose*
- May result in more rapid reduction of galactose-1-phosphate concentrations

any form of soy-based formula is appropriate to recommend for infants. Infants fed soy formula do very well and the red blood cell (RBC) galactose-1-phosphate concentration decreases within a couple of months. Occasionally an infant's RBC galactose-1-phosphate can take up to 6 months to decrease within treatment range, and the metabolic team may suggest a change from soy to an elemental formula to eliminate all galactose [14, 17]. However, it is not known if RBC galactose-1-phosphate concentrations decrease faster if an infant is initially treated with an elemental formula compared to a soy formula or if an elemental formula provides any benefit over soy formula in the short- and long-term care of infants with galactosemia. It is suggested that soy formulas be used with caution in preterm infants [20]. Thus, an elemental formula is recommended for preterm infants with galactosemia.

Isoflavones may be found in small amounts in soy-based infant formulas [15]. Isoflavones are found in whole soybeans and products including tofu, tempeh, and soymilk. Isoflavones are classified as both phytoestrogens (plant estrogens) and selective estrogen receptor modulators. However, studies have found no long-term complications associated with isoflavone ingestion in infants fed soy-based formulas during infancy [15, 21].

The primary source of galactose in the diet is lactose found in dairy products; therefore, most dairy products must be avoided by individuals with galactosemia. However, during food processing, the lactose content of dairy products often decreases. During cheese production, for example, the whey and casein proteins are separated. Since lactose is water-soluble, it is found primarily in the whey fraction. Various whey proteins are often used in commercial food production and contain a significant amount of lactose. The casein fraction (curds) is used to produce cheese and contains a significant amount of residual lactose; however, the lactose content of cheese decreases during production. Several factors determine the final galactose content of cheese, including the type of bacterial cultures used, processing temperature, and length of aging time. Thus, some aged cheeses contain minimal or no galactose in the final product [22, 23]. Sodium and calcium caseinate are added to many processed foods as emulsifiers and stabilizers [24]. Caseinates are produced from casein, but the extensive precipitation and washing results in minimal galactose in the final product [23].

Box 24.4: Bound and Free Galactose

Bound Galactose

- Found in the plant cell wall of many fruits, vegetables, nuts, seeds and legumes
- Cannot be digested in the human gastrointestinal tract because of the absence of the enzyme alpha-galactosidase
- Does not add to the free galactose pool in the body
- Can be released by ripening, heating and fermentation thereby increasing the galactose available for absorption

Free Galactose

- Most abundant in dairy products as part of lactose
- Found in smaller quantities in organ meats and many plants, including fruits, vegetables, nuts, seeds and legumes
- Readily absorbed in the digestive tract and adds to the free galactose pool in the body

Smaller amounts of galactose are found in many plant products as either free or bound galactose [25, 26] (Box 24.4). Galactose is trapped or "bound" in the cell wall of many fruits, vegetables, nuts, seeds, and legumes. Bound galactose cannot be digested in the human gastrointestinal tract because the enzyme alpha-galactosidase required for digestion is not present. For this reason, bound galactose does not add to the free galactose pool in the body. Food processing techniques such as heating and fermentation can release free galactose from bound sources in foods thus increasing the galactose available for absorption [27, 28].

Despite the dietary restriction of galactose, the concentrations of galactose metabolites in blood and urine remain elevated in individuals with galactosemia. There is a negative, nonlinear correlation between RBC galactose-1-phosphate concentrations and residual GALT activity [29]. This phenomenon is believed to be due, in part, to endogenous production of galactose

Endogenous Galactose

Endogenous galactose refers to the galactose that is naturally produced by the body every day. The amount of endogenous galactose produced depends on how old you are.

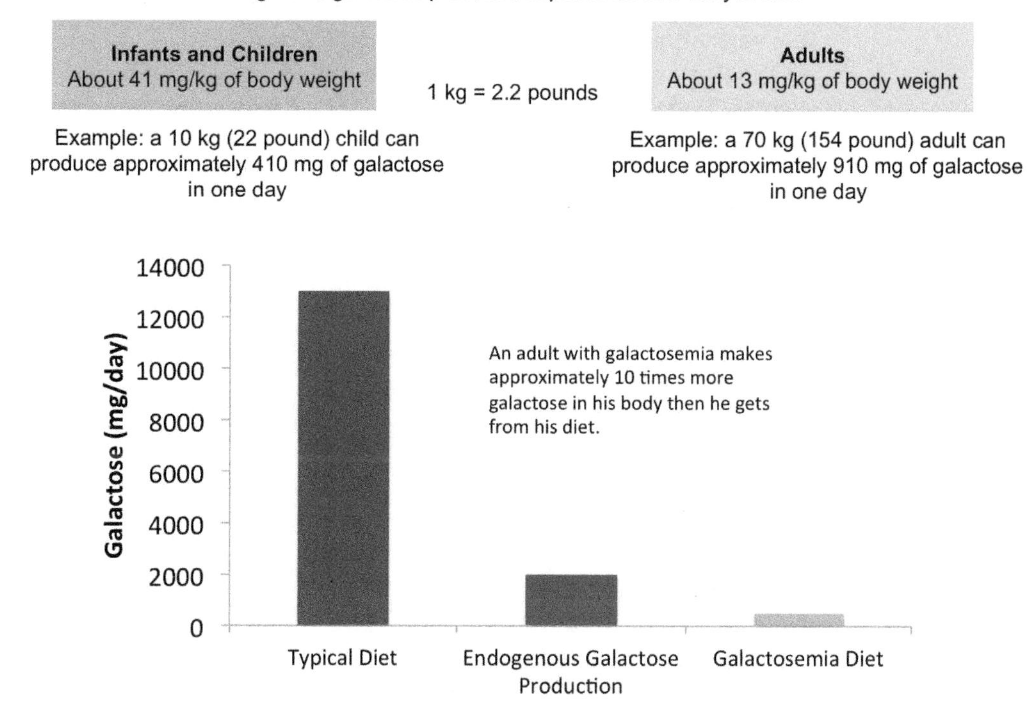

[1] Approximate galactose content of a typical diet including 2 cups of milk and 3 servings of fruits and vegetables with a galactose content >20 mg galactose/100 g food.

[2] Approximate amount of endogenous galactose produced by an adult with galactosemia.

[3] Approximate galactose content of a typical galactose-restricted diet including 3 servings of fruits and vegetables with a galactose content >20 mg galactose/100 g food.

Berry & Elsas, J Inherit Metab Dis, 2011

Fig. 24.2 Comparison of the galactose content in a typical diet, galactose produced endogenously, and the galactose content in the diet for galactosemia [30, 31].

(i.e., galactose that is produced by the body) (Fig. 24.2) [30].

The endogenous production of galactose is age-dependent with greater amounts produced per kg body weight in infants compared with adults [32]. Using a stable isotope tracer of D-galactose in a continuous intravenous infusion, the endogenous galactose production rate in three healthy, unaffected men and three patients with classical galactosemia was measured [33]. The galactose synthesis rate in both subjects and controls ranged from 0.53 to 1.05 mg/kg per hour resulting in production of gram quantities of galactose per day. Endogenous production of galactose may be an important factor in the long-term complications that are seen in older individuals with GALT deficiency [33–35]. Currently, there is not a difference in the quantity of galactose allowed in the diet, regardless of a patient's age [8, 36].

Compared to endogenous production, the quantity of galactose consumed from plant-based foods is quite small (Fig. 24.3). A study published in 1991 indicating that tomatoes contained free galactose [37] was the catalyst for many metabolic clinics to recommend restriction of

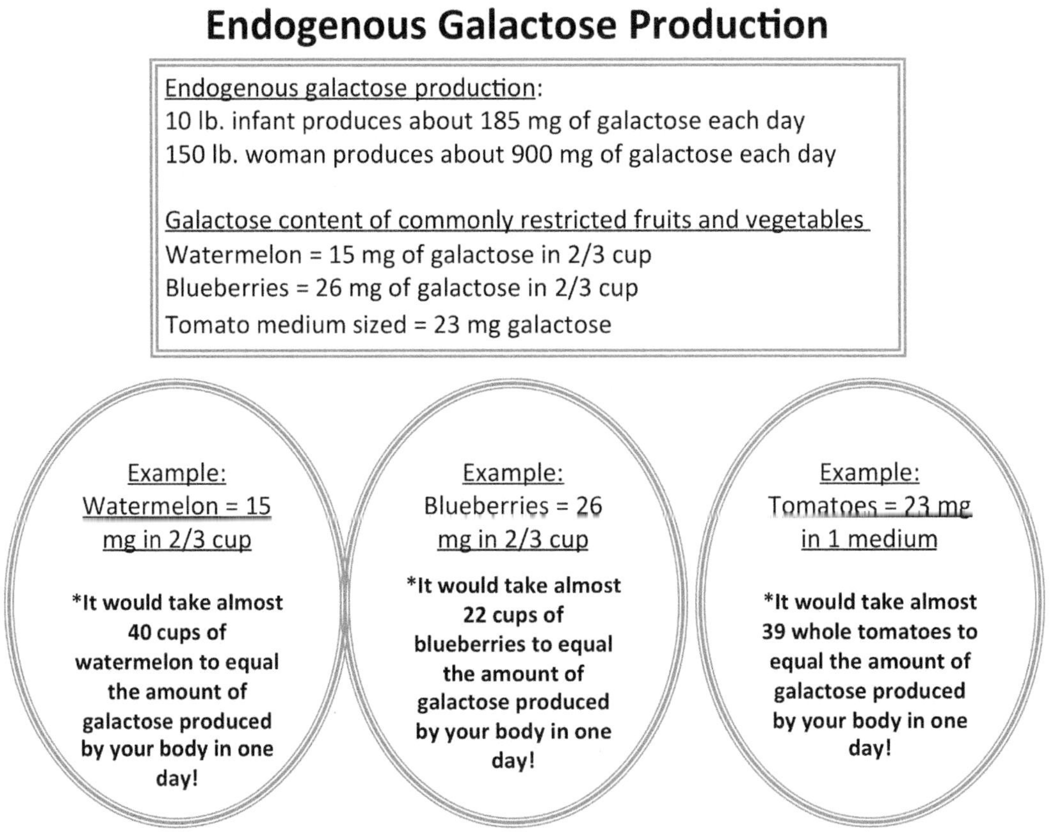

Endogenous Galactose Production

Endogenous galactose production:
10 lb. infant produces about 185 mg of galactose each day
150 lb. woman produces about 900 mg of galactose each day

Galactose content of commonly restricted fruits and vegetables
Watermelon = 15 mg of galactose in 2/3 cup
Blueberries = 26 mg of galactose in 2/3 cup
Tomato medium sized = 23 mg galactose

Example:
Watermelon = 15 mg in 2/3 cup
***It would take almost 40 cups of watermelon to equal the amount of galactose produced by your body in one day!**

Example:
Blueberries = 26 mg in 2/3 cup
***It would take almost 22 cups of blueberries to equal the amount of galactose produced by your body in one day!**

Example:
Tomatoes = 23 mg in 1 medium
***It would take almost 39 whole tomatoes to equal the amount of galactose produced by your body in one day!**

Fig. 24.3 The amount of watermelon, blueberries, or tomatoes that an adult with galactosemia weighing 150 pounds would need to consume to equal the approximate amount of galactose produced endogenously in one day [31]

tomatoes and other fruits, vegetables, and legumes with a higher free galactose content [36]. However, subsequent studies did not demonstrate improved outcomes in patients who eliminated such foods from the diet [8], and some clinics offered fruits and vegetables freely without report of complications (Fig. 24.3) [31].

Additionally, various legumes were found to contain less free galactose than originally reported and avoiding these foods is not necessary [23]. However, the fermentation process used to produce various soy-based products releases free galactose from the bound galactose in legumes and, thus, relatively higher quantities of free galactose have been found in fermented soy products [36]. Fermented products include soy sauce, miso, natto, tempeh, and sufu (fermented soy cheese). However, the amount of these products consumed in the diet is typically small. This needs to be considered in the decision to include these products in the diet. In addition, products such as Beano® contain the enzyme α-galactosidase which does breakdown bound sources of galactose from plant-based foods in the gastrointestinal tract. Thus, use of these over-the-counter products needs to be avoided.

The "Allowed" list of various foods and ingredients includes all fruits, vegetables, legumes, non-fermented soy products, caseinates, and a number of aged cheeses (Table 24.1) [36, 38].

24.3 Monitoring

The primary biochemical marker to evaluate the treatment of galactosemia is RBC galactose-1-phosphate. Periodic monitoring during the first year of life is suggested with subsequent yearly

Table 24.1 Allowed and restricted foods and ingredients for individuals with classical galactosemia

Allowed foods and ingredients
Soy-based infant formulas containing soy protein isolate, amino acid-based elemental infant formulas
All fruits, vegetables and their juices, pickled fruits and vegetables
All legumes (e.g., navy beans, kidney beans, garbanzo beans, soybeans)
Soy-based products that are not fermented (soy milk, tofu, textured soy protein, hydrolyzed vegetable protein, soy protein concentrate, meat analogs, unfermented soy sauce[a])
Mature Cheeses[b] (with galactose content <25 mg/100 g): Jarlsberg, Emmentaler, Swiss, Gruyere, Tilsiter, Parmesan aged >10 months, grated 100% Parmesan cheese, sharp cheddar cheese
Sodium and calcium caseinate
All cocoa products except milk chocolate
Additional ingredients: natural and artificial flavorings, all gums including carrageenan
Foods used in moderation
Offal (organ meats)–galactose content unknown but there is no direct evidence of harm
Soy products that are fermented[c] (e.g., miso, natto, tempeh, sufu)
Meat-by-products
Restricted foods and ingredients
Breast milk, all milk-based infant formulas
All milk-based foods and beverages except for caseinates and aged cheeses, listed above
Milk-based ingredients including buttermilk solids, casein, dry milk protein, dry milk solids, hydrolyzed whey protein, hydrolyzed casein protein, lactose, lactalbumin, whey
All cheese and cheese-based products except those listed above

[a]Soy sauce that has not been fermented is made from hydrolyzed soy protein
[b]Galactose content of allowed cheeses may vary in different countries
[c]These fermented soy products are typically used as condiments or ingredients in foods. The amount of these products in the diet needs to be considered when determining acceptability

measurements until an individual's baseline has been established [38]. RBC galactose-1-phosphate analysis can be helpful to evaluate an increase in galactose intake if it is compared with the individual's baseline concentrations. The usefulness of routine measurement of blood or urine galactitol is limited [38].

Some children and adolescents with galactosemia develop osteopenia of the lumbar spine with abnormal concentrations of various markers of bone resorption and formation, despite reporting dietary intake that meets the established requirements for calcium, magnesium, zinc, vitamin D, and protein [39–41]. Poor nutritional intake, an intrinsic defect in collagen formation, and abnormal sex steroid concentrations in females have been implicated in the decline in bone mineral density observed in this population [42, 43]. In adults with galactosemia, body mass index was correlated with bone density [43]. International guidelines suggest initially measuring bone mineral density using dual energy X-ray absorptiometry (DXA) at age 8–10 years. If the z-score is ≤ -2, follow-up is advised [38]. If there is no evidence of reduced bone density at this age, a repeat DXA is not recommended until the completion of puberty [38, 43]. While the mechanism of decreased bone density in patients with galactosemia is not well understood, ensuring adequate intake of nutrients associated with proper bone development and maintenance can prevent nutrient deficiencies that could exacerbate the development of osteoporosis.

In 2011, the Institute of Medicine revised the recommended Dietary Reference Intakes (DRI) for calcium and vitamin D [44]. Periodic monitoring of total 25-hydroxyvitamin D to maintain serum concentrations of at least 20–32 ng/mL (50–80 nmol/L) coupled with an annual diet assessment of both calcium and vitamin D intake is recommended [38, 45, 46]. With the increased availability of calcium-fortified foods and the addition of allowed dairy products to the diet, patients with classical galactosemia may now be at lower risk for calcium and vitamin D deficiency (Box 24.5).

Box 24.5: Nutrition Monitoring of a Patient with Classical Galactosemia

- Routine assessments including anthropometrics, dietary intake, physical findings
- Laboratory Monitoring
  - Diagnosis-specific biochemical data
    Galactose-1-phosphate (GAL-1-P) in erythrocytes
    Galactitol in urine
  - Nutrition-related laboratory monitoring of patients on a galactose-restricted diet includes serum total 25-hydroxyvitamin D
- Bone mineral density

24.4 Summary

Newborn screening and the early introduction of a galactose-restricted diet has reduced mortality in infants with classical galactosemia, but the long-term efficacy of the galactose-restricted diet is limited, and patients with galactosemia remain at risk for developmental and neurological complications. Endogenous production of galactose contributes significantly to the total free galactose pool and avoidance of small amounts of galactose from plant-based foods is no longer recommended. Recommendations include the avoidance of dairy products that are abundant in galactose; however, some dairy products, such as certain cheeses and sodium or calcium caseinate, contain negligible amounts of galactose and are allowed in the diet. Experience remains limited with regard to evidence to support the safety of discontinuing the galactose-restricted diet in adults.

References

1. Acosta PB. Nutrition management of patients with inherited metabolic disorders. Sudbury: Jones and Bartlett Publishers, LLC; 2010.
2. Calderon FR, Phansalkar AR, Crockett DK, Miller M, Mao R. Mutation database for the galactose-1-phosphate uridyltransferase (GALT) gene. Hum Mutat. 2007;28(10):939–43.
3. Bosch AM, Ijlst L, Oostheim W, Mulders J, Bakker HD, Wijburg FA, et al. Identification of novel mutations in classical galactosemia. Hum Mutat. 2005;25(5):502.
4. Pasquali M, Yu C, Coffee B. Laboratory diagnosis of galactosemia: a technical standard and guideline of American College of Medical Genetics (ACMG). Genet Med. 2018;20(1):3–11.
5. Shils ME, Shike M. Modern nutrition in health and disease. 10th ed. Philadelphia: Lippincott Williams & Wilkins; 2006. xxv, 2069 p.
6. Waggoner DD, Buist NR, Donnell GN. Long-term prognosis in galactosaemia: results of a survey of 350 cases. J Inherit Metab Dis. 1990;13(6):802–18.
7. Hermans ME, Welsink-Karssies MM, Bosch AM, Oostrom KJ, Geurtsen GJ. Cognitive functioning in patients with classical galactosemia: a systematic review. Orphanet J Rare Dis. 2019;14(1):226.
8. Frederick AB, Cutler DJ, Fridovich-Keil JL. Rigor of non-dairy galactose restriction in early childhood, measured by retrospective survey, does not associate with severity of five long-term outcomes quantified in 231 children and adults with classic galactosemia. J Inherit Metab Dis. 2017;40(6):813–21.
9. Shaw KA, Mulle JG, Epstein MP, Fridovich-Keil JL. Gastrointestinal health in classic galactosemia. JIMD Rep. 2017;33:27–32.
10. Coelho AI, Rubio-Gozalbo ME, Vicente JB, Rivera I. Sweet and sour: an update on classic galactosemia. J Inherit Metab Dis. 2017;40(3):325–42.
11. Gross W, Schnarrenberger C. Purification and characterization of a galactose-1-phosphate: UDP-glucose uridyltransferase from the red alga Galdieria sulphuraria. Eur J Biochem. 1995;234(1):258–63.
12. Welsink-Karssies MM, Ferdinandusse S, Geurtsen GJ, Hollak CEM, Huidekoper HH, Jansen MCH, et al. Deep phenotyping classical galactosemia: clinical outcomes and biochemical markers. Brain Comm. 2020;2(1):fcaa006.
13. Welsink-Karssies MM, Schrantee A, Caan MWA, Hollak CEM, Janssen MCH, Oussoren E, et al. Gray and white matter are both affected in classical galactosemia: an explorative study on the association between neuroimaging and clinical outcome. Mol Genet Metab. 2020;131(4):370–9.
14. Zlatunich CO, Packman S. Galactosaemia: early treatment with an elemental formula. J Inherit Metab Dis. 2005;28(2):163–8.
15. Vandenplas Y, De Greef E, Devreker T, Hauser B. Soy infant formula: is it that bad? Acta Paediatr. 2011;100(2):162–6.
16. ESPGHAN Committee on Nutrition, Agostoni C, Axelsson I, Goulet O, Koletzko B, Michaelsen KF, et al. Soy protein infant formulae and follow-on formulae: a commentary by the ESPGHAN committee on nutrition. J Pediatr Gastroenterol Nutr. 2006;42(4):352–61.

17. Ficicioglu C, Hussa C, Yager C, Segal S. Effect of galactose free formula on galactose-1-phosphate in two infants with classical galactosemia. Eur J Pediatr. 2008;167(5):595–6.
18. Turck D. Soy protein for infant feeding: what do we know? Curr Opin Clin Nutr Metab Care. 2007;10(3):360–5.
19. Joint FAO/WHO Expert Committee on Food Additives. Evaluation of certain veterinary drug residues in food. Fiftieth report of the joint FAO/WHO expert committee on food additives. World Health Organ Tech Rep Ser. 1999;888:i-vii,:1–95.
20. Bhatia J, Greer F. American Academy of Pediatrics Committee on Nutrition. Use of soy protein-based formulas in infant feeding. Pediatrics. 2008;121(5):1062–8.
21. Mendez MA, Anthony MS, Arab L. Soy-based formulae and infant growth and development: a review. J Nutr. 2002;132(8):2127–30.
22. Portnoi PA, MacDonald A. Determination of the lactose and galactose content of cheese for use in the galactosaemia diet. J Hum Nutr Diet. 2009;22(5):400–8.
23. Van Calcar SC, Bernstein LE, Rohr FJ, Yannicelli S, Berry GT, Scaman CH. Galactose content of legumes, caseinates, and some hard cheeses: implications for diet treatment of classic galactosemia. J Agric Food Chem. 2014;62(6):1397–402.
24. Southward CR. Casein products: chemical processes in New Zealand. Palmerston North: New Zealand Dairy Research Institute; 1998. p. 1–13.
25. Wright EM, Martin MG, Turk E. Intestinal absorption in health and disease--sugars. Best Pract Res Clin Gastroenterol. 2003;17(6):943–56.
26. Upreti VV, Khurana M, Cox DS, Eddington ND. Determination of endogenous glycosaminoglycans derived disaccharides in human plasma by HPLC: validation and application in a clinical study. J Chromatogr B Analyt Technol Biomed Life Sci. 2006;831(1–2):156–62.
27. Kim HO, Hartnett C, Scaman CH. Free galactose content in selected fresh fruits and vegetables and soy beverages. J Agric Food Chem. 2007;55(20): 8133–7.
28. Hartnett C, Kim HO, Scaman CH. Effect of processing on galactose in selected fruits. Can J Diet Pract Res. 2007;68(1):46–50.
29. Yuzyuk T, Viau K, Andrews A, Pasquali M, Longo N. Biochemical changes and clinical outcomes in 34 patients with classic galactosemia. J Inherit Metab Dis. 2018;41(2):197–208.
30. Berry GT, Elsas LJ. Introduction to the Maastricht workshop: lessons from the past and new directions in galactosemia. J Inherit Metab Dis. 34(2):249–55.
31. Bernstein LE. Galactosemia: the diet. Aurora: Children's Hospital Colorado; 2014.
32. Schadewaldt P, Kamalanathan L, Hammen HW, Wendel U. Age dependence of endogenous galactose formation in Q188R homozygous galactosemic patients. Mol Genet Metab. 2004;81(1):31–44.
33. Berry GT, Nissim I, Lin Z, Mazur AT, Gibson JB, Segal S. Endogenous synthesis of galactose in normal men and patients with hereditary galactosaemia. Lancet. 1995;346(8982):1073–4.
34. Berry GT, Moate PJ, Reynolds RA, Yager CT, Ning C, Boston RC, et al. The rate of de novo galactose synthesis in patients with galactose-1-phosphate uridyltransferase deficiency. Mol Genet Metab. 2004;81(1):22–30.
35. Berry GT, Reynolds RA, Yager CT, Segal S. Extended [13C]galactose oxidation studies in patients with galactosemia. Mol Genet Metab. 2004;82(2): 130–6.
36. Van Calcar SC, Bernstein LE, Rohr FJ, Scaman CH, Yannicelli S, Berry GT. A re-evaluation of life-long severe galactose restriction for the nutrition management of classic galactosemia. Mol Genet Metab. 2014;112(3):191–7.
37. Gross KC, Acosta PB. Fruits and vegetables are a source of galactose: implications in the planning the diets of patients with galactosemia. J Inherit Metab Dis. 1991;14:253–8.
38. Welling L, Bernstein LE, Berry GT, Burlina AB, Eyskens F, Gautschi M, et al. International clinical guideline for the management of classical galactosemia: diagnosis, treatment, and follow-up. J Inherit Metab Dis. 2017;40(2):171–6.
39. Panis B, Forget PP, van Kroonenburgh MJ, Vermeer C, Menheere PP, Nieman FH, et al. Bone metabolism in galactosemia. Bone. 2004;35(4):982–7.
40. Rubio-Gozalbo ME, Hamming S, van Kroonenburgh MJ, Bakker JA, Vermeer C, Forget PP. Bone mineral density in patients with classic galactosaemia. Arch Dis Child. 2002;87(1):57–60.
41. Gajewska J, Ambroszkiewicz J, Radomyska B, Chelchowska M, Oltarzewski M, Laskowska-Klita T, et al. Serum markers of bone turnover in children and adolescents with classic galactosemia. Adv Med Sci. 2008;53(2):214–20.
42. Van Erven B, Welling L, Van Calcar SC, Doulgeraki A, Eyskens F, Gribbon J, et al. Bone health in classical galactosemia: systematic review and meta-analysis. JIMD Reports. 2017;35:87–96.
43. Batey LA, Welt CK, Rohr F, Wessel A, Anastasoaie V, Feldman HA, et al. Skeletal health in adult patients with classic galactosemia. Osteoporos Int. 2013;24(2):501–9.
44. Ross AC, Manson JE, Abrams SA, Aloia JF, Brannon PM, Clinton SK, et al. The 2011 dietary reference intakes for calcium and vitamin D: what dietetics practitioners need to know. J Am Diet Assoc. 2011;111(4):524–7.
45. Bachrach LK, Sills IN, Section on Endocrinology Clinical report-bone densitometry in children and adolescents. Pediatrics. 2011;127(1): 189–94.
46. Panis B, van Kroonenburgh MJ, Rubio-Gozalbo ME. Proposal for the prevention of osteoporosis in paediatric patients with classical galactosaemia. J Inherit Metab Dis. 2007;30(6):982.

Glycogen Storage Diseases

25

Aditi Korlimarla, Rebecca Gibson, and Priya S. Kishnani

Contents

A. Korlimarla (✉) · R. Gibson · P. S. Kishnani
Division of Medical Genetics, Pediatrics, Duke University School of Medicine, Durham, NC, USA
e-mail: aditi.korlimarla@duke.edu; rebecca.a.gibson@duke.edu; priya.kishnani@duke.edu

L. E. Bernstein et al. (eds.), *Nutrition Management of Inherited Metabolic Diseases*, https://doi.org/10.1007/978-3-030-94510-7_25

Core Messages

- In glycogen storage diseases (GSDs), there is excessive glycogen build-up in the muscle, liver, and/or heart.
- There are over 15 types of glycogen storage diseases, which are mainly categorized by the type of tissue involved:
  - Types I, III, IV, VI, and IX primarily affect the liver.
  - Types II, V, and VII primarily affect the muscle.
  - Type II can affect both the liver and heart.

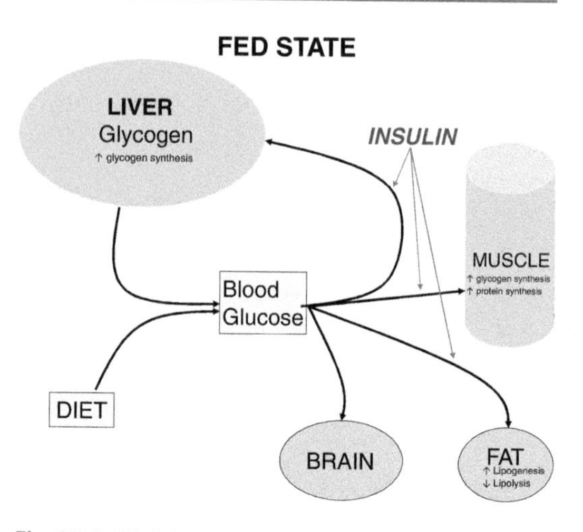

Fig. 25.1 High insulin concentrations suppress lipolysis, glycogenolysis, and stimulate lipogenesis

25.1 Background

Glycogen is the main storage form of glucose. It consists of highly branched chains of glucose molecules bonded together in α-1,4 linkages, with branching points in α-1,6 linkages. Glycogen is formed after an ingestion of carbohydrates, and is broken down to glucose when there is a high glucose demand in the body or when the dietary availability is low. Liver is the main reservoir of glycogen which releases glucose to other tissues that are unable to synthesize sufficient glucose for energy. Skeletal muscles also contains large amounts of glycogen, which are used as the primary source of energy during high-intensity muscular activities.

In the fed state, immediately after a meal, glucose is absorbed, and stored as glycogen. The ingestion of carbohydrates elevates the glucose concentrations in the blood. High blood glucose concentrations trigger the release of insulin, which then up-regulates the GLUT4 glucose transporters, and results in the entry of glucose into the muscle and adipose tissue. High insulin concentrations suppress lipolysis. Excess glucose is converted to lipid via lipogenesis and glycogen via glycogenesis in adipose tissue and muscle, respectively. Liver uses glucose from the bloodstream, and it is taken up using an insulin-independent transporter (GLUT2). At high glucose and insulin concentrations, the liver produces glycogen (glycogen synthesis) (Fig. 25.1). The brain continuously uses glucose in the bloodstream through the insulin-independent GLUT1 transporter.

During the fasting state, blood glucose concentrations gradually decrease. After a sufficiently long fasting period, low insulin concentrations and elevated glucagon levels stop the uptake of glucose into the muscle tissues, and the glycogen synthesis in the liver. Low glucose and insulin concentrations result in two processes that occur simultaneously: glycogen breakdown in the liver (glycogenolysis), and the production of glucose from protein (gluconeogenesis), which result in glucose release, and maintenance of normal glucose concentrations for organs that are dependent on glucose such as red blood cells and brain. As the fasting period extends, adrenaline and cortisol are released, resulting in lipolysis, and fat tissues release free fatty acids and glycerol. These fatty acids are the main source of energy for the muscle tissues as glucose sources decrease. Liver tissue also uses fatty acids for energy, but when fatty acid concentrations are high, the liver will generate ketones from the metabolism of fatty acids. Ketones can then be used by various tissues, including the brain, by adding or replacing glucose as the main fuel source for energy generation. Lactate (Cori cycle) and released amino acids, such as alanine (amino acid catabolism) from muscle, and glycerol from lipolysis provide substrate to the liver for gluconeogenesis (Fig. 25.2). Lactate and the glucogenic amino acids generate pyruvate, and beta oxidation of fatty acids generate ATP. Pyruvate and ATP are the main substrates for gluconeogenesis in the liver.

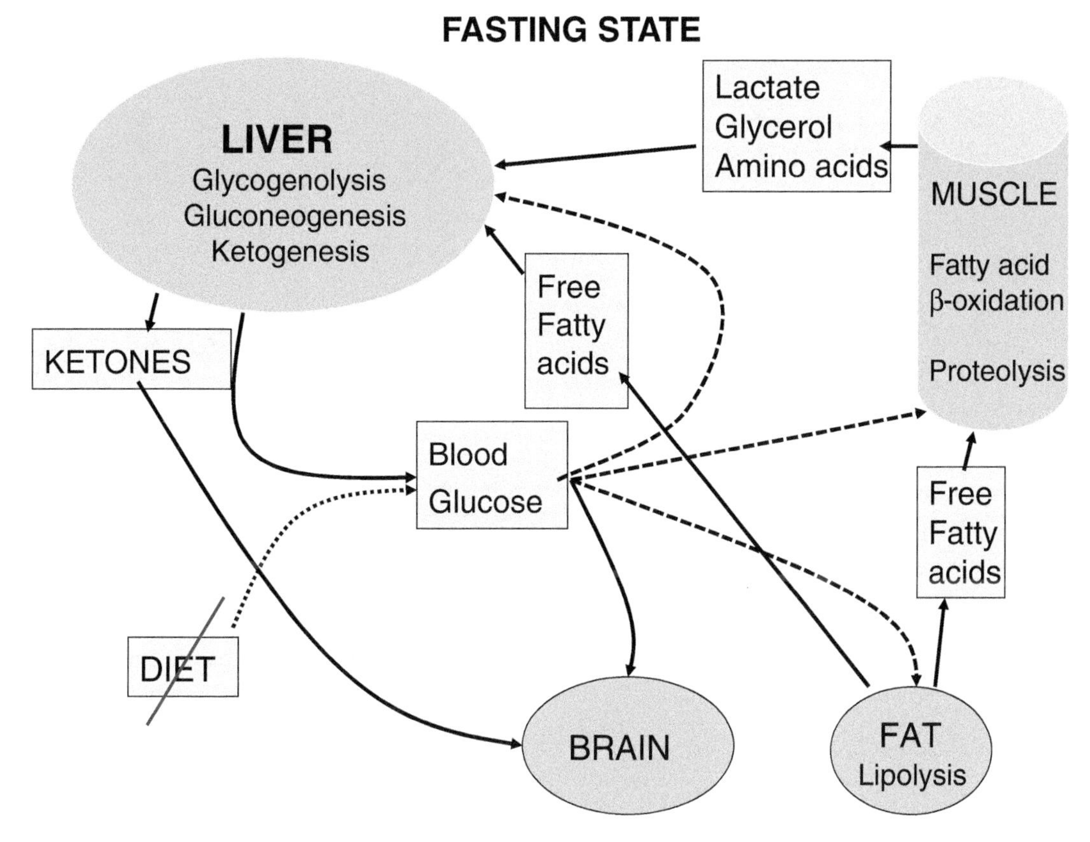

Fig. 25.2 During the fasting state, glucose and insulin concentrations decrease, and glycogenolysis, lipolysis, and ketone production occur to provide energy

The timing of the transition from the fed state to the fasting state has important consequences for clinical care. Absorption of carbohydrates from food takes 3–4 hours after a regular meal. During this absorptive stage, glycogen synthesis is ongoing. As absorption completes, and glucose concentrations become lower and glycogenolysis starts aided by gluconeogenesis. This provides glucose homeostasis from 4 hours to 12–15 hours after a meal. When fasting for 12–15 hours after a meal, glucose and insulin concentrations decrease enough to allow lipolysis to occur. Lipolysis and fatty acid oxidation become the major fuel sources from 15 to 18 hours of fasting and longer, while gluconeogenesis continues (Fig. 25.3).

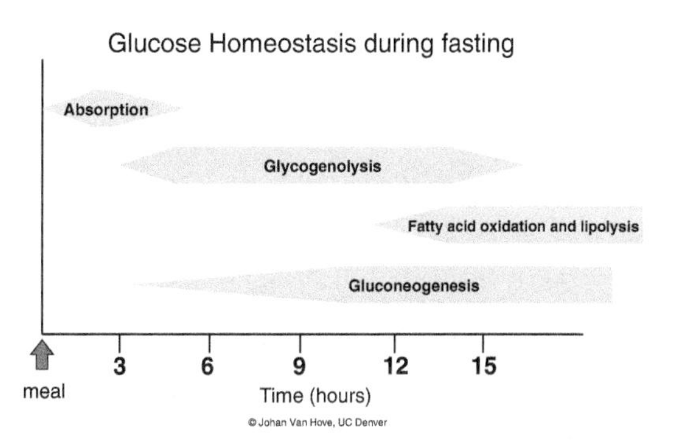

Fig. 25.3 During the fasting state, glucose homeostasis is maintained first by post-prandial glucose absorption, then glycogenolysis and gluconeogenesis, and then ultimately by fatty acid oxidation and ketone production as energy sources

Normal pre-prandial concentrations of glucose are between 3.9 and 6.7 mmol/L, free fatty acids are <0.5 mmol/L, and the ketones 3-hydroxybutyrate and acetoacetate are less than 0.5 mmol/L. The normal ratio of 3-hydroxybutyrate to acetoacetate is >1 after an overnight fast, and <1 in the fed state. Standardized fasting tests in children show the timing of these metabolic and endocrine changes in the postprandial period (Table 25.1) [1].

Table 25.1 Age-wise distribution of biochemical markers during fasting [1]

Age		Infants (≤12 months)			1–7 years			7–15 years		
Biomarker		Glucose	Free fatty acids	Ketones	Glucose	Free fatty acids	Ketones	Glucose	Free fatty acids	Ketones
Pre-prandial		3.9–6.7	<0.5	<0.5	3.9–6.7	<0.5	<0.4	3.9–6.7	<0.5	<0.5
During fasting state	12–hours		Inconsistently elevated			Inconsistently elevated			Inconsistently elevated	
	15–hours	3.9–5.3	0.5–1.6	0.1–1.5	3.5–4.8	0.6–1.5	0.15–2.0	4.4–4.9	0.2–1.1	<0.1–0.5
	20–hours	3.5–4.6	0.6–1.3	0.6–3.2	2.8–4.3	0.9–2.6	1.2–3.7	3.8–4.9	0.6–1.3	0.1–1.3
	24–hours	2.7–4.5	1.1–1.6	1.5–3.9	2.8–3.8	1.1–2.8	2.2–5.8	3.0–4.3	1.0–1.8	0.7–3.7

All units are in millimoles per liter (mmol/L) [1]

Glycogen is broken down into glucose in two steps. First, upon activation by phosphorylase kinase, outer glucose moieties are released by the enzyme phosphorylase, and transferred onto phosphate to form glucose-1-phosphate. Phosphoglucomutase then converts glucose-1-phosphate into glucose-6-phosphate. At the end of phosphorylation, the glycogen core has four glucose moieties at its branching point. This structure is called α-limit dextrin. At that point, debranching enzyme works in two sequential reactions. First, the glycosyltransferase activity of debranching enzyme transfers the outer three glucose molecules to a nearby chain in an α-1,4 linkage, leaving only the glucose molecule that is attached by the α-1,6 linkage. This last glucose molecule is then hydrolyzed to glucose by the α-1,6 glycosidase function of debranching enzyme to free glucose, thus completing the removal of the α-1,6 branch. Glucose-6-phosphate in the liver is converted to glucose by glucose-6-phosphatase for endogenous secretion in the bloodstream during hepatic glycogenolysis. Therefore, deficiency of glucose-6-phosphatase affects both gluconeogenesis and glycogenolysis [1–3].

25.2 Glycogen Storage Diseases

Glycogen Storage Diseases (GSDs) affect glycogen synthesis or breakdown. GSDs that affect the glycogen pool in the liver cause disturbances of glucose homeostasis in the blood. GSDs that affect the glycogen use in skeletal muscles cause muscle symptoms. GSDs that affect the glycogen use in the heart muscle cause cardiac symptoms. As red blood cells are completely dependent on glycolysis, disorders of the glycolytic pathway often involve hemolysis.

Glucose in excess can make glycogen, or glucose can be derived from glycogen in the fasting state. Glucose can also be metabolized to pyruvate in the glycolytic pathway, and from there, to acetyl-CoA for use in the Krebs cycle. Glucose can also be made from precursors in the reverse of the glycolytic pathway during gluconeogenesis. Other carbohydrates such as fructose and galactose can be metabolized to glucose-6-phosphate, and hence into glucose for use in multiple organs. Galactose is converted from galactose-1-phosphate into UDP-galactose, and from there into UDP-glucose, and hence into glucose-1-phosphate entering the pathway of glycogen metabolism. Fructose is metabolized into fructose-1-phosphate which is broken down by aldolase into dihydroxyacetone-phosphate and glyceraldehyde which is then metabolized to glyceraldehyde-3-phosphate, both joining the glycolytic/gluconeogenic pathway.

In GSDs in which glycogen breakdown is blocked, such as phosphorylase deficiency, there will be a shortage of glucose, even if gluconeogenesis is still intact. In the GSDs primarily affecting the liver, this will result in hypoglycemia, and in the GSDs primarily affecting the muscle, this will result in muscle cramping and rhabdomyolysis. Gluconeogenesis occurs mostly in the liver; though it can occur in smaller amounts in the kidney and small intestine.

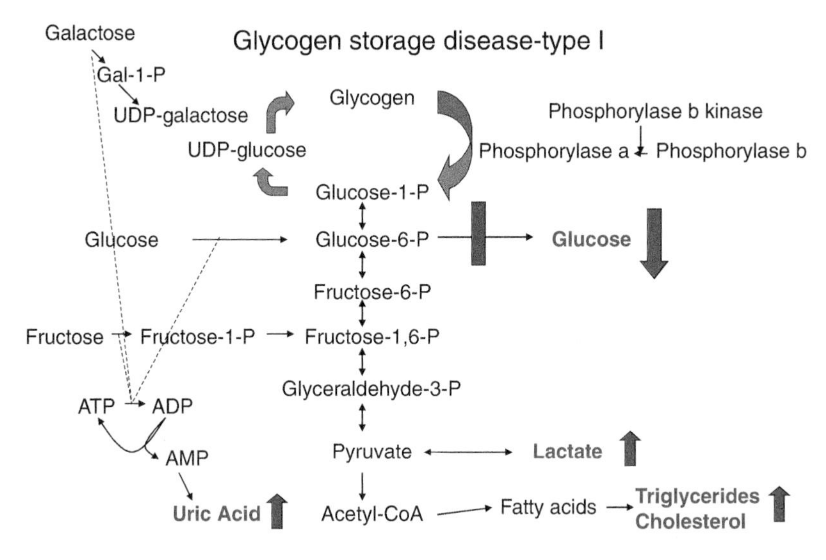

Fig. 25.4 Metabolic pathway of glycogen storage disease-type I

Disorders of gluconeogenesis will also result in a shortage of glucose, and hence, there can be hypoglycemia upon fasting for about 12 hours when glycogen stores are depleted, and will also result in the accumulation of the precursor product pyruvate, which is in equilibrium with lactate. Thus, in isolated gluconeogenetic conditions such a fructose-1,6-bis-phosphatase deficiency, the often-mild hypoglycemia will be accompanied by lactic acidosis. Finally, in glucose-6-phosphatase deficiency, the release of glucose from glucose-6-phosphate is not possible, resulting in an impairment of both glycogenolysis and gluconeogenesis. Due to the combined block of both pathways, hypoglycemia occurs early and is severe. Hypoglycemia is accompanied by lactic acidosis from the accumulation of gluconeogenic precursors (Fig. 25.4).

Key clinical features of GSDs relate to the organ in which the enzyme is deficient (Table 25.2). Hepatic glycogen is used for the homeostasis of blood glucose concentrations. Hepatic GSDs present with hypoglycemia, usually upon fasting.

Disorders of gluconeogenesis present with hypoglycemia, but lactic acidosis is present as well. In conditions where both glycogenolysis and gluconeogenesis are impaired, there is pronounced hepatomegaly reflecting abnormal glycogen storage and steatosis (a fatty change in the liver). The onset of hypoglycemia is dependent on the severity of the condition and the age of the patient. Defects of gluconeogenesis only typically present with hypoglycemia after 8–12 hours fasting. Defects where glycogenolysis is mainly affected, such as in GSD III, VI, and IX, or disorders where there are defects of both glycogenolysis and gluconeogenesis, such as glucose-6-phosphatase deficiency, hypoglycemia can present as soon as the absorptive phase is over, usually 4 hours after a meal.

Table 25.2 Key clinical presentations of GSDs

Involving liver	Hypoglycemia Hepatomegaly Hyperlipidemia Elevated liver transaminases Lactic acidosis (when enzymatic deficiency affects both glycogenolysis and gluconeogenesis pathways) Hepatic fibrosis, cirrhosis
Involving muscle	Weakness, wasting, hypotonia Exercise intolerance Rhabdomyolysis (Type V)
Involving heart	Hypertrophic cardiomyopathy Arrhythmias
Red blood cells	Glycolytic defect: hemolytic anemia

During exercise, muscle uses energy provided by glucose from the bloodstream and aerobic mitochondrial metabolism. However, during short bursts of intense exercise, muscle

Table 25.3 Glycogen storage diseases

Glycogen storage diseases primarily involving the liver:
Type I (glucose-6-phosphatase complex deficiency, von Gierke disease)
Type VI (hepatic phosphorylase deficiency, Hers disease)
Type IX (subtypes α2 and γ2; phosphorylase kinase (PhK) deficiency)
Others: Type 0 (liver glycogen synthase deficiency), Type XI (Fanconi–Bickel syndrome)
Glycogen storage diseases affecting both liver and muscle:
Type III (amylo-1,6-glucosidase deficiency, debrancher deficiency, limit dextrinosis, Cori disease, Forbes disease)
Type IX (subtype β; phosphorylase kinase (PhK) deficiency)
Type IV (brancher deficiency, amylopectinosis, amylo-1,4–1,6-transglucosidase deficiency, Andersen disease)
Glycogen storage diseases primarily involving the muscles:
Type II (Lysosomal acid α-glucosidase deficiency, Pompe disease, acid maltase deficiency, α-1,4-glucosidase deficiency)
Type V (muscle phosphorylase deficiency, McArdle disease, myophosphorylase deficiency, PYGM deficiency)
Type VII (muscle phosphofructokinase deficiency, Tarui disease)
Others: Muscle phosphorylase kinase deficiency, glycogenin-1 deficiency, and other enzyme deficiencies of phosphoglycerate kinase, phosphoglycerate mutase, lactate dehydrogenase, fructose-1,6-bisphosphate aldolase A, and β-enolase
Glycogen storage diseases primarily with cardiac involvement:
PRKAG2 syndrome
Danon disease

uses energy provided by glucose from glycogen. Therefore, in patients with a GSD that affects muscle, there is energy failure leading to painful cramping and rhabdomyolysis, muscle weakness, wasting, and hypotonia. Hemolysis can occur in certain glycolytic defects since the red blood cell is uniquely dependent on glycolysis for its energy needs. Finally, different GSDs can result in accumulation of glycogen in hepatocytes, muscle wasting, cardiac involvement resulting in cardiomyopathy, and neuropathy. Based on these differences GSDs can be broadly categorized (Table 25.3) [4].

25.2.1 Glycogen Storage Diseases Primarily Involving the Liver

25.2.1.1 Glycogen Storage Disease Type I

Biochemistry GSD-I is characterized by deficient activity of the glucose-6-phosphatase enzyme complex. The enzyme complex is comprised of a translocase subunit (glucose-6-phosphate translocase) and a catalytic subunit (glucose-6-phosphatase alpha). The translocase subunit acts as a carrier (gene *SLC37A4*) to transport glucose-6-phosphate from the cytoplasm into the endoplasmic reticulum (ER). Once transported into the ER, the catalytic subunit (gene *G6PC*) helps to convert glucose-6-phosphate to glucose. Deficiency of the catalytic enzyme glucose-6-phosphatase is called GSD-Ia, and deficiency of the glucose-6-phosphate transporter is called GSD-Ib. A defect in either of these two functions will result in deficient activity of glucose-6-phosphatase, and hence lack of release of glucose derived from either glycogen breakdown or from gluconeogenesis. This results in severe hypoglycemia which occurs early in the postprandial period, about 3–4 hours after a meal for young children. During the attempt to generate glucose, the glucose-6-phosphate that cannot be released will be metabolized through the glycolytic pathway resulting in accumulation of pyruvate, and hence, increase in the levels of lactate and acetyl-CoA; which results in the synthesis of triglycerides and cholesterol. Both fructose and galactose cannot be metabolized into glucose but contribute to the accumulation of glucose-6-phosphate, which results in a conversion of ATP to ADP, and then to AMP that leads to increased production of uric acid. Thus, the characteristic biochemical profile of GSD-I consists of hypoglycemia, lactic acidosis, hyperuricemia, hypertriglyceridemia, hypercholesterolemia, and hepatic steatosis in addition to hepatic glycogen accumulation.

Clinical Manifestations Clinical manifestations of GSD-I usually appear in the first 6 months of life (mostly at the time of weaning from breastfeeding), and the infant comes to medical attention either because of marked hepatomegaly or symptoms of hypoglycemia (especially when they

Table 25.4 Signs and symptoms of GSD-I

GSD Ia: deficiency of glucose-6-phosphatase (catalytic subunit)
GSD Ib: deficiency of glucose-6-phosphate transporter (translocase subunit)
Impairment of glycogenolysis and gluconeogenesis
Symptoms:
Hepatomegaly; nephromegaly
Hypoglycemia: early and severe in infancy
Lactic acidosis
Hypertriglyceridemia
Hypercholesterolemia
Hyperuricemia
Short stature, doll-like face
Neutropenia (Ib): Increased propensity of infections and chronic inflammatory bowel disease causing severe diarrhea and malnutrition, periodontal disease, increased risk of autoimmune hypothyroidism

sleep through the night). Untreated, the children have short stature and a doll-like face. There is pronounced hepatomegaly and nephromegaly, but the spleen and heart are of normal size (Table 25.4).

Patients with GSD-Ib have the same biochemical abnormalities as described above for patients with GSD-Ia. The glucose-6-phosphate in the ER is also the precursor for reducing equivalents in the neutrophils, which are essential for the generation of the oxidative burst and the killing of bacteria. Therefore, patients with GSD-Ib have additionally variable neutropenia, and impaired neutrophil function with reduced chemotaxis and killing. This results in increased propensity for infections such as with *Staphylococci*, and for chronic inflammatory bowel disease, which can lead to severe diarrhea and malnutrition.

Historically, the diagnosis of GSD-I was typically made by lack of glucose-6-phosphatase enzyme activity in a liver biopsy, in addition to accumulation of hepatic glycogen and lipids. In GSD-Ib, the deficient activity is only present in fresh tissue, and it normalizes with freezing and thawing. In GSD-Ia, the activity is deficient in fresh, frozen and thawed tissues. This diagnostic method is now replaced by sequencing of the genes *G6PC* and *SLC37A4*. Many genetic variants have been reported in both genes.

Complications Several complications are noted over time. The main long-term complications of GSD-I are renal and hepatic. The kidney has elevated renal blood flow and hyperfiltration, and patients can develop focal segmental glomerulosclerosis leading to renal failure. Once significant proteinuria begins (>1 g/day), the disease progresses, and patients may develop renal failure. Many patients require dialysis or renal transplantation. There is a high risk for kidney stones. Hypercalciuria and hypocitraturia are contributing risk factors. Rare renal complications such as renal amyloidosis can occur particularly in GSD-Ib.

The liver shows a tendency to form hepatic adenomas that may cause acute intrahepatic bleeding. Hepatic adenomas tend to regress with improved treatment, yet there are factors outside of metabolic control. There is a substantial risk for hepatic carcinoma, most commonly developing in the third or fourth decade, although earlier cases are known. Other complications include pancreatitis (severe hypertriglyceridemia), pulmonary hypertension, gout (severe hyperuricemia), and significant osteoporosis with pathological fractures.

Some patients have a von Willebrand disease-like defect which causes platelet dysfunction, and can result in nose bleeds, easy bruising, menorrhagia, and increased risk of bleeding during surgeries. Polycystic ovaries can occur in women; however, many women have had successful pregnancies.

Management Patients with GSD-I require good glycemic control, along with additional medications to avoid metabolic complications [5]. The primary goal of nutritional management of GSD-I is to maintain blood glucose above a concentration that invokes glycogen breakdown and gluconeogenesis, thus preventing the abnormal biochemical response. Complex carbohydrates should be given to maintain plasma glucose concentrations above 70–80 mg/dL. Good glycemic control will result in near normalization of lactate concentrations and substantial reduction in triglyceride and uric acid concentrations. During planned interventions such as surgery with risk for bleeding, ensuring that patients are in good metabolic control is necessary because some patients with GSD-I have platelet dysfunction. Patients should be admitted prior to the procedure and receive intravenous glucose. For acute bleeding, desmopressin acetate (DDAVP®

Ferring Pharmaceuticals, Parsippany-Troy Hills, NJ) or a fibrinolytic inhibitor, such as ε-aminocaproic acid (Amicar®, Pfizer Pharmaceutical, NY), can be used.

Overtreatment is as challenging as undertreatment. Overtreatment can lead to increased lactate, uric acid, and other biomarkers due to an increased concentration of the substrate glucose-6-phosphate. Overtreatment can also result in hypoglycemia due to development of hyperinsulinism. Therefore, routine monitoring of the laboratory biomarkers is key in the management of patients with GSD-I.

Maintenance of Glucose Concentrations To maintain normal levels, continuous supply of glucose needs to be provided. This can be achieved with frequent meals throughout the day, and, at night, either continuous gastric tube feeding or feedings in the middle of the night. Acute hypoglycemia should be treated with oral or intravenous glucose, and patients should be provided with an emergency room letter, and wear a medical alert bracelet (or similar) to warn the healthcare providers of the risk of life-threatening hypoglycemia. Dislodgement of a gastric feeding tube should be suspected if there is unforeseen hypoglycemia.

In infancy, overnight fasting is avoided by feeding infants every 3–4 hours or by overnight gastric feeding using nasogastric or surgically placed gastrostomy tubes. Introduction to solids by age 4–6 months of age includes cereals, vegetables, and meat.

Uncooked cornstarch is introduced between 9 and 12 months when children have attained sufficient pancreatic maturation. The complex nature of uncooked cornstarch requires extended time to digest by human pancreatic amylase, and hence results in a prolonged absorptive phase, often up to 4–6 hours. Dosing of uncooked cornstarch has to be gradually advanced over several months to allow for the pancreas to adjust to this more-difficult-to-digest carbohydrate. Ultimately, a regimen of uncooked cornstarch every 3–4 hours and up to 6 hours, along with meals and snacks (provided an hour before the cornstarch starts to wane), can achieve good glycemic control. For younger children, pancreatic enzymes such as pancrelipase (lipase, protease, and amylase) can be used intermittently, in conjunction with cornstarch. Foods containing galactose, sucrose, fructose, and lactose should be avoided. Limiting dietary fat intake can help reduce hypertriglyceridemia. These dietary restrictions can cause deficiency of vitamin D and calcium, and supplements are recommended (Chap. 26).

Medications may be required to control excessive hypertriglyceridemia and, therefore, the use of fibrates and HMG-CoA reductase inhibitors is recommended for some patients. Most patients who develop substantial hyperuricemia from insufficiently controlled dietary measures should be treated with allopurinol or similar uric acid-reducing agents. For patients with GSD-Ib, neutropenia will respond to treatment with granulocyte-colony stimulating factor (G-CSF). The dose should be carefully controlled as massive splenomegaly with hypersplenism has been reported with high doses. Careful monitoring for infections and use of antibiotics with intracellular killing should be instituted when concern for invasive infections arises. Severe inflammatory bowel disease may require management similar to that of the medical management of Crohn's disease, although fistulas do not tend to occur. Vitamin E use has been reported to improve neutrophil function. The glucose-lowering SGLT2 inhibitor, empagliflozin (or EMPA; used for type 2 diabetes), can be used to treat neutropenia and neutrophil dysfunction in GSD-Ib without causing symptomatic hypoglycemia [6]. The incidences of hepatic adenoma/carcinoma and renal focal segmental glomerulosclerosis are reduced with strict life-long chronic treatment. For patients with a tendency toward proteinuria, treatment with angiotensin-converting enzyme (ACE) inhibitors is advised. It is believed that the secondary biochemical alterations of high lactate and triglycerides strongly contribute to these long-term complications. Thus, the management of adults with GSD-I should not solely focus on the easily achieved avoidance of hypoglycemia but rather on the global control of biochemical abnormalities with normalization of lactate and triglyceride concentrations.

Table 25.5 Monitoring of the adult patient with GSD-I

Metabolic markers
Lactate: < 4 μmol
Glucose
Cholesterol, triglycerides
Liver
Transaminases (AST, ALT)
Hepatic adenomas, fatty steatosis, hepatic carcinoma
MRI
Kidney
Blood pressure
Glomerular filtration rate
Proteinuria
Stones: calcuria, citraturia
Bone
DEXA scan
25-OH vitamin D
Gout
Uric acid <8 mg/dL

Finally, indications of liver transplantation include hepatic carcinoma, an increase in size and/or number of adenomas, medically intractable complications, or poor quality of life with difficult to maintain medical treatment. However, the renal disease can progress in these patients, and in some instances, a combined liver and kidney transplantation may be needed.

Monitoring of treatment of GSD-I includes the measurement of glucose and lactate, cholesterol, triglyceride, and uric acid concentrations. Use of a continuous glucose monitoring system is a safe and reliable method to monitor and maintain normal glucose concentrations with concurrent dietary adjustments [7]. Annual imaging studies of the liver, preferably by MRI, as well as annual evaluation of kidney function by measuring urinary protein, calcium, and citrate is recommended. Osteoporosis monitoring includes periodic DEXA scans for measurement of bone mineral content and monitoring of calcium and vitamin D status (Table 25.5) [5, 7–11].

25.2.1.2 Glycogen Storage Diseases Type VI

Biochemistry GSD-VI is caused by a deficiency of the hepatic phosphorylase kinase enzyme, which prevents the breakdown of glycogen to glucose in the liver. Notably, the phosphorylase activity is usually only partially deficient and hepatic gluconeogenesis is intact.

Clinical Manifestations GSD-VI represents a spectrum of involvement with hypoglycemia, hyperlipidemia, and hyperketosis. Patients usually present in infancy or early childhood with hepatomegaly, distended abdomen, and growth retardation [12]. There is a variable clinical course. Some patients develop significant hepatomegaly and ketosis, recurrent severe hypoglycemia, and failure to thrive. Patients with significant liver disease progression can develop progressive liver fibrosis, and an increased risk of liver cirrhosis [13–15].

Management Treatment is similar to GSD-III. Small, frequent feeds with uncooked cornstarch can reduce hypoglycemia. Since gluconeogenesis is intact, a high protein diet is recommended. Routine screening and long-term follow up of liver status is recommended in all patients with GSD-VI [13, 16].

25.2.2 Glycogen Storage Diseases Involving Both Liver and Muscle

25.2.2.1 Glycogen Storage Disease Type III: Debranching Enzyme Deficiency

Biochemistry The debranching enzyme has two enzymatic activities: a glycosyltransferase and an α-1,6 glycosidase. Both these enzymatic activities are required for the complete breakdown (catalytic activity) of glycogen to glucose. Based on the tissue-specific nature of debranching enzyme deficiency, there are two subtypes of GSD-III. In GSD-IIIa (85% of patients), the enzyme is deficient in both liver and muscle, whereas in GSD-IIIb (15% of patients), the enzyme is only deficient in liver but is normal in muscle. In GSD-IIIb, the preservation of the muscle enzyme activity is caused by genetic variants in exon 2 where a muscle promoter allows for translation using a secondary start site after the genetic variation.

Clinical Manifestations The initial presentation of GSD-III is similar to that of GSD-I with hypoglycemia, hepatomegaly, growth retardation, and elevated triglycerides and cholesterol, but the lactate and uric acid concentrations tend to be normal. In addition, patients with GSD-IIIa present with variable skeletal myopathy, cardiomyopathy, elevated transaminases, and elevated creatine kinase. The hypoglycemia is usually associated with fasting ketosis. Symptoms of liver disease occur from the damage to hepatocytes from accumulated abnormal glycogen. Liver fibrosis, cirrhosis, hepatic carcinoma, and hepatic adenomas can develop [17]. Other severe complications in adulthood include progressive myopathy and cardiomyopathy. Polycystic ovaries are noted in women, but fertility is not affected.

Management Initial treatment of GSD-III is similar to that of GSD-I with frequent meals and supplemental uncooked cornstarch. Continuous glucose monitoring can be effective to monitor hypoglycemia in symptomatic patients and to detect asymptomatic hypoglycemia in patients [7]. Since gluconeogenesis is not impaired in GSD-III, foods with galactose and fructose need not be avoided. Patients may have a progressive cardiomyopathy, and must be specifically evaluated for cardiac conduction defects and arrhythmias. A high protein diet is indicated to stimulate gluconeogenesis, and has been reported to improve cardiomyopathy and myopathy. Similar to GSD-I, liver transplantation will not improve the clinical manifestations in patients with GSD III, because there will be progression of muscle disease and life-threatening cardiac arrhythmias. Additionally, cardiac transplantation may be needed in some instances [7, 17–21]. Regular physical therapy evaluations of muscle strength and endurance, and supervised, individualized exercise programs are recommended over time.

25.2.2.2 Glycogen Storage Diseases Type IX

Biochemistry GSD-IX is caused by a deficiency of the phosphorylase kinase enzyme (PhK). During the fasted state, the release of glucagon and epinephrine activates PhK to facilitate the phosphorylation of glycogen phosphorylase, which helps to metabolize glycogen to glucose-1-phosphate. Deficiency of PhK causes glycogen accumulation, mainly in the liver. PhK is a complex, hetero-tetrameric enzyme comprised of four subunits—α, β, γ, and δ. The γ subunit provides the catalytic activity, which is regulated by phosphorylation of α and β subunits. The δ subunit is calmodulin. There are several tissue-specific isoforms encoded by different genes for each subunit [22, 23]. The gene *PHKA1* encodes the muscle-specific isoform of the α1 PhK subunit, and is associated with the muscle subtype of GSD IX (GSD IX α1). The gene *PHKB* encodes the muscle and liver isoform of the β PhK subunit, and is associated with a muscle and liver GSD IX subtype (GSD IX β). The genes *PHKA2* and *PHKG2* encode the liver-specific isoforms of the α2 and γ2 PhK subunits, respectively, and are associated with the liver GSD IX subtypes *PHKA2* GSD IX (GSD IX α2) and *PHKG2* (GSD IX γ2). The most common subtype is the X-linked variant in the *PHKA2* gene (GSD IX α2). The most severe subtype is GSD IX γ2 (pathogenic variants in the PHKG2 gene).

Clinical Manifestations The enzymatic deficiency in patients with GSD IX prevent the adequate breakdown of glycogen into glucose, leading to hypoglycemia, increased glycogen in the liver, and associated hepatomegaly, growth delay, and elevated liver enzymes [13, 24, 25]. Presenting symptoms generally improve during puberty. However, in GSD IX types α2 and γ2, deficiency of liver PhK leads to severe, progressive liver disease. In one study, about 80% of patients with GSD IX γ2 received a liver biopsy of which 96% of pathology reports identified liver fibrosis and/or cirrhosis [26]. Ultimately, individuals with GSD IX types α2 and γ2 are at high risk for developing severe progressive liver disease, advancing from liver fibrosis, cirrhosis, to liver failure, and death [27, 28]. The subtypes of GSD IX with muscle involvement are very rare, and the onset of clinical features is from childhood to adulthood. Patients typically experience exercise intolerance, myalgia, muscle cramps, myoglobinuria, and progressive muscle weakness.

Management The nutrition management of individuals with GSD IX emphasizes high protein meals with supplements of uncooked cornstarch. High protein intake provides repletion of protein precursors necessary for maintaining gluconeogenesis. Dietary modification provides symptomatic improvement of hypoglycemic episodes but does not address the continued buildup of glycogen in the liver, which is the underlying pathophysiology of the disease. In patients with GSD IX $\gamma 2$, persistent liver glycogen accumulation leads to progressive liver fibrosis, elevated liver enzymes, and decline in liver function, potentially necessitating liver transplant [13, 16, 25, 29]. In patients with muscle subtypes, regular physical therapy evaluations and interventions based on physical status are advised.

25.2.2.3 Glycogen Storage Disease Type IV: Branching Enzyme Deficiency

Biochemistry GSD-IV is caused by genetic variants in the *GBE1* gene, leading to a deficiency in the glycogen branching enzyme (GBE). As a result, an abnormal form of glycogen resembling the structures of amylopectin or polyglucosan accumulates in the body.

Clinical Manifestations GSD-IV is a heterogeneous disorder with hepatic and neuromuscular forms, and each form has a wide clinical spectrum. The hepatic forms include two broad subtypes, classic and non-progressive. The classic progressive hepatic subtype presents in the first 18 months of life with failure to thrive, hepatosplenomegaly progressing to severe liver disease, cirrhosis, hepatocellular carcinoma, end-stage liver failure, and death by 5 years of age [30, 31]. The non-progressive hepatic subtype presents with hepatomegaly, liver dysfunction, myopathy, and hypotonia, but is unlikely to progress to severe liver disease. There is an overlap between manifestations within the two forms of GSD-IV, and long-term studies are needed to better understand the clinical course.

The neuromuscular form of GSD-IV includes four subtypes based on age of onset. The four subtypes include perinatal, congenital, childhood, and adult. Patients with the perinatal form present in utero with fetal akinesia, decreased fetal movements, polyhydramnios, and fetal hydrops. Patients with the congenital form present in the newborn period with hypotonia, muscle weakness, respiratory distress, and dilated cardiomyopathy. For patients with the perinatal and congenital form, death usually occurs in early infancy. Patients with the childhood form have a more variable presentation and course, commonly presenting with muscle weakness, cardiomyopathy, and neuropathy in adolescence, progressing either as a mild disease or to a more progressive course leading to death. Patients with the adult form, also known as adult polyglucosan body disease (APBD), present with isolated myopathy and/or diffuse central and peripheral nervous system dysfunction accompanied by accumulation of polyglucosan bodies in the nervous system. Neuronal symptoms include neurogenic bladder, leukodystrophy, and mild cognitive impairment.

Management The diagnosis is made by the identification of biallelic pathogenic variants in the GBE1 gene. In certain cases, GBE activity is measured in liver, muscle, leukocytes, nerves, or skin fibroblasts. Histopathology can also support the diagnosis with markedly enlarged hepatocytes that contain periodic acid-Schiff (PAS)-positive and diastase-resistant polyglucosan bodies. There is no definitive treatment for GSD-IV. Patients with the neuromuscular form require symptomatic treatment for gait abnormalities and bladder dysfunction. Patients with the progressive hepatic subtype will require liver transplantation for cirrhosis and end-stage liver failure. Notably, the extrahepatic manifestations such as cardiomyopathy and nervous system dysfunction may manifest, even after liver transplantation [30–33].

25.2.3 Selected Glycogen Storage Disease Primarily Involving the Muscle

25.2.3.1 Glycogen Storage Diseases Type II (Pompe Disease, Acid α-1,4 Glucosidase Deficiency)

Biochemistry GSD-II (Pompe disease) is caused by a genetic variant in the *GAA* gene, which results in the deficiency of the enzyme acid alpha glucosidase. This enzyme is required to hydrolyze glycogen to glucose, and its absence results in glycogen accumulation within lysosomes. With disease progression, excess glycogen leaks out of the lysosome and accumulates in the cytoplasm as well. Laboratory values such as liver transaminases (AST and ALT), creatine kinase, and urine glucose tetrasaccharide (urine Glc4) are often elevated, and these are used as biomarkers to monitor disease progression.

Clinical Manifestations GSD-II is now recognized as a multi-systemic disorder affecting skeletal and smooth muscles, cardiac, respiratory, and the nervous systems. Due to a wide clinical spectrum, it is broadly classified as infantile and late-onset Pompe disease [34]. In the classic infantile form, infants present with hypotonia, generalized muscle weakness with a "floppy baby" appearance, developmental delay, a significant hypertrophic cardiomyopathy, macroglossia, and feeding difficulties within the first few days to weeks of life. If untreated, these infants die in the first 2 years due to progressive cardiorespiratory failure.

Patients with the late-onset form can present in the first year of life or as late as the sixth decade. These patients present with progressive proximal and distal skeletal muscle weakness with reduced exercise tolerance. If untreated, these patients have significant gait impairment (requiring ambulatory devices), severe respiratory insufficiency (requiring artificial ventilation), and oropharyngeal muscle weakness [35, 36]. Other complications include cerebral aneurysms, aortic abnormalities, and hemorrhages (brain), arrhythmias (cardiac), peripheral neuropathy and paresthesias (nervous system), chronic bowel disorders (gastrointestinal and genitourinary).

Management GSD-II is now part of the recommended uniform screening panel (RUSP) for newborns in the United States. Newborn screening (NBS) for Pompe disease has been initiated in over 30 states [37]. Across the disease spectrum, early diagnosis is crucial to allow for timely intervention. Blood-based assays to detect the deficient (or absent) enzyme activity and genetic testing are widely used to confirm the diagnosis.

The only definitive treatment for GSD-II is enzyme replacement therapy (ERT), which includes biweekly or weekly intravenous infusion of alglucosidase alfa, a recombinant acid α-glucosidase (rhGAA) or avalglucosidase alfa. ERT has increased the survival rate of the infantile-form and improved morbidity in late-onset forms of the disease. Other adjunctive treatment options include dietary modifications with a high protein diet, submaximal aerobic exercises, and respiratory muscle training (RMT). Night-time ventilatory support in patients with a late-onset form improves the quality of life and is beneficial during periods of respiratory decompensation. Gene therapy is another novel approach to treat patients, and clinical trials are ongoing [34].

25.2.3.2 Glycogen Storage Disease Type V (Muscle Phosphorylase Deficiency, McArdle Disease)

Biochemistry During exercise, the enzyme myophosphorylase promotes muscle glycogenolysis to provide glucose as an energy source to the muscle. In GSD-V, there is a deficiency of myophosphorylase as a result of a genetic defect in the *PYGM* gene, which causes glycogen accumulation in the skeletal muscle.

Clinical Manifestations The clinical onset of GSD-V is heterogenous, but primarily occurs in the first decade of life. Patients present with exercise-induced muscle fatigue, pain, and skeletal muscle damage, which lead to myoglobinuria and renal failure.

Management Diagnosis requires the identification of biallelic pathogenic variants in the *PYGM* gene. For certain cases with negative genetic testing or single allele pathogenic variants, enzymatic assay can be done. Patients have found symptomatic relief with lifestyle and dietary modifications. Moderate intensity aerobic exercise, oral sucrose ingestion prior to exercise, ramipril, low dose creatine, and a carbohydrate-rich diet have proven beneficial. Symptoms often precipitate from high intensity activity, such as sprinting or carrying heavy loads and/or less intense but sustained activity, such as climbing stairs or walking uphill. Pre-exercise ingestion of carbohydrates prevents exercise intolerance as skeletal muscle is able to take advantage of increased glucose concentrations in the blood [38]. During exercise, patients should rest when they start becoming symptomatic. After a few minutes of rest, some patients may experience the "second wind" phenomenon and are able to continue the activity. This is a characteristic feature of GSD V. To date, there is no cure for GSD-V. There have been promising trials of gene therapy in GSD-V animal models [39, 40].

25.3 Summary

In glycogen storage diseases (GSDs), there is excessive glycogen build-up in the muscle, liver, and/or heart. This leads to a number of clinical manifestations with a variable spectrum. The GSDs are broadly classified based on the type of tissues involved. Types I, VI, and IX (subtypes α2 and γ2) primarily affect the liver. Types II, V, and VII primarily affect the muscle. Type a III, IV, and IX (subtype β) can affect both the liver and muscle. There are over 15 types of GSDs. Nutrition plays a key in the management guidelines for all GSDs.

Acknowledgments Thank you to Johan Van Hove of Children's Hospital of Colorado for his contributions to this chapter's content, including all figures, from the first Edition of Nutrition Management of Inherited Metabolic Diseases. We also thank Surekha Pendyal, MSc, MEd, RD, Ghada Hijazi, MD, MRCPCH, FCCMG, and Rebecca L. Koch, PhD, RDN, LDN for providing their expertise during the final revision of this chapter.

References

1. Bonnefont JP, Specola NB, Vassault A, Lombes A, Ogier H, de Klerk JB, et al. The fasting test in paediatrics: application to the diagnosis of pathological hypo- and hyperketotic states. Eur J Pediatr. 1990;150(2):80–5.
2. Costa CC, de Almeida IT, Jakobs C, Poll-The BT, Duran M. Dynamic changes of plasma acylcarnitine levels induced by fasting and sunflower oil challenge test in children. Pediatr Res. 1999;46(4):440–4.
3. van Veen MR, van Hasselt PM, de Sain-van der Velden MG, Verhoeven N, Hofstede FC, de Koning TJ, et al. Metabolic profiles in children during fasting. Pediatrics. 2011;127(4):e1021–7.
4. Kishnani P, Chen Y. Disorders of carbohydrate metabolism. In: Pyeritz RE, Korf BR, Grody WW, editors. Emery and Rimoin's principles and practice of medical genetics and genomics. 7th ed. Academic Press; 2021. p. 105–56.
5. Kishnani PS, Austin SL, Abdenur JE, Arn P, Bali DS, Boney A, et al. Diagnosis and management of glycogen storage disease type I: a practice guideline of the American College of Medical Genetics and Genomics. Genet Med. 2014;16(11):e1.
6. Wortmann SB, Van Hove JLK, Derks TGJ, Chevalier N, Knight V, Koller A, et al. Treating neutropenia and neutrophil dysfunction in glycogen storage disease type Ib with an SGLT2 inhibitor. Blood. 2020;136(9):1033–43.
7. Herbert M, Pendyal S, Rairikar M, Halaby C, Benjamin RW, Kishnani PS. Role of continuous glucose monitoring in the management of glycogen storage disorders. J Inherit Metab Dis. 2018;41(6):917–27.
8. Boers SJ, Visser G, Smit PG, Fuchs SA. Liver transplantation in glycogen storage disease type I. Orphanet J Rare Dis. 2014;9:47.
9. Jun HS, Weinstein DA, Lee YM, Mansfield BC, Chou JY. Molecular mechanisms of neutrophil dysfunction in glycogen storage disease type Ib. Blood. 2014;123(18):2843–53.
10. Chen YT, Van Hove JL. Renal involvement in type I glycogen storage disease. Adv Nephrol Necker Hosp. 1995;24:357–65.
11. Franco LM, Krishnamurthy V, Bali D, Weinstein DA, Arn P, Clary B, et al. Hepatocellular carcinoma in glycogen storage disease type Ia: a case series. J Inherit Metab Dis. 2005;28(2):153–62.
12. Koeberl Y, et al. Glycogen storage diseases. In: Scriver C, Beaudet AL, Sly WS, Valle D, Childs BH, Kinzler KW, et al., editors. The online metabolic and molecular bases of inherited disease. New York: McGraw-Hill; 2002.
13. Roscher A, Patel J, Hewson S, Nagy L, Feigenbaum A, Kronick J, et al. The natural history of glycogen storage disease types VI and IX: long-term outcome from the largest metabolic center in Canada. Mol Genet Metab. 2014;113(3):171–6.
14. Manzia TM, Angelico R, Toti L, Cillis A, Ciano P, Orlando G, et al. Glycogen storage disease type Ia and VI associated with hepatocellular carcinoma: two case reports. Transplant Proc. 2011;43(4):1181–3.
15. Ogawa A, Ogawa E, Yamamoto S, Fukuda T, Sugie H, Kohno Y. Case of glycogen storage disease type VI (phosphorylase deficiency) complicated by focal nodular hyperplasia. Pediatr Int. 2010;52(3):e150–3.
16. Kishnani PS, Goldstein J, Austin SL, Arn P, Bachrach B, Bali DS, et al. Diagnosis and management of

glycogen storage diseases type VI and IX: a clinical practice resource of the American College of Medical Genetics and Genomics (ACMG). Genet Med. 2019;21(4):772–89.
17. Korlimarla A, et al. Hepatic manifestations in glycogen storage disease type III. Curr Pathobiol Rep. 2018;6(4):233–40.
18. Kishnani PS, Austin SL, Arn P, Bali DS, Boney A, Case LE, et al. Glycogen storage disease type III diagnosis and management guidelines. Genet Med. 2010;12(7):446–63.
19. Slonim AE, Coleman RA, Moses WS. Myopathy and growth failure in debrancher enzyme deficiency: improvement with high-protein nocturnal enteral therapy. J Pediatr. 1984;105(6):906–11.
20. Demo E, Frush D, Gottfried M, Koepke J, Boney A, Bali D, et al. Glycogen storage disease type III-hepatocellular carcinoma a long-term complication? J Hepatol. 2007;46(3):492–8.
21. Shen JJ, Chen YT. Molecular characterization of glycogen storage disease type III. Curr Mol Med. 2002;2(2):167–75.
22. Brushia RJ, Walsh DA. Phosphorylase kinase: the complexity of its regulation is reflected in the complexity of its structure. Front Biosci. 1999;4:D618–41.
23. Venien-Bryan C, Jonic S, Skamnaki V, Brown N, Bischler N, Oikonomakos NG, et al. The structure of phosphorylase kinase holoenzyme at 9.9 angstroms resolution and location of the catalytic subunit and the substrate glycogen phosphorylase. Structure. 2009;17(1):117–27.
24. Willems PJ, Gerver WJ, Berger R, Fernandes J. The natural history of liver glycogenosis due to phosphorylase kinase deficiency: a longitudinal study of 41 patients. Eur J Pediatr. 1990;149(4):268–71.
25. Li C, Huang L, Tian L, Chen J, Li S, Yang Z. PHKG2 mutation spectrum in glycogen storage disease type IXc: a case report and review of the literature. J Pediatr Endocrinol Metab. 2018;31(3):331–8.
26. Fernandes SA, Cooper GE, Gibson RA, Kishnani PS. Benign or not benign? Deep phenotyping of liver glycogen storage disease IX. Mol Genet Metab. 2020;131(3):299–305.
27. Burwinkel B, Tanner MS, Kilimann MW. Phosphorylase kinase deficient liver glycogenosis: progression to cirrhosis in infancy associated with PHKG2 mutations (H144Y and L225R). J Med Genet. 2000;37(5):376–7.
28. Bali DS, Goldstein JL, Fredrickson K, Rehder C, Boney A, Austin S, et al. Variability of disease spectrum in children with liver phosphorylase kinase deficiency caused by mutations in the PHKG2 gene. Mol Genet Metab. 2014;111(3):309–13.
29. Herbert M, Goldstein JL, Rehder C, Austin S, Kishnani PS, Bali DS. Phosphorylase kinase deficiency. In: Adam MP, Ardinger HH, Pagon RA, Wallace SE, Bean LJH, Mirzaa G, et al., editors. GeneReviews((R)). Seattle: University of Washington,Seattle; 1993.
30. Magoulas PL, El-Hattab AW. Glycogen storage disease type IV. In: Adam MP, Ardinger HH, Pagon RA, Wallace SE, Bean LJH, Mirzaa G, et al., editors. GeneReviews((R)). Seattle: University of Washington, Seattle;1993.
31. Szymanska E, Szymanska S, Truszkowska G, Ciara E, Pronicki M, Shin YS, et al. Variable clinical presentation of glycogen storage disease type IV: from severe hepatosplenomegaly to cardiac insufficiency. Some discrepancies in genetic and biochemical abnormalities. Arch Med Sci. 2018;14(1):237–47.
32. Davis MK, Weinstein DA. Liver transplantation in children with glycogen storage disease: controversies and evaluation of the risk/benefit of this procedure. Pediatr Transplant. 2008;12(2):137–45.
33. Matern D, Starzl TE, Arnaout W, Barnard J, Bynon JS, Dhawan A, et al. Liver transplantation for glycogen storage disease types I, III, and IV. Eur J Pediatr. 1999;158 Suppl 2:S43–8.
34. Disease AWGoMoP, Kishnani PS, Steiner RD, Bali D, Berger K, Byrne BJ, et al. Pompe disease diagnosis and management guideline. Genet Med. 2006;8(5):267–88.
35. Chan J, Desai AK, Kazi ZB, Corey K, Austin S, Hobson-Webb LD, et al. The emerging phenotype of late-onset Pompe disease: a systematic literature review. Mol Genet Metab. 2017;120(3):163–72.
36. Wokke JH, Escolar DM, Pestronk A, Jaffe KM, Carter GT, van den Berg LH, et al. Clinical features of late-onset Pompe disease: a prospective cohort study. Muscle Nerve. 2008;38(4):1236–45.
37. Kronn DF, Day-Salvatore D, Hwu WL, Jones SA, Nakamura K, Okuyama T, et al. Management of confirmed newborn-screened patients with Pompe disease across the disease spectrum. Pediatrics. 2017;140(Suppl 1):S24–45.
38. Vissing J, Haller RG. The effect of oral sucrose on exercise tolerance in patients with McArdle's disease. N Engl J Med. 2003;349(26):2503–9.
39. Nogales-Gadea G, Santalla A, Brull A, de Luna N, Lucia A, Pinos T. The pathogenomics of McArdle diseaseDOUBLEHYPHENgenes, enzymes, models, and therapeutic implications. J Inherit Metab Dis. 2015;38(2):221–30.
40. McKusick V, et al. Glycogen storage disease V. Online Mendelian Inheritance in Man (OMIM). 2015.

Nutrition Management of Glycogen Storage Disease

26

Mary Sowa

Contents

M. Sowa (✉)
Division of Medical Genetics, CHOC Children's,
Orange, CA, USA
e-mail: MSowa@choc.org

L. E. Bernstein et al. (eds.), *Nutrition Management of Inherited Metabolic Diseases*,
https://doi.org/10.1007/978-3-030-94510-7_26

Core Messages for GSD Type I

- Glycogen storage disease type I is characterized by fasting hypoglycemia and elevated lactic acid, uric acid and triglycerides. Patients with GSD type Ib are also at risk of neutropenia and inflammatory bowel disease.
- Nutrition management of GSD type I includes providing supplemental uncooked cornstarch as a source of glucose, avoidance of dietary galactose and fructose, and a moderate restriction of fat. Vitamin and mineral supplementation are needed to prevent deficiencies.
- Frequent home monitoring of blood glucose and adjustments in the diet are needed to prevent hypo and hyperglycemia.
- Glycosade® is a cornstarch derivative that may extend fasting time.

26.1 GSD Background

Glycogen storage diseases (GSD) are inherited metabolic disorders in the synthesis or degradation of glycogen. Symptoms may appear at any age. GSDs can be categorized based on the organs affected, primarily liver and/or muscle tissue (Table 26.1) [1, 2]. In liver GSDs, hypoglycemia is the primary symptom caused by impaired mobilization of glucose during fasting. In muscle GSDs, muscle weakness and exercise intolerance are primary symptoms caused by the inability to utilize muscle glycogen stores [3]. The focus of this chapter is the nutrition management of GSD Type Ia and b and Type IIIa.

26.2 GSD Type I Background

Glycogen storage disease (GSD) type I, also called Von Gierke disease, results from a deficiency of glucose-6-phosphatase (Type Ia) or

Table 26.1 Glycogen-storage diseases

Type	Defective enzyme	Organ affected	Glycogen in the affected organ	Clinical features
I Von Gierke	Glucose 6-phosphatase or transport system	Liver and kidney	Increased amount; normal structure	Massive enlargement of the liver. Failure to thrive. Severe hypoglycemia, ketosis, hyperuricemia, hyperlipidemia
II Pompe	α-1,4-Glucosidase (lysosomal)	All organs	Massive increase in amount; normal structure.	Cardiorespiratory failure causes death, usually before age 2
III Cori	Amylo-1,6-glucosidase (debranching enzyme)	Muscle and liver	Increased amount; short outer branches.	Hepatomegaly, less severe hypoglycemia but may have more severe ketoacidosis without high lactate or uric acid. Increased AST; normal blood lactate and uric acid
IV Andersen	Branching enzyme (α-1,4 - α-1,6)	Liver and spleen	Normal amount; very long outer branches.	Progressive cirrhosis of the liver. Liver failure causes death, usually before age 2
V McArdle	Phosphorylase	Muscle	Moderately increased amount; normal structure	Limited ability to perform strenuous exercise because of painful muscle cramps Otherwise, patient is clinically normal
VI Hers	Hepatic phosphorylase deficiency	Liver	Increased amount.	Less severe although some patients experience significant hypoglycemia, usually occurring during fasting with hyperketosis; blood lactate is normal but may be elevated postprandially
VII	Phosphofructo-kinase	Muscle	Increased amount; normal structure.	Like type V
VIII	Phosphorylase kinase	Liver	Increased amount; normal structure	Mild liver enlargement. Mild hypoglycemia

Adapted from Berg et al. [1] and Kishnani et al. [2]
Note: Types I through VII are inherited as autosomal recessive. Type VIII is sex-linked

glucose-6-phosphatase translocase (Type Ib), preventing the production of glucose from glycogen stores during periods of fasting leading to severe hypoglycemia, if untreated [4]. The majority (80%) of individuals affected with GSD type I have type Ia and 20% of individuals have type Ib. [4] The primary clinical symptoms and laboratory abnormalities of both types include hypoglycemia, hepatomegaly, failure to thrive, short stature, lactic acidosis, hypertriglyceridemia, and hyperuricemia [4]. Individuals with Type Ib can also develop neutropenia and are at high risk for inflammatory bowel disease (IBD) [4]. Guidelines for the diagnosis and management of GSD type I were published in 2014 [4]. The goals of nutrition management of patients with GSD Type I are to maintain glucose concentrations between 75 and 100 mg/dL (4.2 and 5.6 mmol/L), to prevent or correct metabolic derangements and to provide optimal nutrition to support growth and development [4] (Fig. 26.1).

26.3 Nutrition Management GSD Type I

26.3.1 Diet Principles for Infants

The primary principle of nutrition management is to prevent low blood glucose and elevated lactic acid concentrations [4, 5]. Before the age of 6 months, the infant with GSD type I may need to feed as frequently as every 1.5–2 hours. After 9 months, cornstarch therapy can be introduced (Sect. 26.3.5). Recommended formulas for infants with GSD type I do not contain sucrose (fructose) or lactose. A soy formula without sucrose (i.e., Prosobee®) is typically recommended, but if this is not tolerated, a sucrose-free hydrolyzed or elemental formula (i.e., Nutramigen®, Pregestimil®, Neocate Infant®) is also appropriate (Table 26.2). Feedings of glucose polymers are not recommended to avoid spikes in blood sugar and excessive production of insulin, which can increase

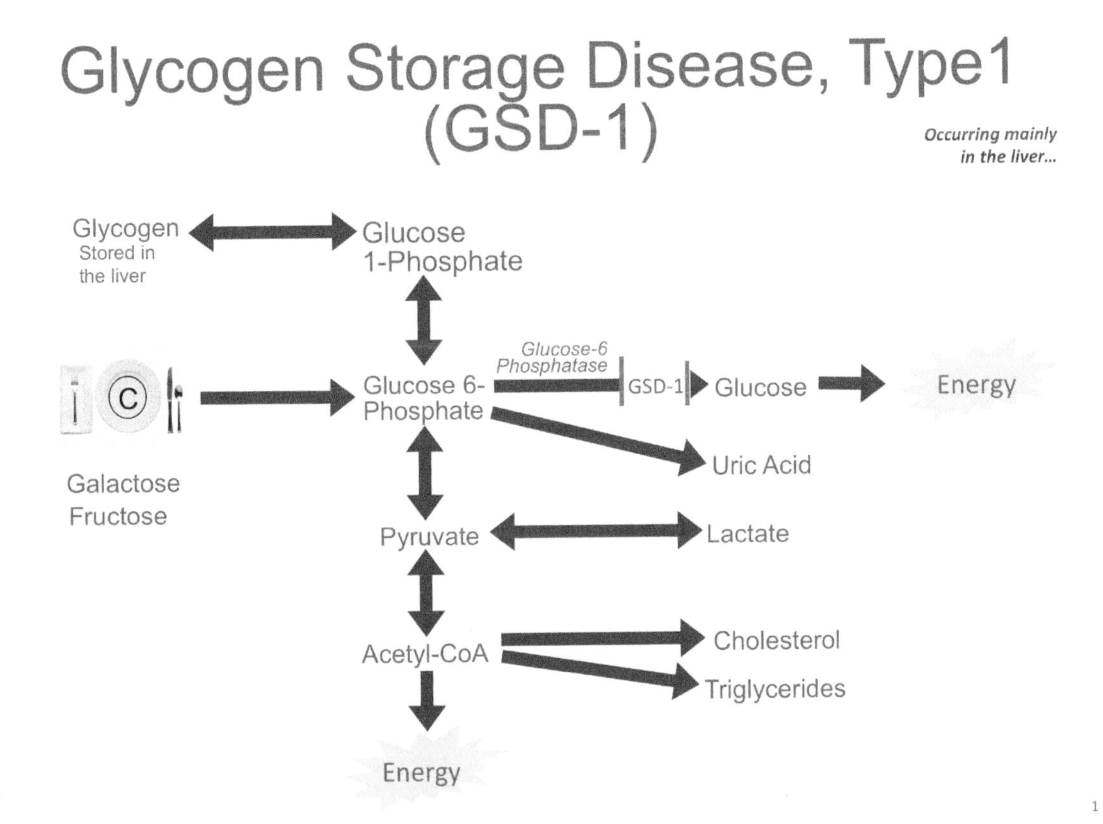

Fig. 26.1 Metabolic pathway of glycogen storage disease type I

Table 26.2 Formulas for GSD type I

Infant formula	Toddler formulas	Adult formulas
Abbott Nutrition		
Elecare® (for infants)	Elecare® Jr. (unflavored) PediaSure® Peptide1.0 (unflavored)	Osmolite®
Mead Johnson		
Enfamil® Prosobee® Nutramigen® Pregestimil® PurAmino™	Nutramigen® Toddler	
Nestle Health Science		
Alfamino® Infant	Alfamino® Junior Peptamen® Junior (unvlavored) Vivonex® Pediatric	Glytrol® (unflavored) Isosource® HN (unflavored) Peptamen® (unflavored) Vivonex® Plus/TEN Tolerex®
Nutricia		
Neocate® Infant	Neocate® Jr.	

Adapted from, email posting, Saavedra, H. July 2019 PNO-METAB-L@listserv.cc.emory.edu

glycogen production [4–6]. Solid foods can be introduced at 4–6 months of age, in accordance with the diet restrictions discussed in the next section. However, many infants with GSD type I develop an aversion to oral feeding and can fall behind in feeding skills. A developmental assessment should be completed and treatment provided for any infant not meeting age-appropriate feeding milestones. In some patients, a nutritionally complete formula will need to be continued after 1 year of age as they transition off of infant formula. The same nutrition principles apply for formula selection for children and adults with GSD type I (Table 26.2).

26.3.2 Nutrition Assessment and Diet Composition

For individuals with GSD type I, estimated energy needs can be based on standard calculations considering age, weight, height, and activity level and adjusted based on weight gain or maintenance goals [7]. The recommended macronutrient composition of the diet includes 60–70% of total energy needs from carbohydrate, 10–15% from protein and the remaining from fat sources with <30% of energy recommended for those over the age of 2 years [4]. Calories from cornstarch (3.8 kcal/g) are included in the total carbohydrate prescription. The monosaccharides fructose and galactose cannot be converted to glucose in patients with GSD type I. Therefore, food sources of both must be avoided or severely limited in the diet. As fructose is a component of the disaccharide sucrose, and galactose is a component of the disaccharide lactose, food sources of sucrose and lactose must also be limited. Table 26.3 provides a list of foods allowed and not allowed in the diet for GSD type I.

In older individuals, carbohydrate is restricted at meals and snacks to avoid excessive glycogen storage, weight gain, and laboratory abnormali-

Table 26.3 Foods allowed and foods not allowed in GSD type 1 [2]

Food group	Foods allowed	Foods not allowed
Dairy	Limit to one serving per day: 1 cup low-fat milk (ideally soy or almond) 1 cup low-fat sugar-free yogurt 1.5 oz hard cheese	Ice cream Sweetened yogurt with milk Sweetened milk
Cereals	Dry and cooked cereal with no added sugar	Cereals with fruit or added sugar
Breads	White, wheat, or rye breads Crackers, matzo English muffins Dinner rolls, biscuits Pita bread	Raisin bread Muffins Sweet rolls Pies Cakes Sweet breads Waffles and pancakes made with sugar
Starches	Brown and white rice Pasta Popcorn Tortillas White potatoes	Any starches with added sugar, milk, cheese Sweet potatoes

Table 26.3 (continued)

Food group	Foods allowed	Foods not allowed
Vegetables	All non-starchy vegetables including asparagus, cabbage, spinach, squash, onion, green beans, turnips, greens	Any with added milk, sugar, cheese Corn, peas, and carrots have more sugar than the others
Fruit	Lemons and limes Avocados	All other fresh, canned, dried, and dried fruits Tomatoes
Meat	Lean poultry, beef, pork, fish	Organ meats Fatty and processed meats
Legumes/ Nuts	All beans and nuts	Any beans, nuts, or seeds with sugar added.
Soups	Broth soups made with allowed meats, starches and vegetables	Creamed soups
Fats	Canola and olive oil Corn, safflower, canola, and soybean oil-based condiments Reduced-fat condiments	*Trans* fatty acids Saturated fats
Sweets	Sugar substitutes, sucralose Dextrose 100% corn syrup, rice syrup Sugar-free Jell-O and pudding Candies made with dextrose	All other sugars, sweets, syrups, high-fructose corn syrup, honey, molasses, sorbitol, and cane sugar, juice, and syrups

ties [6]. Recommended limits for carbohydrate include 15 g at meals and 5 g for snacks (Appendix J) [6]. In addition, simple sugar is restricted to <5 g per meal (equivalent to 2.5 g fructose or galactose) and 2–3 g per snack [5, 6]. Meals and snacks should be separated from cornstarch feedings to provide optimal metabolic control and to not interfere with appetite. Alcohol can lead to hypoglycemia and, thus, should also be avoided (Box 26.1) [4].

A cookbook written specifically for GSD is available from the Association for Glycogen Storage Disease (www.agsdus.org) and additional recipes are available at https://www.vitaflousa.com/. Educational resources for the nutrition management of GSD are available at https://gmdi.org/ under Clinical Practice Tools.

Box 26.1: Recommended Macronutrient Composition of the Diet for a Patient with GSD Type I

- Carbohydrates (60–70% of energy)
  - Cornstarch calories are included
  - Use complex carbohydrates
    Limit to 15 g meal/5 g snack
  - Avoid fructose (limit to 2.5 g/meal)
    Avoid fruit
    Limited vegetables
  - Limit galactose and lactose
    1 serving/day dairy allowed
- Protein (10–15% of energy)
  - Offer lean sources of protein
  - Include protein of high biological value
- Fat (<30% of energy)
  - Limit saturated sources
  - Include mono- and polyunsaturated sources
  - Assure essential fatty acid intake

26.3.3 Fasting and Overnight Feedings

Fasting time is limited in individuals with GSD. Intervals between feedings of 2–3.5 hours for children under the age of 2 and 3–5 hours in older children and adults are typically recommended for GSD type I [4]. Bolus feeds or continuous drip feeds, usually via a gastrostomy tube, are often necessary to meet these fasting recommendations overnight. A meta-analysis of published cases suggested that intermittent administration of uncooked cornstarch (UCCS) at night prevented hypoglycemia better than continuous nocturnal feedings of dextrose [8]. While UCCS feedings during the night is inconvenient, it precludes the problem of pump malfunction which can lead to severe hypoglycemia. If a continuous overnight tube feeding must be used, a glucose infusion rate (GIR) of 8–10 mg/kg/min for infants and 4–8 mg/kg/min for older children can be used as a starting point [4] (Appendix I). Practice varies from clinic to clinic and further research is needed before a definitive recommendation for overnight feeds can be made [9]. Monitoring of blood glucose concentrations at the end of a continuous night-time drip feeding helps determine the correct feeding rate required to prevent hypoglycemia. Additionally, a formula feeding (in infants) or UCCS dose should be given about 30 minutes before the overnight drip feeding ends to prevent hypoglycemia that can be caused by high concentrations of insulin at the end of a feeding cycle [4]. The use of Glycosade® to extend night-time fasting will be discussed later in the chapter.

26.3.4 Supplements for GSD Type I

With the diet restrictions required for an individual with GSD type I, nutritional supplements are needed. A sugar-free multivitamin/mineral supplement is recommended to meet the Dietary Reference Intake (DRI) for most vitamin and minerals (Appendix D). A sugar-free calcium supplement is also recommended to meet the DRI for the individual's age, as most multivitamin/mineral supplements do not contain an adequate amount of calcium. Additional vitamin D_3 may be necessary if the diet is not meeting the DRI and/or if total 25-hydroxyvitamin D concentration is low. Serum total 25-hydroxyvitamin D concentrations can be below normal even in individuals prescribed supplements meeting DRI recommendations [4]. For individuals with GSD type Ib, additional supplements may include probiotics to help manage IBD and vitamin E for neutropenia [4, 5].

26.3.5 Cornstarch Therapy for GSD Type I

Uncooked cornstarch (UCCS) has been used in the treatment of GSD type I since the 1980s. As a slowly digested starch, UCCS provides a sustained source of glucose that lasts longer than any food source [10]. UCCS is not introduced before 9–12 months of age as younger infants do not have sufficient pancreatic amylase activity to adequately digest the starch, leading to gastrointestinal distress [11, 12]. The Bier equation (Box 26.2) can be used to determine ideal dosing of cornstarch for children under 8 years of age [6]. However, this equation is not appropriate for individuals weighing >30 kg, during puberty, or for adults [6]. When initiating UCCS, start with 1 g per dose, increasing by 1 g increments each week until the optimal dose is achieved [5]. Ideally UCCS should be weighed on a gram scale; if using household measures, one tablespoon of UCCS weighs approximately 8 g. Gastrointestinal side effects can be prevented if UCCS doses are increased gradually. UCCS can be added to an infant's formula prior to each formula feeding. If the infant develops gastrointestinal distress, the introduction of UCCS can be delayed or some clinics have prescribed pancreatic enzymes for a short period of time [4] (Box 26.2).

Box 26.2: Calculating Glucose Needs for Individuals Under Age 8 Years with GSD Type I

$$Y = 0.0014X^3 - 0.214X^2 + 10.411X - 9.084$$

$$Y = \text{mg glucose per minute}$$

$$X = \text{weight in kg}$$

i.e., $X = 10$ kg; $Y = 75$ mg/min (4.5 g/h)

For individuals over the age of 8 years, dosing by body weight is not recommended as over treatment can lead to excessive weight gain, glycogen storage, insulin resistance, and elevated lactate concentrations [6]. For individuals over the age of 8 years, initial doses of UCCS providing 10–11 g of glucose per hour are recommended with further adjustments in dose based on blood glucose and lactate concentrations [4]. In a retrospective study of 112 individuals with GSD 1a over the age of 10 years, the mean total daily prescribed UCCS was 272–337 g/d, providing 11.3–14 g glucose/hour (with doses decreasing with age) divided into a mean of 6 doses per day (range, 4–8 doses/d) [13].

UCCS should not be heated or added to acidic beverages since both heat and acid will degrade the starch molecule and reduce its effectiveness [4]. Additionally, citrate solutions (i.e., Bicitra®) increase starch digestion and, thus, should not be given with UCCS [4]. For older individuals, water or sugar-free drinks (given in a ratio of 2–3 mL liquid to 1 g UCCS solution) is recommended [4]. UCCS should be given after meals to reduce its negative effect on appetite and to extend its effectiveness to maintain optimal blood glucose. Other food starches that have been tried when cornstarch (90% carbohydrate) is not tolerated include tapioca (86% carbohydrate), arrowroot (88% carbohydrate), and cassava (88% carbohydrate) [5]. A greater amount of these starches may be needed to provide the same blood sugar results (Box 26.3) [4, 14].

Box 26.3: Cornstarch Therapy for GSD Type I

- Weigh cornstarch with a gram scale, if possible; otherwise use a household measurement.
- One tablespoon of cornstarch weighs 8 g and provides 7.2 g of carbohydrate.
- Mix cornstarch into a sucrose, lactose-free formula, water or diet drink.
- Add 1 g of cornstarch to 2–3 mL of fluid.
- Do not mix into acidic beverages.
- Do not cook.
- Consume immediately after mixing into the liquid.
- Store dry cornstarch at room temperature.
- Cornstarch may only be good for 2–4 weeks after opening a container depending on environmental conditions.
- Argo® is the cornstarch recommended in the United States [3, 13].

26.3.6 Glycosade® Therapy for GSD Type I

Glycosade® (Vitaflo USA) is a cornstarch derivative with a high amylopectin content that has the potential to increase overnight fasting time for individuals with GSD types 0, I, III, VI, and IX [15]. In one study, Glycosade® was more effective than cornstarch in 88% of individuals with GSD type I [16]. Overnight fasting tolerance increased from 4.1 to 7.8 hours [16]. However, Glycosade® was not as effective in individuals with GSD type Ib due to malabsorption related to IBD [16]. In the United States, Glycosade® is currently labeled for night-time use and for individuals over 5 years of age [15]. Day time use is being investigated. Glycosade® can be mixed in a 1 g–2 mL solution in water or an individual's usual cold beverage [15]. A detailed guideline, *A practical guide for overnight use of Glycosade® in hepatic Glycogen Storage Diseases,* to initiate treatment for individuals with GSD type I is available from Vitaflo USA [15] (Box 26.4).

Box 26.4: Glycosade® Dosing Recommendations [15]

GSD Type I

Age	Dose (g)
5–6 years	60–75
7–8 years	75–90
Pre-pubertal	90–120
Pubertal	135–150
Adults	120–150

Glycosade® is available in 60 g packet; 211 calories (3.5 kcal/g) and 53 g carbohydrate

26.4 Nutrition Management in Special Circumstances

26.4.1 Exercise

During periods of physical activity, additional glucose sources are needed to meet the greater energy demand. Hypoglycemia can develop quickly so extra precautions are needed. To help determine the best management strategy, glucose concentrations should be checked before, during, and after exercise. Additional UCCS (1 hour's dose) can be incorporated into the diet plan about 30 minutes before exercise, although gastrointestinal distress may be a problem for some [5]. Frequent glucose monitoring is needed to determine the best strategy for each patient.

26.4.2 Treating Hypoglycemia and Illness

Recommendations for treating low blood glucose (<70 mg/dl or < 4 mmol/L) in a patient who is asymptomatic include providing 5 g of a carbohydrate from food (i.e., pretzels, crackers) and rechecking glucose in 10 minutes. Repeat this treatment if the patient's glucose remains <70 mg/dl [5]. If a patient is symptomatic, give 10 g dextrose (i.e., glucose gels, glucose tablets, Smarties®) plus food or 1 h of usual UCCS dosing. Retest in 10 minutes, and if blood glucose is still low, repeat treatment [5].

An illness can exacerbate the need for glucose and increases the risk of developing hypoglycemia. During minor illnesses, increasing the frequency of UCCS feedings may be sufficient or provide a high carbohydrate formula (i.e., Tolerex®) as a continuous drip feeding to help maintain adequate blood glucose. However, because of the high risk of developing hypoglycemia during illness, there should be a low threshold for emergency evaluation and/or admission. Intravenous dextrose (usually 10% or 12.5% concentration to meet GIR requirements) provided by peripheral line with appropriate electrolytes is typically recommended. It is important that the patient be able to consume carbohydrate and UCCS by mouth or gastrostomy tube before IV sources are gradually decreased to avoid decreasing blood glucose concentrations [11].

All families should be provided with an emergency letter explaining the treatment necessary to avoid hypoglycemia, medications that are contraindicated, and laboratory measures to evaluate the individual's status. Families are encouraged to prepare an "emergency kit" that contains a source of glucose (i.e., Instaglucose®), carbohydrate-containing foods (i.e., pretzels, crackers), a glucometer, cornstarch, and water. All individuals with GSD type I should also carry a form of emergency identification, such as a medical alert bracelet.

26.4.3 Monitoring

Careful monitoring is important as poor metabolic control can lead to several co-morbidities in GSD type I. Renal disease and hepatic adenomas have been described in individuals with poor metabolic control [4]. Gout is a complication of high uric acid levels [4]. Poor bone mineralization has been noted due to insufficient intake of calcium and vitamin D along with the effects of chronically elevated lactic acid [4]. Screening labs and assessments should be obtained on an annual basis, or more frequently as needed (Box 26.5). More details on disease complications,

Box 26.5: Nutrition Monitoring of a Patient with GSD Type I

- Routine assessments including anthropometrics, dietary intake, and physical findings
- Laboratory Monitoring
  - Diagnosis-specific
    - Glucose
    - Lactic Acid
    - Uric Acid
    - Triglycerides
    - Cholesterol
    - Liver Function Tests
  - Nutrition monitoring
    - Nutritional anemia (hemoglobin, hematocrit, MCV, serum vitamin B_{12} and/or methylmalonic acid, total homocysteine, ferritin, iron, folate, total iron binding capacity)
    - Vitamin and mineral status (25-hydroxy vitamin D, zinc, trace minerals)
    - Others as clinically indicated

monitoring, and adjunct/new therapies are discussed in Chap. 25.

26.5 GSD Type III Background

Glycogen storage disease type III, also called Cori or Forbes disease, results from a deficiency of amylo-1,6-glucosidase (glycogen debranching enzyme) leading to incomplete breakdown of glycogen and excessive glycogen storage [17]. The guidelines for GSD type III recognize two forms, a and b [17]. The majority (85%) of individuals with GSD type III have type a, affecting both muscle and liver, 15% of individuals have type b, affecting the liver only [17]. Hypoglycemia, hepatomegaly, hyperlipidemia, short stature, and eventual muscle involvement (including cardiomyopathy) are disease complications of GSD type IIIa (Table 26.1) [17]. This section focuses on diet management of type IIIa. Guidelines for the diagnosis and management of GSD type III were published in 2010 [17]. Chapter 25 further describes the biochemical and clinical features of GSD.

Core Messages for GSD Type IIIa

- Glycogen storage disease type IIIa is not as prone to hypoglycemia as in GSD type I because gluconeogenesis is intact.
- Nutrition management of GSD type IIIa includes providing a high protein, low carbohydrate and moderate fat diet.
- Vitamin and mineral supplementation should be assessed for each individual.
- Home monitoring of blood glucose and adjustments in the diet are needed for proper management.
- Glycosade® is a cornstarch derivative that may extend fasting time.

26.6 Nutrition Management GSD Type III

The primary goal of nutrition management for infants and young children with GSD type III is to prevent hypoglycemia [17]. This can be achieved with frequent feedings and the use of cornstarch (described for GSD I), especially for those with more severe forms of GSD III. However, since gluconeogenesis remains intact in GSD III allowing for production of glucose from amino acids, fatty acids, and other metabolites, there are fewer diet restrictions than for patients with GSD type I. For example, galactose and fructose do not need to be restricted and specific infant formulas are not required [17]. However, limiting intake of simple sugars to prevent excessive energy intake that can lead to increased glycogen storage is recommended [17]. Higher protein intake is an important part of the treatment since amino acids can be used for gluconeogenesis in this disorder. Recommendations for macronutrient distribution are 35–55% of energy intake from carbohydrates, 20–30% of energy from protein and limiting fat intake to 20–35% of total energy [17]. A protein intake goal of 3 g/kg/d has been recommended to normalize serum protein markers (albumin, prealbumin) and creatine kinase (CK) concentrations [4]. Higher protein intakes of up to 4 g/kg/d are suggested by some clinics [5, 6]. The addition of protein supplements (i.e., Unjury®, Beneprotein®) can help meet these higher protein needs. In addition to providing substrates for gluconeogenesis, a high protein intake may improve muscle function and reduce excessive glycogen storage by reducing carbohydrate intake [4]. To help improve overnight fasting tolerance, a high protein bedtime snack (+/− UCCS or Glycosade®) should be recommended; however, an additional night-time feeding may still be indicated in severe cases [17]. Alcohol impedes gluconeogenesis and can impair judgment, and thus should be avoided [6].

26.6.1 Cornstarch Therapy for GSD Type III

Required doses of UCCS are usually less than the amount needed for individuals with GSD type I. A dose of 1 g/kg every 4 hours may be sufficient to prevent low blood glucose, although some individuals with a severe form of type GSD IIIa may require higher doses and a frequency similar to GSD type I [17]. Concerns for initiating cornstarch in GSD type I are the same for type III. Slow and gradual increases in UCCS dose is recommended to minimize gastrointestinal distress. UCCS can be mixed in milk or yogurt to provide an additional source of protein.

26.6.2 Glycosade® Therapy for GSD Type III

Glycosade® use has been studied in the ketotic forms of GSD, including type III. Patients with ketotic forms of GSD (types 0, III, VI, and IX) are able to make ketones and utilize them as a source of energy. If patients are developing low glucose or increased ketones after an overnight fast, Glycosade® may improve overall metabolic control [18]. One study found overnight fasting increased from 4.9 to 9.6 hours on Glycosade® [18]. Recommended bed-time doses for the ketotic forms of GSD range from 30 to 75 g [15].

26.6.3 Supplements for GSD Type III

Vitamin and mineral supplements may not be needed in GSD type III as there are fewer specific diet restrictions than for GSD type I. Decreased bone mineralization has been reported, so calcium intake and vitamin D status should be evaluated [17].

26.6.4 Adjunct Therapy

Musculoskeletal disease can be progressive and significant in this population. It was once thought to develop in adults but is now recognized in the younger population [17]. Modified Atkins and ketogenic diets have been prescribed in a limited number of published cases with improvement in cardiomyopathy, muscle function, and other metabolic parameters noted [19–21].

26.7 Blood Glucose Monitoring

A mainstay for management of GSD type I and III is home monitoring of blood glucose to maintain concentrations within the treatment range throughout a 24-hour period. Indeed, in a multi-center questionnaire, the primary safety concern was developing severe hypoglycemia because of the failure of patients or caregivers to wake up to an alarm during the night [22]. Setting more than one alarm is helpful to avoid catastrophic outcomes related to missed UCCS dosing. Glucometers designed for diabetes management are traditionally recommended for checking blood glucose in the morning prior to cornstarch dosing or at the end of continuous feedings, before meals or cornstarch doses during the day, and after exercise. Caregivers and patients should record glucose measurements and time of meals, cornstarch doses, and activity to help fine-tune each individual's plan.

Continuous glucose monitoring (CGM) is a more recently available tool that provides information about trends in blood glucose over 24 hours. This monitoring system was originally designed for diabetes management but has been adapted for GSD care. Glucose levels from CGM are recorded every 5 minutes and information can be downloaded and viewed on cell phones in "real time" [23]. However, in CGM, glucose is measured in interstitial fluid and thus is not equivalent to a measurement from a glucometer [23]. This needs to be considered when interpreting CGM data to adjust treatment. However, CGM monitoring is useful to detect trends in blood glucose control which allows for fine-tuning of maximum fasting times, UCCS/Glycosade® doses, and carbohydrate feedings [23, 24].

In GSD type I, measuring blood lactate concentrations may also be helpful since lactic acidosis can be present even when glucose concentrations are normal and, thus, may provide a more sensitive marker of metabolic control in this disorder [4, 25]. A lactate meter can be used to check blood lactate at similar times as recommended for glucose monitoring with the goal of maintaining normal lactate concentrations [26]. If elevations are frequently detected, then the diet and UCCS or Glycosade® doses need to be reevaluated. In GSD type III, blood ketone monitoring may be useful to assess metabolic control in response to fasting [17].

26.8 Summary

The overall goal for nutrition management in GSD type I and III is to prevent hypoglycemia and minimize metabolic disturbances. By maintaining blood glucose concentrations of 75–100 mg/dl (4.2 and 5.6 mmol/L), along with normal lactate and ketone levels, an individual with GSD can minimize complications and co-morbidities. The nutrition management of GSD includes a galactose-and fructose-restricted diet for type I, a high protein diet for type III and avoidance of fasting, use of UCCS and/or Glycosade,® and careful blood glucose monitoring for both disorders. The clinical outcome for individuals with GSD type I and III will continue to improve as further adjunct therapies are developed, including gene therapy.

26.9 Diet Calculation Example

The following nutrition calculations provide an example of the steps to determine a nutrition plan for a 6-year-old boy with glycogen storage disease, type Ia. His weight is 21.5 kg.

- *Step 1. Determine nutrient goals*
  Energy: 85 kcal/kg = 1800 kcal/day.
  - The recommended distribution of macronutrients:
  - Carbohydrate: 60% of total kcal: 1080 kcal ÷ 4 kcal/g = 270 g CHO (cornstarch is included in total CHO intake)
  - Protein: 12% of total kcal: 216 kcal ÷ 4 kcal/g = 54 g protein
  - Fat: 28% of total kcal: 504 kcal ÷ 9 kcal/kg = up to 56 g fat
- *Step 2. Glucose needed based on the Bier equation* [6]
  - $Y = 0.0014X^3 - 0.214X^2 + 10.411X - 9.084$
  - Y = mg glucose per minute
  - X = weight in kg
  - X = 21.5 kg, From Bier equation: Y = 130 mg/min; 130 mg/min × 60 min/1000 mg = 7.8 g/h
- Assuming the uncooked cornstarch (UCCS) will be provided every 3 hours around the clock, give 7.8 g/h × 3 h = 23.4 g (Divide by 0.9 (CHO/g powder) = 26 g UCCS (round down to 25 g) at each feeding. There are 8 three-hour periods in a day, therefore this child will get 8 feedings × 25 g/feed = 200 g UCCS.
- *Step 3. Determine the number of calories provided by UCCS*
  - UCCS 200 g × 3.8 kcal/g = 760 kcal
- *Step 4. Determine the grams of CHO provided by the UCCS*
  - 760 kcal/4 kcal per gram = 190 g CHO
- *Step 5. Determine the amount of CHO remaining that will be allowed from food sources*
  - 270 g CHO goal – 190 g CHO from UCCS = 80 g CHO from food
- *Step 6. Determine a feeding schedule that distributes complex CHO and cornstarch doses evenly throughout the day*
  - To use an exchange system, 1 serving = 15 g of complex CHO
  - 80 g total CHO from food ÷ 15 g CHO/exchange = 5.3 exchanges/day (round to 5 servings)
  - Meals: Breakfast and Lunch, 1 serving each; Dinner, 2 servings;
  - Snacks: 1 exchange or15 g; 5 g in each snack × 3 servings
  - *Providing UCCS every 3 h day and night will not be possible for every family. Some alternative suggestions:

1. Provide the equivalent grams of carbohydrate for a 6–8-hour period via an overnight gastrostomy feeding.
   - Ex. 7.8 g/h × 6 h period = 46.8 g glucose
   - Select a GSD type I formula (Table 26.2)
   - PediaSure® Peptide 1.0, unflavored, CHO content 31.7 g/237 ml
   - 46.8 g glucose/ 31.7 g = 1.48 × 237 ml = 350 ml
   - Feeding tube rate; 350 ml/ 6 h = 58 ml/h

2. Glycosade® (Recommended Dosing Box 26.4)
   Provide 70 g Glycosade® at bedtime- 9 pm, this dose was trialed and lasted 7 hours (the Glycosade® dose needs to be verified for each patient as the length of time that a dose of Glycosade® will prevent low blood glucose will vary between individuals.)
   Cornstarch to resume at 4 am, provide 25 g UCCS and continue with every 3-hour dosing throughout the day

Acknowledgments Thank you to Sandy van Calcar of Oregon Health & Science University for her contributions to this chapter's content in the first Edition of Nutrition Management of Inherited Metabolic Diseases.

References

1. Berg JM, Tymoczko JL, Stryer L. Biochemistry. 7th ed. New York: W.H. Freeman; 2012. xxxii, 1054, 43, 41, 48 p.
2. Kishnani PS, Austin SL, Abdenur JE, Arn P, Bali DS, Boney A, et al. Diagnosis and management of glycogen storage disease type 1: a practical guideline of the American College of Medical Genetics and Genomics. Genet Med. 2014;16:1–29.
3. Baumgartner MR, Saudubray J-M, Walter JH. Inborn metabolic diseases : diagnosis and treatment. Berlin/Heidelberg: Springer: Imprint: Springer; 2016.
4. Weinstein DA, Steuerwald U, De Souza CFM, Derks TGJ. Inborn errors of metabolism with hypoglycemia: glycogen storage diseases and inherited disorders of gluconeogenesis. Pediatr Clin N Am. 2018;65(2):247–65.
5. Saavedra H, editor. Management of glycogen storage disease type I & IIIf. Vitaflo metabolic RD summit. San Diego; 2020.
6. Ross KM, Ferrecchia IA, Dahlberg KR, Dambska M, Ryan PT, Weinstein DA. Dietary management of the glycogen storage diseases: evolution of treatment and ongoing controversies. Adv Nutr. 2020;11(2):439–46.
7. Institute of Medicine (U.S.). Panel on Macronutrients., Institute of Medicine (U.S.). Standing Committee on the Scientific Evaluation of Dietary Reference Intakes. Dietary reference intakes for energy, carbohydrate, fiber, fat, fatty acids, cholesterol, protein, and amino acids. Washington, DC: National Academies Press; 2005. xxv, 1331 p.
8. Shah KK, O'Dell SD. Effect of dietary interventions in the maintenance of normoglycaemia in glycogen storage disease type 1a: a systematic review and meta-analysis. J Hum Nutr Diet. 2013;26(4):329–39.
9. Derks TG, Martens DH, Sentner CP, van Rijn M, de Boer F, Smit GP, et al. Dietary treatment of glycogen storage disease type Ia: uncooked cornstarch and/or continuous nocturnal gastric drip-feeding? Mol Genet Metab. 2013;109(1):1–2.
10. Sidbury JB, Chen YT, Roe CR. The role of raw starches in the treatment of type I glycogenosis. Arch Intern Med. 1986;146(2):370–3.
11. Saudubray JM, Van den Berghe G, Walter J. Inborn metabolic diseases: diagnosis and treatment. 5th ed. Berlin: Springer; 2012. xxv, 656 p.
12. Blau N, Duran M, Gibson KM, Vici C D. Physician's guide to the treatment and follow-up of metabolic diseases. New York: Springer; 2014.
13. Dahlberg KR, Ferrecchia IA, Dambska-Williams M, Resler TE, Ross KM, Butler GL, et al. Cornstarch requirements of the adult glycogen storage disease Ia population: a retrospective review. J Inherit Metab Dis. 2020;43(2):269–78.
14. Nalin T, Venema K, Weinstein DA, de Souza CF, Perry ID, van Wandelen MT, et al. In vitro digestion of starches in a dynamic gastrointestinal model: an innovative study to optimize dietary management of patients with hepatic glycogen storage diseases. J Inherit Metab Dis. 2015;38(3):529–36.
15. Vitaflo. A practical guide for overnight use of glycosade in hepatic glycogen storage disease. Bridgewater: Vitaflo USA, LLC; 2020.
16. Ross KM, Brown LM, Corrado MM, Chengsupanimit T, Curry LM, Ferrecchia IA, et al. Safety and efficacy of chronic extended release cornstarch therapy for glycogen storage disease type I. JIMD Rep. 2016;26:85–90.
17. Kishnani PS, Austin SL, Arn P, Bali DS, Boney A, Case LE, et al. Glycogen storage disease type III diagnosis and management guidelines. Genet Med. 2010;12(7):446–63.
18. Ross KM, Brown L, Corrado MM, Chengsupanimit T, Curry LM, Ferrecchia IA, et al. Safety and efficacy of long-term use of extended release cornstarch therapy for glycogen storage disease types 0, III, VI, and IX. J Nutr Ther. 2015;4(4):137–42.
19. Olgac A, Inci A, Okur I, Biberoglu G, Oguz D, Ezgu FS, et al. Beneficial effects of modified Atkins diet in glycogen storage disease type IIIa. Ann Nutr Metab. 2020;76(4):233–41.
20. Francini-Pesenti F, Tresso S, Vitturi N. Modified Atkins ketogenic diet improves heart and skeletal muscle function in glycogen storage disease type III. Acta Myol. 2019;38(1):17–20.
21. Marusic T, Zerjav Tansek M, Sirca Campa A, Mezek A, Berden P, Battelino T, et al. Normalization of obstructive cardiomyopathy and improvement of hep-

atopathy on ketogenic diet in patient with glycogen storage disease (GSD) type IIIa. Mol Genet Metab Rep. 2020;24:100628.
22. Steunenberg TAH, Peeks F, Hoogeveen IJ, Mitchell JJ, Mundy H, de Boer F, et al. Safety issues associated with dietary management in patients with hepatic glycogen storage disease. Mol Genet Metab. 2018;125(1–2):79–85.
23. Herbert M, Pendyal S, Rairikar M, Halaby C, Benjamin RW, Kishnani PS. Role of continuous glucose monitoring in the management of glycogen storage disorders. J Inherit Metab Dis. 2018;41(6):917–27.
24. White FJ, Jones SA. The use of continuous glucose monitoring in the practical management of glycogen storage disorders. J Inherit Metab Dis. 2011;34(3):631–42.
25. Daublin G, Schwahn B, Wendel U. Type I glycogen storage disease: favourable outcome on a strict management regimen avoiding increased lactate production during childhood and adolescence. Eur J Pediatr. 2002;161(Suppl 1):S40–5.
26. Saunders AC, Feldman HA, Correia CE, Weinstein DA. Clinical evaluation of a portable lactate meter in type I glycogen storage disease. J Inherit Metab Dis. 2005;28(5):695–701.

Appendix A. Nutrient Composition of Frequently Used Parenteral Fluids

Carbohydrate

Carbohydrate is provided as IV dextrose.

Dextrose contains 3.4 kcal/g.

Dextrose solutions range from 5% (D5W) to 25% (D25W) by weight.

Solutions containing 12.5% dextrose and higher cannot be given peripherally and require a central line (peripherally inserted central catheter or PICC, port or central access).

Percent solution	CHO content (g/100 mL)	kcal/100 mL
D5W (5%)	5	17
D10W (10%)	10	34
D25W (25%)	25	85

Protein

Protein is provided as crystalline amino acid solutions.

Trophamine 6% and 10% (B. Braun) and Aminosyn-PF 7% (Hospira) are frequently used solutions. Amino acid solutions provide 4 kcal/g.

Percent solution (%)	Amino acid content (g/100 mL)	kcal/100 mL
3.0	3	12
3.5	3.5	14
5.0	5	20
10	10	40

Fat

Fat is provided as a lipid emulsion.

Intralipid 10% and Intralipid 20% are frequently used lipid emulsions.

Percent solution of fat emulsion	kcal/100 mL
10%	1.1 kcal/mL
20%	2.0 kcal/mL

SMOFlipid (Fresenius Kabi, Zurich Switzerland) contains 0.2 g lipid/mL and is a mixture of soybean oil, medium-chain triglycerides (MCTs), olive oil, and fish oil.

L. E. Bernstein et al. (eds.), *Nutrition Management of Inherited Metabolic Diseases*, https://doi.org/10.1007/978-3-030-94510-7

Appendix B. Maintenance Fluid Requirements

The Holliday-Segar nomogram is a common method used in approximating water loss and calculating the fluid requirement [1].

Fluid Requirement Calculation

1. 100 mL/kg for the first 10 kg of weight +
2. 50 mL/kg for the second 10 kg of weight +
3. 20 mL/kg for remaining kg of weight =
4. Total daily fluid requirement

Example: A child weighing 25 kg would require:

1. 100 mL × first 10 kg = 1000 mL +
2. 50 mL × second 10 kg = 500 mL+
3. 20 mL × remaining 5 kg =100 mL =
4. Total fluid requirement of 1600 mL/day

Fluid requirements are typically thought of on a 24-hour basis, while administration is based on an hourly infusion rate via the delivery pump. To approximate the hourly rate, the "4-2-1" formula can be used [2].

Hourly Maintenance Fluid Infusion Calculation (Using 4-2-1 Formula)

1. 4 mL/kg/hour for the first 10 kg +
2. 2 mL/kg/hour for the second 10 kg +
3. 1 mL/kg/hour for the remaining kg =
4. Total hourly infusion rate

Example: For a 25 kg child, the maintenance fluid rate would be:

1. 4 mL/kg/hour × first 10 kg = 40 mL/hour +
2. 2 mL/kg/hour × second 10 kg = 20 mL/hour +
3. 1 mL/kg/hour × remaining 5 kg = 5 mL/hour =
4. Total hourly infusion = 65 mL/hour =1560 mL

References

1. Holliday MA, SEGAR WE. The maintenance need for water in parenteral fluid therapy. Pediatrics. 1957;19(5):823–32.
2. Kalia A. Maintenance fluid therapy in children. Fluids Electrol. 2008 [cited 2014 October 8]; Available from: http://www.utmb.edu/pedi_ed/CORE/Fluids&Electyrolytes/page_04.htm.

L. E. Bernstein et al. (eds.), *Nutrition Management of Inherited Metabolic Diseases*, https://doi.org/10.1007/978-3-030-94510-7

Appendix C. Energy Needs Required for Anabolism During Acute Illness

Age	Weight	Height	Total energy needs	Carbo-hydrates (D10)	Daily Fluids	Fluid rate	GIR	Energy from glucose	Intralipid®	Energy from Intralipid®	Total energy (glucose + lipid)	Fraction of required
	Kg	M	kcal	X maintenance	mL/day	mL/h	mg/kg/min	kcal	g/kg/day	kcal	kcal	%
Infant (0–3 mo)	3.5	NA	387	1.5	525	22	10.5	179	4	140	319	82%
Infant (0–3 mo)	3.5	NA	387	1× D20	350	14.6	13.9	238	4	140	378	98%
Infant (4–6 mo)	7	NA	579	1.5	1050	44	10.5	357	3	210	567	98%
									4	280	637	110%
Infant (7–12 mo)	10	NA	812	1.5	1500	63	10.5	510	1	100	610	75%
									3	300	810	100%
									4	400	910	112%
Toddler (13–36 mo)	15	NA	1255	1.5	1875	78	8.7	638	2	300	938	75%
									3	450	1088	87%
Male Child (6 yr)	20	1.15	1310	1.5	2250	94	7.85	765	2	400	1165	89%
									3	600	1365	104%
Female Child (6 yr)	20	1.15	1245	1.5	2250	94	7.85	765	2	400	1165	94%
									3	600	1365	110%
Male adolescent (10 yr)	30	1.35	1515	1.5	2550	106	5.9	867	2	600	1467	97%
Female adolescent (10 yr)	30	1.35	1413	1.5	2550	106	5.9	867	2	600	1467	104%
Male older adolescent (16 yr)	60	1.7	2260	1.5	3450	144	4.0	1173	1	600	1773	78%
									2	1200	2373	105%
Female older adolescent (16 yr)	55	1.625	1735	1.5	3300	138	4.2	1122	1	550	1672	96%
									2	1100	2222	128%

Abbreviations used: D10 = glucose 10%, D20 = glucose 20%, GIR = glucose infusion rate, yr = year.

Kimberly A.Kripps[ab]Peter R.BakerII[a]Janet A.Thomas[a]Heather E.Skillman[c]LaurieBernstein[a]SommerGaughan[a]CaseyBurns[a]Curtis R.CoughlinII[a]Shawn E.McCandless[a]Austin A.Larson[a]AainaKochar[a]Chelsey F.Stillman[de]Erica M.Wymore[f]Ellie G.Hendricks[g]MichaelWoontner[a]Johan L.K.Van Hove[a] REVIEW: Practical strategies to maintain anabolism by intravenous nutritional management in children with inborn metabolic diseases. Molecular Genetics and Metabolism: Available online 7 May 2021

L. E. Bernstein et al. (eds.), *Nutrition Management of Inherited Metabolic Diseases*,
https://doi.org/10.1007/978-3-030-94510-7

Appendix D. Dietary Reference Intakes

Dietary Reference Intakes (DRIs): Estimated Average Requirements
Food and Nutrition Board, Institute of Medicine, National Academies

Life Stage Group	Calcium (mg/d)	CHO (g/d)	Protein (g/kg/d)	Vit A (μg/d)[a]	Vit C (mg/d)	Vit D (μg/d)	Vit E (mg/d)[b]	Thiamin (mg/d)	Riboflavin (mg/d)	Niacin (mg/d)[c]	Vit B_6 (mg/d)	Folate (μg/d)[d]	Vit B_{12} (μg/d)	Copper (μg/d)	Iodine (μg/d)	Iron (mg/d)	Magnesium (mg/d)	Molybdenum (μg/d)	Phosphorus (mg/d)	Selenium (μg/d)	Zinc (mg/d)
Infants																					
0 to 6 mo																					
6 to 12 mo			1.0													6.9					2.5
Children																					
1–3 y	500	100	0.87	210	13	10	5	0.4	0.4	5	0.4	120	0.7	260	65	3.0	65	13	380	17	2.5
4–8 y	800	100	0.76	275	22	10	6	0.5	0.5	6	0.5	160	1.0	340	65	4.1	110	17	405	23	4.0
Males																					
9–13 y	1,100	100	0.76	445	39	10	9	0.7	0.8	9	0.8	250	1.5	540	73	5.9	200	26	1,055	35	7.0
14–18 y	1,100	100	0.73	630	63	10	12	1.0	1.1	12	1.1	330	2.0	685	95	7.7	340	33	1,055	45	8.5
19–30 y	800	100	0.66	625	75	10	12	1.0	1.1	12	1.1	320	2.0	700	95	6	330	34	580	45	9.4
31–50 y	800	100	0.66	625	75	10	12	1.0	1.1	12	1.1	320	2.0	700	95	6	350	34	580	45	9.4
51–70 y	800	100	0.66	625	75	10	12	1.0	1.1	12	1.4	320	2.0	700	95	6	350	34	580	45	9.4
> 70 y	1,000	100	0.66	625	75	10	12	1.0	1.1	12	1.4	320	2.0	700	95	6	350	34	580	45	9.4
Females																					
9–13 y	1,100	100	0.76	420	39	10	9	0.7	0.8	9	0.8	250	1.5	540	73	5.7	200	26	1,055	35	7.0
14–18 y	1,100	100	0.71	485	56	10	12	0.9	0.9	11	1.0	330	2.0	685	95	7.9	300	33	1,055	45	7.3
19–30 y	800	100	0.66	500	60	10	12	0.9	0.9	11	1.1	320	2.0	700	95	8.1	255	34	580	45	6.8
31–50 y	800	100	0.66	500	60	10	12	0.9	0.9	11	1.1	320	2.0	700	95	8.1	265	34	580	45	6.8
51–70 y	1,000	100	0.66	500	60	10	12	0.9	0.9	11	1.3	320	2.0	700	95	5	265	34	580	45	6.8
> 70 y	1,000	100	0.66	500	60	10	12	0.9	0.9	11	1.3	320	2.0	700	95	5	265	34	580	45	6.8
Pregnancy																					
14–18 y	1,000	135	0.88	530	66	10	12	1.2	1.2	14	1.6	520	2.2	785	160	23	335	40	1,055	49	10.5
19–30 y	800	135	0.88	550	70	10	12	1.2	1.2	14	1.6	520	2.2	800	160	22	290	40	580	49	9.5
31–50 y	800	135	0.88	550	70	10	12	1.2	1.2	14	1.6	520	2.2	800	160	22	300	40	580	49	9.5
Lactation																					
14–18 y	1,000	160	1.05	885	96	10	16	1.2	1.3	13	1.7	450	2.4	985	209	7	300	35	1,055	59	10.9
19–30 y	800	160	1.05	900	100	10	16	1.2	1.3	13	1.7	450	2.4	1,000	209	6.5	255	36	580	59	10.4
31–50 y	800	160	1.05	900	100	10	16	1.2	1.3	13	1.7	450	2.4	1,000	209	6.5	265	36	580	59	10.4

NOTE: An Estimated Average Requirement (EAR) is the average daily nutrient intake level estimated to meet the requirements of half of the healthy individuals in a group. EARs have not been established for vitamin K, pantothenic acid, biotin, choline, chromium, fluoride, manganese, or other nutrients not yet evaluated via the DRI process.

[a] As retinol activity equivalents (RAEs). 1 RAE = 1 μg retinol, 12 μg β-carotene, 24 μg α-carotene, or 24 μg β-cryptoxanthin. The RAE for dietary provitamin A carotenoids is two-fold greater than retinol equivalents (RE), whereas the RAE for preformed vitamin A is the same as RE.

[b] As α-tocopherol. α-Tocopherol includes *RRR*-α-tocopherol, the only form of α-tocopherol that occurs naturally in foods, and the *2R*-stereoisomeric forms of α-tocopherol (*RRR*-, *RSR*-, *RRS*-, and *RSS*-α-tocopherol) that occur in fortified foods and supplements. It does not include the *2S*-stereoisomeric forms of α-tocopherol (*SRR*-, *SSR*-, *SRS*-, and *SSS*-α-tocopherol), also found in fortified foods and supplements.

[c] As niacin equivalents (NE). 1 mg of niacin = 60 mg of tryptophan.

[d] As dietary folate equivalents (DFE). 1 DFE = 1 μg food folate = 0.6 μg of folic acid from fortified food or as a supplement consumed with food = 0.5 μg of a supplement taken on an empty stomach.

SOURCES: *Dietary Reference Intakes for Calcium, Phosphorous, Magnesium, Vitamin D, and Fluoride* (1997); *Dietary Reference Intakes for Thiamin, Riboflavin, Niacin, Vitamin B₆, Folate, Vitamin B₁₂, Pantothenic Acid, Biotin, and Choline* (1998); *Dietary Reference Intakes for Vitamin C, Vitamin E, Selenium, and Carotenoids* (2000); *Dietary Reference Intakes for Vitamin A, Vitamin K, Arsenic, Boron, Chromium, Copper, Iodine, Iron, Manganese, Molybdenum, Nickel, Silicon, Vanadium, and Zinc* (2001); *Dietary Reference Intakes for Energy, Carbohydrate, Fiber, Fat, Fatty Acids, Cholesterol, Protein, and Amino Acids* (2002/2005); and *Dietary Reference Intakes for Calcium and Vitamin D* (2011). These reports may be accessed via www.nap.edu.

L. E. Bernstein et al. (eds.), *Nutrition Management of Inherited Metabolic Diseases*,
https://doi.org/10.1007/978-3-030-94510-7

Dietary Reference Intakes (DRIs): Recommended Dietary Allowances and Adequate Intakes, Vitamins

Food and Nutrition Board, Institute of Medicine, National Academies

Life Stage Group	Vitamin A (μg/d)[a]	Vitamin C (mg/d)	Vitamin D (μg/d)[b,c]	Vitamin E (mg/d)[d]	Vitamin K (μg/d)	Thiamin (mg/d)	Riboflavin (mg/d)	Niacin (mg/d)[e]	Vitamin B$_6$ (mg/d)	Folate (μg/d)[f]	Vitamin B$_{12}$ (μg/d)	Pantothenic Acid (mg/d)	Biotin (μg/d)	Choline (mg/d)[g]
Infants														
0 to 6 mo	400*	40*	10	4*	2.0*	0.2*	0.3*	2*	0.1*	65*	0.4*	1.7*	5*	125*
6 to 12 mo	500*	50*	10	5*	2.5*	0.3*	0.4*	4*	0.3*	80*	0.5*	1.8*	6*	150*
Children														
1–3 y	**300**	**15**	**15**	**6**	30*	**0.5**	**0.5**	**6**	**0.5**	**150**	**0.9**	2*	8*	200*
4–8 y	**400**	**25**	**15**	**7**	55*	**0.6**	**0.6**	**8**	**0.6**	**200**	**1.2**	3*	12*	250*
Males														
9–13 y	**600**	**45**	**15**	**11**	60*	**0.9**	**0.9**	**12**	**1.0**	**300**	**1.8**	4*	20*	375*
14–18 y	**900**	**75**	**15**	**15**	75*	**1.2**	**1.3**	**16**	**1.3**	**400**	**2.4**	5*	25*	550*
19–30 y	**900**	**90**	**15**	**15**	120*	**1.2**	**1.3**	**16**	**1.3**	**400**	**2.4**	5*	30*	550*
31–50 y	**900**	**90**	**15**	**15**	120*	**1.2**	**1.3**	**16**	**1.3**	**400**	**2.4**	5*	30*	550*
51–70 y	**900**	**90**	**15**	**15**	120*	**1.2**	**1.3**	**16**	**1.7**	**400**	**2.4**[h]	5*	30*	550*
> 70 y	**900**	**90**	**20**	**15**	120*	**1.2**	**1.3**	**16**	**1.7**	**400**	**2.4**[h]	5*	30*	550*
Females														
9–13 y	**600**	**45**	**15**	**11**	60*	**0.9**	**0.9**	**12**	**1.0**	**300**	**1.8**	4*	20*	375*
14–18 y	**700**	**65**	**15**	**15**	75*	**1.0**	**1.0**	**14**	**1.2**	**400**[i]	**2.4**	5*	25*	400*
19–30 y	**700**	**75**	**15**	**15**	90*	**1.1**	**1.1**	**14**	**1.3**	**400**[i]	**2.4**	5*	30*	425*
31–50 y	**700**	**75**	**15**	**15**	90*	**1.1**	**1.1**	**14**	**1.3**	**400**[i]	**2.4**	5*	30*	425*
51–70 y	**700**	**75**	**15**	**15**	90*	**1.1**	**1.1**	**14**	**1.5**	**400**	**2.4**[h]	5*	30*	425*
> 70 y	**700**	**75**	**20**	**15**	90*	**1.1**	**1.1**	**14**	**1.5**	**400**	**2.4**[h]	5*	30*	425*
Pregnancy														
14–18 y	**750**	**80**	**15**	**15**	75*	**1.4**	**1.4**	**18**	**1.9**	**600**[j]	**2.6**	6*	30*	450*
19–30 y	**770**	**85**	**15**	**15**	90*	**1.4**	**1.4**	**18**	**1.9**	**600**[j]	**2.6**	6*	30*	450*
31–50 y	**770**	**85**	**15**	**15**	90*	**1.4**	**1.4**	**18**	**1.9**	**600**[j]	**2.6**	6*	30*	450*
Lactation														
14–18 y	**1,200**	**115**	**15**	**19**	75*	**1.4**	**1.6**	**17**	**2.0**	**500**	**2.8**	7*	35*	550*
19–30 y	**1,300**	**120**	**15**	**19**	90*	**1.4**	**1.6**	**17**	**2.0**	**500**	**2.8**	7*	35*	550*
31–50 y	**1,300**	**120**	**15**	**19**	90*	**1.4**	**1.6**	**17**	**2.0**	**500**	**2.8**	7*	35*	550*

NOTE: This table (taken from the DRI reports, see www.nap.edu) presents Recommended Dietary Allowances (RDAs) in **bold type** and Adequate Intakes (AIs) in ordinary type followed by an asterisk (*). An RDA is the average daily dietary intake level; sufficient to meet the nutrient requirements of nearly all (97-98 percent) healthy individuals in a group. It is calculated from an Estimated Average Requirement (EAR). If sufficient scientific evidence is not available to establish an EAR, and thus calculate an RDA, an AI is usually developed. For healthy breastfed infants, an AI is the mean intake. The AI for other life stage and gender groups is believed to cover the needs of all healthy individuals in the groups, but lack of data or uncertainty in the data prevent being able to specify with confidence the percentage of individuals covered by this intake.

[a] As retinol activity equivalents (RAEs). 1 RAE = 1 μg retinol, 12 μg β-carotene, 24 μg α-carotene, or 24 μg β-cryptoxanthin. The RAE for dietary provitamin A carotenoids is two-fold greater than retinol equivalents (RE), whereas the RAE for preformed vitamin A is the same as RE.

[b] As cholecalciferol. 1 μg cholecalciferol = 40 IU vitamin D.

[c] Under the assumption of minimal sunlight.

[d] As α-tocopherol. α-Tocopherol includes *RRR*-α-tocopherol, the only form of α-tocopherol that occurs naturally in foods, and the *2R*-stereoisomeric forms of α-tocopherol (*RRR-*, *RSR-*, *RRS-*, and *RSS*-α-tocopherol) that occur in fortified foods and supplements. It does not include the *2S*-stereoisomeric forms of α-tocopherol (*SRR-*, *SSR-*, *SRS-*, and *SSS*-α-tocopherol), also found in fortified foods and supplements.

[e] As niacin equivalents (NE). 1 mg of niacin = 60 mg of tryptophan; 0–6 months = preformed niacin (not NE).

[f] As dietary folate equivalents (DFE). 1 DFE = 1 μg food folate = 0.6 μg of folic acid from fortified food or as a supplement consumed with food = 0.5 μg of a supplement taken on an empty stomach.

[g] Although AIs have been set for choline, there are few data to assess whether a dietary supply of choline is needed at all stages of the life cycle, and it may be that the choline requirement can be met by endogenous synthesis at some of these stages.

[h] Because 10 to 30 percent of older people may malabsorb food-bound B$_{12}$, it is advisable for those older than 50 years to meet their RDA mainly by consuming foods fortified with B$_{12}$ or a supplement containing B$_{12}$.

[i] In view of evidence linking folate intake with neural tube defects in the fetus, it is recommended that all women capable of becoming pregnant consume 400 μg from supplements or fortified foods in addition to intake of food folate from a varied diet.

[j] It is assumed that women will continue consuming 400 μg from supplements or fortified food until their pregnancy is confirmed and they enter prenatal care, which ordinarily occurs after the end of the periconceptional period—the critical time for formation of the neural tube.

SOURCES: *Dietary Reference Intakes for Calcium, Phosphorous, Magnesium, Vitamin D, and Fluoride* (1997); *Dietary Reference Intakes for Thiamin, Riboflavin, Niacin, Vitamin B$_6$, Folate, Vitamin B$_{12}$, Pantothenic Acid, Biotin, and Choline* (1998); *Dietary Reference Intakes for Vitamin C, Vitamin E, Selenium, and Carotenoids* (2000); *Dietary Reference Intakes for Vitamin A, Vitamin K, Arsenic, Boron, Chromium, Copper, Iodine, Iron, Manganese, Molybdenum, Nickel, Silicon, Vanadium, and Zinc* (2001); *Dietary Reference Intakes for Water, Potassium, Sodium, Chloride, and* Sulfate (2005); and *Dietary Reference Intakes for Calcium and Vitamin D* (2011). These reports may be accessed via www.nap.edu.

Dietary Reference Intakes (DRIs): Recommended Dietary Allowances and Adequate Intakes, Elements

Food and Nutrition Board, Institute of Medicine, National Academies

Life Stage Group	Calcium (mg/d)	Chromium (μg/d)	Copper (μg/d)	Fluoride (mg/d)	Iodine (μg/d)	Iron (mg/d)	Magnesium (mg/d)	Manganese (mg/d)	Molybdenum (μg/d)	Phosphorus (mg/d)	Selenium (μg/d)	Zinc (mg/d)	Potass-ium (g/d)	Sodium (g/d)	Chloride (g/d)
Infants															
0 to 6 mo	200*	0.2*	200*	0.01*	110*	0.27*	30*	0.003*	2*	100*	15*	2*	0.4*	0.12*	0.18*
6 to 12 mo	260*	5.5*	220*	0.5*	130*	**11**	75*	0.6*	3*	275*	20*	**3**	0.7*	0.37*	0.57*
Children															
1–3 y	**700**	11*	**340**	0.7*	**90**	**7**	**80**	1.2*	**17**	**460**	**20**	**3**	3.0*	1.0*	1.5*
4–8 y	**1,000**	15*	**440**	1*	**90**	**10**	**130**	1.5*	**22**	**500**	**30**	**5**	3.8*	1.2*	1.9*
Males															
9–13 y	**1,300**	25*	**700**	2*	**120**	**8**	**240**	1.9*	**34**	**1,250**	**40**	**8**	4.5*	1.5*	2.3*
14–18 y	**1,300**	35*	**890**	3*	**150**	**11**	**410**	2.2*	**43**	**1,250**	**55**	**11**	4.7*	1.5*	2.3*
19–30 y	**1,000**	35*	**900**	4*	**150**	**8**	**400**	2.3*	**45**	**700**	**55**	**11**	4.7*	1.5*	2.3*
31–50 y	**1,000**	35*	**900**	4*	**150**	**8**	**420**	2.3*	**45**	**700**	**55**	**11**	4.7*	1.5*	2.3*
51–70 y	**1,000**	30*	**900**	4*	**150**	**8**	**420**	2.3*	**45**	**700**	**55**	**11**	4.7*	1.3*	2.0*
> 70 y	**1,200**	30*	**900**	4*	**150**	**8**	**420**	2.3*	**45**	**700**	**55**	**11**	4.7*	1.2*	1.8*
Females															
9–13 y	**1,300**	21*	**700**	2*	**120**	**8**	**240**	1.6*	**34**	**1,250**	**40**	**8**	4.5*	1.5*	2.3*
14–18 y	**1,300**	24*	**890**	3*	**150**	**15**	**360**	1.6*	**43**	**1,250**	**55**	**9**	4.7*	1.5*	2.3*
19–30 y	**1,000**	25*	**900**	3*	**150**	**18**	**310**	1.8*	**45**	**700**	**55**	**8**	4.7*	1.5*	2.3*
31–50 y	**1,000**	25*	**900**	3*	**150**	**18**	**320**	1.8*	**45**	**700**	**55**	**8**	4.7*	1.5*	2.3*
51–70 y	**1,200**	20*	**900**	3*	**150**	**8**	**320**	1.8*	**45**	**700**	**55**	**8**	4.7*	1.3*	2.0*
> 70 y	**1,200**	20*	**900**	3*	**150**	**8**	**320**	1.8*	**45**	**700**	**55**	**8**	4.7*	1.2*	1.8*
Pregnancy															
14–18 y	**1,300**	29*	**1,000**	3*	**220**	**27**	**400**	2.0*	**50**	**1,250**	**60**	**12**	4.7*	1.5*	2.3*
19–30 y	**1,000**	30*	**1,000**	3*	**220**	**27**	**350**	2.0*	**50**	**700**	**60**	**11**	4.7*	1.5*	2.3*
31–50 y	**1,000**	30*	**1,000**	3*	**220**	**27**	**360**	2.0*	**50**	**700**	**60**	**11**	4.7*	1.5*	2.3*
Lactation															
14–18 y	**1,300**	44*	**1,300**	3*	**290**	**10**	**360**	2.6*	**50**	**1,250**	**70**	**13**	5.1*	1.5*	2.3*
19–30 y	**1,000**	45*	**1,300**	3*	**290**	**9**	**310**	2.6*	**50**	**700**	**70**	**12**	5.1*	1.5*	2.3*
31–50 y	**1,000**	45*	**1,300**	3*	**290**	**9**	**320**	2.6*	**50**	**700**	**70**	**12**	5.1*	1.5*	2.3*

NOTE: This table (taken from the DRI reports, see www.nap.edu) presents Recommended Dietary Allowances (RDAs) in **bold type** and Adequate Intakes (AIs) in ordinary type followed by an asterisk (*). An RDA is the average daily dietary intake level; sufficient to meet the nutrient requirements of nearly all (97-98 percent) healthy individuals in a group. It is calculated from an Estimated Average Requirement (EAR). If sufficient scientific evidence is not available to establish an EAR, and thus calculate an RDA, an AI is usually developed. For healthy breastfed infants, an AI is the mean intake. The AI for other life stage and gender groups is believed to cover the needs of all healthy individuals in the groups, but lack of data or uncertainty in the data prevent being able to specify with confidence the percentage of individuals covered by this intake.

SOURCES: *Dietary Reference Intakes for Calcium, Phosphorous, Magnesium, Vitamin D, and Fluoride* (1997); *Dietary Reference Intakes for Thiamin, Riboflavin, Niacin, Vitamin B$_6$, Folate, Vitamin B$_{12}$, Pantothenic Acid, Biotin, and Choline* (1998); *Dietary Reference Intakes for Vitamin C, Vitamin E, Selenium, and Carotenoids* (2000); and *Dietary Reference Intakes for Vitamin A, Vitamin K, Arsenic, Boron, Chromium, Copper, Iodine, Iron, Manganese, Molybdenum, Nickel, Silicon, Vanadium, and Zinc* (2001); *Dietary Reference Intakes for Water, Potassium, Sodium, Chloride, and* Sulfate (2005); and *Dietary Reference Intakes for Calcium and Vitamin D* (2011). These reports may be accessed via www.nap.edu.

Dietary Reference Intakes (DRIs): Recommended Dietary Allowances and Adequate Intakes, Total Water and Macronutrients

Food and Nutrition Board, Institute of Medicine, National Academies

Life Stage Group	*Total* Water[a] (L/d)	Carbohydrate (g/d)	Total Fiber (g/d)	Fat (g/d)	Linoleic Acid (g/d)	α-Linolenic Acid (g/d)	Protein[b] (g/d)
Infants							
0 to 6 mo	0.7*	60*	ND	31*	4.4*	0.5*	9.1*
6 to 12 mo	0.8*	95*	ND	30*	4.6*	0.5*	**11.0**
Children							
1–3 y	1.3*	**130**	19*	ND[c]	7*	0.7*	**13**
4–8 y	1.7*	**130**	25*	ND	10*	0.9*	**19**
Males							
9–13 y	2.4*	**130**	31*	ND	12*	1.2*	**34**
14–18 y	3.3*	**130**	38*	ND	16*	1.6*	**52**
19–30 y	3.7*	**130**	38*	ND	17*	1.6*	**56**
31–50 y	3.7*	**130**	38*	ND	17*	1.6*	**56**
51–70 y	3.7*	**130**	30*	ND	14*	1.6*	**56**
> 70 y	3.7*	**130**	30*	ND	14*	1.6*	**56**
Females							
9–13 y	2.1*	**130**	26*	ND	10*	1.0*	**34**
14–18 y	2.3*	**130**	26*	ND	11*	1.1*	**46**
19–30 y	2.7*	**130**	25*	ND	12*	1.1*	**46**
31–50 y	2.7*	**130**	25*	ND	12*	1.1*	**46**
51–70 y	2.7*	**130**	21*	ND	11*	1.1*	**46**
> 70 y	2.7*	**130**	21*	ND	11*	1.1*	**46**
Pregnancy							
14–18 y	3.0*	**175**	28*	ND	13*	1.4*	**71**
19–30 y	3.0*	**175**	28*	ND	13*	1.4*	**71**
31–50 y	3.0*	**175**	28*	ND	13*	1.4*	**71**
Lactation							
14–18	3.8*	**210**	29*	ND	13*	1.3*	**71**
19–30 y	3.8*	**210**	29*	ND	13*	1.3*	**71**
31–50 y	3.8*	**210**	29*	ND	13*	1.3*	**71**

NOTE: This table (take from the DRI reports, see www.nap.edu) presents Recommended Dietary Allowances (RDA) in **bold type** and Adequate Intakes (AI) in ordinary type followed by an asterisk (*). An RDA is the average daily dietary intake level; sufficient to meet the nutrient requirements of nearly all (97-98 percent) healthy individuals in a group. It is calculated from an Estimated Average Requirement (EAR). If sufficient scientific evidence is not available to establish an EAR, and thus calculate an RDA, an AI is usually developed. For healthy breastfed infants, an AI is the mean intake. The AI for other life stage and gender groups is believed to cover the needs of all healthy individuals in the groups, but lack of data or uncertainty in the data prevent being able to specify with confidence the percentage of individuals covered by this intake.

[a] *Total* water includes all water contained in food, beverages, and drinking water.

[b] Based on g protein per kg of body weight for the reference body weight, e.g., for adults 0.8 g/kg body weight for the reference body weight.

[c] Not determined.

SOURCE: *Dietary Reference Intakes for Energy, Carbohydrate, Fiber, Fat, Fatty Acids, Cholesterol, Protein, and Amino Acids* (2002/2005) and *Dietary Reference Intakes for Water, Potassium, Sodium, Chloride, and Sulfate* (2005). The report may be accessed via www.nap.edu.

Dietary Reference Intakes (DRIs): Acceptable Macronutrient Distribution Ranges

Food and Nutrition Board, Institute of Medicine, National Academies

Macronutrient	Range (percent of energy) Children, 1–3 y	Children, 4–18 y	Adults
Fat	30–40	25–35	20–35
n-6 polyunsaturated fatty acids[a] (linoleic acid)	5–10	5–10	5–10
n-3 polyunsaturated fatty acids[a] (α-linolenic acid)	0.6–1.2	0.6–1.2	0.6–1.2
Carbohydrate	45–65	45–65	45–65
Protein	5–20	10–30	10–35

[a] Approximately 10 percent of the total can come from longer-chain *n*-3 or *n*-6 fatty acids.

SOURCE: *Dietary Reference Intakes for Energy, Carbohydrate, Fiber, Fat, Fatty Acids, Cholesterol, Protein, and Amino Acids* (2002/2005). The report may be accessed via www.nap.edu.

Dietary Reference Intakes (DRIs): Acceptable Macronutrient Distribution Ranges

Food and Nutrition Board, Institute of Medicine, National Academies

Macronutrient	Recommendation
Dietary cholesterol	As low as possible while consuming a nutritionally adequate diet
Trans fatty Acids	As low as possible while consuming a nutritionally adequate diet
Saturated fatty acids	As low as possible while consuming a nutritionally adequate diet
Added sugars[a]	Limit to no more than 25 % of total energy

[a]Not a recommended intake. A daily intake of added sugars that individuals should aim for to achieve a healthful diet was not set.

SOURCE: *Dietary Reference Intakes for Energy, Carbohydrate, Fiber, Fat, Fatty Acids, Cholesterol, Protein, and Amino Acids* (2002/2005). The report may be accessed via www.nap.edu.

Dietary Reference Intakes (DRIs): Tolerable Upper Intake Levels, Vitamins

Food and Nutrition Board, Institute of Medicine, National Academies

Life Stage Group	Vitamin A (μg/d)[a]	Vitamin C (mg/d)	Vitamin D (μg/d)	Vitamin E (mg/d)[b,c]	Vitamin K	Thiamin	Riboflavin	Niacin (mg/d)[c]	Vitamin B_6 (mg/d)	Folate (μg/d)[c]	Vitamin B_{12}	Pantothenic Acid	Biotin	Choline (g/d)	Carotenoids[d]
Infants															
0 to 6 mo	600	ND[e]	25	ND	ND	ND	ND	ND	ND	ND	ND	ND	ND	ND	ND
6 to 12 mo	600	ND	38	ND	ND	ND	ND	ND	ND	ND	ND	ND	ND	ND	ND
Children															
1–3 y	600	400	63	200	ND	ND	ND	10	30	300	ND	ND	ND	1.0	ND
4–8 y	900	650	75	300	ND	ND	ND	15	40	400	ND	ND	ND	1.0	ND
Males															
9–13 y	1,700	1,200	100	600	ND	ND	ND	20	60	600	ND	ND	ND	2.0	ND
14–18 y	2,800	1,800	100	800	ND	ND	ND	30	80	800	ND	ND	ND	3.0	ND
19–30 y	3,000	2,000	100	1,000	ND	ND	ND	35	100	1,000	ND	ND	ND	3.5	ND
31–50 y	3,000	2,000	100	1,000	ND	ND	ND	35	100	1,000	ND	ND	ND	3.5	ND
51–70 y	3,000	2,000	100	1,000	ND	ND	ND	35	100	1,000	ND	ND	ND	3.5	ND
> 70 y	3,000	2,000	100	1,000	ND	ND	ND	35	100	1,000	ND	ND	ND	3.5	ND
Females															
9–13 y	1,700	1,200	100	600	ND	ND	ND	20	60	600	ND	ND	ND	2.0	ND
14–18 y	2,800	1,800	100	800	ND	ND	ND	30	80	800	ND	ND	ND	3.0	ND
19–30 y	3,000	2,000	100	1,000	ND	ND	ND	35	100	1,000	ND	ND	ND	3.5	ND
31–50 y	3,000	2,000	100	1,000	ND	ND	ND	35	100	1,000	ND	ND	ND	3.5	ND
51–70 y	3,000	2,000	100	1,000	ND	ND	ND	35	100	1,000	ND	ND	ND	3.5	ND
> 70 y	3,000	2,000	100	1,000	ND	ND	ND	35	100	1,000	ND	ND	ND	3.5	ND
Pregnancy															
14–18 y	2,800	1,800	100	800	ND	ND	ND	30	80	800	ND	ND	ND	3.0	ND
19–30 y	3,000	2,000	100	1,000	ND	ND	ND	35	100	1,000	ND	ND	ND	3.5	ND
31–50 y	3,000	2,000	100	1,000	ND	ND	ND	35	100	1,000	ND	ND	ND	3.5	ND
Lactation															
14–18 y	2,800	1,800	100	800	ND	ND	ND	30	80	800	ND	ND	ND	3.0	ND
19–30 y	3,000	2,000	100	1,000	ND	ND	ND	35	100	1,000	ND	ND	ND	3.5	ND
31–50 y	3,000	2,000	100	1,000	ND	ND	ND	35	100	1,000	ND	ND	ND	3.5	ND

NOTE: A Tolerable Upper Intake Level (UL) is the highest level of daily nutrient intake that is likely to pose no risk of adverse health effects to almost all individuals in the general population. Unless otherwise specified, the UL represents total intake from food, water, and supplements. Due to a lack of suitable data, ULs could not be established for vitamin K, thiamin, riboflavin, vitamin B_{12}, pantothenic acid, biotin, and carotenoids. In the absence of a UL, extra caution may be warranted in consuming levels above recommended intakes. Members of the general population should be advised not to routinely exceed the UL. The UL is not meant to apply to individuals who are treated with the nutrient under medical supervision or to individuals with predisposing conditions that modify their sensitivity to the nutrient.

[a]As preformed vitamin A only.

[b]As α-tocopherol; applies to any form of supplemental α-tocopherol.

[c]The ULs for vitamin E, niacin, and folate apply to synthetic forms obtained from supplements, fortified foods, or a combination of the two.

[d]β-Carotene supplements are advised only to serve as a provitamin A source for individuals at risk of vitamin A deficiency.

[e]ND = Not determinable due to lack of data of adverse effects in this age group and concern with regard to lack of ability to handle excess amounts. Source of intake should be from food only to prevent high levels of intake.

SOURCES: *Dietary Reference Intakes for Calcium, Phosphorous, Magnesium, Vitamin D, and Fluoride* (1997); *Dietary Reference Intakes for Thiamin, Riboflavin, Niacin, Vitamin B_6, Folate, Vitamin B_{12}, Pantothenic Acid, Biotin, and Choline* (1998); *Dietary Reference Intakes for Vitamin C, Vitamine E, Selenium, and Carotenoids* (2000); *Dietary Reference Intakes for Vitamin A, Vitamin K, Arsenic, Boron, Chromium, Copper, Iodine, Iron, Manganese, Molybdenum, Nickel, Silicon, Vanadium, and Zinc* (2001); and *Dietary Reference Intakes for Calcium and Vitamin D* (2011). These reports may be accessed via www.nap.edu.

Dietary Reference Intakes (DRIs): Tolerable Upper Intake Levels, Elements
Food and Nutrition Board, Institute of Medicine, National Academies

Life Stage Group	Arsenic[a]	Boron (mg/d)	Calcium (mg/d)	Chromium	Copper (μg/d)	Fluoride (mg/d)	Iodine (μg/d)	Iron (mg/d)	Magnesium (mg/d)[b]	Manganese (mg/d)	Molybdenum (μg/d)	Nickel (mg/d)	Phosphorus (g/d)	Selenium (μg/d)	Silicon[c]	Vanadium (mg/d)[d]	Zinc (mg/d)	Sodium (g/d)	Chloride (g/d)
Infants																			
0 to 6 mo	ND[e]	ND	1,000	ND	ND	0.7	ND	40	ND	ND	ND	ND	ND	45	ND	ND	4	ND	ND
6 to 12 mo	ND	ND	1,500	ND	ND	0.9	ND	40	ND	ND	ND	ND	ND	60	ND	ND	5	ND	ND
Children																			
1–3 y	ND	3	2,500	ND	1,000	1.3	200	40	65	2	300	0.2	3	90	ND	ND	7	1.5	2.3
4–8 y	ND	6	2,500	ND	3,000	2.2	300	40	110	3	600	0.3	3	150	ND	ND	12	1.9	2.9
Males																			
9–13 y	ND	11	3,000	ND	5,000	10	600	40	350	6	1,100	0.6	4	280	ND	ND	23	2.2	3.4
14–18 y	ND	17	3,000	ND	8,000	10	900	45	350	9	1,700	1.0	4	400	ND	ND	34	2.3	3.6
19–30 y	ND	20	2,500	ND	10,000	10	1,100	45	350	11	2,000	1.0	4	400	ND	1.8	40	2.3	3.6
31–50 y	ND	20	2,500	ND	10,000	10	1,100	45	350	11	2,000	1.0	4	400	ND	1.8	40	2.3	3.6
51–70 y	ND	20	2,000	ND	10,000	10	1,100	45	350	11	2,000	1.0	4	400	ND	1.8	40	2.3	3.6
> 70 y	ND	20	2,000	ND	10,000	10	1,100	45	350	11	2,000	1.0	3	400	ND	1.8	40	2.3	3.6
Females																			
9–13 y	ND	11	3,000	ND	5,000	10	600	40	350	6	1,100	0.6	4	280	ND	ND	23	2.2	3.4
14–18 y	ND	17	3,000	ND	8,000	10	900	45	350	9	1,700	1.0	4	400	ND	ND	34	2.3	3.6
19–30 y	ND	20	2,500	ND	10,000	10	1,100	45	350	11	2,000	1.0	4	400	ND	1.8	40	2.3	3.6
31–50 y	ND	20	2,500	ND	10,000	10	1,100	45	350	11	2,000	1.0	4	400	ND	1.8	40	2.3	3.6
51–70 y	ND	20	2,000	ND	10,000	10	1,100	45	350	11	2,000	1.0	4	400	ND	1.8	40	2.3	3.6
> 70 y	ND	20	2,000	ND	10,000	10	1,100	45	350	11	2,000	1.0	3	400	ND	1.8	40	2.3	3.6
Pregnancy																			
14–18 y	ND	17	3,000	ND	8,000	10	900	45	350	9	1,700	1.0	3.5	400	ND	ND	34	2.3	3.6
19–30 y	ND	20	2,500	ND	10,000	10	1,100	45	350	11	2,000	1.0	3.5	400	ND	ND	40	2.3	3.6
61–50 y	ND	20	2,500	ND	10,000	10	1,100	45	350	11	2,000	1.0	3.5	400	ND	ND	40	2.3	3.6
Lactation																			
14–18 y	ND	17	3,000	ND	8,000	10	900	45	350	9	1,700	1.0	4	400	ND	ND	34	2.3	3.6
19–30 y	ND	20	2,500	ND	10,000	10	1,100	45	350	11	2,000	1.0	4	400	ND	ND	40	2.3	3.6
31–50 y	ND	20	2,500	ND	10,000	10	1,100	45	350	11	2,000	1.0	4	400	ND	ND	40	2.3	3.6

NOTE: A Tolerable Upper Intake Level (UL) is the highest level of daily nutrient intake that is likely to pose no risk of adverse health effects to almost all individuals in the general population. Unless otherwise specified, the UL represents total intake from food, water, and supplements. Due to a lack of suitable data, ULs could not be established for vitamin K, thiamin, riboflavin, vitamin B_{12}, pantothenic acid, biotin, and carotenoids. In the absence of a UL, extra caution may be warranted in consuming levels above recommended intakes. Members of the general population should be advised not to routinely exceed the UL. The UL is not meant to apply to individuals who are treated with the nutrient under medical supervision or to individuals with predisposing conditions that modify their sensitivity to the nutrient.

[a] Although the UL was not determined for arsenic, there is no justification for adding arsenic to food or supplements.

[b] The ULs for magnesium represent intake from a pharmacological agent only and do not include intake from food and water.

[c] Although silicon has not been shown to cause adverse effects in humans, there is no justification for adding silicon to supplements.

[d] Although vanadium in food has not been shown to cause adverse effects in humans, there is no justification for adding vanadium to food and vanadium supplements should be used with caution. The UL is based on adverse effects in laboratory animals and this data could be used to set a UL for adults but not children and adolescents.

[e] ND = Not determinable due to lack of data of adverse effects in this age group and concern with regard to lack of ability to handle excess amounts. Source of intake should be from food only to prevent high levels of intake.

SOURCES: *Dietary Reference Intakes for Calcium, Phosphorous, Magnesium, Vitamin D, and Fluoride* (1997); *Dietary Reference Intakes for Thiamin, Riboflavin, Niacin, Vitamin B_6, Folate, Vitamin B_{12}, Pantothenic Acid, Biotin, and Choline* (1998); *Dietary Reference Intakes for Vitamin C, Vitamin E, Selenium, and Carotenoids* (2000); *Dietary Reference Intakes for Vitamin A, Vitamin K, Arsenic, Boron, Chromium, Copper, Iodine, Iron, Manganese, Molybdenum, Nickel, Silicon, Vanadium, and Zinc* (2001); *Dietary Reference Intakes for Water, Potassium, Sodium, Chloride, and Sulfate* (2005); and *Dietary Reference Intakes for Calcium and Vitamin D* (2011). These reports may be accessed via www.nap.edu.

Appendix E. Carnitine in Inherited Metabolic Diseases

Carnitine

- Is synthesized by the body from the substrate trimethyllysine (itself a product of lysine and methionine). The synthesis of carnitine also requires iron, vitamins B_1, B_6, and C.
- Transports long-chain fatty acids into the mitochondria so they can be oxidized to produce energy.
- Transports potentially toxic compounds (e.g., short-chain organic acids) out of the mitochondria to prevent their accumulation and allows for excretion of acylcarnitines in the urine.

L. E. Bernstein et al. (eds.), *Nutrition Management of Inherited Metabolic Diseases*,
https://doi.org/10.1007/978-3-030-94510-7

The Carnitine Shuttle

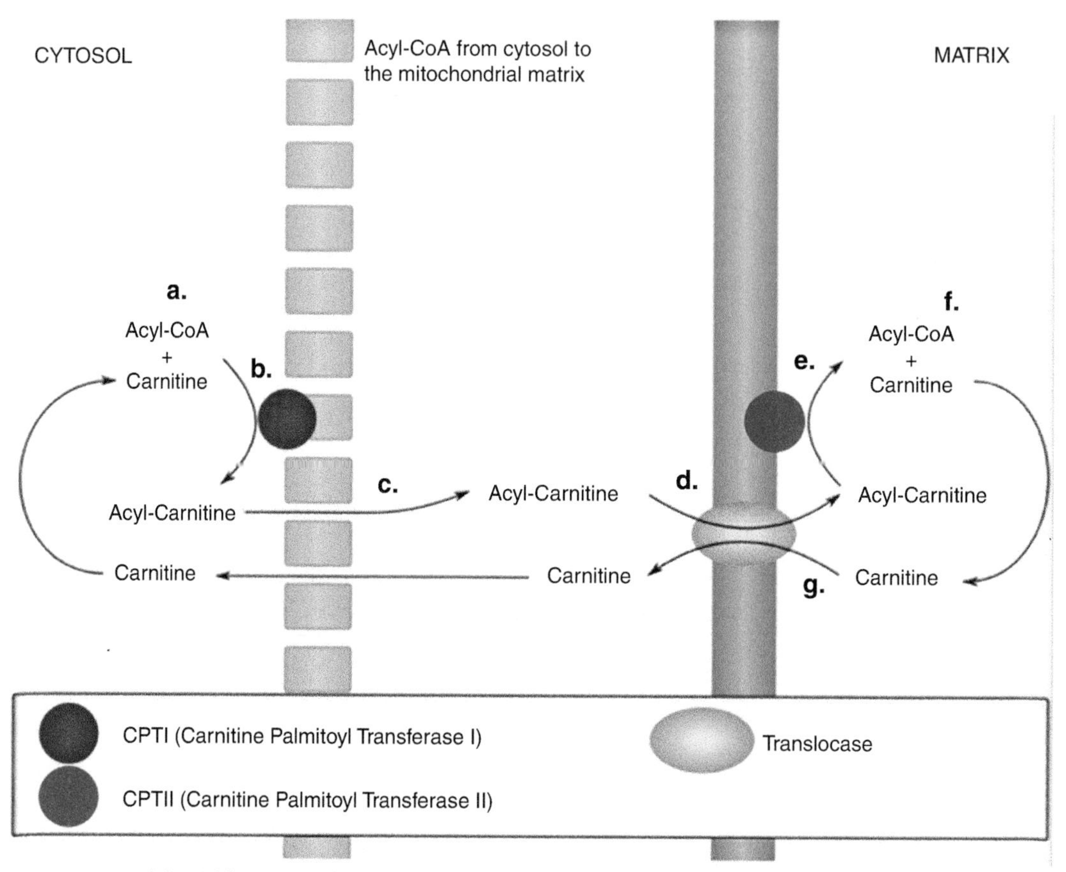

Adapted from https://en.wikipedia.org/wiki/Carnitine-acylcarnitine translocase

(a) In the cytosol, fatty acids (released from triglycerides during lipolysis) are esterified to form acyl-CoAs.
(b) An acyl-CoA is conjugated with carnitine to form an acylcarnitine. This requires the enzyme carnitine palmitoyl transferase 1 (CPT1) (red dot).
(c) The acylcarnitine moves through the outer mitochondrial membrane (yellow dashed line) to the intermembrane space.
(d) The acylcarnitine is transported through the inner mitochondrial membrane (blue line) into the mitochondrial matrix using the enzyme carnitine acylcarnitine translocase (CACT) (yellow oval).
(e) The acylcarnitine is unconjugated back into free carnitine and acyl-CoA using the enzyme carnitine palmitoyl transferase 2 (CPT2) (blue dot).
(f) The acyl-CoA is trapped inside the mitochondrial matrix and undergoes beta-oxidation.
(g) The free carnitine is shuttled back through the inner mitochondrial membrane (requiring CACT) and then moves freely into the cytosol where it can conjugate with another acyl-CoA.
(h) The carnitine in the inner mitochondrial matrix is sometimes conjugated to organic acids or fatty acids that have accumulated and transports these metabolites out of the mitochondria.

L-Carnitine Food Sources and Supplementation

- Foods high in carnitine include red meats, other meats to a lesser extent, and dairy products.
- Good vegan sources are tempeh, avocados, whole wheat products, and peanut butter, but these contain much less carnitine than animal sources.
- Medical foods for inherited metabolic disorders (IMD) often contain added L-carnitine.
- Carnitine is present in sufficient amounts (from the diet and biosynthesis) for most people; however, those with medical conditions such as prematurity, malnutrition, liver, and renal disease often are carnitine-deficient and require supplementation with L-carnitine (the active form of carnitine).
- In some IMD, L-carnitine supplementation may be needed (Table 1).
- Supplementation is considered to be safe, yet large doses (>3 g/day) can cause nausea, vomiting, and diarrhea and/or a "fishy" odor. The latter occurs when intestinal bacteria metabolize carnitine to form trimethylamine-N-oxide (TMAO), a compound that might increase the risk of cardiovascular disease [1] .
- In long-chain fatty acid oxidation disorders, supplemental L-carnitine may cause accumulation of acylcarnitines that are potentially cardiotoxic. This is based on a study in mice, and the relevance to humans is not known [2].

Table 1 L-Carnitine supplementation in inherited metabolic diseases

Disease	Supplementation (divided into 2–4 doses/day)	Rationale
Primary carnitine deficiency [3]	Standard therapy 100–200 mg/kg/d	Corrects deficiency
Glutaric acidemia type 1 [4] Isovaleric acidemia [5]	Standard therapy 100 mg/kg/d	Binds with toxic organic acids
Methylmalonic acidemia Propionic acidemia [6]	Often recommended 100–200 mg/kg/d	Corrects secondary deficiency
Medium chain Acyl-CoA Dehydrogenase deficiency [7]	No consensus 25–100 mg/kg/day If free carnitine is low	Binds with acyl groups Corrects secondary deficiency
Long-chain fatty acid oxidation Disorders [8]	No consensus 25 mg/kg/day If free carnitine <10 μmol/L	

Table 2 Plasma carnitine profile

Species	Description	Normal range [9] (nmol/mL)	
		Age (years)	Range
Total carnitine	All carnitine species: both free carnitine and carnitine bound to acyl-CoA	<1	23–68
		1–10	35–83
		11–18	34–77
		>18	34–78
Free carnitine	Carnitine species that are not bound to acyl-CoA	<1	12–49
		1–10	24–66
		11–18	22–65
		>18	35–54
Acyl (or esterified) carnitine	Carnitine species that are bound to acyl-CoA	<1	7–19
		1–10	4–32
		11–18	4–29
		>18	5–30

References

1. Office of Dietary Supplements: Carnitine Fact Sheet for Professionals. https://ods.od.nih.gov/factsheets/Carnitine-HealthProfessionals. Accessed 3/8/21.
2. Primassin S, et al. Carnitine supplementation induces acylcarnitine production in tissues of very long-chain acyl-CoA dehydrogenase-deficient mice, without replenishing low free carnitine. Pediatr Res. 2008;63(6):632–7.
3. Longo N, et al Carnitine transport and fatty acid oxidation. Biochim Biophys Acta. 2016;1863(10):2422–35.
4. Boy N, et al. Proposed recommendations for diagnosing and managing individuals with glutaric aciduria type I: second revision. J Inherit Metab Dis. 2017;40(1):75–101.
5. Schlune A, et al. Aspects of newborn screening in isovaleric acidemia. Int J Neonatal Screen. 2018;4(1):7.
6. Baumgartner MR, et al. Proposed guidelines for the diagnosis and management of methyl-

malonic and propionic acidemia. Orphanet J Rare Dis. 2014;9:130.
7. Merritt JL 2nd, et al. In: Adam MP, Ardinger HH, Pagon RA, Wallace SE, Bean LJH, Stephens K, Amemiya A, editors. GeneReviews® [Internet]. Seattle: University of Washington, Seattle; 1993–2020.
8. van Calcar SC, et al. Nutrition management guideline for very-long chain acyl-CoA dehydrogenase deficiency (VLCAD): an evidence- and consensus-based approach. Mol Genet Metab. 2020;131(1–2):23–7.
9. Mayo Clinic Test ID:CARN Carntine, Plasma.https://www.mayocliniclabs.com/test-catalog/Clinical+and+Interpretive/8802. Accessed 3/8/21.

Appendix F. Quick Guide to Acylcarnitine Profiles

Carnitine ester	Acylcarnitine name	Clinical correlate*
C0	Free carnitine	Primary carnitine deficiency, CPT1
C3	Propionylcarnitine	PA, MMAs, mitochondrial
C3-DC	Malonylcarnitine	Malonic aciduria
C4	Butyrylcarnitine	SCAD, IBD, MADD (GA II)
C4-OH	3-hydroxybutyrylcarnitine	SCHADD
C5:1	Tiglylcarnitine	BKT, MHBDD
C5	Isovalerylcarnitine 3-Methyl-butyrylcarnitine	IVA, SBCAD, MADD
C5-OH	Hydroxyisovalerylcarnitine 2-Methyl-3-hydroxybutyrylcarnitine	3MCC, holocarboxylase, biotinidase, BKT, HMG-CoA lyase, 3MGA
C5-DC	Glutarylcarnitine	GA I, MADD
C8	Octanoylcarnitine	MCADD, MADD
C14:1	Tetradecanoylcarnitine	VLCADD
C16	Hexadecanoylcarnitine	CPT II, CACT
C16-OH	Hydroxyhexadecanoylcarnitine	LCHADD/TFP

L. E. Bernstein et al. (eds.), *Nutrition Management of Inherited Metabolic Diseases*, https://doi.org/10.1007/978-3-030-94510-7

Appendix G. Simplified Diet

Simplified Diet

Uncounted Fruits

- Apples – fresh and dry
- Apricots – fresh and dry
- Bananas
- Berries (all varieties)
- Cherries
- Cranberries – fresh and dry
- Dates
- Figs
- Grapefruit
- Grapes
- Guava
- Jackfruit
- Kiwi
- Lemons
- Limes
- Mango
- Melon (all varieties)
- Olives
- Oranges
- Papaya
- Peaches
- Pears – dry and fresh
- Pineapple
- Plantains
- Plums
- Pomegranates
- Prunes
- Raisins

Uncounted Vegetables

- Acorn Squash
- Beets
- Bok Choy
- Butternut Squash
- Cabbage
- Carrots
- Cauliflower
- Celery
- Chayote Squash
- Cucumber
- Green Beans
- Eggplant
- Jicama
- Leeks
- Lettuce
- Okra
- Onions
- Parsnips
- Peppers (all varieties)
- Pumpkin
- Radishes
- Rutabaga
- Sauerkraut
- Spaghetti Squash
- Summer Squash (zucchini and yellow)
- Tomatoes
- Turnips
- Yucca (Cassava Root)

Please remember your NO foods are still NO foods

For any questions on specific items, please contact your metabolic dietitian.
Developed by IMD Nutrition, Children's Hospital Colorado

L. E. Bernstein et al. (eds.), *Nutrition Management of Inherited Metabolic Diseases*,
https://doi.org/10.1007/978-3-030-94510-7

Simplified Diet

Measure and Count Phe/Protein

- Dried Fruit (except apples, apricots, craisins, pears, prunes, raisins)

- Artichokes
- Arugula
- Asparagus
- Avocado
- Broccoli
- Brussels Sprouts
- Corn
- Kale, mustard greens, Swiss chard
- Mushrooms
- Peas
- Potatoes
- Seaweed/Nori
- Sundried Tomatoes
- Spinach
- Yams/Sweet Potatoes

Do Not Measure and Count Phe/Protein

- Fruits and vegetables that have less than 75 mg phe per 100 grams of food weight(see separate sheet for specific list)
- Low protein foods less than 20 mg of phe per serving size. See package for serving size.
- Foods that contain ≤ 0.4 grams of protein per serving.

Please remember your NO foods are still NO foods

For any questions on specific items, please contact your metabolic dietitian.
Developed by IMD Nutrition, Children's Hospital Colorado

Appendix H. Interpreting Quantitative Fatty Acid Profiles

Courtesy of Dr. Melanie Gillingham, PhD, RD, Oregon Health & Science University, Portland, Oregon

L. E. Bernstein et al. (eds.), *Nutrition Management of Inherited Metabolic Diseases*,
https://doi.org/10.1007/978-3-030-94510-7

Example Fatty Acid Profile			
COMPOUND	REFERENCE	PATIENT	
C 8:0	8-47	43	
C10:1	1.8-5.0	7.8	H
C10:0	2-18	70	H
C12:1	1.4-6.6	6	
C12:0	6-90	22	
C14:2	0.8-5.0	6.8	H
C14:1	3-64	30	
C14:0 Myristic Acid	**30-450**	**98**	
C16:2	10-48	18	
C16:1n-9	25-105	86	
C16:1n-7	110-1130	269	
C16:0 Palmitic Acid	**1480-3730**	**1426**	**L**
C18:3n-6	16-150	18	
C18:3n-3 Linolenic Acid	**50-130**	**37**	**L**
C18:2n-6 Linoleic Acid	**2270-3850**	**1207**	**L**
C18:1n-9	650-3500	872	
C18:1n-7	280-740	207	L
C18:0 Stearic Acid	**590-1170**	**648**	
C20:5n-3 Eicosapentaenoic acid (EPA)	**14-100**	**31**	
C20:4n-6 Arachidonic Acid	**520-1490**	**316**	**L**
C20:3n-9	7-30	7	
C20:3n-6	50-250	43	L
C20:0 Arachidic acid	**50-90**	**46**	**L**
C22:6n-3 Docosahexaenoic acid (DHA)	**50-250**	**29**	**L**
C22:5n-6	10-70	13	
C22:5n-3	20-210	38	
C22:4n-6	10-80	11	
C22:1	4-13	5	
C22:0	0.0-96.3	36.5	
C24:1n-9	60-100	82	
C24:0	0.0-91.4	38.8	
C26:1	0.3-0.7	1	
C26:0	0.00-1.30	0.78	
C19:B	0.00-2.98	0.04	
C20:B	0.00-9.88	0.5	
HOLMAN RATIO	0.010-0.038	0.022151899	

1.) Evaluate n-6 status:
a. Low linoleic acid
b. Low arachidonic acid
c. Normal Holman ratio
- The patient is consuming a low fat diet so the Holman ratio is normal because both n-6 and n-9 are low. The Holman ratio may or may not indicate an essential fatty acid deficiency in metabolic patients.

Compound	Reference	Patient	Low
C18:2n-6 Linoleic acid	2270 - 3850	1207	Yes
C20:4n-6 Arachidonic Acid	520-1490	316	Yes
C22:5n-6 Docosapentaenoic acid n-6	10-70	13	No
Holman Ratio	0.010-0.038	0.022	No

2.) Evaluate saturated fatty acids:
a. Low saturated fat acids
- The patient is consuming a low fat diet.

Compound	Reference	Patient	Low
C14:0 Myristic acid	30-450	98	No
C16:0 Palmitic acid	1480-3730	1426	Yes
C18:0 Stearic acid	590-1170	648	No
C20:0 Arachidic acid	50-90	46	Yes

3.) Evaluate n-3 fatty acids:
a. Low linolenic acid
b. Low in DHA
c. ARA:DHA ratio is too high (goal is less than 4)
d. Low C22:5n-6 is another indicator of n-3 deficiency.

Compound	Reference	Patient	Low
C18:3n-3 Linolenic acid	50-130	37	Yes
C20:5n-3 Eicopentaenoic acid (EPA)	14-100	31	No
C22:6n-3 Docosahexaenoic acid (DHA)	30-250	29	Yes
ARA:DHA	2.1-4.6	10.8	-

Nutrition Management Plan:

- **Increase n-6 fatty acid intaketocorrect low linoleic and arachidonic acid concentrations.**
- **Decrease saturated fatty acid intake in order to maintain low dietary fat intake.**
- **Begin DHA supplements to correct low DHA concentrations.**
- **Alpha-linoleic acid is low but as it is primarily needed as a precursor to DHA, additional alpha-linoleic acid is not needed as long as DHA is supplemented in the diet.**

Plasma Fatty Acids

- Free fatty acids are found in plasma in the ionized form. FFA are elevated with fasting and low with feeding.
- Most plasma fatty acids exist as esters in lipoproteins:
  - Triglycerides
  - Phospholipids
- **Fatty acid profiles include both FFA and plasma fatty acids in lipoprotein.**
- Plasma fatty acids are a short-term marker of dietary intake.
- Red blood cell (RBC) fatty acids are a long-term marker of dietary intake.
- Adipose fatty acids reflect dietary intake over years.
- **Plasma and RBC fatty acids are similar in people with repetitive diets such as patients with inherited metabolic diseases.**

- Primary circulating fatty acids include: stearic, palmitic, oleic, palmitoleic, and linoleic acids.
- Arachidonic acid (C20:4n-6) can fall with DHA supplements.
- With regard to the DRI for fatty acids, the Institute of Medicine states, "The linoleic acid: α-linolenic acid ratio is likely most important in diets that are very low or devoid of arachidonic acid" [1].

Shorthand	Abbreviation	Name
C10:0	–	Capric acid
C12:0	–	Lauric acid
C14:0	MA	Myristic acid
C16:0	PA	Palmitic acid
C16:1n7	PO	Palmitoleic acid
C16:1n7t	t-PO	*Trans*-palmitoleic acid
C18:0	SA	Stearic acid
C18:1n9	OA	Oleic acid
C18:1n9t	t-OA	*Trans*-oleic acid
C18:2n6	LA	Linoleic acid
C18:2n6t	t-LA	*Trans*-linoleic acid
C20:0	–	Arachidic acid
C18:3n6	GLA	Gamma linolenic acid

Shorthand	Abbreviation	Name
C20:1n9	–	Eicosenoic acid
C18:3n3	ALA	Alpha linolenic acid
C20:2n6	–	Eicosadienoic acid
C20:3n6	–	Eicosatrienoic acid
C22:0	–	Docosanoic acid
C20:4n6	AA	Arachidonic acid
C24:0	–	Lignoceric acid
C20:5n3	EPA	Eicosapentaenoic acid
C24:1n9	–	Nervonic acid
C22:4n6	DTA	Docosatetraenoic acid
C22:5n6	DPAn6	Docosapentaenoic acid n6
C22:5n3	DPAn3	Docosapentaenoic acid n3
C22:6n3	DHA	Docosahexaenoic acid

Reference

1. Institute of Medicine (USA). Panel on Macronutrients and Institute of Medicine (U.S.). Standing Committee on the Scientific Evaluation of Dietary Reference Intakes., Dietary reference intakes for energy, carbohydrate, fiber, fat, fatty acids, cholesterol, protein, and amino acids. 2005; Washington, DC: National Academies Press. xxv, 1331 p.

Appendix I. Calculation of Glucose Infusion Rate and Cornstarch Dosing for Patients with Glycogen Storage Disease

The main priority for GSD type 1 is to prevent hypoglycemia and suppress lactic acidosis. This is achieved by calculating glucose requirements using the glucose infusion rate. Glucose infusion rate (GIR) is expressed as mg/kg/minute. Glucose can be provided through formula feeding, nocturnal nasogastric drip feeding, or the use of uncooked cornstarch. Nasogastric drip feedings provide a continuous source of glucose, and cornstarch provides a source of glucose that is slowly released and slowly absorbed.

Recommended GIR[a]

0–12 months	7–9 mg/kg/min
1–3 years	7 mg/kg/min
3–6 years	6–7 mg/kg/min
6–14 years	5–6 mg/kg/min
Adolescents	4–5 mg/kg/min
Adults	3–4 mg/kg/min

[a]Fernandes J, Saudubray J-M, van den Berghe G. *Inborn metabolic diseases: diagnosis and treatment*, 3rd ed. Berlin/Heidelbrug/New York: Springer;2000

$$\text{Uncooked cornstarch 1tbsp} = 8\,\text{g} = 7.2\,\text{g carbohydrate (CHO)}$$

Example GIR Calculations

Example 1

Patient weight: 22 kg

Patient age: 5 years

Current cornstarch dose: 36 g at 6:00, 10:00, 14:00, and 18:00

Step 1	7.2 g CHO = 0.9 g CHO per 1 g cornstarch
Step 2	36 g cornstarch × 0.9 g CHO = 32.4 g CHO
Step 3	32.4 g CHO × 1000 mg = 32,400 mg CHO
Step 4	$\frac{32{,}400 \text{ mg CHO}}{22\text{kg}}$ = 1472.7 mg CHO per kg
Step 5	4 hours × 60 min per hour = 240 min
Step 6	$\frac{1472.7\text{mg CHO per kg}}{240\text{min}}$ = **6.13 mg/kg/min**

Example 2

You have a 12-year-old patient weighing 43 kg and is experiencing low blood sugar with his current cornstarch dosing regimen. He currently takes 48 g of cornstarch every 4 hours starting at 10 AM. Calculate the current GIR and the cornstarch dose that is appropriate for a correct GIR.

L. E. Bernstein et al. (eds.), *Nutrition Management of Inherited Metabolic Diseases*,
https://doi.org/10.1007/978-3-030-94510-7

Current Dose

Step 1	7.2 g CHO = 0.9 g CHO per g cornstarch
Step 2	48 g cornstarch × 0.9 g CHO per g cornstarch = 43.2 g CHO
Step 3	43.2 g CHO × 1000 mg/g = 43,200 mg CHO
Step 4	$\frac{43,200 \text{ mg CHO}}{43 \text{ kg}}$ = 1004.6 mg CHO/kg
Step 5	4 hours × 60 min/hour = 240 min
Step 6	$\frac{1004.6 \text{ mg CHO/kg}}{240 \text{ min}}$ = **4.18 mg/kg/min**

New Dose

Step 1	**5.5 mg/kg/min** (this GIR is provided to you by the metabolic physician; the recommended GIR for a 6–14-year-old is 5–6 mg/kg/min)
Step 2	5.5 mg CHO/kg/min × 240 min = 1320 mg CHO/kg
Step 3	1320 mg CHO/kg × 43 kg =56,760 mg CHO
Step 4	56,760 mg CHO ÷ 1000 mg = 56.76 g CHO
Step 5	56.76 g CHO ÷ 0.9 g CHO per 1 g cornstarch = **63 g cornstarch**

Appendix J. Guide to Counting Carbohydrates for Patients with GSD Type 1

Food	Grams food for 1 g CHO	Serving size for 5 g CHO	Grams food for 5 g CHO
Almonds-dry roasted	4	18 almonds	20
Bacon Bits Imitation	3	2.5 Tablespoons	17
Baked Beans	5	1.5 Tablespoons	25
Banana	4	1/4 small banana	21
Cashews-dry roasted	3	8 cashews	15
Chicken McNuggets	7	1 McNugget	34
Chicken Popcorn Chicken (KFC)	5	4 nuggets	24
Corn canned	5	3 Tablespoons	27
Corn Chips	2	5 chips	8
Corn Syrup – light	1	1 tsp	7
Crackers Chicken in a Biscuit	2	3 crackers	9
Crackers Original Cheez It	2	7 crackers	8
Crackers Original Goldfish	2	15 pieces	8
Crackers Triscuit	1	2 crackers	7
Crackers Wheat Thin	2	4 crackers	8
Dill Pickle Spears	24	4 spears	120
Dressing Kraft Buttermilk Ranch	30	5 Tablespoons	150
French Fries – Frozen	4	3 strips	19
FunYuns	2	11 pieces	8
Green Beans – boiled	13	1/2 cup	63
Green Beans – canned	22	3/4 cup	110
Macaroni – Cooked	4	1/8 cup	18
Olives Black	16	16 olives	80
Peanuts-dry roasted	5	23 peanuts	23
Potato Boiled	5	3 Tablespoons	25
Pretzels – Rold Gold	2	1 twist	9
Rice-a-Roni Rice Pilaf	1	3/4 cup	7
Smarties	1	1 roll	6
Strawberries	14	1/3 cup sliced	71
Tortilla Chips Santitas	1	3 chips	7
Waffles Eggos Buttermilk	3	1 waffle	13
Food	Grams food for 1 g CHO	Serving size for 5 g CHO	Grams food for 5 g CHO

L. E. Bernstein et al. (eds.), *Nutrition Management of Inherited Metabolic Diseases*,
https://doi.org/10.1007/978-3-030-94510-7

Appendix K: At-A-Glance

L. E. Bernstein et al. (eds.), *Nutrition Management of Inherited Metabolic Diseases*,
https://doi.org/10.1007/978-3-030-94510-7

K-1 Glutaric Aciduria

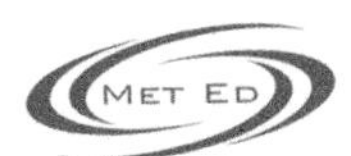

At a Glance
Glutaric Acidemia Type 1 (GA-1)

Deficient enzyme: Glutaryl-CoA dehydrogenase

Metabolites*: Elevated concentrations of 3-hydroxyglutaric acid, glutaric acid, glutaconic acid and glutaryl carnitine

Restricted Amino Acid: Lysine

Clinical presentation, in untreated patients: brain atrophy, macrocephaly, striatal necrosis, dystonia, hypotonia

Goal Treatment Range: Plasma lysine-maintain at low end of normal range
Plasma free carnitine-maintain within normal range

*Boy N, et al. Proposed recommendations for diagnosing and managing individuals with glutaric aciduria type 1: second revision. J Inherit Metab Dis (2017) 40: 75-101

Nutrient Needs by Age*

Age	Lysine mg/kg/d	Total Protein g/d
0-6 mo.	65-100	2.75-3.0
6-12 mo.	55-90	2.5-3.0
1-4 yrs.	50-80	1.8-2.6
4-6 yrs.	40-70	1.6-20
>6 yrs.	Consider liberalization of protein intake to age-appropriate DRIs**	

* Bernstein, LE. Nutrition Management of Glutaric Acidemia Type 1. In LE Bernstein, F Rohr, S van Calcar (Eds.) *Nutrition Management of Inherited Metabolic Diseases(2nd Edition).* Springer: 2021

**Boy N, et al. Proposed recommendations for diagnosing and managing individuals with glutaric aciduria type 1: second revision. J Inherit Metab Dis (2017) 40: 75-101

Illness in GA-1*

Emergency treatment is often needed at the <u>first sign</u> of illness such asdecreased intake, fever, vomitingor diarrhea.Delaying emergency treatment is associated with significant risk for aneurologic crisis.Patients should be counseled to call their metabolic team for guidance at the first sign of illness.

* Bernstein, LE. Nutrition Management of Glutaric Acidemia Type 1. In LE Bernstein, F Rohr, S van Calcar (Eds.) *Nutrition Management of Inherited Metabolic Diseases (2nd Edition).* Springer: 2021

Starting a GA-1Diet

1. Determine goals for Lysine(mg),Total Protein (g), Energy (kcal)
   - to estimatemg of lysine from grams of protein use the conversion 35mglysine = ~1 g protein
2. Calculate amount of intact protein source(breast milk, infant formula, food) needed to meet lysine goal.
3. Calculate amount of medical food needed in addition to the intact protein source to meet total protein goal.
4. Calculate energy intake from intact protein and medical food sources to ensure total energygoalsare met.

Glutaric Acidemia (GA-1)

Medical Food Therapy

	Abbott abbottnutrition.com	Mead Johnson Hcp.meadjohnson.com	Nutricia NutriciaMetabolics.com	Vitaflo www.VitafloUSA.com
Infant (0-1 yr)	Glutarex® -1	GA	GA-1 Anamix® Early Years	
Toddler & Young Children	Glutarex® -1 Glutarex® -2	GA	GA-1 Anamix® Early Years GlutarAde™ Junior GA-1Drink Mix GlutarAde™ Essential GA-1 Drink Mix GlutarAde™ Amino Acid Blend	GA gel™ GA express® 15
Older Children & Adults	Glutarex® -2	GA	GlutarAde™ Junior GA-1 Drink Mix GlutarAde™ Essential GA-1 Drink Mix GlutarAde™ Amino Acid Blend	GA express® 15

Nutrition Supplementation*

L-Carnitine-100 mg/kg/d

L-Arginine
  -Supplied by medical food, no evidence for benefit of additionalsupplementation
Riboflavin
  -No standard protocol for evaluating responsiveness although certain individuals may show biochemical improvement

*Boy N, et al. Proposed recommendations for diagnosing and managing individuals with glutaric aciduria type 1: second revision. J Inherit Metab Dis (2017) 40: 75-101

Laboratory Monitoring*

Plasma Amino Acids[1, 2]
Carnitine[1, 2]
Albumin[3]
CBC[3]
Calcium[3]
Phosphorus[3]
Ferritin[3]
B12[3]

[1]Every 3 months until age 1 yr.
[2]Every 6 months until age 6 yrs., then annually thereafter
[3]As indicated

*Boy N, et al. Proposed recommendations for diagnosing and managing individuals with glutaric aciduria type 1: second revision. J Inherit Metab Dis (2017) 40: 75-101

K-2 Homocystinuria

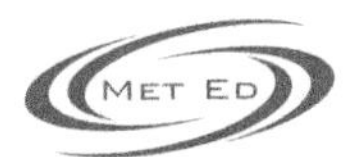

At a Glance
Homocystinuria (HCU)

Deficient enzyme: Cystathionine Beta-Synthase (CBS)

Cofactor: Pyridoxine (Vitamin B_6)

Toxic Metabolite: Homocysteine

Restricted Amino Acid: Methionine

Clinical presentation, in untreated patients: Ectopic lentis, skeletal abnormalities, intellectualdisabilities seizures, thromboembolic disease

***Goal Treatment Range**: Plasma Total Homocysteine(tHcy):

Keep the tHcy concentration as close to normal as possible:

<50 μmol/L for pyridoxine-responsive patients

<100 μmol/L for pyridoxine-unresponsive patients

Plasma Methionine: <1000 μmol/L

Plasma Cystine: normal range

*Morris et al. Guidelines for the diagnosis and management of cystathionine beta-synthase deficiency. JInherit Metab Dis 2017, 40: 49-74.

Nutrient Needs by Age*†

Age	Methionine mg/kg	Cystine mg/d	Intact Protein	Total Protein	Energy DRI/EER
0-6 mo	15-60	85-150	60-100% DRI based on plasma tHCY and methionine	100-140% DRI or 120-140% DRI for those on medical food	80-120% based on growth trend
6-12 mo	12-43	85-150			
1-4 yr	9-28	60-100			
4-7 yr	7-22	50-80			
7-11 years	7-22	30-50			

*Roberts, AM. Nutrition Management of Homocystinuria and Cobalamin Disorders. In LE Bernstein, F Rohr, S van Calcar (Eds.) *Nutrition Management of Inherited Metabolic Diseases* (2nd Edition). Springer: 2021

†For ages >11 years, see book chapter

Simplified Diet

1. At 4-6 months of age, when solid food is introduced, consider implementing a simplified diet
2. Reduce Met allowance (from whole protein source) by 30% (40% in those with more restrictive Met allowances).
3. Allow unmeasured intake of "free foods." These are fruits, vegetables, foods with <20 mg Met/100g
4. Monitor blood Met per clinic protocol

Starting a HCU Diet
(in individuals with CBS deficiency who arenon-responsive to vitamin B_6 therapy)

1. Determine goals for Methionine(mg), Cystine (mg), Intact Protein (g), Total Protein (g), Energy (kcal)
   -use 20 mg Met = 1 g protein to calculate mg of methionine from grams of protein
2. Calculate amount of whole protein source (breast milk, infant formula, food) needed to meet Methgoal.
3. Calculate amount of medical food needed in addition to the whole protein source to meet total protein goal.
4. Calculate energy intake from whole protein and medical food sources to ensure total calorie needs are met.

Homocystinuria (HCU)

Medical Food Therapy					
	Abbott abbottnutrition.com	**Cambrooke** Cambrooke.com	**Mead Johnson** Hcp.meadjohnson.com	**Nutricia** NutriciaMetabolics.com	**Vitaflo** www.vitafloUSA.com
Infant (0-1 yr)	Hominex® -1		HCY 1	HCU Anamix® Early Years	
Toddler & Young Children	Hominex® -1 Hominex® -2	Homactin™ AA Plus Powder 15	HCY 1 HCY 2	HCU Anamix® Early Years HCU Anamix® Next	HCU gel™ HCU express® 15 HCU cooler® 15
Older Children & Adults		Homactin™ AA Plus Powder 15	HCY 2	HCU Anamix® Next XMet Maxamum® HCU Lophlex® LQ	HCU express® 15, 20 HCU cooler® 15

Nutritional Supplementation (dose may vary based on blood laboratory results)*

Vitamin B_6 (used as sole therapy in individuals who are pyridoxineresponsive)
-recommended starting dose to assess responsiveness: 100 mg/d
-maintain unrestricted diet and correct folate and vitamin B_{12} deficiencies prior to assessingresponse

Correct folate deficiencies (5-10 mg/d folate or 1-5 mg/d folinic acid)
Correct vitamin B_{12} deficiency (dose varies)

*Roberts, AM. Nutrition Management of Homocystinuria and Cobalamin Disorders. In LE Bernstein, F Rohr, S van Calcar (Eds.) *Nutrition Management of Inherited Metabolic Diseases* (2nd Edition). Springer: 2021
*Morris et al. Guidelines for the diagnosis and management of cystathionine beta-synthase deficiency. JInherit Metab Dis 2017, 40: 49-74

Medical Therapy

Cystadane® (betaine anhydrous) www.recordati.com
*Recommended starting dose:
Children-50 mg/kg twice daily
Adults-3 g twice daily

*Morris et al. Guidelines for the diagnosis and management of cystathionine beta-synthase deficiency. JInherit Metab Dis 2017, 40: 49-74

Laboratory Monitoring

Total Homocysteine[1]	B_{12}[2]	Zinc, Ferritin, Copper, Selenium[2]
Plasma Methionine[1]	Folate[2]	Essential Fatty Acids[2]
Plasma Amino Acids[2]	Albumin[2]	25-OH Vitamin D[2]

[1]Weekly in infancy, weekly to monthly thereafter
[2]At least annually; if deficiency identified, provide supplementation and repeat in 3-6 months

*Morris et al. Guidelines for the diagnosis and management of cystathionine beta-synthase deficiency. JInherit Metab Dis 2017, 40: 49-74

K-3 Maple Syrup Urine Disease

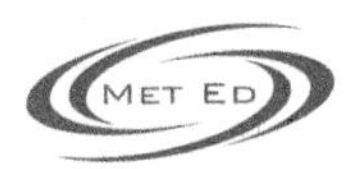

At a Glance
Maple Syrup Urine Disease(MSUD)

Deficient enzyme: Branched-chain keto acid dehydrogenase enzyme complex

Toxic Metabolite: Leucine and its keto acid (2-oxo-isocaproic acid)

Restricted Amino Acid: Branched-chain amino acids (BCAA)

Clinical presentation, in untreated patients:

Classic: neonatal onset, poor feeding, lethargy, altered tone, ketoacidosis, seizures, developmental delays

Intermediate: failure to thrive, ketoacidosis, developmental delays, classic symptoms during catabolic illness

Intermittent: normal development, episodic ataxia, ketoacidosis

***Goal Treatment Range**: Maintain plasma BCAA as close to normal as possible. Acceptable ranges:

Leucine: 100-300 μmol/L
Isoleucine: 100-300 μmol/L
Valine: 200-400 μmol/L

*van Calcar, S. Nutrition Management of Maple Syrup Urine Disease. In LE Bernstein, F Rohr, S van Calcar (Eds.) *Nutrition Management of Inherited Metabolic Diseases (2nd Edition)*. Springer: 2021

Nutrient Needs by Age*

Age	Leucine mg/kg/d	Isoleucine mg/kg/d	Valine mg/kg/d	Intact Protein† g/kg/d	Total Protein g/kg/d	Energy kcal/kg/d
0-6 months	40-100	36-100	40-95	1.0-1.6	2.5-3.5	95-145
7-12 months	40-75	30-70	30-80	0.8-1.4	2.5-3.0	80-135
1-3 years	40-70	20-70	30-70	0.6-1.2	1.5-2.5	80-130
4-8 years	35-65	20-30	30-50	0.4-0.9	1.3-2.0	50-120
9-13 years	30-60	20-30	25-40	5.0-8.0 g/day	1.2-1.8	40-90
14-18 years	15-50	10-30	15-30	5.0-8.0 g/day	1.2-1.8	35-70
19+ years	15-50	10-30	15-30	5.0-8.0 g/day	1.1-1.7	35-45

*van Calcar, S. Nutrition Management of Maple Syrup Urine Disease. In LE Bernstein, F Rohr, S van Calcar (Eds.) *Nutrition Management of InheritedMetabolic Diseases (2nd Edition)*. Springer: 2021 †SERN/GMDI MSUD Management Guidelines; https://southeastgenetics.org/ngp/guidelines.php

Starting a MSUD Diet*

1. Determine goals for Leucine (mg), Intact Protein (g), Total Protein (g), Energy (kcal)
   - if estimating mg of leucinefrom grams of protein: 60 mgleucineis ~1 g protein
2. Calculate amount of intact protein source (breast milk, infant formula, food) needed to meet Leu goal.
3. Calculate amount of medical food needed in addition to the intact protein source to meet total protein goal.
4. Calculate energy intake from intact protein and medical food sources to ensure total calorie needs are met.

Diet During Illness

In consultation with the medical team, if the patient's plasma leucine is significantly elevated:

1. Reduce intact protein by 50-100%,depending on the leucine levels and severity of illness,until plasma leucine is in the treatment range. With holding all intact protein for extended periods maylead to catabolism.
2. Increase medical food and non-protein energy sources to support anabolism.
3. Add L-isoleucine and L-valine supplements (20-120 mg/kg/d of each) to maintain plasma isoleucine and valine higher than the normal treatment range. Goal is 400-800 μmol/L.

*van Calcar, S. Nutrition Management of Maple Syrup Urine Disease. In LE Bernstein, F Rohr, S van Calcar(Eds.) *Nutrition Management ofInherited Metabolic Diseases (2nd Edition)*. Springer: 2021

Maple Syrup Urine Disease (MSUD)

	Abbott abbottnutrition.com	Mead Johnson hcp.meadjohnson.com	Nutricia NutriciaMetabolics.com	Vitaflo www.vitafloUSA.com
Infant (0-1 yr)	Ketonex® -1	BCAD 1	MSUD Anamix® Early Years	
Toddler & Young Children	Ketonex® -1 Ketonex® -2	BCAD 1 BCAD 2	MSUD Anamix® Early Years Complex Junior MSD Drink Mix Complex Essential MSD Drink Mix Complex MSD Amino Acid Blend	MSUD gel™ MSUD express® 15 MSUD cooler® 15
Older Children & Adults	Ketonex® -2	BCAD 2	Complex Essential MSD Drink Mix Complex MSD Amino Acid Blend MSUD Maxamum® MSUD Lophlex® LQ	MSUD express® 15 MSUD cooler® 15

Nutrition Supplementation

Thiamine*

-Trial of 100-1,000 mg/d to determine responsiveness (only effective in variant forms of MSUD)

L-isoleucine and L-valine*

-given to maintain plasma ILE and VAL in treatment range(dose varies)
-used during metabolic crisis to decrease plasma leucine (see Diet During Illness)

*van Calcar, S. Nutrition Management of Maple Syrup Urine Disease. In LE Bernstein, F Rohr, S van Calcar(Eds.) *Nutrition Management of Inherited Metabolic Diseases (2nd Edition)*. Springer: 2021

Laboratory Monitoring

Plasma Leucine[1,2]
Plasma Amino Acids[1,2]
Ketones[1,2]

Prealbumin[3]
Albumin[3]

Ferritin[3]
CBC[3]

[1]Daily until stable, weekly to twice weekly until 6 months old
[2]Monthly after 24 months of age
[3]Every 6 months

*SERN/GMDI MSUD Management Guidelines; https://southeastgenetics.org/ngp/guidelines.php

K-4 Methylmalonic acidemia/ Propionic acidemia

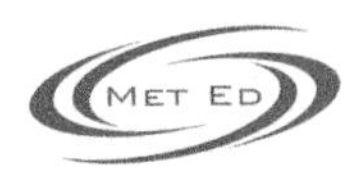

At a Glance
Methylmalonic/Propionic Acidemia

Deficient enzyme: MMA-methylmalonyl-CoA mutase (mut^0 or mut-)
PROP-propionyl-CoA carboxylase

Cofactor: MMA-Adenosylcobalamin (Vitamin B_{12})
PROP-Biotin

Toxic Metabolite: MMA-Methylmalonic Acid
PROP-Propionic Acid

Restricted Amino Acids: Valine, Isoleucine, Methionine, Threonine

Clinical presentation in untreated patients: acute: poorfeeding, vomiting, lethargy, tachypnea, acidosis, respiratory distress, coma; longer-term: neurologic complications, optic atrophy, renal dysfunction (MMA), cardiomyopathy(PROP)

***Goal Treatment Range**: Plasma amino acids-maintain within normal range

Nutrient Needs by Age*			
Age	**Intact Protein g/kg/d**	**TotalProtein g/kg/d**	**Energy kcal/kg/d**
0-3 mo	0.9–1.5	1.5–1.8	72-109
3-6 mo	0.9–1.5	1.5–1.8	72-109
7-12 mo	0.7–1.2	1.2–1.4	64-97
1-3 yrs	0.6–1.05	1.0–1.2	66-99
4-8 yrs	0.57–0.95	0.95–1.1	56-88

*SERN/GMDI PROP Nutrition Management Guidelines; https://southeastgenetics.org/ngp/guidelines.php

Starting a Diet

1. Determine goals for Intact Protein (g), Total Protein (g), Energy (kcal)
2. Calculate amount of intactprotein source (breast milk, infant formula, food) needed to meet Intact Protein (g) goal.
3. Calculate amount of medical food required to provide remaining protein to meet total protein goal.
4. Calculate energy intake from intactprotein and medical food sources to ensure total calorie needs are met.

Methylmalonic/Propionic Acidemia

	Abbott abbottnutrition.com	Mead Johnson hcp.meadjohnson.com	Nutricia NutriciaMetabolics.com	Vitaflo www.vitafloUSA.com
Infant (0-1 yr)	Propimex®-1	OA1	MMA/PA Anamix® Early Years	
Toddler & Young Children	Propimex®-1 Propimex®-2	OA1 OA2	MMA/PA Anamix® Early Years MMA/PA Anamix® Next	MMA/PA gel™ MMA/PA express®15 MMA/PA cooler®15
Older Children & Adults	Propimex®-2	OA2	MMA/PA Anamix® Next XMTVI Maxamum®	MMA/PA express®15 MMA/PA cooler®15

Nutrition Supplementation (dose may vary based on blood laboratory results)

L-Carnitine: 100-300 mg/kg/d; divided two to four times per day

*MMA-Hydroxycobalamin: 1.0-2.0 mg daily to weekly for those who are vitamin B_{12} responsive (these patients may need little to no dietary restriction)

To determine responsiveness: 1.0 mg (IM or IV) hydroxycobalamin x 5 days; reduction in MMA levels of ≥50% indicates responsiveness

**PROP-Biotin: 5-40 mg/dto determine responsiveness and if a non-responder, stop biotin

*Sowa, M. Nutritional Management of Propionic and Methylmalonic Acidemia. In LE Bernstein, F Rohr, S van Calcar (Eds.) Nutritional Management of Inherited Metabolic Diseases (2nd Edition). Springer: 2021
**Jurecki E et al. Nutrition management guideline for propionic acidemia: An evidence-and consensus-based approach.Mol Genet Metab.2019;126(4):341-54

Medical Therapy
Carbaglu (carglumicacid) (www.recordati.com)
Maintenance dose for chronic hyperammonemia (pediatric and adults) 10-100 mg/kg/d

Laboratory Monitoring*

Plasma Amino Acids[1]
Serum Methylmalonic Acid[1]
Carnitine (Free and Acyl)[1]
Ketones[1] (continue monthly in PROP

CBC, Albumin[2]
Prealbumin[2]
Propionic Acid[3]

Urine organic acids[3]
25-OH Vitamin D[4]
Folate, ferritin, B_{12}, B_6, zinc, selenium
Complete Metabolic Panel (CMP)[4]

[1]Monthly in infancy; every 3-6 months thereafter
[2]Every 6 months in infancy; annually thereafter
[3]Every 6 months in infancy; then annually as indicated
[4]Annually

*SERN/GMDI PROP Nutrition Management Guidelines; https://southeastgenetics.org/ngp/guidelines.php

K-5 Phenylketonuria

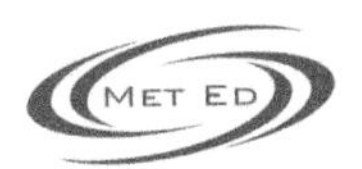

At a Glance
Phenylketonuria (PKU)

Deficient enzyme: Phenylalanine hydroxylase (PAH); converts phenylalanine to tyrosine

Enzyme Cofactor: Tetrahydrobiopterin (BH_4)

Toxic Metabolite: Phenylalanine (Phe)

Clinical Presentation, if untreated: irreversible intellectual disabilities, seizures, behavioral abnormalities eczema, "musty" odor, hypopigmentation (skin, hair, iris)

Goal Treatment Range: Blood Phenylalanine: 120-360 µmol/L (2-6 mg/dL)
(to convert mg/dL to µmol/L multiply by 60)
Blood Tyrosine: normal for lab

Nutrient Needs by Age*

Age	Phe mg/d	Phe mg/kg/d	Tyr mg/d	Protein g/kg/d	Energy
0-3 mo	130-430	25-70	1100-1300	2.5-3.0	Age appropriate DRI
3-6 mo	135-400	20-45	1400-2100	2.0-3.0	
6-9 mo	145-370	15-35	2500-3000	2.0-2.5	
9-12 mo	135-330	10-35	2500-3000	2.0-2.5	
1-4 yrs	200-320	-	2800-3500	1.5-2.1	
>4 yrs to adult	200-1100	-	4000-6000	120-140% DRI	

*SERN/GMDI PKU Management Guidelines;https://southeastgenetics.org/ngp/guidelines.php

Starting a PKU Diet

1. Determine goals for Phe (mg), Protein (g) Tyrosine (mg), Energy (kcal)
   - use 50 mg Phe = 1 g protein to calculate mg of phenylalanine from grams of protein.
2. Calculate amount of whole protein source (breast milk, infant formula, food) needed to meet Phe goal.
3. Calculate amount of medical food needed, in addition to the whole protein source to meet total protein goal.
4. Calculate energy intake from whole protein and medical food sources to ensure total calorie needs are met.
5. Calculate tyrosine intake from whole protein and medical food sources.

Implementing the Simplified PKU Diet*

1. At 4-6 months of age, when solid food is introduced, consider implementing the Simplified PKU Diet.
2. Reduce phe allowance (from whole protein source) by 30% (40% in those with more restrictive Phe allowances).
3. Allow unmeasured intake of "uncountedfoods." These are fruits, vegetables, foods with <75 mg Phe/100g and all other foods with <20 mg Pheor <0.4 g protein per serving.
4. Monitor blood Phe weekly for the first 4 weeks, without making diet changes.

*Bernstein LE, et al. Multiclinic Observations on the Simplified Diet in PKU. JNutrMetab.2017.

Phenylketonuria (PKU)

Medical Foods for PKU

	Abbott abbottnutrition.com	Cambrooke Cambrooke.com	Mead Johnson hcp.meadjohnson.com	Nutricia NutriciaMetabolics.com	Vitaflo www.vitafloUSA.com
Infant (0-1 yr)	Phenex™ -1		Phenyl-Free® 1	PKU Periflex® Early Years	PKU explore™ 5, 10
Toddler & Young Children	Phenex™-1 Phenex™-2	*Glytactin® BetterMilk 15 *Glytactin® RTD 10, 15 *Glytactin® BUILD 10, 20/20 *Glytactin® COMPLETE 10 Bar *Glytactin® RESTORE 10 *Glytactin® RESTORE Powder *Glytactin® SWIRL 15	Phenyl-Free® 1 Phenyl-Free® 2	PKU Periflex® Junior Plus PhenylAde® EssentialDrink Mix *PhenylAde® GMP Drink Mix *PhenylAde® GMP Ready *PhenylAde® GMP Mix-In *PhenylAde® GMP Ready *PhenylAde® GMP Ultra	PKU gel™ PKU trio™ PKU express® 15 PKU cooler® 10, 15 *PKU sphere® 15 *PKU sphere® liquid
Children thru Adult	Phenex™ -2	*Glytactin® BetterMilk 15, Lite *Glytactin® RTD 10, 15, Lite *Glytactin® BUILD 10, 20/20 *Glytactin® RESTORE 10, Lite *Glytactin® RESTORE Powder 5, Lite 10 *Glytactin® COMPLETE 10 Bar *Glytactin® SWIRL 15	Phenyl-Free® 2 Phenyl-Free® 2HP	Periflex® Advance Periflex® LQ Phenylade® EssentialDrink Mix Phenylade® Drink Mix40, 60 Phenylade® MTE Amino Acid Blend *PhenylAde® GMP Drink Mix *PhenylAde® GMP Ready *PhenylAde® GMP Ultra *PhenylAde® GMP Mix-In PKU Lophlex® LQ & Powder XPhe Maxamum® Phlexy-10® Tablets, Drink Mix **PhenylAde® PheBLOC™ LNAA	PKU express® 15, 20 PKU cooler® 10, 15, 20 PKU Air® 20 *PKU sphere® 15, 20 *PKU sphere® liquid

*A Glycomacropeptide (GMP) product **Product used for Large Neutral Amino Acid therapy

Medical Therapy (www.biomarin.com)

Kuvan (sapropterin dihydrochloride): synthetic form of BH4 (PAH cofactor) Dose: 5-20 mg/kg/d

Palynziq (pegvaliase): phenylalanine ammonia lyase (enzyme substitution for PAH) Dose:20-60mg/d

Laboratory Monitoring* Biomarin Pharmaceutical, Inc. www.biomarin.com

Blood Phenylalanine[1]	Prealbumin[2]	Zinc, Copper[3]
Blood Tyrosine[1]	25-OH Vitamin D[2]	Vitamin B_{12}[3]
Plasma Amino Acids[2]	CBC[2]	Essential Fatty Acids[3]

[1]Weeklyin infancy, weekly to monthly thereafter
[2] Every 6-12 months
[3]As indicated

*www.gmdi.org/Resources/Nutrition-Guidelines/Phenylketonuria-PKU

K-6 Tyrosinemia

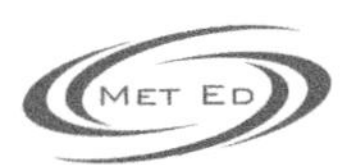

At a Glance
Hereditary Tyrosinemia Type 1 (HT-1)

Deficient enzyme: FumarylacetoacetateHydrolase(FAH)

Toxic Metabolite: Succinylacetoneand succinylacetoacetate

Clinical presentation, if untreated: failure to thrive, rickets, hepatic failure, renalfailure,neurologic comorbidities

Restricted Amino Acids: Phenylalanine and Tyrosine

***Goal Treatment Range**:

Plasma Phenylalanine: 20-80 μmol/L
Plasma Tyrosine: 200-600 μmol/L

*Chinsky JM, et al. Diagnosis and treatment of tyrosinemia type 1: a US and Canadian consensus group review and recommendations. Genetics in Medicine, Aug 2017.

Nutrient Needs by Age*

Age	Phenylalanine plus Tyrosi mg/kg/d	TotalProtein g/kg/d	Energy kcal/kg/d
0-3 mo	65 - 155	3.0 - 3.5	120 (95-145)
3-6 mo	55 - 135	3.0 - 3.5	120 (95-145)
6-9 mo	50 - 120	2.5 - 3.0	110 (80-135)
9-12 mo	40 - 105	2.5 - 3.0	105 (80-135)
1-4 yrs	380–800 mg/d	>/= 30 g/d	1300 (900-1800)

*Acosta PB. Nutrition Support Protocols: The Ross Metabolic Formula System. Abbot Laboratories, 2001

Starting a HT-1 Diet

1. Determine goals for Phenylalanine (mg) plus Tyrosine (mg), Total Protein (g), and Energy (kcal)
   -use 50 mg Phe = 1 g protein to calculate milligrams of phe from protein
2. Calculate amount of whole protein source (breast milk, infant formula, food) needed to meet phe + tyrgoal.
3. Calculate amount of medical food needed in addition to the whole protein source to meet total protein goal.
4. Calculate energy intake from whole protein and medical food sources to ensure total calorie needs are met.

Hereditary Tyrosinemia Type 1 (HT-1)

Medical Food Therapy

	Abbott abbottnutrition.com	Cambrooke Cambrooke.com	Mead Johnson hcp.meadjonson.com	Nutricia NutriciaMetabolics.com	Vitaflo www.vitafloUSA.com
Infant (0-1 yr)	Tyrex® -1		Tyros 1	TYR Anamix® Early Years	
Toddler & Young Children	Tyrex® -1 Tyrex® -2	*Tylactin® Complete 15 Bar Tylactin® RTD15 Tylactin® RESTORE 10 Tylactin® RESTORE Powder 5 Tylactin® BUILD20	Tyros 1 Tyros 2	TYR Anamix® Early Years TYR Anamix® Next *TYR Lophlex® GMP Mix-In	TYR gel™ TYR express® 15 TYR cooler® 15 *TYR sphere® 20
Older Children & Adults	Tyrex®-2	*Tylactin® Complete 15 Bar Tylactin® RTD 15 Tylactin® RESTORE 10 Tylactin® RESTORE Powder 5 Tylactin® BUILD 20	Tyros 2	TYR Anamix® Next *TYR Lophlex® GMP Mix-In TYR Lophlex® LQ	TYR express® 15, 20 TYR coole® 15 *TYR sphere™ 20

*Product contains GMP

Medical Therapy*

Nitisinone (NTBC)

Orfadin® www.orfadin.com

NITYR™ www.cyclepharma.com

-Starting dose:1 mg/kg/d, increase to 2 mg/kg/d for those inacute severe liver failure

-Goal blood NTBC concentration-30-70 μmol/L

*Chinsky JM, et al. Diagnosis and treatment of tyrosinemia type 1: a US and Canadian consensus group review and recommendations. Genetics in Medicine, Aug 2017.

Laboratory Monitoring

Plasma succinylacetone[1,4,7]
Plasma Amino Acids[1,4,7]
Blood NTBC concentration[3,4,7]
Serum AFP concentration[1,5,7]
PT/PTT[1,6]
Bicarbonate[8]
BUN/Creat[8]
Calcium[8]
Phosphorous[8]
ALT/AST[2,6]
CBC[2,6]

[1] At initiation of treatment, then monthly for the first year of life
[2] At initiation of treatment, then every 3 months for the first year of life
[3] Monthly for the first year of life
[4] Every 3 months from age 1 year thru 5 years
[5] Every 6 months from age 1 year thru 5 years
[6] Annually after 1 year of age
[7] Every 6 months after age 5 years
[8] At initiation then annually

**Chinsky JM, et al. Diagnosis and treatment oftyrosinemia type 1: a US and Canadian consensus group review and recommendations. Genetics in Medicine, Aug 2017.

K-7 Urea Cycle Disorder

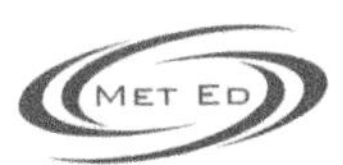

At a Glance
Urea Cycle Disorders (UCD)

Deficient enzyme: NAGS-N-acetylglutamate synthetase
CPS-Carbamoyl phosphate synthetase
OTC-Ornithine transcarbamylase
ASS (Citrullinemia I)-Argininosuccinic acid synthetase
ASL-Argininosuccinic acid lyase
Argininemia-Arginase

Toxic Metabolites: Ammonia
Argininosuccinic acid-in ASL deficiency
Arginine-in arginase deficiency

Treatment: prevent catabolism, limit intact protein and provide essential amino acid medical food, supplement citrulline or arginine (except in arginase deficiency), provide nitrogen scavenging medications

Clinical presentation in untreated patients: hyperammonemia caused neurotoxicity, poor feeding, growth failure vomiting, seizures, lethargy, liver dysfunction, coma, death; late identified adolescents/adults-chronic neurological symptoms and dietary history of self-restricting dietary protein.

Goal Treatment Range*: Ammonia-normal (<35 µmol/L; <60 mcg/dL)
Plasma amino acids-maintain all within normal range

*MacLeod, E. Nutrition Management of Urea Cycle Disorders. In LE Bernstein, F Rohr, S van Calcar (Eds.) *Nutrition Management of Inherited Metabolic Diseases* (2nd Edition). Springer: 2021

Nutrient Needs by Age*

Age	Intact Protein g/kg/d	Essential Amino Acid (medical food; g/kg/d)	Total Protein g/kg/d
0-1 yr	0.8-1.1	0.4-1.1	1.2-2.2
1-7 yr	0.7-0.8	0.3-0.7	1.0-1.2
7-19 yr	0.3-1.0	0.4-0.7	0.8-1.4
>19 yr	0.6-0.7	0.2-0.5	0.8-1.0

*MacLeod, E. Nutrition Management of Urea Cycle Disorders. In LE Bernstein, F Rohr, S van Calcar (Eds.) *Nutrition Management of Inherited Metabolic Diseases* (2nd Edition). Springer: 2021

Starting a Diet

1. Determine goals for total protein (g) and percentage to be provided by intact protein vs essential amino acids (medical food). Consider 30-50% from essential amino acids for initial diet.
2. Calculate amount of intactprotein source (breast milk, infant formula, food) and amount of medical food required to meet total protein (g)goal.
3. Calculate energy (kcals) provided by intact protein and medical food sources to ensure DRI for energy needs are met. Consider addition of protein-free calorie modular as needed to meet energy needs.
4. Consider use of enteral nutrition support in this population as anorexia is a common complication.
5. Patients with severe forms of UCD may require placement of a gastrostomy tube.

Urea Cycle Disorders (UCD)

Medical Food Therapy				
	Abbott abbottnutrition.com	**Mead Johnson** hcp.meadjohnson.com	**Nutricia** NutriciaMetabolics.com	**Vitaflo** www.VitafloUSA.com
Infant (0-1 yr)	Cyclinex-1®	WND 1		
Toddler & Young Children	Cyclinex-1® Cyclinex-2®	WND 1 WND 2	UCD Anamix® Junior Essential Amino Acid Mix	UCD trio™ EAA supplement™
Older Children & Adults	Cyclinex-2®	WND 2	UCD Anamix® Junior Essential Amino Acid Mix	UCD trio™ EAA supplement™
Protein Free Modular	Pro-Phree®	PFD Toddler PFD 2	Duocal® Polycal™	S.O.S™ 20, 25

Supplementation*

L-Arginine (ASS and ASL deficiency): 100-300 mg/kg/d(100 mg/kg/dmay be sufficient in ASL)

L-Citrulline (OTC and CPS deficiency): 100-200 mg/kg/d

*MacLeod, E. Nutrition Management of Urea Cycle Disorders. In LE Bernstein, F Rohr, S van Calcar (Eds.) *Nutrition Management of Inherited Metabolic Diseases* (2nd Edition). Springer: 2021

Medical Therapy*

Nitrogen scavenging medications – use alternative pathways to remove nitrogen to prevent hyperammonemia while allowing for greater protein tolerance. Monitor branched chain amino acids.

Sodium Benzoate-binds with glycine to form hippurate, removes one nitrogen atom, then is excreted in urine

Sodium Phenylacetate-binds with glutamine to form phenylacetylglutamine, removes two nitrogen atoms, then is excreted in urine

Buphenyl® (Horizon Pharma-www.horizonpharma.com)

Glycerol Phenylacetate-same mechanism of action as sodium phenylacetate

Ravicti® (Horizon Pharma-www.horizonpharma.com)

Sodium Phenylacetate + Sodium Benzoate (IV only)

Ammonul® (Ucyclyd Pharma, Inc-www.ucyclyd.com)

Carglumic acid-asynthetic form of N-acetylglutamate synthase used for NAGS deficiency

CARBAGLU® (www.recordati.com)

*MacLeod, E. Nutrition Management of Urea Cycle Disorders. In LE Bernstein, F Rohr, S van Calcar (Eds.) *Nutrition Management of Inherited Metabolic Diseases* (2nd Edition). Springer: 2021

Laboratory Monitoring

Plasma Amino Acids[1] (especially glutamine)
Ammonia[1]
Prealbumin[2]
25-OH Vitamin D[2]
CBC[2]
Ferritin, iron, folate, zinc[2]

[1] Weekly in infancy, monthly thereafter
[2] At least annually

*MacLeod, E. Nutrition Management of Urea Cycle Disorders. In LE Bernstein, F Rohr, S van Calcar (Eds.) *Nutrition Management of Inherited Metabolic Diseases* (2nd Edition). Springer: 2021

K-8 Very Long-Chain Acyl-CoA Dehydrogenase Deficiency

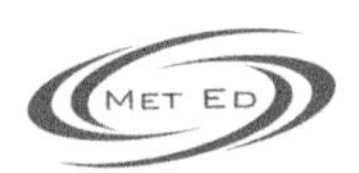

At a Glance
Very Long ChainAcyl Co-A Dehydrogenase Deficiency
(VLCAD)

Deficient enzyme: Very long chain acyl-CoA dehydrogenase

Restrict: Dietary long chain fat(LCF)

Clinical presentation, in untreated patients:*

Mild: asymptomatic beyond infancy, tolerates catabolic stressors without decompensation, potential for rhabdomyolysis

Moderate: asymptomatic at diagnosis, hypoketotic hypoglycemia, rhabdomyolysis due to catabolic illness, fasting or exercise

Severe: symptomatic at diagnosis or within first months of life, hypertrophic or dilated cardiomyopathy, pericardial effusion, hypotonia, hepatomegaly, intermittent hypoglycemia rhabdomyolysis

* SERN/GMDI VLCAD Management; https://southeastgenetics.org/ngp/guidelines.php
https://southeastgenetics.org/ngp/guidelines.php

Nutrient Needs by Age (VLCAD)*

Age	Disease Severity	Total Fat (% of total energy)	Long-Chain Fat (% of total energy)	Medium-Chain Fat (% of total energy)
0-6 months	Severe	40-55	10-15	30-45
	Moderate		15-30	10-30
	Mild		30-55	0-20
7-12 months	Severe	35-42	10-15	25-30
	Moderate		15-30	10-25
	Mild		30-40	0-10
1-3 years	Severe	30-40	10-15	10-30
	Moderate		20-30	10-20
	Mild		20-40	0-10
4-18 years	Severe	25-35	10	15-25
	Moderate		15-25	10-20
	Mild		20-35	0-10
>19 years	Severe	20-35	10	10-25
	Moderate		15-20	10-20
	Mild		20-35	0-10

*SERN/GMDI VLCADManagement Guidelines; https://southeastgenetics.org/ngp/guidelines.php

Starting a VLCAD Diet
(asymptomatic individuals with mild VLCADmay not need a fat-restricted diet)

1. Determine goals forLCF, MCT, Total Fat, Protein (g), Energy (kcal)
2. Calculate amount of LCF (breast milk, infant formula, food) needed to meet LCFgoal.
3. Calculate amount of MCT neededto meet total fatgoal.
4. Calculate energy intake from protein and fat sources to ensure total energyneeds are met.

Very Long Chain Acyl Co-A Dehydrogenase Deficiency(VLCAD)

Medical Food Therapy			
	Mead Johnson hcp.meadjohnson.com	**Nutricia** NutriciaMetabolics.com	**Vitaflo** www.VitafloUSA.com
Infant (0-1 yr)	Enfaport®		
Toddler & Young Children		Monogen® Liquigen®	LIPIstart™ MCTprocal® Betaquik®
Older Children & Adults		Monogen® Liquigen®	LIPIstart® MCTprocal® Betaquik®

Nutrition Supplementation*

Medium chain triglycerides (MCT): dosedepends on severity of disease and LCF restriction

-Medical foods (above)contain varying amounts of MCT. MCT oil is also available.These sources of MCT contain even-chain fatty acids with 6 to 10 carbons.

Docosahexaenoic acid (DHA): 60 mg/d-for patients <20 kg; 100 mg/d-for patients >20 kgifnormal plasma or RBC DHA concentrations cannot be achieved by diet modification

*SERN/GMDI VLCAD Management Guidelines; https://southeastgenetics.org/ngp/guidelines.php

Medical Management

Triheptanoin (Dojolvi®) Ultragenyx Pharmaceutical (Novato, CA): An odd-chain fatty acid containing 7 carbons, used instead of even-chain MCT. Dose: 35% of total energy intake.www.dojolvi.com

Fasting Precautions*

Times between feedings forawell patient; lower end of the range applies to patients with severe VLCAD:

0-4 months: 3-4 hours
4-<6 months: 4-6 hours
6-<9 months: 6-8 hours
9-<12 months: 8-10 hours
>12 months: 10-12 hours

*SERN/GMDI VLCAD Management Guidelines; https://southeastgenetics.org/ngp/guidelines.php

Laboratory Monitoring

Creatine Kinase[1, 2]
Plasma Carnitine[1, 2]
Plasma Acylcarnitine[1, 2]
Essential Fatty Acids[2]
B-natriuretic protein (BNP)[3]
25-OH Vitamin D[3]
CMP[3]
CBC[3]

[1] Every 3 months
[2] Every 6 months after 1 yr.of age
[3] As indicated

*SERN/GMDIVLCADManagement Guidelines; https://southeastgenetics.org/ngp/guidelines.php

Index

L. E. Bernstein et al. (eds.), *Nutrition Management of Inherited Metabolic Diseases*, https://doi.org/10.1007/978-3-030-94510-7